THIRTEENTH EDITION

Junqueira's
Basic Histology

TEXT AND ATLAS

Anthony L. Mescher, PhD

Professor of Anatomy and Cell Biology

Indiana University School of Medicine

Bloomington, Indiana

McGraw Hill Education | Medical

Junqueira's Basic Histology, Thirteenth Edition
International Edition 2013

10 09 08 07 06 05 04
20 15 14
CTP   MPM

NOTICE

Medicine is an ever-changing science. As new research and clinical experience broaden our knowledge, changes in treatment and drug therapy are required. The authors and the publisher of this work have checked with sources believed to be reliable in their efforts to provide information that is complete and generally in accord with the standards accepted at the time of publication. However, in view of the possibility of human error or changes in medical sciences, neither the authors nor the publisher nor any other party who has been involved in the preparation or publication of this work warrants that the information contained herein is in every respect accurate or complete, and they disclaim all responsibility for any errors or omissions or for the results obtained from use of the information contained in this work. Readers are encouraged to confirm the information contained herein with other sources. For example and in particular, readers are advised to check the product information sheet included in the package of each drug they plan to administer to be certain that the information contained in this work is accurate and that changes have not been made in the recommended dose or in the contraindications for administration. This recommendation is of particular importance in connection with new or infrequently used drugs.

The Figure Credit section for this book begins on page 515 and is considered an extension of the copyright page.

When ordering this title, use ISBN 978-1-259-07232-1 or MHID 1-259-07232-0

Printed in Singapore

Contents

Key Features of
Junqueira's Basic Histology,
Thirteenth Edition:

- **Recognized for more than three decades** as the most authoritative, comprehensive, and effective approach to understanding medical histology

- **Unmatched** in its ability to explain the relationship between cell and tissue structure and their function in the human body

- **Updated** to the latest research and developments on each topic

- **New and additional Medical Applications** throughout each chapter provide clinical relevance for every subject

- **New design** incorporates full color for each figure and table in addition to color micrographs of each cell and tissue

- **Figure legends** summarize and provide easy access to key points of each topic

- **Author Anthony L. Mescher, Ph.D.** has over 30 years' experience teaching cell biology and histology to medical students

- **Summaries of Key Points** at the end of each chapter list main points concisely for very easy review

- **Many new tables** help integrate each histological topic with relevant physiological aspects of the system

- **New, detailed tables of contents** within each chapter.

1,500+ illustrations bring important concepts to life

Student-suggested detailed legends

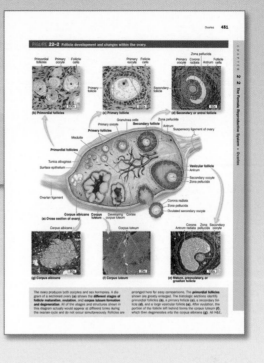

State-of-the art micrographs are the core of an all-new art program

Medical Applications are incorporated into every chapter

Visit www.LangeTextbooks.com

Preface

Now in its 13th edition, *Junqueira's Basic Histology* continues as the preeminent source of **concise yet thorough** information on human tissue structure and function. For over 40 years this educational resource has met the needs of learners for a well-organized and concise presentation of **cell biology and histology** that integrates the material with that of **biochemistry and physiology** and provides an excellent foundation for subsequent studies in **pathology**. The text is prepared specifically for students of medicine and other health-related professions, as well as for advanced undergraduate courses in tissue biology. As a result of its value and appeal to students and instructors alike, *Junqueira's Basic Histology* is used worldwide in nearly a dozen different languages.

For this edition I have revised the text and shortened each chapter while adding new information and expanding coverage of specific topics as needed. Study is also facilitated by a **new style and page design**. Inserted throughout each chapter are more numerous, short paragraphs that indicate how the information presented can be used medically and which emphasize the foundational relevance of the material learned. Prompted by student requests, I also now close each chapter with a list of the **key points** summarizing that chapter. More figures and **summary tables** organizing the information to facilitate student learning have also been added to each chapter.

Additional **new art** and other figures are present in each chapter, with the goal to simplify learning and integration with related material. The McGraw-Hill medical illustrations now used throughout the text, supplemented by numerous animations in the electronic version of the text, are the most useful, thorough, and attractive of any similar medical textbook. Electron and light micrographs have been replaced throughout the book as needed, and again they make up a complete atlas of cell, tissue, and organ structures fully compatible with the students' own collection of glass or digital slides. A **virtual microscope** with over 150 slides of all human tissues and organs is available: http://medsci.indiana.edu/junqueira/virtual/junqueira.htm.

As with the previous edition, the book facilitates learning by its **organization**:

- An opening chapter reviews how the structures of cells and tissues are studied.
- Two chapters then summarize the structural and functional organization of the human cell cytoplasm and nucleus.
- The next seven chapters cover the four basic tissues that make up our organs: epithelia, connective tissue (and its major subtypes), nervous tissue, and muscle.
- Remaining chapters explain the organization and functional significance of these tissues in each of the body's organ system, closing with up-to-date consideration of cells in the eye and ear.

For student review and rapid assimilation of the material in *Junqueira's Basic Histology*, McGraw-Hill has published a set of 200 full-color *Basic Histology Flash Cards*, both as actual cards and as an app for smart phone, tablet, or computer use, with each card having key structures to identify a summary of important facts and a clinical comment.

With these new features, I am confident that *Junqueira's Basic Histology* will continue as one of the most useful and widely used educational resources in histology.

Anthony L. Mescher
mescher@indiana.edu

Acknowledgments

I wish to thank the students at Indiana University with whom I have studied histology for over 30 years and from whom I have learned how to present the basic concepts most effectively. I am especially grateful to my colleagues Dr Matt Allan, Dr Vince Gattone, and Dr James C. Williams, who contributed extremely valuable expertise, critiques, and original photographs for this edition. Useful illustrations were also provided at my request by many other scientific experts who are acknowledged in the legend of the figures they contributed.

I also thank those teachers, students, and other users worldwide who have made valuable suggestions for improvements. The help of Sue Childress and Dr Mark Braun was invaluable in slide preparation and presentation of histology slides on the virtual microscope, respectively. Finally, I thank the staff of McGraw-Hill Medical, especially editors Michael Weitz and Brian Kearns, whose work made possible publication of this new edition of *Junqueira's Basic Histology*.

1 Histology & Its Methods of Study

Histology is the study of the tissues of the body and how these tissues are arranged to constitute organs. The Greek root *histo* can be translated as either "tissue" or "web," both of which are appropriate because tissues are usually webs of interwoven filaments and fibers, both cellular and noncellular, with membranous linings. Histology involves all aspects of tissue biology, with the focus on how cells' structure and arrangement optimize functions specific to each organ.

Tissues have two interacting components: cells and extracellular matrix (ECM). The ECM consists of many kinds of macromolecules, most of which form complex structures, such as collagen fibrils and basement membranes. The ECM supports the cells and the fluid that transports nutrients to the cells, and carries away their catabolites and secretory products. The cells produce the ECM and are also influenced and sometimes controlled by matrix molecules. Cells and matrix interact extensively, with many components of the matrix recognized by and attaching to cell surface receptors. Many of these protein receptors span the cell membranes and connect to structural components inside the cells. Thus, cells and ECM form a continuum that functions together and reacts to stimuli and inhibitors together.

The fundamental tissues of the body are each formed by several types of cell-specific associations between cells and ECM. These characteristic associations facilitate the recognition of the tissue types by students. Organs are formed by an orderly combination of several tissues, and the precise combination of these tissues allows the functioning of each organ and of the organism as a whole.

The small size of cells and matrix components makes histology dependent on the use of microscopes and molecular methods of study. Advances in biochemistry, molecular biology, physiology, immunology, and pathology are essential for a better knowledge of tissue biology. Familiarity with the tools and methods of any branch of science is essential for a proper understanding of the subject. This chapter reviews several of the more common methods used to study cells and tissues, focusing on microscopic approaches.

› PREPARATION OF TISSUES FOR STUDY

The most common procedure used in histologic research is the preparation of tissue sections or slices that can be studied with the light microscope. Under the light microscope, tissues are examined visually in a beam of transmitted light. Because most tissues and organs are too thick for light to pass through them, they must be sliced to obtain thin, translucent sections that are attached to glass slides for microscopic examination.

The ideal microscopic preparation is preserved so that the tissue on the slide has the same structure and molecular

FIGURE **1–1** Sectioning fixed and embedded tissue.

(a)   Fixation   Dehydration   Clearing   Infiltration   Embedding

52°-60°C

Drive wheel

Block holder

Paraffin block

Tissue

Steel knife

b

Most tissues studied histologically are prepared as shown, with this sequence of steps **(a)**:

- **Fixation:** Small pieces of tissue are placed in solutions of chemicals that preserve by cross-linking proteins and inactivating degradative enzymes.
- **Dehydration:** The tissue is transferred through a series of increasingly concentrated alcohol solutions, ending in 100%, which removes all water.
- **Clearing:** Alcohol is removed in toluene or other agents in which both alcohol and paraffin are miscible.
- **Infiltration:** The tissue is then placed in melted paraffin until it becomes completely infiltrated with this substance.
- **Embedding:** The paraffin-infiltrated tissue is placed in a small mold with melted paraffin and allowed to harden.
- **Trimming:** The resulting paraffin block is trimmed to expose the tissue for sectioning (slicing) on a microtome.

Similar steps are used in preparing tissue for transmission electron microscopy (TEM), except special fixatives and dehydrating solutions are used with smaller tissue samples and embedding involves epoxy resins which become harder than paraffin to allow very thin sectioning.

(b) A **microtome** is used for sectioning paraffin-embedded tissues for light microscopy. The trimmed tissue specimen is mounted in the paraffin block holder, and each turn of the drive wheel by the histologist advances the holder a controlled distance, generally between 1 and 10 μm. After each forward move, the tissue block passes over the steel knife edge and a section is cut at a thickness equal to the distance the block advanced. The paraffin sections are placed on glass slides and allowed to adhere, deparaffinized, and stained for light microscope study. For TEM, sections less than 1 μm thick are prepared from resin-embedded cells using an ultramicrotome with a glass or diamond knife.

composition as it had in the body. However, as a practical matter, this is seldom feasible, and artifacts, distortions, and loss of components due to the preparation process are often present. The basic steps used in tissue preparation for light microscopy are shown in Figure 1–1.

Fixation

To avoid tissue digestion by enzymes present within the cells (autolysis) or bacteria and to preserve cell and tissue structure, pieces of organs begin to be treated as soon as possible after removal from the body. The initial treatment—**fixation**—usually involves immersion in solutions of stabilizing or cross-linking compounds called **fixatives**. Because a fixative must fully diffuse through the tissues to preserve all cells, tissues are usually cut into small fragments before fixation to facilitate penetration and better ensure tissue preservation. Intravascular perfusion of fixatives can be used with some organs or laboratory animals. Because the fixative in this case rapidly reaches the tissues through the blood vessels, fixation is improved.

One fixative widely used for light microscopy is formalin, a buffered isotonic solution of 37% formaldehyde. The chemistry of the process involved in fixation of many tissue components is complex and not always well understood. Both formaldehyde and glutaraldehyde, a fixative often used for electron microscopy, react with the amine groups (NH_2) of tissue proteins, preventing their degradation. Glutaraldehyde reinforces this fixing activity by being a dialdehyde capable also of cross-linking proteins.

With the greater magnification and resolution of very small structures in the electron microscope, fixation must be done carefully to preserve "ultrastructural" detail. Toward that end, a double-fixation procedure, using a buffered glutaraldehyde solution followed by immersion in buffered osmium tetroxide, is a standard method to prepare tissue for such studies. Osmium tetroxide preserves (and stains) membrane lipids as well as proteins.

Embedding & Sectioning

Tissues are embedded in a solid medium to facilitate sectioning. In order to cut very thin sections, tissues must be infiltrated after fixation with embedding material that imparts a rigid consistency to the tissue. Embedding materials include paraffin and plastic resins; paraffin is used routinely for light microscopy, resins for both light and electron microscopy.

Paraffin embedding, or tissue impregnation, is preceded by two other main steps: **dehydration** and **clearing**. In dehydration, water is extracted from the fixed tissues by successive transfer through a graded series of ethanol and water mixtures, usually from 70% to 100% ethanol. The ethanol is then replaced by an organic solvent miscible with both alcohol and the embedding medium. As the solvent infiltrates the tissues, they become more transparent (undergo clearing). The fully cleared tissue is then placed in melted paraffin in an oven at 52°-60°C. At such temperatures the clearing solvent evaporates and the tissue is filled with liquid paraffin. The impregnated tissue then hardens in a small container of paraffin at room temperature. Tissues to be embedded with plastic resin are also dehydrated in ethanol and—depending on the kind of resin used—subsequently infiltrated with plastic solvents. The ethanol or solvents are later replaced by plastic solutions that harden with the addition of cross-linking polymerizers. Plastic embedding avoids the higher temperatures needed for paraffin embedding, which helps avoid shrinkage and major distortion of the tissue.

A hardened block containing tissue and paraffin is placed in an instrument called a **microtome** (Figure 1–1) and sliced by the steel blade into extremely thin sections. Paraffin sections are generally cut at 1-10 μm thickness, while the glass or diamond knives of ultramicrotomes produce sections of less than 1 μm for electron microscopy. One micrometer (1 μm) equals 1/1000 of a millimeter (mm) or 10^{-6} m. Other spatial units commonly used in histology include the nanometer (1 nm = 0.001 μm = 10^{-6} mm = 10^{-9} m) and angstrom (1 Å = 0.1 nm or 10^{-4} μm). The very thin sections are placed on glass slides and stained for light microscopy or on special grids for electron microscopic staining and examination.

Staining

Most cells and extracellular material are completely colorless, and to be studied microscopically sections must typically be stained (dyed). Methods of staining have been devised that not only make the various tissue components conspicuous but also permit distinctions to be made between them. Dyes stain tissue components more or less selectively, with many behaving like acidic or basic compounds and forming electrostatic (salt) linkages with ionizable radicals of molecules in tissues. Cell components such as nucleic acids with a net negative charge (anionic) stain more readily with basic dyes and are termed **basophilic**; cationic components, such as proteins with many ionized amino groups, have affinity for acidic dyes and are termed **acidophilic**.

Examples of basic dyes are toluidine blue, alcian blue, and methylene blue. Hematoxylin behaves like a basic dye, staining basophilic tissue components. The main tissue components that ionize and react with basic dyes do so because of acids in their composition (DNA, RNA, and glycosaminoglycans). Acid dyes (eg, eosin, orange G, and acid fuchsin) stain the acidophilic components of tissues such as mitochondria, secretory granules, and collagen.

Of all staining methods, the simple combination of **hematoxylin and eosin (H&E)** is used most commonly. Hematoxylin produces a dark blue or purple color, staining DNA in the cell nucleus and other acidic structures (such as RNA-rich portions of the cytoplasm and the matrix of cartilage). In contrast, eosin stains other cytoplasmic components and collagen

FIGURE **1–2** Hematoxylin and eosin (H&E) and periodic acid-Schiff (PAS) staining.

Micrograph of epithelium lining the small intestine, **(a)** stained with H&E, and **(b)** stained with the PAS reaction for glycoproteins. With H&E, basophilic cell nuclei are stained purple while cytoplasm stains pink. Cell regions with abundant oligosaccharides on glycoproteins, such as the ends of the cells at the lumen (**L**) or the scattered mucus-secreting goblet cells (**G**), are poorly stained. With PAS, however, cell staining

is most intense at the lumen, where projecting microvilli have a prominent layer of glycoproteins at the lumen (**L**) and in the mucin-rich secretory granules of goblet cells. Cell surface glycoproteins and mucin are PAS-positive because of their high content of oligosaccharides and polysaccharides respectively. The PAS-stained tissue was counterstained with hematoxylin to show the cell nuclei. Both X300.

pink (Figure 1–2a). Other dyes, such as the trichromes (eg, Mallory stain, Masson stain), are used in more complex histologic procedures. The trichromes, besides showing the nuclei and cytoplasm very well, help to distinguish extracellular tissue components better than H&E.

The chemical basis of other staining procedures is more complicated than that of the electrostatic interactions underlying basophilia and acidophilia. DNA can be specifically identified and quantified in nuclei using the Feulgen reaction, in which deoxyribose sugars are hydrolyzed by mild hydrochloric acid, followed by treatment with **periodic acid-Schiff (PAS) reagent**. This PAS reaction is based on the transformation of 1,2-glycol groups present in the sugars into aldehyde residues, which then react with Schiff reagent to produce a purple or magenta color.

Polysaccharides constitute a heterogeneous group in tissues, occurring either in a free state or bound to proteins and lipids. Because of their hexose sugar content, many polysaccharides can also be demonstrated by the PAS reaction. A very common free polysaccharide in animal cells is **glycogen**, which can be demonstrated by PAS in liver, striated muscle, and other tissues where it accumulates.

Short branched chains of sugars (oligosaccharides) are attached to specific amino acids of **glycoproteins**, making most glycoproteins PAS-positive. Figure 1–2b shows an example of cells stained by the PAS reaction. **Glycosaminoglycans** (GAGs) are anionic, unbranched long-chain polysaccharides containing aminated sugars. Many GAGs are synthesized while attached to a core protein and are part of a class of macromolecules called **proteoglycans**, which upon secretion make up important parts of the ECM (see Chapters 5 and 7). GAGs and many acidic glycoproteins do not undergo the PAS reaction, but because of their high content of anionic carboxyl and sulfate groups, they show a strong electrostatic interaction with alcian blue and other basic stains.

Basophilic or PAS-positive material can be further identified by **enzyme digestion**, pretreatment of a tissue section with an enzyme that specifically digests one substrate. For example, pretreatment with ribonuclease will greatly reduce cytoplasmic basophilia with little overall effect on the nucleus, indicating the importance of RNA for the cytoplasmic staining. Similarly, free polysaccharides are digested by amylase, which can therefore be used to distinguish glycogen from glycoproteins in PAS-positive material.

In many staining procedures certain structures such as nuclei become visible, but other parts of cells remain color-free. In such cases a **counterstain** is used to give additional information. A counterstain is usually a single stain that is applied separately to allow better recognition of nuclei and other structures. In H&E staining, eosin is the counterstain to hematoxylin.

Lipid-rich structures of cells are best revealed with **lipid-soluble dyes** and avoiding the processing steps that remove lipids such as treatment with heat, organic solvents, or paraffin. Typically, frozen sections are stained in alcohol solutions saturated with a lipophilic dye such as **Sudan black**, which dissolves in lipid-rich structures of cells. Specialized methods for the localization of cholesterol, phospholipids, and glycolipids are useful in diagnosis of metabolic diseases in which there are intracellular accumulations of these different lipids. In addition to staining tissues with dyes, **metal impregnation techniques** usually using solutions of silver salts are a common method of visualizing certain ECM fibers and specific cellular elements in nervous tissue.

The whole procedure, from fixation to observing a tissue in a light microscope, may take from 12 hours to 2½ days, depending on the size of the tissue, the fixative, the embedding medium, and the method of staining. The final step before microscopic observation is mounting a protective glass coverslip on the slide with clear adhesive.

❯ LIGHT MICROSCOPY

Conventional bright-field microscopy, as well as fluorescence, phase-contrast, differential interference, confocal, and polarizing microscopy are all based on the interaction of light with tissue components and are used to reveal and study tissue features in different ways.

Bright-Field Microscopy

With the **bright-field microscope**, widely used by students of histology, stained preparations are examined by means of ordinary light that passes through the specimen. The microscope includes an optical system and mechanisms to move and focus the specimen (Figure 1–3). The optical components consist of three lenses. The **condenser** collects and focuses a cone of light that illuminates the object to be observed. The **objective** lens enlarges and projects the image of the object in the direction of the eyepiece. The **eyepiece** or ocular lens further magnifies this image and projects it onto the viewer's retina or a charge-coupled device (CCD) highly sensitive to low light levels with a monitor and camera. The total magnification is obtained by multiplying the magnifying power of the objective and ocular lenses.

The critical factor in obtaining a crisp, detailed image with a light microscope is its **resolving power**, defined as the smallest distance between two particles at which they can be seen as separate objects. The maximal resolving power of

FIGURE **1–3** Components and light path of a bright-field microscope.

Photograph of a bright-field light microscope showing mechanical components and the pathway of light from the substage lamp to the eye of the observer. The optical system has three sets of lenses:

- The **condenser** collects and focuses a cone of light that illuminates the tissue slide on the stage.
- **Objective** lenses enlarge and project the illuminated image of the object toward the eyepiece. Interchangeable objectives with different magnifications routinely used in histology include X4 for observing a large area (field) of the tissue at low magnification; X10 for medium magnification of a smaller field; and X40 for high magnification of more detailed areas.
- The two **eyepieces** or oculars magnify this image another X10 and project it to the viewer, yielding a total magnification of X40, X100, or X400.

(*With permission, from Nikon Instruments.*)

the light microscope is approximately 0.2 μm, a power that permits good images magnified 1000-1500 times. Objects smaller or thinner than 0.2 μm (such as a ribosome, a membrane, or a filament of actin) cannot be distinguished with this instrument. Likewise, two structures such as mitochondria will be seen as only one object if they are separated by less than 0.2 μm. The quality of the image—its clarity and richness of detail—depends on the microscope's resolving power. The magnification is of value only when accompanied by high resolution. The resolving power of a microscope depends mainly on the quality of its objective lens. The eyepiece lens enlarges only the image obtained by the objective; it does not improve resolution. For this reason, when objectives of different magnifications are compared, those providing higher magnification also have higher resolving power.

Digital cameras highly sensitive to light enhance the power of the bright-field and other light microscopes by allowing the capture of images suitable for quantitative analysis and immediate printing. The frontiers of light microscopy have been redefined by the use of digital cameras, and image-enhancement programs (eg, to improve contrast) allow objects that may not be directly visible through the eyepieces to be analyzed on the video screen. Such systems are also useful for studying living cells for long periods of time because they use low-intensity light that avoids damaging the cells with heat from more intense illumination. Software developed for image analysis allows rapid measurements and quantitative study of microscopic structures.

Fluorescence Microscopy

When certain cellular substances are irradiated by light of a proper wavelength, they emit light with a longer wavelength—a phenomenon called **fluorescence**. In **fluorescence microscopy**, tissue sections are usually irradiated with ultraviolet (UV) light and the emission is in the visible portion of the spectrum. The fluorescent substances appear brilliant on a dark background. For this method, the microscope has a strong UV light source and special filters that select rays of different wavelengths emitted by the substances.

Fluorescent compounds with affinity for specific cell macromolecules may be used as fluorescent stains. Acridine orange, which binds both DNA and RNA, is an example. When observed in the fluorescence microscope, these nucleic acids emit slightly different fluorescence, allowing them to be localized separately in cells (Figure 1–4a). Other compounds

---

FIGURE 1–4 **Appearance of cells with fluorescent microscopy.**

Components of cells are often stained with compounds visible by fluorescence microscopy.

(a) Acridine orange binds nucleic acids and causes DNA in cell nuclei (**N**) to emit yellow light and the RNA-rich cytoplasm (**R**) to appear orange in these cells of a kidney tubule.

(b) Cultured cells stained with DAPI (4′,6-diamino-2-phenylindole) that binds DNA and with fluorescein-phalloidin

that binds actin filaments show nuclei with blue fluorescence and actin filaments stained green. Important information such as the greater density of microfilaments at the cell periphery is readily apparent. Both X500.

(Figure 1–4b, contributed with permission, from Drs Claire E. Walczak and Rania Risk, Indiana University School of Medicine, Bloomington.)

such as DAPI and Hoechst stain specifically bind DNA and are used to stain cell nuclei, emitting a characteristic blue fluorescence under UV. Another important application of fluorescence microscopy is achieved by coupling compounds such as fluorescein to molecules that will specifically bind to certain cellular components and thus allow the identification of these structures under the microscope (Figure 1–4b). Antibodies labeled with fluorescent compounds are extremely important in immunohistologic staining. (See section on Visualizing Specific Molecules.)

Phase-Contrast Microscopy

Unstained cells and tissue sections, which are usually transparent and colorless, can be studied with these modified light microscopes. Cellular detail is normally difficult to see in unstained tissues because all parts of the specimen have roughly similar optical densities. **Phase-contrast microscopy**, however, uses a lens system that produces visible images from transparent objects and, importantly, can be used with living, cultures cells (Figure 1–5).

Phase-contrast microscopy is based on the principle that light changes its speed when passing through cellular and extracellular structures with different refractive indices. These changes are used by the phase-contrast system to cause the structures to appear lighter or darker in relation to each other. Because they allow the examination of cells without fixation or staining, phase-contrast microscopes are prominent tools in all cell culture laboratories. A modification of phase-contrast microscopy is **differential interference microscopy** with Nomarski optics, which produces an image of living cells with a more apparent three-dimensional (3D) aspect (Figure 1–5c).

Confocal Microscopy

With a regular bright-field microscope, the beam of light is relatively large and fills the specimen. Stray (excess) light reduces contrast within the image and compromises the resolving power of the objective lens. Confocal microscopy (Figure 1–6) avoids these problems and achieves high resolution and sharp focus by using (1) a small point of high-intensity light, often from a laser, and (2) a plate with a pinhole aperture in front of the image detector. The point light source, the focal point of the lens, and the detector's pinpoint aperture are all optically conjugated or aligned to each other in the focal plane (confocal), and unfocused light does not pass through the pinhole. This greatly improves resolution of the object in focus and allows the localization of specimen components with much greater precision than with the bright-field microscope.

Confocal microscopes include a computer-driven mirror system (the beam splitter) to move the point of illumination across the specimen automatically and rapidly. Digital images captured at many individual spots in a very thin plane of focus are used to produce an "optical section" of that plane. Creating such

FIGURE 1–5 Unstained cells' appearance in three types of light microscopy.

Living neural crest cells growing in culture appear differently with various techniques of light microscopy. Here the *same field* of unstained cells, including two differentiating pigment cells, is shown using three different methods (all X200):

(a) Bright-field microscopy: Without fixation and staining, only the two pigment cells can be seen.

(b) Phase-contrast microscopy: Cell boundaries, nuclei, and cytoplasmic structures with different refractive indices affect in-phase light differently and produce an image of these features in *all* the cells.

(c) Differential interference microscopy: Cellular details are highlighted in a different manner using Nomarski optics. Phase-contrast microscopy, with or without differential interference, is widely used to observe live cells grown in tissue culture.

(With permission, from Dr Sherry Rogers, Department of Cell Biology and Physiology, University of New Mexico, Albuquerque, NM.)

FIGURE **1–6** Principle of confocal microscopy.

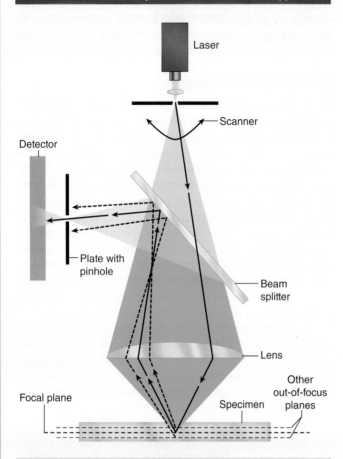

Although a very small spot of light originating from one plane of the section crosses the pinhole and reaches the detector, rays originating from other planes are blocked by the blind. Thus, only one very thin plane of the specimen is focused at a time. The diagram shows the practical arrangement of a confocal microscope. Light from a laser source hits the specimen and is reflected. A beam splitter directs the reflected light to a pinhole and a detector. Light from components of the specimen that are above or below the focused plane is blocked by the blind. The laser scans the specimen so that a larger area of the specimen can be observed.

optical sections at a series of focal planes through the specimen allows them to be digitally reconstructed into a 3D image.

Polarizing Microscopy

Polarizing microscopy allows the recognition of stained or unstained structures made of highly organized subunits. When normal light passes through a **polarizing** filter, it exits vibrating in only one direction. If a second filter is placed in the microscope above the first one, with its main axis perpendicular to the first filter, no light passes through. If, however, tissue structures containing oriented macromolecules are located between the two polarizing filters, their repetitive structure rotates the axis of the light emerging from the polarizer and they appear

FIGURE **1–7** Tissue appearance with bright-field and polarizing microscopy.

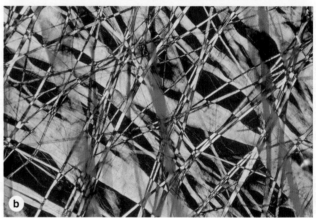

Polarizing light microscopy produces an image only of material having repetitive, periodic macromolecular structure; features without such structure are not seen. Pieces of thin, unsectioned mesentery were stained with red picrosirius, orcein, and hematoxylin, placed on slides and observed by bright-field **(a)** and polarizing **(b)** microscopy.

(a) With bright-field microscopy collagen fibers appear red, with thin elastic fibers and cell nuclei darker.

(b) With polarizing microscopy, only the collagen fibers are visible and these exhibit intense yellow or orange birefringence (a: X40; b: X100).

as bright structures against a dark background (Figure 1–7). The ability to rotate the direction of vibration of polarized light is called **birefringence** and is a feature of crystalline substances or substances containing highly oriented molecules, such as cellulose, collagen, microtubules, and actin filaments.

❯ ELECTRON MICROSCOPY

Transmission and scanning electron microscopes are based on the interaction of tissue components with beams of electrons. The wavelength in the electron beam is much shorter than that of light, allowing a 1000-fold increase in resolution.

Transmission Electron Microscopy

The **transmission electron microscope (TEM)** is an imaging system that permits resolution around 3 nm. This high resolution allows magnifications of up to 400,000 times to be viewed in detail. Unfortunately, this level of magnification applies only to isolated macromolecules or particles. Very thin tissue sections can be observed with details at magnifications of up to about 120,000 times.

As shown in Figure 1–8a, in the TEM a metallic filament cathode emits electrons that move toward an anode, a metal plate with a central hole that forms a beam of electrons passing through it. The voltage difference between cathode and anode can be varied between roughly 60 and 120 kV, producing electron beams of different wavelengths. The beam is focused by passing through electromagnets whose strength is also variable.

The first lens is a condenser focusing the beam of electrons on a section of the specimen. Some electrons interact with atoms in the section and their course is modified, while others simply cross the specimen without interacting.

FIGURE 1–8 Electron microscopes.

(a) Transmission electron microscope

(b) Scanning electron microscope

Electron microscopes are large instruments generally housed in a specialized EM facility.

(a) Schematic view of the major components of a transmission electron microscope (TEM), which is configured rather like an upside-down light microscope. With the microscope column in a vacuum, a metallic (usually tungsten) filament (cathode) at the top emits electrons that travel to an anode with an accelerating voltage between 60 and 120 kV. Electrons passing through a hole in the anode form a beam that is focused electromagnetically by circular electric coils in a manner analogous to the effect of optical lenses on light.

The first lens is a condenser focusing the beam on the section. Some electrons interact with atoms in the section, being absorbed or scattered to different extents, while others are simply transmitted through the specimen with no interaction. Electrons reaching the objective lens form an image that is then magnified and finally projected on a fluorescent screen or a charge-coupled device (CCD) monitor and camera.

In a TEM image areas of the specimen through which electrons passed appear bright (electron lucent), while denser areas or those that bind heavy metal ions during specimen preparation absorb or deflect electrons and appear darker (electron dense). Such images are therefore always black, white, and shades of gray.

(b) The scanning electron microscope (SEM) has many similarities to a TEM. However, here the focused electron beam does not pass through the specimen, but rather is moved sequentially (scanned) from point to point across its surface similar to the way an electron beam is scanned across a television tube or screen. For SEM specimens are coated with metal atoms with which the electron beam interacts, producing reflected electrons and newly emitted secondary electrons. All of these are captured by a detector and transmitted to amplifiers and processed to produce a black-and-white image on the monitor. The SEM shows only surface views of the coated specimen but with a striking 3D, shadowed quality. The inside of organs or cells can be analyzed after sectioning to expose their internal surfaces.

Electrons transmitted through the specimen reach the objective lens, which forms a focused, magnified image that is then magnified further through other lenses and captured on a viewing screen. The image of the specimen shows areas of white, black, and shades of gray corresponding to areas through which electrons passed readily (appearing brighter or electron lucent) and areas where electrons were absorbed or deflected (appearing darker or more electron dense). To improve contrast and resolution in TEM, compounds with **heavy metal ions** are often added to the fixative or dehydrating solutions used to prepare the tissue. These include osmium tetroxide, lead citrate, and uranyl compounds, which bind cellular macromolecules, increasing their electron density and visibility.

TEM normally requires very thin sections (40-90 nm); therefore tissue is embedded in a hard epoxy and sectioned with a glass or diamond knife. Sections are collected on small metal grids that are placed in the microscope column for analysis.

Cryofracture and **freeze etching** are techniques that allow TEM study of cells without fixation or embedding. Cryofracture has been particularly useful in the study of membrane structure. In these methods very small tissue specimens are rapidly frozen in liquid nitrogen and either fractured or cut with a knife. A replica of the frozen exposed surface is produced in a vacuum by applying thin coats of vaporized platinum or other metal atoms. After removal of the organic material, the replica of the cut surface can be examined by EM. With membranes the random fracture planes often split the lipid bilayers, exposing protein components whose size, shape, and distribution are difficult to study by other methods.

Scanning Electron Microscopy

Scanning electron microscopy (SEM) provides a high-resolution view of the surfaces of cells, tissues, and organs. Like the TEM, this microscope produces and focuses a very narrow beam of electrons, but in this instrument the beam does not pass through the specimen (Figure 1–8b). Instead, the surface of the specimen is first dried and spray-coated with a very thin layer of heavy metal (often gold) through which electrons do not pass readily. When the beam is scanned from point to point across the specimen, it interacts with the metal atoms and produces reflected electrons or secondary electrons emitted from the metal. These are captured by a detector, and the resulting signal is processed to produce a black-and-white image on a monitor. SEM images are usually easy to interpret because they present a 3D view that appears to be illuminated from above, in the same way that large objects are seen with highlights and shadows caused by light from above.

〉 AUTORADIOGRAPHY

Microscopic **autoradiography** is a method of localizing newly synthesized macromolecules (DNA, RNA, protein, glycoproteins, and polysaccharides) in cells or tissue sections. Radioactively labeled metabolites (nucleotides, amino acids, sugars) incorporated into the macromolecules emit weak radiation that is restricted to the specific regions where the molecules are located. Slides with radiolabeled cells or tissue sections are coated in a darkroom with photographic emulsion containing silver bromide crystals, which act as microdetectors of the radiation in the same way that they respond to light in photographic film. After an adequate exposure time in lightproof boxes, the slides are developed photographically. Silver bromide crystals reduced by the radiation produce small black grains of metallic silver, which under either the light microscope or TEM indicate the locations of radiolabeled macromolecules in the tissue (Figure 1–9).

Much information becomes available by autoradiography of cells or tissues. If a radioactive precursor of DNA (such as tritium-labeled thymidine) is used, it is possible to know which cells in a tissue (and how many) are replicating DNA and preparing to divide. Dynamic events may also be analyzed. For example, if one wishes to know where in the cell protein is produced, if it is secreted, and its path in the cell before being secreted, several animals are injected with a radioactive amino acid and tissues collected at different times after the injections. Autoradiography of the tissues from the sequential times will indicate the migration of the radioactive proteins.

〉 CELL & TISSUE CULTURE

Live cells and tissues can be maintained and studied outside the body in culture (in vitro). In the organism (in vivo) cells are bathed in fluid derived from blood plasma, containing many different molecules required for survival and growth. Cell culture has been invaluable in studying the functions of these molecules. It also allows the direct observation of cellular behavior under a phase-contrast microscope. Many experiments technically not possible to perform in the living animal can be accomplished in vitro.

The cells and tissues are grown in complex solutions of known composition (salts, amino acids, vitamins) to which serum components or specific growth factors are added. In preparing cultures from a tissue or organ, cells must be dispersed mechanically or enzymatically. Once isolated, the cells can be cultivated in a clear dish to which they adhere, usually as a single layer of cells (Figure 1–5). Cultures of cells isolated in this way are called **primary cell cultures**. Many cell types, once isolated from normal or pathologic tissue, can be maintained in vitro for long periods because they become immortalized and constitute a permanent **cell line**. Most cells obtained from normal tissues have a finite, genetically programmed life span. Certain changes, however (some related to oncogenes; see Chapter 3), can promote cell immortality, a process called **transformation**, and are similar to the initial changes in a normal cell's becoming a cancer cell. Because of improvements in culture technology, most cell types can now be maintained in the laboratory. All procedures with living cells and tissues must be performed in a sterile area, using sterile solutions and equipment, to avoid contamination with microorganisms.

FIGURE **1–9** Microscopic autoradiography.

Autoradiographs are tissue preparations in which particles called **silver grains** indicate the cells or regions of cells in which specific macromolecules were synthesized just prior to fixation. Shown here are autoradiographs from the salivary gland of a mouse injected with ³H-fucose 8 hours before tissue fixation. Fucose was incorporated into oligosaccharides, and the free ³H-fucose was removed during fixation and sectioning of the gland. Autoradiographic processing and microscopy reveal locations of newly synthesized glycoproteins containing that sugar.

(a) Black grains of silver from the light-sensitive material coating the specimen are visible over cell regions with secretory granules and the duct indicating glycoprotein locations. X1500.

(b) The same tissue prepared for TEM autoradiography shows silver grains with a coiled or amorphous appearance again localized mainly over the granules (**G**) and in the gland lumen (**L**). X7500.

(*Figure 1–9b, with permission, from Drs Ticiano G. Lima and A. Antonio Haddad, School of Medicine, Ribeirão Preto, Brazil.*)

As shown in Chapter 2, incubation of living cells in vitro with a variety of new fluorescent compounds that are sequestered and metabolized in specific compartments of the cell provides a new approach to understanding these compartments both structurally and physiologically. Other histologic techniques applied to cultured cells have been particularly important for understanding the locations and functions of microtubules, microfilaments, and other components of the cytoskeleton.

›› MEDICAL APPLICATION

Cell culture is very widely used to study molecular changes that occur in cancer; to analyze infectious viruses, mycoplasma, and some protozoa; and for many routine genetic or chromosomal analyses. Cervical cancer cells from a patient later identified as Henrietta Lacks, who died from the disease in 1951, were used to establish one of the first cell lines, called **HeLa cells**, which are still used in research on cellular structure and function throughout the world.

› ENZYME HISTOCHEMISTRY

Enzyme histochemistry (cytochemistry) is a method for localizing cellular structures using a specific enzymatic activity present in those structures. To preserve these enzymes, histochemical procedures usually use unfixed or mildly fixed tissue, which is sectioned on a cryostat to avoid adverse effects of heat and organic solvents on enzymatic activity. Enzyme histochemistry involves the following: (1) Tissue sections are immersed in a solution containing the substrate of the enzyme to be localized; (2) the enzyme is allowed to act on its substrate; (3) at this stage or later, the section is put in contact with a marker compound that reacts with a product of the enzymatic action on the substrate; (4) the final product from the marker, which must be insoluble and visible by light or electron microscopy by having color or electron density, precipitates over the site of the enzymes, allowing the region to be localized microscopically.

Examples of enzymes that can be detected histochemically include the following:

- **Phosphatases**, which split the bond between a phosphate group and phosphorylated molecules. Both alkaline phosphatases (those with maximum activity at an alkaline pH) and acid phosphatases can be detected (Figure 1–10).
- **Dehydrogenases**, which remove hydrogen ions from one substrate and transfer them to another, are localized by incubating tissue sections in a substrate solution containing a molecule that receives hydrogen and precipitates as an insoluble colored compound. Mitochondria can be specifically identified by this method, because dehydrogenases are among the citric acid (Krebs) cycle enzymes of this organelle.

FIGURE **1–10** Enzyme histochemistry.

(a) Micrograph of cross sections of kidney tubules treated histochemically to demonstrate alkaline phosphatases shows strong activity of this enzyme at the apical surfaces of the cells at the lumens (**L**) of the tubules. X200.

(b) TEM image of a kidney cell in which acid phosphatase has been localized histochemically in three lysosomes (**Ly**) near the nucleus (**N**). The dark material within these structures is lead phosphate that precipitated in places with acid phosphatase activity. X25,000.

(*Figure 1–10b, with permission, from Dr Eduardo Katchburian, Department of Morphology, Federal University of São Paulo, Brazil.*)

- **Peroxidase**, which promotes the oxidation of substrates with the transfer of hydrogen ions to hydrogen peroxide, forming water molecules, is commonly localized by histochemistry. Cell or tissue sections are incubated in a solution containing hydrogen peroxide and 3,3′-diaminoazobenzidine (DAB), which is oxidized in the presence of peroxidase to produce an insoluble, brown, electron-dense precipitate.

>> **MEDICAL APPLICATION**

Many enzyme histochemical procedures are used in the medical laboratory, including Perls' Prussian blue reaction for iron (used to diagnose the iron storage diseases, hemochromatosis and hemosiderosis), the PAS-amylase and alcian blue reactions for glycogen and GAGs (to detect glycogenosis and mucopolysaccharidosis), and reactions for lipids and sphingolipids (to detect sphingolipidosis).

› VISUALIZING SPECIFIC MOLECULES

A specific macromolecule present in a tissue section may sometimes be identified by using tagged compounds or macromolecules that bind *specifically* with the molecule of interest. The compounds that interact with the molecule must be visible with the light or electron microscope, often by being tagged with a detectible label. The most commonly used labels are fluorescent compounds, radioactive atoms that can be detected with autoradiography, molecules of peroxidase or other enzymes that can be detected with histochemistry, and metal (usually gold) particles that can be observed with light and electron microscopy. These methods can be used to detect and localize specific sugars, proteins, and nucleic acids.

Examples of molecules that interact specifically with other molecules include the following:

- **Phalloidin** is a compound extracted from a mushroom, *Amanita phalloides*, and interacts strongly with actin. Tagged with fluorescent dyes, phalloidin is commonly used to demonstrate actin filaments in cells (Figure 1-4b).
- **Protein A** is obtained from *Staphylococcus aureus* bacteria and binds to the Fc region of immunoglobulin (antibody) molecules. Labeled protein A can therefore be used to localize naturally occurring or applied antibodies bound to cell structures.
- **Lectins** are proteins or glycoproteins, derived mainly from plant seeds, that bind to carbohydrates with high affinity and specificity. Different lectins bind to specific sugars or sequences of sugar residues. Fluorescently labeled lectins are used to stain specific glycoproteins, proteoglycans, and glycolipids and are used to characterize membrane components with specific sequences of sugar residues.

Immunohistochemistry

A highly specific interaction between molecules is that between an antigen and its antibody. For this reason, histologic methods using labeled antibodies are extremely useful in identifying and localizing many specific proteins, not just those with enzymatic activity that can be demonstrated by histochemistry.

The body's immune cells interact with and produce **antibodies** against other macromolecules—called **antigens**—that are recognized as "foreign," not a normal part of the organism, and potentially dangerous. Antibodies belong to the **immunoglobulin** family of glycoproteins, produced by lymphocytes. These molecules normally bind specifically to their provoking antigens and help eliminate them.

For both diagnostic and research purposes, **immunohistochemistry** is very widely used to detect specific proteins (or other molecules) of interest in cells and tissues. This technique requires an antibody against the protein that is to be detected, which means that the protein must have been previously purified using biochemical or molecular approaches so that antibodies against it can be produced. To produce antibodies against protein x of a certain animal species (eg, a human or rat), the isolated protein is injected into an animal of another species (eg, a rabbit or a goat). If the protein's amino acid sequence is sufficiently different for this animal to recognize it as foreign—that is, as an antigen—the animal will produce antibodies against the protein.

In immunohistochemistry a tissue section (or cells in culture) that one believes contains the protein of interest is incubated in a solution containing labeled antibody to this protein. The antibody binds specifically to the protein, whose location in

the tissue or cell can then be seen with either the light or electron microscope, depending on how the antibody was labeled. Antibodies are commonly tagged with fluorescent compounds, with peroxidase or alkaline phosphatase for histochemical detection, or with electron-dense gold particles for TEM.

Different groups (clones) of lymphocytes in the injected animal recognize different parts of protein x and each clone produces an antibody against that part. These antibodies are collected from the animal's plasma and constitute a mixture of **polyclonal antibodies**, each capable of binding a different region of protein x.

It is also possible, however, to inject protein x into a mouse and a few days later isolate the activated lymphocytes and place them into culture. Growth and activity of these cells can be prolonged indefinitely by fusing them with lymphocytic tumor cells to produce hybridoma cells. Different hybridoma clones produce different antibodies against the several parts of protein x and each clone can be isolated and cultured separately so that the different antibodies against protein x can be collected separately. Each of these antibodies is a **monoclonal antibody**. An advantage to using a monoclonal antibody rather than polyclonal antibodies is that it can be selected to be highly specific and to bind strongly to the protein to be detected, with less nonspecific binding to other proteins that are similar to the one of interest.

There are **direct and indirect methods of immunocytochemistry** (Figure 1–11). In the direct method the antibody (either monoclonal or polyclonal) is itself tagged with an appropriate label. A tissue section is incubated with the antibody for some time so that the antibody interacts with and

---

FIGURE **1–11** Immunocytochemistry.

Immunocytochemistry (or immunohistochemistry) can be direct or indirect. **Direct immunocytochemistry** (left) uses an antibody made against the tissue protein of interest and tagged directly with a label such as a fluorescent compound or peroxidase. When placed with the tissue section on a slide, these labeled antibodies bind specifically to the protein (antigen) against which they were produced and can be visualized by the appropriate method. **Indirect immunocytochemistry** (right) uses first a **primary antibody** made against the protein (antigen) of interest and applied to the tissue section to bind

its specific antigen. Then a **labeled secondary antibody** is obtained that was (1) made in another species against immunoglobulin proteins (antibodies) from the species in which the primary antibodies were made and (2) labeled with a fluorescent compound or peroxidase. When the labeled secondary antibody is applied to the tissue section, it specifically binds the primary antibodies, indirectly labeling the protein of interest on the slide. Because more than one labeled secondary antibody can bind each primary antibody molecule, labeling of the protein of interest is amplified by the indirect method.

binds to protein *x*. The section is then washed to remove the unbound antibody, processed by the method appropriate for the label, and examined microscopically to study the location or other aspects of protein *x*.

Indirect immunohistochemistry involves sequential application of two antibodies and additional washing steps. The (primary) antibody specifically binding protein *x* is not labeled. The detectible tag is conjugated to a **secondary antibody** made in an animal species different ("foreign") from that which made the primary antibody. For example, primary antibodies made by mouse lymphocytes (such as most monoclonal antibodies) are specifically recognized and bound by antibodies made in a rabbit or goat injected with mouse antibody immunoglobulin.

The indirect method is used more widely in research and pathologic tests because it is more sensitive, with the extra level of antibody binding serving to amplify the visible signal. Moreover, the same preparation of labeled secondary antibody can be used in studies with different primary antibodies (specific for different antigens) as long as all these are made in the same species. There are other indirect methods that involve the use of other intermediate molecules, such as the biotin-avidin technique, which are also used to amplify detection signals.

Examples of indirect immunocytochemistry are shown in Figure 1–12, demonstrating the use of this method with cells in culture or after tissue sectioning for both light microscopy and TEM.

FIGURE 1–12 Cells and tissues stained by immunohistochemistry.

throughout the cytoplasm. Primary antibodies against the filament protein desmin and fluorescein isothiocyanate (FITC)–labeled secondary antibodies were used in the indirect staining technique, with the nucleus counterstained blue with DAPI. X650.

(b) A section of small intestine treated with an antibody against the enzyme lysozyme. The secondary antibody labeled with peroxidase was then applied and the localized brown color produced histochemically with the peroxidase substrate 3,3′-diamino-azobenzidine (DAB). The method demonstrates lysozyme-containing structures in scattered macrophages and in the large clusters of cells. Nuclei were counterstained with hematoxylin. X100.

(c) A section of pancreatic cells in a TEM preparation incubated with an antibody against the enzyme amylase and then with protein A coupled with gold particles. Protein A has high affinity toward antibody molecules and the resulting image reveals the presence of amylase with the gold particles localized as very small black dots over dense secretory granules and developing granules (left). With specificity for immunoglobulin molecules, labeled protein A can be used to localize any primary antibody. X5000.

(Figure 1–12c, with permission, from Dr Moise Bendayan, Departments of Pathology and Cell Biology, University of Montreal, Montreal, Canada.)

Immunocytochemical methods to localize specific proteins can be applied to either light microscopic or TEM preparations using a variety of labels.

(a) A single cultured uterine cell stained fluorescently to reveal a meshwork of intermediate filaments (green)

TABLE **1–1**	Examples of specific antigens with diagnostic importance.
Antigens	**Diagnosis**
Specific cytokeratins	Tumors of epithelial origin
Protein and polypeptide hormones	Certain endocrine tumors
Carcinoembryonic antigen (CEA)	Glandular tumors, mainly of the digestive tract and breast
Steroid hormone receptors	Breast duct cell tumors
Antigens produced by viruses	Specific virus infections

❯❯ MEDICAL APPLICATION

Because cells in some diseases, including many cancer cells, often produce proteins unique to their pathologic condition, immunohistochemistry can be used by pathologists to diagnose many diseases, including certain types of tumors and some virus-infected cells. Table 1–1 shows some applications of immunocytochemistry routinely used in clinical practice.

Hybridization Techniques

Hybridization usually implies the specific binding between two single strands of nucleic acid, which occurs under appropriate conditions if the strands are complementary. The greater the similarities of their nucleotide sequences, the more readily the complementary strands form "hybrid" double-strand molecules. Hybridization at stringent conditions allows the specific identification of sequences in genes or RNA. This occurs readily with complementary nucleic acids in solution, but hybridization also occurs when nucleic acid sequences in solution are applied directly to prepared cells and tissue sections, a procedure called *in situ* **hybridization** (ISH).

This technique is ideal for (1) determining if a cell has a specific sequence of DNA, such as a gene or part of a gene (Figure 1–13), (2) identifying the cells containing specific messenger RNAs (mRNAs) (in which the corresponding gene is being transcribed), or (3) determining the localization of a gene in a specific chromosome. DNA and RNA of the cells must be initially denatured by heat or other agents to become completely single-stranded. The nucleotide sequences of interest are detected with **probes** consisting of single-stranded complementary DNA (cDNA). The probe may be obtained by cloning, by polymerase chain reaction (PCR) amplification of the target sequence, or by chemical synthesis if the desired sequence is short. The probe is tagged with nucleotides containing a radioactive isotope (localized by autoradiography) or modified with a small compound such as digoxigenin (identified by immunocytochemistry). A solution containing the probe is placed over the specimen for a period of time and under conditions necessary for hybridization. After the excess unbound probe is washed off, the localization of the hybridized probe is revealed through its label.

FIGURE **1–13** Cells stained by in situ hybridization (ISH).

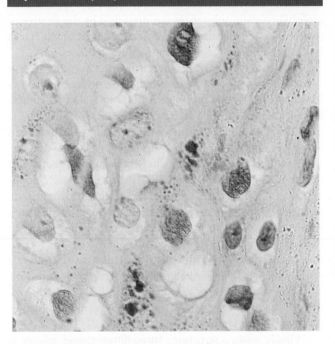

ISH of this tissue section reveals that many cells contain the human papilloma virus (HPV). The section was incubated with a solution containing a digoxigenin-labeled complementary DNA (cDNA) probe for the HPV DNA. The probe was then visualized by direct immunohistochemistry using peroxidase-labeled antibodies against digoxigenin. This procedure stains brown only those cells containing HPV. X400. H&E.

(*With permission, from Dr Jose E. Levi, Virology Lab, Institute of Tropical Medicine, University of São Paulo, Brazil.*)

❯❯ MEDICAL APPLICATION

Warts on the skin of the genitals and elsewhere are due to infection with the human papilloma virus (HPV) which causes the characteristic benign proliferative growth. As shown in Figure 1-13 such virus-infected cells can often be demonstrated by ISH. Certain cancer cells with unique or elevated expression of specific genes are also localized in tumors and studied microscopically by ISH.

❯ INTERPRETATION OF STRUCTURES iN TISSUE SECTIONS

In studying and interpreting stained tissue sections, it is important to remember that microscopic preparations are the end result of a series of processes that began with collecting the tissue and ended with mounting a coverslip on the slide. Certain steps in this procedure may distort the tissues slightly, producing minor structural abnormalities called **artifacts** not present in the living tissue.

One such distortion is minor shrinkage of cells or tissue regions produced by the fixative, by the ethanol, or by the heat needed for paraffin embedding. Shrinkage can create artificial spaces between cells and other tissue components. Such spaces can also result from the loss of lipids, glycogen, or low-molecular-weight substances not preserved by the fixative or removed by the dehydrating and clearing fluids. Slight cracks in sections also appear as large spaces in the tissues.

Other artifacts may include small wrinkles in the section (which the novice may confuse with linear structures such as blood capillaries) and precipitates from the stain (which may be confused with cellular structures such as cytoplasmic granules). Students must be aware of the existence of artifacts and able to recognize them.

Another difficulty in the study of histologic sections is the impossibility of differentially staining all tissue components on one slide. A single stain can seldom demonstrate well nuclei, mitochondria, lysosomes, basement membranes, elastic fibers, etc. With the light microscope, it is necessary to examine preparations stained by different methods before an idea of the whole composition and structure of a cell or tissue can be obtained. The TEM allows the observation of cells with all its internal structures and surrounding ECM components, but only a few cells in a tissue can be conveniently studied in these very small samples.

Finally, when a structure's **three-dimensional** volume is cut into very thin sections, the sections appear microscopically to have only two dimensions: length and width. When examining a section under the microscope, the viewer must always keep in mind that components are missing in front of and behind what is being seen because many tissue structures are thicker than the section. Round structures seen microscopically may be portions of spheres or tubes. Because structures in a tissue have different orientations, their two-dimensional (2D) appearance will also vary depending on the plane of section. A single convoluted tube will appear histologically as many separate rounded or oval structures (Figure 1-14).

FIGURE **1–14** Interpretation of 3D structures in 2D sections.

In thin sections 3D structures appear to have only two dimensions. Such images must be interpreted correctly to understand the actual structure of tissue and organ components. For example, blood vessels and other tubular structures appear in sections as round or oval shapes whose size and shape depend on the transverse or oblique angle of the cut. A highly coiled tube will appear as several round and oval structures. In TEM sections of cells, round structures may represent spherical organelles or transverse cuts through tubular organelles such mitochondria. It is important to develop such interpretive skill to understand tissue and cell morphology in microscopic preparations.

Histology & Its Methods of Study SUMMARY OF KEY POINTS

Preparation of Tissues for Study

- Chemical **fixatives** such as formalin are used to **preserve tissue structure** by cross-linking and denaturing proteins, inactivating enzymes, and preventing cell autolysis or self-digestion.
- **Dehydration** of the fixed tissue in alcohol and clearing in organic solvents prepare it for **embedding** and **sectioning**.
- Embedding in paraffin wax or epoxy resin allows the tissue to be cut into very thin sections (slices) with a **microtome**.
- Sections are mounted on glass slides for **staining**, which is required to reveal specific cellular and tissue components with the microscope.
- The most commonly used staining method is a combination of the stains **hematoxylin and eosin (H&E)**, which act as basic and acidic dyes, respectively.
- Cell substances with a net negative (anionic) charge, such as DNA and RNA, react strongly with hematoxylin and basic stains; such material is said to be "**basophilic**."
- Cationic substances, such as collagen and many cytoplasmic proteins, react with eosin and other acidic stains and are said to be "**acidophilic**."

Light Microscopy

- **Bright-field microscopy**, the method most commonly used by both students and pathologists, uses ordinary light and the colors are imparted by tissue staining.
- **Fluorescence microscopy** uses ultraviolet light, under which only fluorescent molecules are visible, allowing localization of fluorescent probes which can be much more specific than routine stains.
- **Phase-contrast microscopy** uses the differences in refractive index of various natural cell and tissue components to produce an image without staining, allowing observation of living cells.
- **Confocal microscopy** involves scanning the specimen at successive focal planes with a focused light beam, often from a laser, and produces a 3D reconstruction from the images.

Electron Microscopy

- With wavelengths much shorter than those of light, electron beams allow very-high-resolution images at high magnification, called **ultrastructural images**.
- **Transmission EM** sends an electromagnetically focused beam of electrons at very high voltage through ultrathin sections of tissue.
- Tissue preparation for TEM involves adding **heavy metal ions** that associate at different electron densities with cell and tissue components, improving contrast in the resulting image.
- **Cryofracture** and freeze etching allow TEM study of unfixed frozen cells, with fractured membranes or cut surfaces coated with carbon and heavy metal to make a replica of the surface for analysis.
- **Scanning EM** scans an electron beam across a specimen coated with a thin layer of heavy metal; reflected and secondary electrons from the specimen are processed into a 3D ultrastructural image.

Autoradiography

- This process localizes cell components synthesized using **radioactive precursors** by detecting silver grains produced by weakly emitted radiation in a photographic emulsion coating the tissue section or cells.
- With either light microscopy or TEM, autoradiography permits unique studies of processes such as tissue growth (using radioactive DNA precursors) or cellular pathways of macromolecular synthesis.

Cell & Tissue Culture

- Cells can be grown in vitro from newly **explanted** tissues (primary cultures) or as long established cell lines and can be examined in the living state by phase-contrast light microscopy.

Enzyme Histochemistry

- **Histochemical (or cytochemical) techniques** use specific enzymatic activities in lightly fixed or unfixed tissue sections to produce visible products in the specific enzyme locations.
- Fixation and paraffin embedding denatures most enzymes, so histochemistry usually uses frozen tissue sectioned with a **cryostat**.
- Enzyme classes for which histochemical study is useful include phosphatases, dehydrogenases, and peroxidases, with peroxidase often conjugated to antibodies used in immunohistochemistry.

Visualizing Specific Molecules

- Some substances specifically bind certain targets in cells.
- **Immunohistochemistry** is based on specific reactions between an antigen and antibodies labeled with visible markers, often fluorescent compounds or peroxidase for light microscopy and gold particles for TEM.
- If the cell or tissue antigen of interest is detected by directly binding a labeled **primary antibody** specific for that antigen, the process is considered **direct immunohistochemistry**.
- **Indirect immunohistochemistry** uses an unlabeled primary antibody that is detected bound to its antigen with labeled **secondary antibodies**.
- The indirect immunohistochemical method is more commonly used because the added level of antibody binding amplifies the signal detected and provides greater technical flexibility.
- Specific gene sequences or mRNAs of cells can be detected microscopically using labeled complementary DNA (cDNA) probes in a technique called **in situ hybridization (ISH)**.

Interpretation of Structures in Tissue Sections

- Many steps in tissue processing, slide preparation, and staining can introduce minor **artifacts** such as spaces and precipitates that are not normally present in the living tissue and must be recognized.
- Sections of cells or tissues are essentially 2D planes through 3D structures, and understanding this fact is needed for their correct interpretation and study.

CHAPTER

2 The Cytoplasm

Cells and extracellular material together comprise all the tissues that make up the organs of multicellular animals. In all tissues, cells themselves are the basic structural and functional units, the smallest living parts of the body. Animal cells are **eukaryotic** (Gr. *eu*, good, + *karyon*, nucleus), with distinct membrane-limited nuclei surrounded by cytoplasm containing various membrane-limited organelles. In contrast, the smaller prokaryotic cells of bacteria typically have a cell wall around the plasmalemma and lack other membranous structures, including an envelope around their DNA. In multicellular organisms, different cells become specialized by concentrating specific organelles and specializing in various basic cellular activities generally found to more limited extents in all eukaryotic cells.

› CELL DIFFERENTIATION

The human organism consists of hundreds of different cell types, all derived from the zygote, the single cell formed by the merger of a spermatozoon with an oocyte at fertilization. The first zygotic cellular divisions produce cells called **blastomeres**, and as part of the early embryo's inner cell mass blastomeres give rise to all tissue types of the fetus. Explanted to tissue culture cells of the inner call mass are called **embryonic stem cells**. During their specialization process, called **cell differentiation**, cells synthesize increased quantities of specific proteins and become very efficient in specialized functions, often changing their shape accordingly. For example, muscle cell precursors elongate into fiber-like cells containing large arrays of actin and myosin. All animal cells contain and use actin filaments and myosins, but muscle cells are specialized for using these proteins to convert chemical energy into forceful contractions.

Major cellular functions performed by specialized cells in the body are listed in Table 2–1. It is important to understand that the functions listed there can be performed by most cells of the body; specialized cells have greatly expanded their capacity for one or more of these functions during differentiation. Changes in cells' microenvironments under normal and pathologic conditions can cause the same cell type to have variable features and activities. Cells that appear similar structurally often have different families of receptors for signaling molecules such as hormones and extracellular matrix (ECM) components, causing them to behave differently. For example, because of their diverse arrays of receptors, breast fibroblasts and uterine smooth muscle cells are exceptionally sensitive to female sex hormones while most other fibroblasts and smooth muscle cells are insensitive.

› CYTOPLASMIC ORGANELLES

The cell is composed of two basic parts: **cytoplasm** (Gr. *kytos*, cell, + *plasma*, thing formed) that surrounds the **nucleus** (L. *nux*, nut). The outermost component of the cell, separating the cytoplasm from its extracellular environment, is the **plasma membrane** (**plasmalemma**). Although the plasma membrane defines the outer limit of the cell, a continuum exists between the interior of the cell and extracellular macromolecules. The plasma membrane contains proteins called **integrins** linked to both cytoplasmic protein filaments and ECM components. These linkages produce a continuous exchange of influences, in both directions, between the ECM and the cytoplasm.

The cytoplasm consists largely of a fluid component, **cytosol**, bathing metabolically active structures, the **organelles**, which

TABLE **2–1**	Differentiated cells typically specialize in one activity.
General Cellular Activity	**Specialized Cell(s)**
Movement	Muscle and other contractile cells
Form adhesive and tight junctions between cells	Epithelial cells
Synthesize and secrete components of the extracellular matrix	Fibroblasts, cells of bone and cartilage
Convert physical and chemical stimuli into action potentials	Neurons and sensory cells
Synthesis and secretion of degradative enzymes	Cells of digestive glands
Synthesis and secretion of glycoproteins	Cells of mucous glands
Synthesis and secretion of steroids	Certain cells of the adrenal gland, testis, and ovary
Ion transport	Cells of the kidney and salivary gland ducts
Intracellular digestion	Macrophages and neutrophils
Lipid storage	Fat cells
Metabolite absorption	Cells lining the intestine

may be membranous (such as mitochondria) or nonmembranous protein complexes (such as ribosomes and proteasomes). In addition to the organelles, there are protein components of the cytoplasmic **cytoskeleton**, which determines the shape and motility of eukaryotic cells. Among the minor cytoplasmic structures are **inclusions** that are generally deposits of carbohydrates, lipids, or pigments.

Cytosol also contains hundreds of enzymes, such as those of the glycolytic pathway, that produce building blocks for larger molecules and break down small molecules to liberate energy. All the machinery converging on the ribosomes for protein synthesis (mRNA, transfer RNA, enzymes, and other factors) is also contained within the cytosol. Oxygen, CO_2, electrolytic ions, low-molecular-weight substrates, metabolites, and waste products all diffuse through cytosol, either freely or bound to proteins, entering or leaving organelles where they are used or produced.

Plasma Membrane

The limiting membranes that envelop all eukaryotic cells are made of phospholipids, cholesterol, proteins, and oligosaccharide chains covalently linked to phospholipid and protein molecules. The plasma membrane (cell membrane) functions as a selective barrier regulating the passage of materials into and out of the cell and facilitating the transport of specific molecules. One important role of the cell membrane is to keep

constant the ion content of cytoplasm, which differs from that of the extracellular fluid. Membranes also carry out a number of specific recognition and signaling functions, playing a key role in the interactions of the cell with its environment.

Membranes range from 7.5 to 10 nm in thickness and consequently are visible only in the electron microscope. The line between adjacent cells sometimes seen faintly with the light microscope is formed by plasma membrane proteins plus extracellular material, which together can reach a dimension visible by light microscopy.

Membrane phospholipids are amphipathic, consisting of two nonpolar (hydrophobic or water-repelling) long-chain fatty acids linked to a charged polar (hydrophilic or water-attracting) head that bears a phosphate group (Figure 2–1a). Phospholipids are most stable when organized into a double layer (bilayer) with the hydrophobic fatty acid chains directed toward the middle away from water and the hydrophilic polar head groups facing the water (Figure 2–1b). Molecules of cholesterol, a sterol lipid, insert at varying densities among the closely-packed phospholipid fatty acids, restricting their movement, and modulating the fluidity and movement of all membrane components. The phospholipids in each half of the bilayer are different. For example, in the well-studied membranes of red blood cells phosphatidylcholine and sphingomyelin are more abundant in the outer half, while phosphatidylserine and phosphatidylethanolamine are more concentrated in the inner layer. Some of the outer lipids, known as **glycolipids**, include oligosaccharide chains that extend outward from the cell surface and contribute to a delicate cell surface coating called the **glycocalyx** (Figures 2-1b and 2–2). With the transmission electron microscope (TEM) the cell membrane—and all other organellar membranes—may exhibit a trilaminar appearance after fixation in osmium tetroxide; osmium binding the polar heads of the phospholipids, the outer sugar chains, and associated membrane proteins produces the two dark outer lines enclosing the light band of osmium-free fatty acids (Figure 2–1b).

Proteins are major constituents of membranes (~50% by weight in the plasma membrane). **Integral proteins** are directly incorporated within the lipid bilayer itself, whereas **peripheral proteins** exhibit a looser association with one of the two membrane surfaces, particularly the inner (Figure 2–2). The loosely bound peripheral proteins can be easily extracted from cell membranes with salt solutions, whereas integral proteins can be extracted only by using detergents to disrupt lipids. The polypeptide chains of many integral proteins span the membrane several times, from one side to the other, and are accordingly called **multipass transmembrane proteins**. Integration of the proteins within the lipid bilayer is mainly the result of hydrophobic interactions between the lipids and nonpolar amino acids present on the outer region of the proteins.

Freeze-fracture electron microscope studies of membranes show that parts of many integral proteins protrude from both the outer or inner membrane surface (Figure 2–2b). Like those of glycolipids, the carbohydrate moieties of glycoproteins project from the external surface of the plasma

FIGURE **2–1** Lipids in membrane structure.

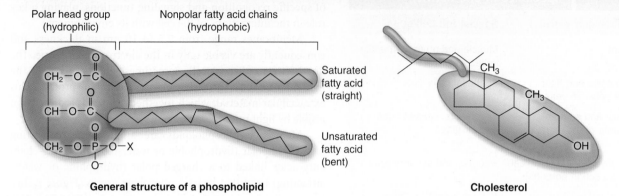

Polar head group (hydrophilic)   Nonpolar fatty acid chains (hydrophobic)

Saturated fatty acid (straight)

Unsaturated fatty acid (bent)

General structure of a phospholipid

CH₃

CH₃

OH

Cholesterol

a

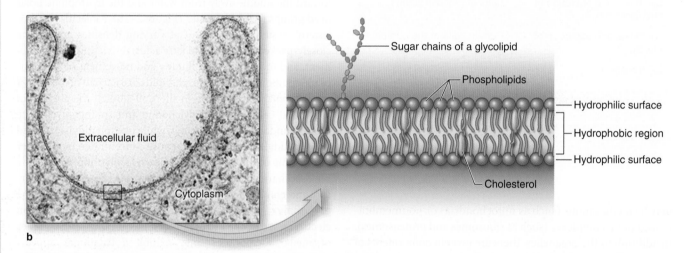

Extracellular fluid

Cytoplasm

b

Sugar chains of a glycolipid

Phospholipids

Hydrophilic surface

Hydrophobic region

Hydrophilic surface

Cholesterol

(a) Membranes of animal cells have as their major lipid components **phospholipids** and **cholesterol**. A phospholipid is amphipathic, with a phosphate group charge on the polar head and two long, nonpolar fatty acid chains, which can be straight (saturated) or kinked (at an unsaturated bond). Membrane cholesterol is present in about the same amount as phospholipid.

(b) The amphipathic nature of phospholipids produces the bilayer structure of membranes as the charged (hydrophilic) polar heads spontaneously form each membrane surface, in direct contact with water, and the hydrophobic nonpolar fatty acid chains are buried in the membrane's middle, away from water. Cholesterol molecules are also amphipathic and are interspersed less evenly throughout the lipid bilayer; cholesterol affects the packing of the fatty acid chains, with a major effect on membrane fluidity. The outer layer of the cell membrane also contains **glycolipids** with extended carbohydrate chains.

Sectioned, osmium-fixed cell membrane may have a faint trilaminar appearance with the transmission electron microscope (TEM), showing two dark (electron-dense) lines enclosing a clear (electron-lucent) band. Reduced osmium is deposited on the hydrophilic phosphate groups present on each side of the internal region of fatty acid chains where osmium is not deposited. The "fuzzy" material on the outer surface of the membrane represents the **glycocalyx** of oligosaccharides of glycolipids and glycoproteins. X100,000.

membrane and contribute to the glycocalyx (Figure 2–3). They are important components of proteins acting as **receptors**, which participate in important interactions such as cell adhesion, cell recognition, and the response to protein hormones. As with lipids, the distribution of membrane polypeptides is different in the two surfaces of the cell membranes. Therefore, all membranes in the cell are asymmetric.

Studies with labeled membrane proteins of cultured cells reveal that many such proteins are not bound rigidly in place and are able to move laterally (Figure 2–4). Such observations as well as data from biochemical, electron microscopic, and other studies showed that membrane proteins comprise a moveable mosaic within the fluid lipid bilayer, the well-established **fluid mosaic model** for membrane structure (see Figure 2–2a).

FIGURE **2–2** Proteins associated with the membrane lipid bilayer.

(a) The fluid mosaic model of membrane structure emphasizes that the phospholipid bilayer of a membrane also contains proteins inserted in it or associated with its surface (peripheral proteins) and that many of these proteins move within the fluid lipid phase. **Integral proteins** are firmly embedded in the lipid layers; those that completely span the bilayer are called **transmembrane proteins**. Hydrophobic amino acids of these proteins interact with the hydrophobic fatty acid portions of the membrane lipids. Both the proteins and lipids may have externally exposed oligosaccharide chains.

(b) When cells are frozen and fractured (**cryofracture**), the lipid bilayer of membranes is often cleaved along the hydrophobic center. Splitting occurs along the line of weakness formed by the fatty acid tails of phospholipids. Electron microscopy of such cryofracture preparation replicas provides a useful method for studying membrane structures. Most of the protruding membrane particles seen (1) are proteins or aggregates of proteins that remain attached to the half of the membrane adjacent to the cytoplasm (P or protoplasmic face). Fewer particles are found attached to the outer half of the membrane (E or extracellular face). Each protein bulging on one surface has a corresponding depression (2) on the opposite surface.

However, unlike the lipids, many membrane proteins are restricted in their lateral diffusion by attachment to cytoskeletal components. In most epithelial cells, tight junctions between the cells (see Chapter 4) also restrict lateral diffusion of unattached transmembrane proteins and outer layer lipids, producing specific membrane domains.

Membrane proteins functioning as components of large enzyme complexes are also less mobile, especially those involved in the transduction of signals from outside the cell. Such protein complexes are located in specialized membrane patches termed **lipid rafts** having higher concentrations of cholesterol and saturated fatty acids which reduce lipid fluidity.

This together with the presence of scaffold proteins that maintain spatial relationships between enzymes and signaling proteins allows the proteins assembled within lipid rafts to remain in close proximity and interact more efficiently.

Transmembrane Proteins & Membrane Transport

The plasma membrane is the site where materials are exchanged between the cell and its environment, with many molecules moving through the membrane by the general mechanisms shown in Figure 2–5. Small, lipophilic (fat-soluble) molecules can pass through lipid bilayers by **simple diffusion**.

FIGURE **2–3** Membrane proteins.

Functions of Plasma Membrane

1. **Physical barrier:** Establishes a flexible boundary, protects cellular contents, and supports cell structure. Phospholipid bilayer separates substances inside and outside the cell
2. **Selective permeability:** Regulates entry and exit of ions, nutrients, and waste molecules through the membrane
3. **Electrochemical gradients:** Establishes and maintains an electrical charge difference across the plasma membrane
4. **Communication:** Contains receptors that recognize and respond to molecular signals

Both protein and lipid components often have covalently attached oligosaccharide chains exposed at the external membrane surface. These contribute to the cell's **glycocalyx**, which provides important antigenic and functional properties to the cell surface. Membrane proteins serve as receptors for various signals coming from outside cells, as parts of intercellular connections, and as selective gateways for molecules entering the cell.

Transmembrane proteins often have multiple hydrophobic regions buried within the lipid bilayer to produce a channel or other active site for specific transfer of substances through the membrane.

Ions such as Na⁺, K⁺, and Ca²⁺ cross membranes by passing through integral membrane proteins that act as **ion channels** or ion pumps. Transmembrane diffusion of water molecules (by **osmosis**) involves their passive movement through multipass transmembrane proteins called **aquaporins**. Other ions and many molecules only cross membranes after binding to carrier or transporter proteins, which are integral membrane proteins in which conformational changes deliver the bound molecule to the other side (Figure 2–5). While simple diffusion is passive (requiring no energy), ion pumps and carrier proteins involve **active transport**, using energy from the breakdown of adenosine triphosphate (ATP). These transport processes are summarized with further details and examples in Table 2–2.

Vesicular Transport: Endocytosis & Exocytosis

Bulk uptake of material also occurs across the plasma membrane in a general process called **endocytosis**, an active process involving folding and fusion of the membrane to form **vesicles** that enclose the material transported. Cells show three general types of endocytosis, summarized in Table 2–2 and Figure 2–6.

1. **Phagocytosis:** Phagocytosis literally means "cell eating." Certain white blood cells, such as macrophages and neutrophils, are specialized for engulfing and removing particulate matter such as bacteria, protozoa, dead cells, and unneeded extracellular constituents. When a bacterium becomes bound to the surface of a neutrophil, cytoplasmic

FIGURE **2–4** Experiment demonstrating the fluidity of membrane proteins.

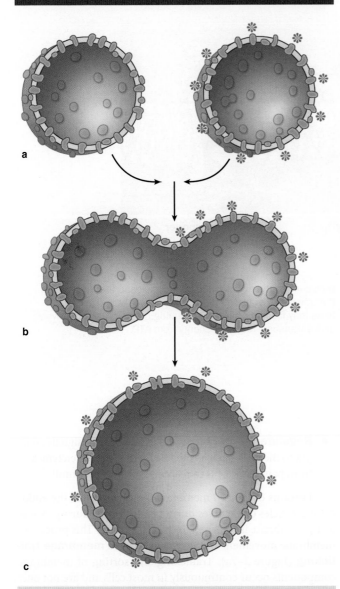

(a) Two types of cells were grown in tissue cultures, one with fluorescently labeled transmembrane proteins in the plasmalemma (right) and one without.

(b) Cells of each type were fused together experimentally into hybrid cells.

(c) Minutes after the fusion of the cell membranes, the fluorescent proteins of the labeled cell spread to the entire surface of the hybrid cells. Such experiments provide important data supporting the fluid mosaic model. However, many membrane proteins show more restricted lateral movements, being anchored in place by links to the cytoskeleton.

extensions are extended from the cell (in an actin-dependent process) and to surround the bacterium. The membranes of these extensions meet and fuse, enclosing the bacterium in an intracellular vacuole called a **phagosome**, which then

fuses with a lysosome for degradation of the contents as discussed later in this chapter.

2. **Fluid-phase endocytosis:** In fluid-phase pinocytosis ("cell drinking"), smaller invaginations of the cell membrane form and entrap extracellular fluid and its dissolved contents. **Pinocytotic vesicles** (~80 nm in diameter) then pinch off inwardly from the cell surface. In most cells such vesicles usually fuse with lysosomes. In many very thin cells, however, pinocytotic vesicles may move to the opposite cell surface where they fuse with the membrane and release their contents outside the cell. This accomplishes bulk transfer of material across the cell in a process termed **transcytosis**.

3. **Receptor-mediated endocytosis:** Receptors for many substances, such as low-density lipoproteins and protein hormones, are integral membrane proteins at the cell surface. High-affinity binding of such ligands to their receptors causes these proteins to aggregate in special membrane regions that then invaginate and pinch off internally as vesicles.

As shown in Figure 2–7, the formation and fate of vesicles emerging from receptor-mediated endocytosis is regulated by specific peripheral membrane coat proteins. The occupied receptors associate with other proteins on the cytoplasmic membrane surface and begin invagination as **coated pits**. The electron-dense coating on the cytoplasmic surface of such pits contains several polypeptides, the major one being **clathrin**. In a coated pit clathrin molecules interact like the struts in a geodesic dome, forming that region of cell membrane into a cage-like invagination that is pinched off into the cytoplasm as a **coated vesicle** (Figure 2–7) containing the ligands and their receptors internally. Another type of receptor-mediated endocytosis very prominent in endothelial cells uses invaginations called **caveolae** (L. *caveolae*, little caves) that involve the membrane protein caveolin.

In all these endocytotic processes, the vesicles or vacuoles produced quickly enter and fuse with the **endosomal compartment**, a dynamic system of membranous vesicles (Figure 2–7) of various sizes and shapes located in the cytoplasm near the cell surface (**early endosomes**) or deeper in the cytoplasm (**late endosomes**). The clathrin molecules separated from the coated vesicles recycle back to the cell membrane to participate in the formation of new coated pits. The membrane of endosomes contains ATP-driven H$^+$ pumps that acidify their interior.

While phagosomes and pinocytotic vesicles soon fuse with lysosomes, molecules penetrating the endosomal compartment after receptor-mediated endocytosis may also be directed down other pathways (Figure 2–7a). The acidic pH of early endosomes causes many ligands to uncouple from their receptors, after which the two molecules are sorted into separate vesicles. The receptors may be returned to the cell membrane to be reused. Low-density lipoprotein receptors, for example, are recycled several times. The ligands typically are transferred to late endosomes. However, some ligands

FIGURE 2–5 Major mechanisms by which molecules cross membranes.

(a) Simple diffusion   **(b) Channel**   **(c) Carrier/transporter**

Lipophilic and some small, uncharged molecules can cross membranes by simple diffusion **(a)**.

Most ions are transported through membranes in proteins whose structure includes an ion-specific channel **(b)**.

Many other larger, water-soluble molecules require binding to sites on selective carrier proteins or transporters, which

then change their conformations and release the molecule to the other side of the membrane **(c)**. Channel and carrier proteins may facilitate diffusion requiring no energy or may involve active transport requiring energy from ATP.

are returned to the extracellular milieu with their receptors and both are used again. An example of this activity is the iron-transport protein transferrin: ferric ions dissociate from transferrin at low endosomal pH and the free protein and the receptor both return to the cell surface. Other endosomes may release their entire contents at a separate domain of the cell membrane (transcytosis), which is especially important in epithelial cells.

Bulk movement of large molecules from inside to outside the cell can involve the form of vesicular transport called **exocytosis**. In this process a membrane-limited cytoplasmic vesicle fuses with the plasma membrane, resulting in the release of its contents into the extracellular space without compromising the integrity of the plasma membrane (Figure 2–7a). Exocytosis is triggered in many cells by transient increase in cytosolic Ca^{2+}. The pathways and process of membrane fusion during exocytosis are highly regulated and involve interactions between several specific membrane proteins. Exocytosis of stored products from epithelial cells usually occurs specifically at the apical domains of cells, constituting a major mechanism of glandular secretion (see Chapter 4).

Protein secretion involving exocytosis may follow two pathways:

■ **Constitutive secretion** is used for products that are released from cells continuously, as soon as synthesis is complete, such as procollagen for the ECM.

■ **Regulated secretion** occurs in response to signals coming to the cells, such as the release of digestive enzymes from pancreatic cells in response to specific stimuli.

Portions of the cell membrane become part of the endocytotic vesicles or vacuoles during endocytosis; during exocytosis, membrane is returned to the cell surface. This process of membrane movement and recycling is called **membrane trafficking** (Figure 2–7a). Trafficking and sorting of membrane components occur continuously in most cells and are not only crucial for maintaining the cell but also for physiologically important processes such as reducing blood lipid levels.

Subpopulations of vacuoles among the early and late endosomes in many cells accumulate small vesicles and tubules *within* their lumens by further invaginations of their limiting membranes, becoming **multivesicular bodies**. While multivesicular bodies may merge with lysosomes for selective degradation of their contents, this organelle may also fuse with the plasma membrane and release the intralumenal vesicles outside the cell. The small (<120 nm diameter) vesicles released (called **exosomes**) allow transfer of membrane proteins and other materials to nearby cells.

Signal Reception & Transduction

Cells in a multicellular organism communicate with one another to regulate tissue and organ development, to control their growth

TABLE **2–2**	Mechanisms of transport across the plasma membrane.	
Process	**Type of Movement**	**Example**
PASSIVE PROCESSES	Movement of substances down a concentration gradient due to the kinetic energy of the substance; no expenditure of cellular energy is required; continues until equilibrium is reached (if unopposed)	
Simple diffusion	Unassisted net movement of small, nonpolar substances down their concentration gradient across a selectively permeable membrane	Exchange of oxygen and carbon dioxide between blood and body tissues
Facilitated diffusion	Movement of ions and small, polar molecules down their concentration gradient; assisted across a selectively permeable membrane by a transport protein	
Channel-mediated	Movement of ion down its concentration gradient through a protein channel	Na^+ moves through Na^+ channel into cell
Carrier-mediated	Movement of small, polar molecule down its concentration gradient by a carrier protein	Transport of glucose into cells by glucose carrier
Osmosis	Diffusion of water across a selectively permeable membrane; direction is determined by relative solute concentrations; continues until equilibrium is reached	Solutes in blood in systemic capillaries "pulls" fluid from interstitial space back into the blood
ACTIVE PROCESSES	Movement of substances requires expenditure of cellular energy	
Active transport	Transport of ions or small molecules across the membrane against a concentration gradient by transmembrane protein pumps	
Primary	Movement of substance up its concentration gradient; powered directly by ATP	Ca^{2+} pumps transport Ca^{2+} out of the cell Na^+/K^+ pump moves Na^+ out of cell and K^+ into cell
Secondary	Movement of a substance up its concentration gradient is powered by harnessing the movement of a second substance (eg, Na^+) down its concentration gradient	
Symport	Movement of substance up its concentration gradient in the same direction as Na^+	Na^+/glucose transport
Antiport	Movement of substance up its concentration gradient in the opposite direction from Na^+	Na^+/H^+ transport
Vesicular transport	Vesicle formed or lost as material is brought into a cell or released from a cell	
Exocytosis	Bulk movement of substance out of the cell by fusion of secretory vesicles with the plasma membrane	Release of neurotransmitter by nerve cells
Endocytosis	Bulk movement of substances into the cell by vesicles forming at the plasma membrane	
Phagocytosis	Type of endocytosis in which vesicles are formed as particulate materials external to the cell are engulfed by pseudopodia	White blood cell engulfing a bacterium
Pinocytosis	Type of endocytosis in which vesicles are formed as interstital fluid is taken up by the cell	Formation of small vesicles in capillary wall to move substances
Receptor-mediated endocytosis	Type of endocytosis in which plasma membrane receptors first bind specific substances; receptor and bound substance then taken up by the cell	Uptake of cholesterol into cells

FIGURE 2–6 Three major forms of endocytosis.

Extracellular fluid

Pseudopodia

Particle

Plasma membrane

Vacuole

Cytoplasm

a Phagocytosis

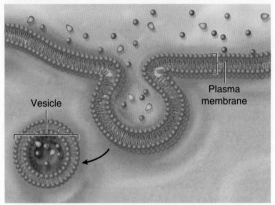

Vesicle

Plasma membrane

b Pinocytosis

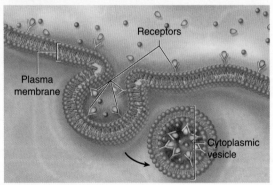

Receptors

Plasma membrane

Cytoplasmic vesicle

c Receptor-mediated endocytosis

There are three general types of endocytosis:

(a) Phagocytosis involves the extension from the cell of large folds called **pseudopodia** that engulf particles, for example bacteria, and then internalize this material into a cytoplasmic vacuole or **phagosome**.

(b) In **pinocytosis** the cell membrane invaginates (dimples inward) to form a pit containing a drop of extracellular fluid. The pit pinches off inside the cell when the cell membrane fuses and forms a pinocytotic vesicle containing the fluid.

(c) Receptor-mediated endocytosis includes membrane proteins called **receptors** that bind specific molecules (ligands). When many such receptors are bound by their ligands, they aggregate in one membrane region, which then invaginates and pinches off to create a vesicle or **endosome** containing both the receptors and the bound ligands.

and division, and to coordinate their functions. Many cells form communicating junctions that couple adjacent cells and allow the exchange of ions and small molecules (see Chapter 4). Through these channels, called **gap junctions**, signals may pass directly from cell to cell without reaching the extracellular fluid.

Cells also use nearly two dozen families of receptor proteins to detect and respond to extracellular molecules and physical stimuli of all types. Only cells with receptors for a specific ligand are **target cells** for that molecule. Each cell type in the body contains a distinctive set of receptor proteins that enable it to respond to a complementary set of signaling molecules in a specific, programmed way. Signal molecules can take different routes:

- In **endocrine signaling**, the signal molecules (called **hormones**) are carried in the blood to target cells throughout the body.
- In **paracrine signaling**, the chemical mediators are rapidly metabolized after release so that they act only on local cells very close to the source.
- In **synaptic signaling**, a special kind of paracrine interaction, neurotransmitters act only on adjacent cells through special contact areas called **synapses** (see Chapter 9).
- In **autocrine signaling**, signals bind receptors on the same cell type that produced the messenger molecule.
- In **juxtacrine signaling**, important in early embryonic tissue interactions, signaling molecules such as proteins remain part of a cell membrane and bind surface receptors of the target cell when the two cells make direct physical contact.

Receptors for **hydrophilic signaling molecules**, including most hormones and neurotransmitters, are usually transmembrane proteins in the plasmalemma of target cells, frequently as part of lipid rafts. Three important functional classes of such receptors are shown in Figure 2–8:

- **Channel-linked receptors** open upon ligand binding to allow ion transfer across the membrane.
- **Enzymatic receptors**, in which ligand binding induces catalytic activity in associated peripheral proteins.
- **G-protein–coupled receptors** upon ligand binding change an associated "G protein" that then binds the guanine nucleotide GTP and is released to activate other cytoplasmic proteins.

›› MEDICAL APPLICATION

Many diseases are caused by defective receptors. For example, **pseudohypoparathyroidism** and one type of **dwarfism** are caused by nonfunctioning parathyroid and growth hormone receptors, respectively. In these two conditions the glands produce the respective hormones, but the target cells cannot respond because they lack normal receptors.

FIGURE **2–7** Receptor-mediated endocytosis involves regulated membrane trafficking.

Major steps during and after endocytosis are indicated diagrammatically in part **a**. Ligands bind at high affinity to specific surface receptors, which then associate with specific cytoplasmic proteins, including clathrin and adaptor proteins, and aggregate in membrane regions to form **coated pits**. Clathrin facilitates invagination of the pits, and another peripheral membrane protein, dynamin, forms constricting loops around the developing neck of the pit, which cause the region to pinch off as a **coated vesicle**. The clathrin lattice of coated pits **(CP)** and vesicles **(CV)** is shown ultrastructurally in part **b**.

The internalized vesicles lose their clathrin coats and usually merge by membrane fusion with other endosomal vesicles. Ligands may have different fates within the endosomal compartment:

■ Receptors and ligands may be carried to late endosomes and then to lysosomes for **degradation**.
■ Ligands may be released internally and the **receptors recycled** to the cell surface.
■ Vesicles may move to and fuse with another cell surface, where the ligands are released again outside the cell **(transcytosis)**.

(Figure 2–7b, with permission, from Dr John Heuser, Department of Cell Biology and Physiology, Washington University School of Medicine, St. Louis, MO.)

The hydrophilic ligands (or first messengers) binding such receptor proteins often begin a process of **signal transduction**, activating a series of intracellular intermediaries producing changes in either the cytoplasm, the nucleus, or both. Channel-mediated ion influx or activation of kinases can activate downstream proteins, amplifying the signal. Activated G proteins target ion channels or other membrane-bound effectors that also propagate the signal further into the cell (Figure 2–8). One such effector protein is the enzyme adenyl cyclase that generates large quantities of second messenger molecules, such as cyclic adenosine monophosphate (cAMP). Other second messengers include 1,2-diacyglycerol (DAG), and inositol 1,4,5-triphosphate (IP_3). The ionic changes or second messengers amplify the first signal and trigger a

FIGURE **2–8** Major types of membrane receptors.

a Channel-linked receptors

b Enzymatic receptors

c G-protein–coupled receptors

Protein and most small ligands are hydrophilic molecules that bind transmembrane protein receptors to initiate changes in the target cell. **(a) Channel-linked receptors** bind ligands such as neurotransmitters and open to allow influx of specific ions. **(b) Enzymatic receptors** are usually protein kinases that are activated to phosphorylate (and usually activate) other proteins upon ligand binding. **(c) G-protein–coupled receptors** bind ligand, changing the conformation of its G-protein subunit, allowing it to bind GTP, and activating and releasing this protein to in turn activate other proteins such as ion channels and adenyl cyclase.

cascade of enzymatic activity, usually including kinases, leading to changes in gene expression or cell behavior. Second messengers may diffuse through the cytoplasm or be retained locally by scaffold proteins for more focused amplification of activity.

Hydrophobic signaling molecules, such as steroids and thyroid hormones, bind reversibly to carrier proteins in the plasma for transport through the body. Such hormones are lipophilic and, once released from their carrier proteins, pass by diffusion through the plasma membrane of the target cell and bind to specific intracellular receptor proteins. With many steroid

hormones, receptor binding activates that protein, enabling the complex to move into the nucleus and bind with high affinity to specific DNA sequences. This generally increases the level of transcription from specific genes. Each steroid hormone is recognized by a different member of a family of homologous receptor proteins.

Ribosomes

Ribosomes are small electron-dense particles, about 20×30 nm in size. Ribosomes found in the cytosol are composed of four

FIGURE 2–9 Polyribosomes: free or bound to the endoplasmic reticulum.

Free polyribosomes (not attached to the endoplasmic reticulum, or ER) synthesize cytosolic and cytoskeletal proteins and proteins for import into the nucleus, mitochondria, and peroxisomes.

Proteins that are to be incorporated into membranes, stored in lysosomes, or eventually secreted from the cell are made on polysomes attached to the membranes of ER. The proteins produced by these ribosomes are segregated during translation into the interior of the ER's membrane cisternae.

In both pathways misfolded proteins are conjugated to ubiquitin and targeted for proteasomal degradation.

segments of rRNA and approximately 80 different proteins. Bound to mRNA, all ribosomes have two subunits of different sizes and act to catalyze the process of protein translation.

In eukaryotic cells, the rRNA molecules of both subunits are synthesized within the nucleus. Their numerous proteins are synthesized in the cytoplasm but then enter the nucleus and associate with rRNAs. The assembled large and small subunits then leave the nucleus and enter the cytoplasm to participate in protein synthesis.

The large and small ribosomal subunits come together by binding an mRNA strand (Figure 2–9), and typically many ribosomes occupy a single mRNA to form **polyribosomes** (or **polysomes**). With the nucleotide sequence of the mRNA specifying the polypeptide sequence being synthesized, ribosomes assemble the protein chain from amino acids ferried in by tRNA. The compact core of each ribosome contains the rRNA molecules that not only provide structural support but also position tRNAs in the correct "reading frame" and catalyze the formation of the peptide bonds. The more peripheral proteins of the ribosome seem to function primarily to stabilize the catalytic RNA core.

Polyribosomes are intensely basophilic because of the numerous phosphate groups of the constituent RNAs that act as polyanions. Thus, cytoplasmic regions that stain intensely with hematoxylin and basic dyes, such as methylene and toluidine blue, indicate sites of active protein synthesis.

Proper folding of new proteins is guided by protein chaperones (often present in chaperonin complexes); denatured proteins or those that cannot be refolded properly are conjugated to the protein ubiquitin that targets them for breakdown by proteasomes (discussed later). As indicated in Figure 2–9, proteins synthesized for use within the cytosol (eg, glycolytic enzymes) or for import into the nucleus and certain other organelles are synthesized on polyribosomes existing as isolated cytoplasmic clusters. Polyribosomes attached via the large subunits to the membranes of the endoplasmic reticulum (ER) translate mRNA coding for membrane proteins of the ER, the Golgi apparatus, or the cell membrane; enzymes to be stored in lysosomes; and proteins to undergo exocytosis from secretory vesicles.

Endoplasmic Reticulum

The cytoplasm of most cells contains a convoluted membranous network called the **endoplasmic reticulum (ER)**. This network (reticulum) extends from the surface of the nucleus to the cell membrane and encloses a series of intercommunicating channels and sacs called **cisternae** (Figure 2–10). With a membrane surface up to 30 times that of the cell membrane, the ER provides a major site for vital cellular activities,

FIGURE 2–10 Rough and smooth endoplasmic reticulum.

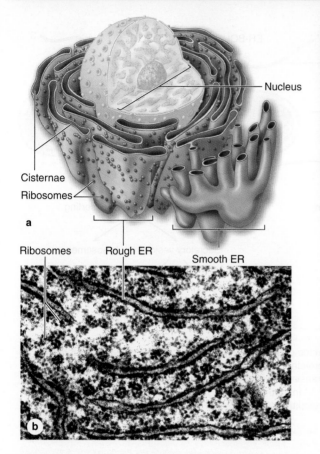

Nucleus

Cisternae

Ribosomes

a

Ribosomes   Rough ER   Smooth ER

b

c

Functions of Endoplasmic Reticulum

1. **Synthesis:** Provides a place for chemical reactions
   a. Smooth ER is the site of lipid synthesis and carbohydrate metabolism
   b. Rough ER synthesizes proteins for secretion, incorporation into the plasma, membrane, and as enzymes within lysosomes
2. **Transport:** Moves molecules through cisternal space from one part of the cell to another, sequestered away from the cytoplasm
3. **Storage:** Stores newly synthesized molecules
4. **Detoxification:** Smooth ER detoxifies both drugs and alcohol

(a) The **endoplasmic reticulum** is an anastomosing network of intercommunicating channels or **cisternae** formed by a continuous membrane, with some regions that bear polysomes appearing rough and other regions appearing smooth. While RER is the site for synthesis of most membrane-bound proteins, three diverse activities are associated with smooth ER: (1) lipid biosynthesis, (2) detoxification of potentially harmful compounds, and (3) sequestration of Ca^{++} ions. Specific cell types with well-developed SER are usually specialized for one of these functions.

(b) By TEM cisternae of RER appear separated, but they actually form a continuous channel or compartment in the cytoplasm. The interconnected membranous cisternae of RER are flattened, while those of SER are frequently tubular. 14,000X.

(c) In a very thin cultured endothelial cell, both ER (green) and mitochondria (orange) can be visualized with vital fluorescent dyes that are sequestered specifically into those organelles. This staining method with intact cells clearly reveals the continuous, lacelike ER present in all regions of the cytoplasm.
(*Figure 2–10c, with permission, from Invitrogen.*)

including biosynthesis of proteins and lipids. In addition, the ER cisternae (L. *cisternae*, reservoirs), which appear as separated spaces in electron microscopic sections, comprise a continuous internal cell compartment that collects newly synthesized proteins for modification and delivery into pathways leading to other organelles and for secretion. In most cells over a quarter of all proteins are imported into the lumen of the ER or integrated into ER membranes.

In many places the cytosolic side of the ER membrane is covered by polyribosomes forming the polypeptides that enter the adjacent cisterna during synthesis. The attached polysomes permit the distinction between the two types of ER: **rough** and **smooth**.

Rough Endoplasmic Reticulum

Rough endoplasmic reticulum (RER) is prominent in cells specialized for protein secretion, such as pancreatic acinar cells (making digestive enzymes), fibroblasts (collagen), and plasma cells (immunoglobulins). The RER consists of saclike as well as parallel stacks of flattened cisternae (Figure 2–10), each limited by membranes that are continuous with the outer membrane of the nuclear envelope. The presence of polyribosomes on the cytosolic surface of the RER confers basophilic staining properties on this organelle when viewed with the light microscope.

Principal activities of the RER include synthesis and segregation of proteins not destined for the cytosol. Additional functions include the initial (core) glycosylation of glycoproteins,

FIGURE **2–11** Movement of polypeptides into the RER.

The newly translated amino terminus of a protein to be incorporated into membranes or sequestered into vesicles contains 15-40 amino acids that include a specific sequence of hydrophobic residues comprising the **signal sequence** or signal peptide. This sequence is bound by a signal-recognition particle (SRP), which then recognizes and binds a receptor on the ER. Another receptor in the ER membrane binds a structural protein of the large ribosomal subunit, more firmly attaching the ribosome to the ER. The hydrophobic signal peptide is translocated through a protein pore (translocon) in the ER membrane, and the SRP is freed for reuse. The signal peptide is removed from the growing protein by a peptidase and translocation of the growing polypeptide continues until it is completely segregated into the ER cisterna.

certain other posttranslational modifications of newly formed polypeptides, and the assembly of multichain proteins. These activities are mediated by resident enzymes of the RER and by protein complexes that act as molecular chaperones guiding the folding of nascent proteins, inhibiting aggregation, and generally monitoring protein quality within the ER.

Protein synthesis begins on polyribosomes in the cytosol. The 5′ ends of mRNAs for proteins destined to be segregated in the ER encode an N-terminal **signal sequence** of 15-40 amino acids that includes a series of six or more hydrophobic residues. As shown in Figure 2–11, the newly translated signal sequence is bound by a protein complex called the **signal-recognition particle (SRP)**, which inhibits further polypeptide elongation. The SRP-ribosome-nascent peptide complex binds to SRP receptors on the ER membrane. SRP then releases the signal sequence, allowing translation to continue with the nascent polypeptide chain transferred to a **translocator complex** (also called a translocon or protein-conducting channel) through the ER membrane (Figure 2–11). Inside the lumen of the RER, the signal sequence is removed by an enzyme, signal peptidase. With the ribosome docked at the ER surface, translation continues with the growing polypeptide pushing itself while chaperones and other proteins serve to "pull" the nascent polypeptide through the translocator complex. Upon release from the ribosome, posttranslational modifications and proper folding of the polypeptides continue.

As mentioned, proteins synthesized in the RER can have several destinations: intracellular storage (eg, in lysosomes and specific granules of leukocytes), provisional intracellular storage of proteins before exocytosis (eg, in the pancreas, some endocrine cells), and as integral membrane proteins. Diagrams in Figure 2–12 show a few cell types with distinct differences in the destinations of their major protein products and how these differences determine a cell's histologic features.

RER has a highly regulated system to prevent nonfunctional proteins being forwarded to the pathway for secretion or to other organelles. New proteins that cannot be folded or assembled properly by chaperones undergo ER-associated degradation (ERAD), in which unsalvageable proteins are translocated back into the cytosol, conjugated to ubiquitin, and then degraded by proteasomes.

>> **MEDICAL APPLICATION**

Quality control during protein production in the RER and properly functioning ERAD to dispose of defective proteins are extremely important and several inherited diseases result from malfunctions in this system. For example, in some forms of **osteogenesis imperfecta** bone cells synthesize and secrete defective procollagen molecules which cannot assemble properly and produce very weak bone tissue.

FIGURE **2–12** Protein localization and cell morphology.

(a) Erythroblast   **(b)** Eosinophilic leukocyte   **(c)** Plasma cell   **(d)** Pancreatic acinar cell

The ultrastructure and general histologic appearance of a cell are determined by the nature of the most prominent proteins the cell is making.

(a) Cells that make few or no proteins for secretion have very little RER, with essentially all polyribosomes free in the cytoplasm.

(b) Cells that synthesize, segregate, and store various proteins in specific secretory granules or vesicles always have RER, a Golgi apparatus, and a supply of granules containing the proteins ready to be secreted.

(c) Cells with extensive RER and a well-developed Golgi apparatus show few secretory granules because the proteins undergo exocytosis immediately after Golgi processing is complete. Many cells, especially those of epithelia, are *polarized*, meaning that the distribution of RER and secretory vesicles is different in various regions or poles of the cell.

(d) Epithelial cells specialized for secretion have distinct polarity, with RER abundant at their basal ends and mature secretory granules at the apical poles undergoing exocytosis into an enclosed extracellular compartment, the lumen of a gland.

Smooth Endoplasmic Reticulum

Regions of ER that lack bound polyribosomes make up the smooth endoplasmic reticulum (SER), which is continuous with RER but frequently less abundant (Figure 2–10). Lacking polyribosomes, SER is not basophilic and is best seen with the TEM. SER cisternae are often more tubular and more likely to appear as interconnected channels of various shapes and sizes than as stacks of flattened cisternae. SER contains some enzymes also found in RER, but is specialized for other distinct functions, including glycogen and lipid metabolism, detoxification reactions, and temporary Ca^{2+} sequestration.

A major role of enzymes in the SER is *phospholipid synthesis*, including the various phospholipids that are major constituents of cellular membranes. The phospholipids are transferred from the SER to other membranes in various ways: (1) by direct communication with the RER, allowing lateral diffusion, (2) by vesicles that detach, move along the cytoskeleton, and fuse with other membranous organelles, and (3) by phospholipid transfer proteins. In cells that secrete steroid hormones (eg, cells of the adrenal cortex), SER occupies a large portion of the cytoplasm and contains enzymes required for *steroid synthesis*.

SER is also abundant in many liver cells, where it contains enzymes responsible for glycogen metabolism, for processing endogenous molecules such as the components of bile, and for the oxidation, conjugation, and methylation reactions

that neutralize potentially toxic exogenous molecules such as alcohol, barbiturates, and other drugs. Important for such *detoxification reactions* are enzymes of the cytochrome P450 family.

Another function of the SER is to *sequester and release Ca^{2+}* in a controlled manner, which is part of the rapid response of cells to various stimuli. This function is very well developed in muscle cells, where the SER has an important role in the contraction process and assumes a specialized form called the **sarcoplasmic reticulum** (see Chapter 10).

›› MEDICAL APPLICATION

Jaundice denotes a yellowish discoloration of the skin and is caused by accumulation in extracellular fluid of bilirubin and other pigmented compounds, which are normally metabolized by SER enzymes in cells of the liver and excreted as bile. A frequent cause of jaundice in newborn infants is an underdeveloped state of SER in liver cells, with failure of bilirubin to be converted to a form that can be readily excreted.

Golgi Apparatus

The dynamic organelle called the **Golgi apparatus**, or Golgi complex, completes posttranslational modifications of proteins synthesized in the RER and then packages and addresses these proteins to proper destinations. Named after histologist Camillo Golgi who discovered it in 1898, the Golgi apparatus is composed of smooth membranous saccules containing enzymes for these functions (Figure 2–13). In polarized secretory cells with apical and basal ends, such as mucus-secreting goblet cells, the Golgi apparatus occupies a characteristic position between the nucleus and the apical plasma membrane.

As shown in Figure 2–13, the Golgi apparatus generally shows two distinct sides structurally and functionally, which reflect the complex traffic of vesicles within cells. Material moves from the RER cisternae to the Golgi apparatus in small, membrane-enclosed carriers called **transport vesicles** that are transported along cytoskeletal polymers by motor proteins. The transport vesicles merge with the Golgi-receiving region, or *cis face*. On the opposite side of the Golgi network, at its shipping or *trans face*, larger saccules or vacuoles accumulate, condense, and generate other vesicles that carry completed protein products to organelles away from the Golgi (Figure 2–13).

Formation of transport vesicles and secretory vesicles is driven by assembly of various coat proteins (including clathrin), which also regulate vesicular traffic to, through, and beyond the Golgi apparatus. Forward movement of vesicles in the *cis* Golgi network of saccules is promoted by the **coat protein COP-II**, while retrograde movements in that region involve **COP-I**. Other membrane proteins important for directed vesicle fusion include **golgins**, which interact with enzymes; receptors and other binding proteins; and fusion-promoting proteins to specify, organize, and shape Golgi membranes. Depending on their protein contents and activity of these proteins, vesicles are directed toward different Golgi regions and they give rise to lysosomes or secretory vesicles for exocytosis.

As indicated in Figure 2–14, Golgi saccules at sequential locations contain different enzymes at different *cis, medial*, and *trans* levels. Enzymes of the Golgi apparatus are important for glycosylation, sulfation, phosphorylation, and limited proteolysis of proteins. Along with these activities, the Golgi apparatus initiates packing, concentration, and storage of secretory products. Protein movements through the Golgi and the control of protein processing are subjects of active research.

Secretory Granules

Originating as condensing vesicles in the Golgi apparatus, **secretory granules** are found in cells that store a product until its release by exocytosis is signaled by a metabolic, hormonal, or neural message (regulated secretion). The granules are surrounded by a membrane and contain a concentrated form of the secretory product (Figure 2–15). The contents of some secretory granules may be up to 200 times more concentrated than those in the cisternae of the RER. Secretory granules with dense contents of digestive enzymes are also referred to as **zymogen granules**.

Lysosomes

Lysosomes are sites of intracellular digestion and turnover of cellular components. Lysosomes (Gr. *lysis*, solution, + *soma*, body) are membrane-limited vesicles that contain about 40 different hydrolytic enzymes and are particularly abundant in cells with great phagocytic activity (eg, macrophages, neutrophils). Although the nature and activity of lysosomal enzymes vary depending on the cell type, the most common are acid hydrolyases such as proteases, nucleases, phosphatase, phospholipases, sulfatases, and β-glucuronidase. As can be seen from this list, lysosomal enzymes are capable of breaking down most macromolecules.

Lysosomes, which are usually spherical, range in diameter from 0.05 to 0.5 μm and present a uniformly granular, electron-dense appearance in the TEM (Figure 2–16). In macrophages and neutrophils, lysosomes are slightly larger and visible with the light microscope, especially after histochemical staining.

Cytosolic components are protected from these enzymes by the membrane surrounding lysosomes and because the enzymes have optimal activity at an acidic pH (~5.0). Any leaked lysosomal enzymes are practically inactive at the pH of cytosol (~7.2) and harmless to the cell.

Lysosomal hydrolases are synthesized and segregated in the RER and then transferred to the Golgi apparatus, where the enzymes are further modified and packaged in vacuoles that form lysosomes. The marker mannose-6-phosphate (M6P) is added by a phosphotransferase in the *cis* Golgi only to the N-linked oligosaccharides of the hydrolases destined for lysosomes. Membrane receptors for M6P-containing proteins in the *trans* Golgi network then bind these proteins and divert them from the secretory pathway for segregation into lysosomes.

Material taken from outside the cell by endocytosis is digested when the membrane of the phagosome or pinocytotic vesicle fuses with a lysosome. This mixes the endocytosed material with the lysosomal enzymes and activates proton pumps in the lysosomal membrane that acidify the contents, allowing digestion. The composite, active organelle is now termed a secondary or **heterolysosome**. Heterolysosomes are generally somewhat larger and have a more heterogeneous appearance in the TEM because of the wide variety of materials they may be digesting (Figure 2–16c).

During this digestion of macromolecules, released nutrients diffuse into the cytosol through the lysosomal membrane. Indigestible material is retained within a small vacuolar remnant called a **residual body** (Figure 2–17). In some long-lived cells (eg, neurons, heart muscle), residual bodies can accumulate over time as granules of **lipofuscin**.

Besides degrading exogenous macromolecules, lysosomes also function in the removal of excess or nonfunctional organelles and other cytoplasmic structures in a process called **autophagy** (Figures 2–17 and 2–18). A membrane from SER forms around the organelle or cytoplasmic portion to be removed, producing an **autophagosome** (Gr. *autos*, self, + *phagein*, to eat, + *soma*). These then fuse with lysosomes

FIGURE **2–13** Golgi apparatus.

The **Golgi apparatus** is a highly plastic, morphologically complex system of membrane vesicles and cisternae in which proteins and other molecules made in the RER undergo further modification and sorting into specific vesicles destined for different roles in the cell.

(a) TEM of the Golgi apparatus provided early evidence about how this organelle functions. To the left is a cisterna of RER and close to it are many small vesicles at the *cis* face **(CF)**, or receiving face, of the Golgi apparatus, merging with the first of several flattened Golgi cisternae. In the center are the characteristic flattened, curved, and stacked medial cisternae of the complex. Cytological and molecular data suggest that other transport vesicles **(TV)** move proteins serially through the cisternae until at the *trans* face **(TF)**, or shipping region, larger condensing secretory vesicles **(SV)** and other vacuoles emerge to carry the modified proteins elsewhere in the cell. Formation and fusion of the vesicles through the Golgi apparatus is controlled by specific membrane proteins. X30,000.
Inset: a small region of a Golgi apparatus in a 1-μm section from a silver-stained cell, demonstrating abundant glycoproteins within cisternae.

(b) Morphological aspects of the Golgi apparatus are revealed more clearly by SEM, which shows a three-dimensional snapshot of the region between RER and the Golgi membrane compartments. Cells may have multiple Golgi apparatuses, each with the general organization shown here and typically situated near the cell nucleus. 30,000X.

(c) The Golgi apparatus location can be clearly seen in intact cultured cells processed by immunocytochemistry using an antibody against golgin-97 to show the many complexes of Golgi vesicles (green), all near the nucleus, against a background of microfilaments organized as stress fibers and stained with fluorescent phalloidin (violet). Because of the abundance of lipids in its many membranes, the Golgi apparatus is difficult to visualize in typical paraffin-embedded, H&E-stained sections. In developing white blood cells with active Golgi complexes, the organelle can sometimes be seen as a faint unstained juxtanuclear region (sometimes called a "Golgi ghost") surrounded by basophilic cytoplasm.

(*Figure 2–13b reproduced, with permission, from Naguro T, Iino A. Prog Clin Biol Res. 1989;295:250; Figure 2–13c, with permission, from Invitrogen.*)

FIGURE 2–14 Summary of functions within the Golgi apparatus.

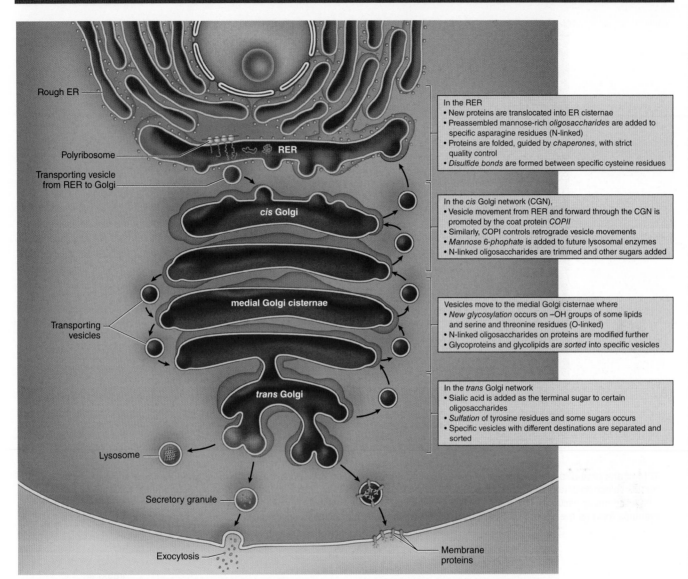

In the RER
- New proteins are translocated into ER cisternae
- Preassembled mannose-rich *oligosaccharides* are added to specific asparagine residues (N-linked)
- Proteins are folded, guided by *chaperones*, with strict quality control
- *Disulfide bonds* are formed between specific cysteine residues

In the *cis* Golgi network (CGN),
- Vesicle movement from RER and forward through the CGN is promoted by the coat protein *COPII*
- Similarly, COPI controls retrograde vesicle movements
- *Mannose 6-phophate* is added to future lysosomal enzymes
- N-linked oligosaccharides are trimmed and other sugars added

Vesicles move to the medial Golgi cisternae where
- *New glycosylation* occurs on –OH groups of some lipids and serine and threonine residues (O-linked)
- N-linked oligosaccharides on proteins are modified further
- Glycoproteins and glycolipids are *sorted* into specific vesicles

In the *trans* Golgi network
- Sialic acid is added as the terminal sugar to certain oligosaccharides
- *Sulfation* of tyrosine residues and some sugars occurs
- Specific vesicles with different destinations are separated and sorted

Rough ER — Polyribosome — RER — Transporting vesicle from RER to Golgi — *cis* Golgi — medial Golgi cisternae — Transporting vesicles — *trans* Golgi — Lysosome — Secretory granule — Exocytosis — Membrane proteins

The main molecular processes are listed at the right, with the major compartments where they occur. In the *trans* Golgi network, the proteins and glycoproteins combine with specific receptors that guide them to the next stages toward their destinations.

that digest the enclosed cytoplasm. Autophagy is enhanced in secretory cells that have accumulated excess secretory granules and in times of nutrient stress, such as starvation. Digested products from autophagosomes are reused in the cytoplasm.

›› MEDICAL APPLICATION

Diseases categorized as *lysosomal storage disorders* stem from defects in one or more of the digestive enzymes present in lysosomes, usually due to a mutation leading to a deficiency of one of the enzymes, or defects due to faulty posttranslational processing. In cells that must digest the substrate of the missing or defective enzyme following autophagocytosis, the lysosomes cannot function properly. Such cells accumulate large secondary lysosomes or residual bodies filled with the indigestible macromolecule. The accumulation of these vacuoles may eventually interfere with normal cell or tissue function, producing symptoms of the disease. A few lysosomal storage diseases are listed in Table 2–3, with the enzyme involved for each and the tissue affected.

FIGURE **2–15** Secretory granules.

TEM of one area of a pancreatic acinar cell shows numerous mature, electron-dense **secretory granules (S)** in association with condensing vacuoles **(C)** of the Golgi apparatus **(G)**. Such granules form as the contents of the Golgi vacuoles become more condensed. In H&E-stained sections secretory granules are often shown as intensely eosinophilic structures, which in polarized epithelial cells are concentrated at the apical region prior to exocytosis. X18,900.

Proteasomes

Proteasomes are very small abundant protein complexes not associated with membrane, each approximately the size of the small ribosomal subunit. They function to degrade denatured or otherwise nonfunctional polypeptides. Proteasomes also remove proteins no longer needed by the cell and provide an important mechanism for restricting activity of a specific protein to a certain window of time. Whereas lysosomes digest organelles or membranes by autophagy, proteasomes deal primarily with free proteins as individual molecules.

As shown in Figure 2–9, the proteasome is a cylindrical structure made of four stacked rings, each composed of seven proteins including proteases. At each end of the cylinder is a regulatory particle that contains ATPase and recognizes proteins with ubiquitin molecules attached. **Ubiquitin** is an abundant cytosolic 76-amino acid protein found in all cells. Misfolded or denatured proteins, or proteins with oxidized amino acids, are recognized by chaperones and targeted for destruction by other enzyme complexes that conjugate a molecule of ubiquitin to a lysine residue in the protein, followed by formation of a multiubiquitin chain. Ubiquinated proteins are recognized by the regulatory particle of proteasomes, unfolded by the ATPase using energy from ATP, and then translocated into the core of the cylindrical structure and degraded into short peptides. These peptides are transferred to the cytosol, and the ubiquitin molecules are released by the regulatory particles for reuse.

The peptides may be broken down further to amino acids or they may have other specialized destinations, such as the antigen-presenting complexes of cells activating an immune response.

FIGURE **2–16** Lysosomes.

Lysosomes are spherical membrane-enclosed vesicles that function as sites of intracellular digestion and are particularly numerous in cells active after the various types of endocytosis. Lysosomes are not well shown on H&E-stained cells but can be visualized by light microscopy after staining with toluidine blue.

(a) Cells in a kidney tubule show numerous purple lysosomes **(L)** in the cytoplasmic area between the basally located nuclei **(N)** and apical ends of the cells at the center of the tubule. Using endocytosis, these cells actively take up small proteins in the lumen of the tubule, degrade the proteins in lysosomes, and then release the resulting amino acids for reuse. X300.

(b) Lysosomes in cultured vascular endothelial cells can be specifically stained using fluorescent dyes sequestered into these organelles (green), which are abundant around the blue Hoechst-stained nucleus. Mitochondria (red) are scattered among the lysosomes.

(c) In the TEM lysosomes **(L)** have a characteristic very electron-dense appearance and are shown here near groups of Golgi cisternae **(G)**. The less electron-dense lysosomes represent heterolysosomes in which digestion of the contents is under way. The cell is a macrophage with numerous fine cytoplasmic extensions (arrows). X15,000.

(Figure 2–16b, with permission, from Invitrogen.)

TABLE **2–3**   Examples of lysosomal storage diseases caused by defective lysosomal enzymes.

Disease	Faulty Enzyme	Main Organs Affected
Hurler syndrome (MPS I)	α-L-Iduronidase	Skeleton and nervous system
McArdle syndrome	Muscle phosphorylase	Skeletal muscles
Tay-Sachs	GM_2-gangliosidase	Nervous system
Gaucher	Glucocerebrosidase	Liver and spleen
I-cell disease	Phosphotransferase for M6P formation	Skeleton and nervous system

FIGURE 2–17 Lysosomal functions.

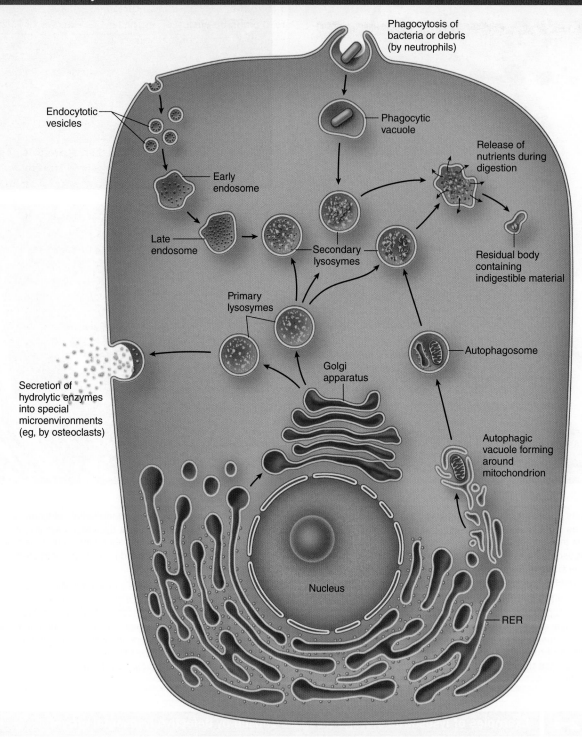

Phagocytosis of bacteria or debris (by neutrophils)

Endocytotic vesicles

Phagocytic vacuole

Release of nutrients during digestion

Early endosome

Late endosome

Secondary lysosymes

Residual body containing indigestible material

Primary lysosymes

Autophagosome

Secretion of hydrolytic enzymes into special microenvironments (eg, by osteoclasts)

Golgi apparatus

Autophagic vacuole forming around mitochondrion

Nucleus

RER

Synthesis of lysosomal enzymes occurs in the RER, with packaging in the Golgi apparatus. Endocytosis produces vesicles that fuse with **endosomes** before merging with **lysosomes**. Phagocytic vacuoles (or phagosomes) fuse with primary lysosomes to become **secondary lysosomes** (or heterolysosomes), in which ingested material is degraded. **Autophagosomes**, such as those depicted here with a mitochondrion in the process of digestion, are formed after nonfunctional or surplus organelles become enclosed with membrane and the resulting structure fuses with a lysosome. The products of lysosomal digestion are recycled to the cytoplasm, but indigestible molecules remain in a membrane-enclosed **residual body**, which may accumulate in long-lived cells as lipofuscin. In some cells, such as osteoclasts, the lysosomal enzymes are secreted into a restricted extracellular compartment.

FIGURE **2–18** Autophagy.

RB

Autophagy is a process in which the cell uses lysosomes to dispose of excess or nonfunctioning organelles or membranes. Membrane that appears to emerge from the SER encloses the organelles to be destroyed, forming an autophagosome that then fuses with a lysosome for digestion of the contents. In this TEM the two autophagosomes at the **upper left** contain portions of RER more electron dense than the neighboring normal RER and one near the **center** contains what may be mitochondrial membranes plus RER. Also shown is a vesicle with features of a residual body **(RB)**. 30,000X.

›› MEDICAL APPLICATION

Failure of proteasomes or other aspects of a cell's protein quality control can allow large aggregates of protein to accumulate in affected cells. Such aggregates may adsorb other macromolecules to them and damage or kill cells. Aggregates released from dead cells can accumulate in the extracellular matrix of the tissue. In the brain this can interfere directly with cell function and lead to neurodegeneration. **Alzheimer disease** and **Huntington disease** are two neurologic disorders caused initially by such protein aggregates.

Mitochondria

Mitochondria (Gr. *mitos*, thread, + *chondros*, granule) are membrane-enclosed organelles with arrays of enzymes specialized for aerobic respiration and production of **adenosine triphosphate (ATP)**, with high-energy phosphate bonds, which supplies energy for most cellular activities. Glycolysis converts glucose anaerobically to pyruvate in the cytoplasm, releasing some energy. The rest of the energy is captured when pyruvate is imported into mitochondria and oxidized to CO_2 and H_2O. Mitochondrial enzymes yield 15 times more ATP than is produced by glycolysis alone. Some of the energy released in mitochondria is not stored in ATP but is dissipated as heat that maintains body temperature.

Mitochondria are usually elongated structures with diameters of 0.5-1 µm and lengths up to 10 times greater. They are highly plastic, rapidly changing shape, fusing with one another and dividing, and are moved through the cytoplasm along microtubules. The number of mitochondria is related to the cell's energy needs: cells with a high-energy metabolism (eg, cardiac muscle, cells of some kidney tubules) have abundant mitochondria, whereas cells with a low-energy metabolism have few mitochondria. Similarly, mitochondria of differentiated cells are concentrated in cytoplasmic regions where energy utilization is more intense.

›› MEDICAL APPLICATION

Myoclonic epilepsy with ragged red fibers (MERRF) is a rare disease occurring in individuals in whom cells of specific tissues, notably regions of skeletal muscle, inherit mitochondrial DNA with a mutated gene for lysine-tRNA, leading to defective synthesis of respiratory chain proteins which can produce structural abnormal in muscle fibers and other cells.

Mitochondria are often large enough to be visible with the light microscope as numerous discrete organelles (Figure 2–19). Under the TEM each mitochondrion is seen to have two separated and very different membranes that together create two compartments: the innermost **matrix** and a narrow **intermembrane space** (Figure 2–20a). Both mitochondrial membranes contain a higher density of protein molecules than other membranes in the cell and have reduced fluidity. The **outer membrane** is sieve-like, containing many transmembrane proteins called **porins** that form channels through which small molecules such as pyruvate and other metabolites readily pass from the cytoplasm to the intermembrane space.

The **inner membrane** is folded to form a series of long infoldings called **cristae**, which project into the matrix and greatly increase this membrane's surface area (Figure 2–20). The number of cristae in mitochondria also corresponds

FIGURE **2–19** Mitochondria in the light microscope.

(a) In certain sectioned cells stained with H&E, mitochondria appear throughout the cytoplasm as numerous eosinophilic structures. The mitochondria usually appear round or slightly elongated and are more numerous in cytoplasmic regions with higher energy demands, such as near the cell membrane in cells undergoing much active transport. The central nuclei are also clearly seen in these cells.

(b) Entire mitochondria can be shown in cultured cells, such as the endothelial cells shown here, and often appear as the elongated structures (shown in yellow or orange here), usually arrayed in parallel along microtubules. Such preparations also show that mitochondrial shape can be quite plastic and variable. Specific mitochondrial staining such as that shown here involves incubating living cells with specific fluorescent compounds that are specifically sequestered into these organelles, followed by fixation and immunocytochemical staining of the microtubules. In this preparation, microtubules are stained green and mitochondria appear yellow or orange, depending on their association with the green microtubules. The cell nucleus was stained with DAPI.

(*Figure 2–19b, with permission, from Invitrogen.*)

to the energy needs of the cell. The lipid bilayer of the inner membrane contains unusual phospholipids and is highly impermeable to ions (Figure 2–20). Integral proteins include various transport proteins that make the inner membrane selectively permeable to the small molecules required by enzymes in the matrix. Matrix enzymes include those that oxidize pyruvate and fatty acids to form acetyl coenzyme A (CoA) and those of the citric acid cycle that oxidize acetyl CoA, releasing CO_2 as waste and small energy-rich molecules that provide electrons for transport along the **electron-transport chain** (or respiratory chain). Enzymes and other components of this chain are embedded in the inner membrane and allow oxidative phosphorylation, which produces most of the ATP in animal cells.

Formation of ATP by oxidative phosphorylation enzymes occurs by a **chemiosmotic process**. Membrane proteins guide the small electron carrier molecules through closely packed enzyme complexes so that the electrons move sequen-tially along the chain. Electron transfer is coupled with oriented proton uptake and release, with protons accumulating in the intermembrane space (Figure 2–20) and producing an **electrochemical gradient** across the inner membrane. Membrane-associated proteins of the **ATP synthase** system form large (10-nm), multisubunit, globular complexes on stalk-like structures that project from the matrix side of the inner membrane (Figure 2–20). Through this enzyme complex runs a hydrophilic pathway that allows protons to flow down the electrochemical gradient, crossing the membrane back into the matrix. Passage of protons through this channel causes rotation of specific polypeptides in the globular ATP synthase complex, converting the energy of proton flow into the mechanical energy of protein movement. Mechanical energy is stored in the new phosphate bond of ATP by other subunit polypeptides binding adenosine diphosphate (ADP) and inorganic phosphate (Figure 2–20). A steady torrent of protons along the gradient allows each of these remarkable synthase complexes to produce more than 100 molecules of ATP per second.

Another role for mitochondria occurs at times of cell stress, when cytochrome c is released from the intermembranous space into the cytoplasm. In the cytoplasm this protein activates sets of proteases that degrade all cellular components in a regulated process called **apoptosis** that results in rapid cell death (see Chapter 3).

New mitochondria originate by growth and division (fission) of preexisting mitochondria. During cell mitosis each daughter cell receives approximately half the mitochondria in the parent cell.

Unlike most organelles mitochondria are partly autonomous of nuclear genes and activities. The mitochondrial matrix contains a small circular chromosome of DNA, ribosomes, mRNA, and tRNA, all with similarities to the corresponding bacterial components. Protein synthesis occurs in mitochondria, but because of the reduced amount of mitochondrial DNA, only a small subset of mitochondrial proteins is produced locally. Most are encoded by nuclear DNA and synthesized on free polyribosomes of the cytosol. These proteins have short terminal amino acid sequences that serve as signals for their uptake across the mitochondrial membranes. The observation that mitochondria have certain bacterial characteristics led with later work to the understanding that mitochondria evolved from an ancestral aerobic prokaryote that lived symbiotically within an ancestral eukaryotic host cell.

Peroxisomes

Peroxisomes are spherical organelles enclosed by a single membrane and named for their enzymes producing and degrading hydrogen peroxide, H_2O_2 (Figure 2–21). **Oxidases** located here oxidize substrates by removing hydrogen atoms that are transferred to molecular oxygen (O_2), producing H_2O_2. Peroxidases such as **catalase** immediately break down H_2O_2, which is potentially damaging to the cell. These enzymes also inactivate various potentially toxic molecules, including some prescription drugs, particularly in the large and abundant peroxisomes of liver and kidney cells.

Other diverse enzymes in peroxisomes complement certain functions of the SER and mitochondria in the metabolism of lipids and other molecules. Thus, the β-oxidation of long-chain fatty acids (18 carbons and longer) is preferentially accomplished by peroxisomal enzymes that differ from their mitochondrial counterparts. Certain reactions leading to the formation of bile acids and cholesterol also occur in peroxisomes.

Peroxisomes form in two ways: budding of precursor vesicles from the ER or growth and division of preexisting peroxisomes. These organelles lack nucleic acids; their enzymes are synthesized on free cytosolic polyribosomes and bear a small signal sequence of amino acids at the carboxyl terminus. This signal is recognized by receptors located in the peroxisomal membrane and the proteins are imported.

>> **MEDICAL APPLICATION**

Several fairly rare disorders arise from defective peroxisomal proteins. **Neonatal adrenoleukodystrophy** is caused by a defective integral membrane protein needed for transport of very-long-chain fatty acids into the peroxisome for β-oxidation. Accumulation of these fatty acids in body fluids can disrupt the myelin sheaths in nerve tissue, causing severe neurologic symptoms. Deficiencies of peroxisomal enzymes cause **Zellweger syndrome** that affects the structure and functions of several organ systems.

❯ THE CYTOSKELETON

The cytoplasmic **cytoskeleton** is a complex array of (1) microtubules, (2) microfilaments (actin filaments), and (3) intermediate filaments. These protein polymers determine the shapes of cells, play an important role in the movements of organelles and cytoplasmic vesicles, and also allow the movement of entire cells. Important properties, functions, and locations of the cytoskeletal components are summarized in Table 2–4.

Microtubules

Within the cytoplasm of all eukaryotic cells are fine tubular structures known as **microtubules** (see Table 2–4; Figure 2–22). Microtubules are also organized into larger arrays called **axonemes** in the cytoplasmic extensions called **cilia** (discussed in Chapter 4) and **flagella**. Each microtubule is hollow, with an outer diameter of 25 nm and a wall 5 nm thick, a structure that confers significant rigidity to help maintain cell shape. Microtubules vary in length, but can become many micrometers long. Two or more microtubules are often linked side-by-side by protein arms or bridges, which are particularly important in cilia and flagella.

As indicated in Table 2–4, the protein subunit of a microtubule is a heterodimer of α and β **tubulin**, each with a molecular mass of about 50 kDa. Under appropriate conditions (in vivo or in vitro), the tubulin heterodimers polymerize to form microtubules, which have a slight spiral organization overall. A total of 13 units are present in one complete turn of the spiral. Aligned subunits make up longitudinal protofilaments, and 13 parallel protofilaments make up the microtubule wall.

Polymerization of tubulins is directed by **microtubule organizing centers (MTOCs)**, which contain tubulin assemblies that act as nucleating sites for polymerization. Microtubules are polarized structures and growth (polymerization) occurs more rapidly at the (+) end of existing microtubules (Figure 2–23). Microtubules show **dynamic instability**, with continuous cycles of polymerization and depolymerization at steady-state conditions, which depend on concentrations of tubulin, Ca^{2+}, Mg^{2+}, and the presence of various **microtubule-associated proteins (MAPs)**. Energy for assembly is

FIGURE **2–20** Mitochondrial structure and ATP formation. (Legend Opposite)

The two mitochondrial membranes and the matrix can be seen in the TEM and diagram.

(a) The **outer membrane** is smooth and the **inner membrane** has many sharp folds called **cristae** that increase its surface area greatly. Cristae are more numerous in mitochondria of highly active cells. The innermost **mitochondrial matrix** is a gel containing numerous enzymes. The inner membrane surface in contact with the matrix is studded with many multimeric protein complexes resembling globular units on short stalks. These contain the ATP synthase complexes that generate most of the cell's ATP.

(b) Metabolites such as pyruvate and fatty acids enter mitochondria via membrane porins and are converted to acetyl CoA by matrix enzymes of the **citric acid cycle** (or Krebs cycle), yielding some ATP and NADH (nicotinamide adenine dinucleotide), a major source of electrons for the electron-transport chain. The movement of electrons through the protein complexes of the inner membrane's **electron-transport system** is accompanied by the directed movement of protons (H^+) from the matrix into the intermembranous space. The inner membrane is impermeable to protons, and the result is an electrochemical gradient across the membrane. The other membrane-associated proteins make up the **ATP synthase** systems, each of which forms a globular complex on a stalk-like structure projecting from the matrix side of the inner membrane. A channel in this enzyme complex allows proton flow down the electrochemical gradient and across the membrane back into the matrix. The channeled movement of protons causes rapid spinning of specific polypeptides in the globular ATP synthase complex, converting the energy of proton flow into mechanical energy. Other subunit proteins of the complex store this energy in the new phosphate bond of ATP which then leaves the mitochondrion for use throughout the cell.

FIGURE **2–21** Peroxisomes.

Peroxisomes are small spherical, membranous organelles, containing enzymes that use O_2 to remove hydrogen atoms from fatty acids, in a reaction that produces hydrogen peroxide (H_2O_2) that must be broken down to water and O_2 by another enzyme, **catalase**.

(a) By TEM peroxisomes (**P**) generally show a matrix of moderate electron density. Aggregated electron-dense particles represent glycogen (G). X30,000.

(b) Peroxisomes (**P**) in most species are characterized by a central, more electron-dense crystalloid aggregate of constituent enzymes, as shown here. X60,000.

(c) A cultured endothelial cell processed by immunocytochemistry shows many peroxisomes (green) distributed throughout the cytoplasm among the vitally stained elongate mitochondria (red) around the DAPI-stained nucleus (blue). Peroxisomes shown here were specifically stained using an antibody against the membrane protein PMP70.

(*Figure 2–21c, with permission, from Invitrogen.*)

TABLE **2–4**	Properties of cytoskeletal components (microtubules, microfilaments, and intermediate filaments).

General Function of Cytoskeleton

1. **Structural:** Provides structural support to cell; stabilizes junctions between cells
2. **Movement:** Assists with cytosol streaming and cell motility; helps move organelles and materials throughout cell; helps move chromosomes during cell division

	Microtubules	Microfilaments	Intermediate filaments
Subunit	Heterodimers of αβ-tubulin	G-actin monomers	Antiparallel tetramers of 2 rod-like dimers
Overall structure	Hollow tube with a wall of 13 parallel protofilaments	2 intertwined filaments of F-actin	Cable of 4 intertwined protofibrils, each consisting of bundled tetramers associated end to end
Diameter	25 nm	5-7 nm	8-10 nm
Monomeric proteins	α and β tubulin (54 kDa)	Globular G-actin (42 kDa)	Various α-helical rod-like proteins (~55 kDa, Table 2–5)
Polarity	+ and − ends	+ and − ends	No apparent polarity
Relative stability	Dynamic in cytoplasm; stable in axonemes	Dynamic	Stable
General locations	Radiating through cytoplasm from concentration at centrosomes; axonemes	Concentrated beneath cell membrane; in cell extensions like microvilli	Arrayed throughout cytoplasm; at desmosomes; inside nuclear envelop
Key functions	Maintain cell's shape and polarity; provide tracks for organelle and chromosome movement; move cilia and flagella	Contract and move cells; change cell shape; cytokinesis; cytoplasmic transport and streaming	Strengthen cell and tissue structure; maintain cell shape; maintain nuclear shape (lamins)

derived from GTP bound to tubulin, and individual microtubules shorten as depolymerization exceeds growth. Microtubule stability varies greatly with cellular location and function; microtubules of cilia are very stable, while those of the mitotic spindle are short-lived.

The dominant MTOC in most somatic cells is the **centrosome**, which is organized around two cylindrical **centrioles**, each about 0.2 μm in diameter and 0.3-0.5 μm in length. Each centriole is composed of nine highly organized microtubular triplets (Figure 2–24). With their long axes at right angles,

FIGURE **2–22** Microtubules and actin filaments in cytoplasm.

FIGURE **2–23** Dynamic instability of microtubules.

(a) Microtubules (MT) and actin microfilaments (MF) can both be clearly distinguished in this TEM of fibroblast cytoplasm, which provides a good comparison of the relative diameters of these two cytoskeletal components. X60,000.

(b) Arrays of microfilaments and microtubules are easily demonstrated by immunocytochemistry using antibodies against their subunit proteins, as in this cultured cell. Actin filaments (red) are most concentrated at the cell periphery, forming prominent circumferential bundles from which finer filaments project into cellular extensions and push against the cell membrane. Actin filaments form a dynamic network important for cell shape changes such as those during cell division, locomotion, and formation of cellular processes, folds, pseudopodia, lamellipodia, microvilli, etc, which serve to change a cell's surface area or give direction to a cell's crawling movements.

Microtubules (green/yellow) are oriented in arrays that generally extend from the centrosome area near the nucleus into the most peripheral extensions. Besides serving to stabilize cell shape, microtubules form the tracks for kinesin-based transport of vesicles and organelles into the cell periphery and dynein-based transport toward the cell nucleus.

(*Figure 2–22b, with permission, from Dr Albert Tousson, University of Alabama—Birmingham High Resolution Imaging Facility, Birmingham.*)

At stable tubulin concentrations some microtubules grow while others shrink, each existing in a condition called dynamic instability. In cytoplasmic areas where the tubulin concentration is high, tubulin GTP is added at a microtubule's (+) end faster than the incorporated GTP can be hydrolyzed. The resulting "GTP cap" stabilizes that end of the microtubule and promotes further rapid growth. As free tubulin concentrations decrease, the rate of growth also decreases, thereby allowing GTP hydrolysis to catch up. The resulting "GDP cap" at the microtubule end is unstable and favors rapid depolymerization (termed "catastrophe"). This increases the local concentration of free, monomeric tubulin that "rescues" the microtubule before it completely disappears and produces another short period of microtubule elongation.

Dynamic instability allows the growing ends of microtubules to explore the cytoplasm and become stabilized when they contact stabilizing structures, such as kinetochores on chromosomes early in mitosis (see Chapter 3).

FIGURE **2–24** Centrosome.

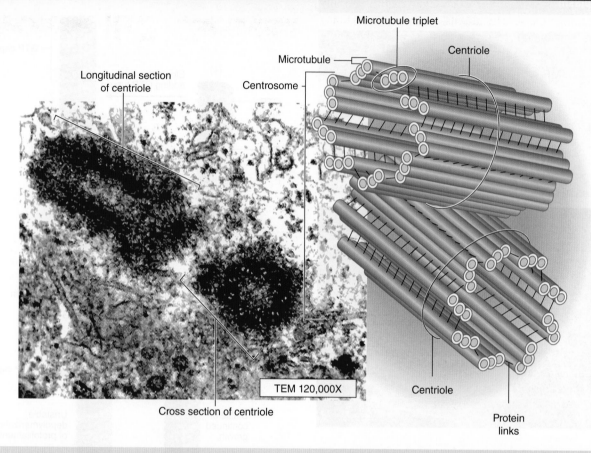

The **centrosome** is the microtubule-organizing center for the mitotic spindle and consists of paired centrioles. The TEM reveals that the two centrioles in a centrosome exist at right angles to each other in a dense matrix of free tubulin subunits and other proteins. Each centriole consists of **nine microtubular triplets**. In a poorly understood process, the centrosome duplicates itself and is divided equally during a cell's interphase, each half having a duplicated centriole pair. At the onset of mitosis, the two daughter centrosomes move to opposite sides of the nucleus and become the two poles of the mitotic spindle of microtubules attaching to chromosomes.

the paired centrioles organize nearby tubulin complexes and other proteins as a pericentriolar matrix found close to the nucleus of nondividing cells. Before cell division, more specifically during the period of DNA replication, each centrosome duplicates itself so that now each centrosome has two pairs of centrioles. During mitosis, the centrosome divide into halves, which move to opposite poles of the cell, and become organizing centers for the microtubules of the mitotic spindle.

Microtubules also form part of the system for intracellular transport of membranous vesicles, macromolecular complexes, and organelles. Well-studied examples include axoplasmic transport in neurons, melanin transport in pigment cells, chromosome movements by the mitotic spindle, and vesicle movements among different cell compartments. In each of these examples, movement is suspended if microtubules are disrupted. Transport along microtubules is under the control of proteins called **motor proteins**, which use ATP in moving the larger structures.

Kinesins carry material away from the MTOC near the nucleus toward the plus end of microtubules (anterograde transport); **cytoplasmic dyneins** carry material along microtubules in the opposite direction (retrograde transport), generally toward the nucleus. Important roles for this system include extending the ER from the nuclear envelope to the plasmalemma and moving vesicles to and through the Golgi apparatus.

>> MEDICAL APPLICATION

Several inhibitory compounds used by cell biologists to study details of microtubule dynamics are also widely used in cancer chemotherapy to block activity of the mitotic spindle in rapidly growing neoplastic cells. Such drugs include **vinblastine**, **vincristine**, and **paclitaxel**, all of which were originally discovered as plant derivatives.

Microfilaments (Actin Filaments)

Microfilaments composed of **actin** allow cellular motility and most contractile activity in cells, by reversible assembly of the actin filaments and interactions between these filaments and the associated protein, **myosin**. Actin filaments are thin (5-7 nm diameter), polarized polymers, shorter and more flexible than microtubules (Figure 2–22). They are composed of globular G-actin monomers that assemble in the presence of K^+ and Mg^{2+} into a double-stranded helix of filamentous F-actin (Table 2–4). G-actin is generally added to preexisting filaments, but new filaments can be formed from a pool of G-actin by the action of nucleation factors such as *formin*.

Actin filaments are also highly dynamic. Monomers are added rapidly at the (+) or barbed end, with hydrolysis of ATP at each addition; at the same time monomers dissociate at the (−) or pointed end. This leads to migration of subunits through the polymer, which occurs rapidly in purified filaments in a process called **treadmilling** (Figure 2–25). In cells both the assembly and disassembly of subunits from F-actin are promoted by other proteins, such as *profilin* and *cofilin*, respectively.

Actin is very abundant in all cells, usually concentrated as networks of actin filaments and abundant free globular G-actin subunits concentrated near the cell membrane (a region sometimes called the **cell cortex**) and in cellular extensions. Microvilli are extensions that increase a cell's surface area for improved cellular absorption, while other protrusions are used in cell motility. In cells attached to firm substrates, actin filaments may be concentrated into parallel bundles called **stress fibers** (see Figure 2–13c).

The physical properties of actin filaments, particularly their lengths and interactions with other proteins, determine the mechanical properties of the local cytoplasm, most notably its viscosity. Cross-linking within networks of F-actin increases cytoplasmic viscosity, while severing (and capping) the filaments tends to decrease viscosity. The lengths and other physical properties of actin filaments are controlled by a large variety of **actin-binding proteins**, a few of which are indicated in Figure 2–26. Important activities of such proteins include the following:

- Severing and/or capping the end of F-actin (eg, *gelsolin*, *capZ*)
- Cross-linking (eg, *filamin*) or bundling (eg, *fimbrin*, α-*actinin*) actin filaments
- Linking F-actin to membrane proteins and other cytoskeletal filaments (eg, *spectrin*)

Just as the molecular motors kinesin and dynein move along microtubules, various **myosin** motors use ATP to transport cargo along F-actin. Movement is usually toward the barbed (+) end of actin filaments; myosin VI is the only known myosin that moves in the other direction. Interactions between F-actin and myosins form the basis for various cell movements:

FIGURE 2–25 Actin filament treadmilling.

(a) Actin filaments or microfilaments are helical two-stranded polymers assembled from **globular actin subunits**.

(b) Assembly of actin filaments (F-actin) is polarized, with G-actin subunits added to the plus (+) end and removed at the minus (−) end. Even actin filaments of a constant length are highly dynamic structures, balancing G-actin assembly and disassembly at the opposite ends, with a net movement or flow along the polymer known as **treadmilling**.

(Figure 2–25a, with permission, from John Heuser, Washington University School of Medicine, St. Louis, MO.)

- Transport of various organelles, vesicles, and granules through the cell (*cytoplasmic streaming*)
- Contractile rings of microfilaments and with myosin II that constrict to produce two cells at the end of mitosis (*cytokinesis*)

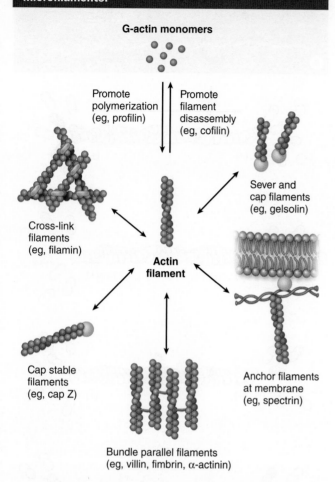

FIGURE **2–26** Roles of major actin-binding proteins in regulating the organization of microfilaments.

G-actin monomers

Promote polymerization (eg, profilin)

Promote filament disassembly (eg, cofilin)

Sever and cap filaments (eg, gelsolin)

Cross-link filaments (eg, filamin)

Actin filament

Cap stable filaments (eg, cap Z)

Anchor filaments at membrane (eg, spectrin)

Bundle parallel filaments (eg, villin, fimbrin, α-actinin)

A large number of proteins regulate the assembly of micro-filaments and the interactions of these filaments with one another. By altering microfilament length and cross-linking, such proteins greatly influence physical properties of the local cytoplasm.

- Membrane-associated molecules of myosin I whose movements along microfilaments are important in the cell surface changes that underlie phagocytosis and pinocytosis
- Contraction of cytoplasm that shortens cells or rapidly retracts cellular extensions

Stabilized arrays of actin filaments integrated with arrays of thicker (16-nm) myosin filaments permit very forceful contractions in specialized cells such as those of muscle (see Chapter 10).

Intermediate Filaments

In addition to microtubules and actin filaments, the cytoskeleton includes class of filaments intermediate in size between the other two and with a diameter averaging 10 nm (Table 2–4). The **intermediate filaments** are much more stable than microtubules and actin filaments. Moreover, these filaments are composed of different protein subunits in different cell types. More than a dozen heterogeneous protein classes, ranging in size from 40 to 230 kDa, forming subunits of intermediate filaments have been identified and localized immunocytochemically. As indicated in Table 2–4, nearly all these subunits are coiled, rod-like dimers that form antiparallel tetramers, which self-assemble into large cable-like bundles or protofibrils stabilized by further lateral interactions. Table 2–5 lists six classes of intermediate filament proteins forming rod-like subunits, their sizes and cell distributions, and diseases that result from their disruption.

Intermediate filament proteins with particular biological, histological, or pathological importance include the following:

- **Keratins** (Gr. *keras*, horn) or cytokeratins are a diverse family of acidic and basic isoforms that compose heterodimer subunits of intermediate filaments in all epithelial cells (see Chapter 4). They are encoded by over 30 related genes and produce filaments with different chemical and immunologic properties for various functions. In epidermal cells, cytokeratins accumulate in the differentiation process termed **keratinization**, which results in an outer layer of nonliving skin cells that reduces dehydration. The evolution of keratins made terrestrial life possible. Keratinization also provides some protection from minor abrasions and produces various hard protective structures of skin, such as nails (as well as feathers, beaks, horns, and the scales of reptiles). Intermediate filaments of keratins form large bundles (tonofibrils) that attach to certain junctions between epithelial cells (Figure 2–27).
- **Vimentin** is the most common class III intermediate filament protein and is found in most cells derived from mesenchyme. Important vimentin-like proteins include **desmin** found in almost all muscle cells and **glial fibrillar acidic protein (GFAP)** found especially in astrocytes, supporting cells of central nervous system tissue. Desmin filaments of a cultured cell are shown immunocytochemically in Figure 1–12a.
- **Neurofilament** proteins of three distinct sizes make heterodimers that form the subunits of the major intermediate filaments of neurons.
- **Lamins** are a family of seven isoforms present in the cell nucleus, where they form a structural framework called the **nuclear lamina** just inside the nuclear envelope (see Chapter 3).

		Major classes and representatives of intermediate filament proteins, their sizes and locations.		
TABLE 2–5				
Class	Protein	Size (kDa)	Cell Distribution	Disease Involvement (If Known)
I	Acidic cytokeratin	40-65	Epithelial cells	Certain skin-blistering disorders
II	Basic cytokeratin	51-68	Epithelial cells	Keratoderma; corneal dystrophy
III	Desmin	53	Muscle cells	Myopathies
	Synemin	190	Muscle cells	
	GFAP	50	Astrocytes (less in other glial cells)	Alexander disease
	Peripherin	57	Neurons	
	Vimentin	54	Mesenchymal cells	
IV	NF-L	68	Neurons	
	NF-M	110	Neurons	
	NF-H	130	Neurons	
	α-internexin	55	Embryonic neurons	
V	Lamins	62-72	Nuclei of all cells	Cardiomyopathy; muscular dystrophies; progeria
VI	Nestin	230	Some stem and embryonic cells	

FIGURE **2–27** Intermediate filaments of keratin.

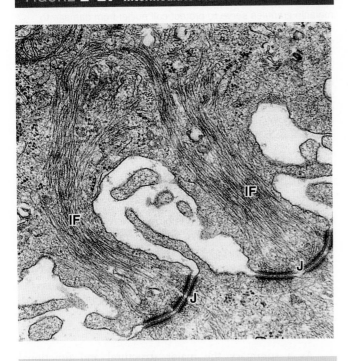

Intermediate filaments (IF) display an average diameter of 8-10 nm, between that of actin filaments and microtubules, and serve to provide mechanical strength or stability to cells. A large and important class of intermediate filaments is composed of **keratin** subunits, which are prominent in epithelial cells. Bundles of keratin filaments called **tonofibrils** associate with certain classes of intercellular junctions **(J)** common in epithelial cells and are easily seen with the TEM, as shown here in two extensions in an epidermal cell bound to a neighboring cell. 60,000X.

›› MEDICAL APPLICATION

The presence of a specific type of intermediate filament in tumors can often reveal the cellular origin of the tumor, information important for diagnosis and treatment of the cancer. Identification of intermediate filament proteins by means of immunocytochemical methods is a routine procedure. One example is the use of GFAP to identify **astrocytomas**, the most common type of brain tumor.

› INCLUSIONS

Cytoplasmic **inclusions** have little or no metabolic activity (which distinguishes them from organelles), but contain accumulated metabolites or other substances not enclosed by membrane. Most kinds of inclusions are transitory cytoplasmic components not enclosed by membrane. Important and commonly seen inclusions include the following:

- **Fat droplets** (Figure 2–28a), accumulations of lipid molecules prominent in adipocytes (fat cells), adrenal cortex cells, liver and other cells.
- **Glycogen granules** (Figure 2–28b), aggregates of the carbohydrate polymer in which glucose is stored, are visible in several cell types, mainly liver cells, in the form of irregular clumps of periodic acid-Schiff (PAS)–positive or electron-dense material.
- **Lipofuscin** is a yellowish-brown pigment visualized by H&E staining in many cells, especially in stable nondividing cells (eg, neurons, cardiac muscle). Sometimes called "wear-and-tear pigment," granules of lipofuscin contain a complex mix of material partly derived from residual bodies after lysosomal digestion.

FIGURE **2–28** Cellular inclusions.

Inclusions are cytoplasmic structures or deposits filled with stored macromolecules and are not present in all cells.

(a) Lipid droplets are abundant in cells of the adrenal cortex and appear with the TEM as small spherical structures with homogenous matrices (L). Mitochondria are also seen here. As aggregates of hydrophobic lipid molecules these inclusions are enclosed by a single monolayer of phospholipids with various peripheral proteins, including enzymes for lipid metabolism. In routine processing of tissue for paraffin sections, fat droplets are generally removed, leaving empty spaces in the cells. Common fat cells have cytoplasm essentially filled with one large lipid droplet. X19,000.

(b) TEM of a liver cell cytoplasm shows numerous individual or clustered electron-dense particles representing **glycogen granules**, although these granules lack membrane. Glycogen granules usually form characteristic aggregates such as those

shown. Glycogen is a ready source of energy, and such granules are often abundant in cells with high metabolic activity. X30,000.

(c) Pigment deposits (PD) occur in many cell types and may contain various complex substances, such as **lipofuscin** or **melanin**. Lipofuscin granules represent an accumulating by-product of lysosomal digestion in long-lived cells, but melanin granules serve to protect cell nuclei from damage to DNA caused by light. Many cells contain pigmented deposits of **hemosiderin granules** containing the protein ferritin, which forms a storage complex for iron. Hemosiderin granules are very electron dense, but with the light microscope they appear brownish and resemble lipofuscin. The liver cells shown have large cytoplasmic regions filled with pigment deposits, which probably represent iron-containing hemosiderin. X400. Giemsa.

■ **Hemosiderin** (Figure 2–28c) is a dense brown aggregate of denatured ferritin proteins with many atoms of bound iron. It occurs in phagocytic cells, especially macrophages of the liver and spleen, where it results from phagocytosis of red blood cells.

>> MEDICAL APPLICATION

A condition termed **hemosiderosis**, in which the iron-containing inclusion **hemosiderin** occurs in cells of organs throughout the body, may be seen with increased uptake

of dietary iron, impaired iron utilization, or with excessive lysis of red blood cells. Hemosiderosis itself does not damage cell or organ function. However, extreme accumulations of iron in cellular hemosiderin can lead to disorders such as hemochromatosis and iron overload syndrome, in which tissues of the liver and other organs are damaged.

As a summary the major structural and functional features of all cytoplasmic components are presented in Table 2–6.

TABLE 2–6	Summary of cellular structural components.

Component	Structure	Major Function	Appearance
Plasma membrane	Phospholipid bilayer containing cholesterol and proteins (integral and peripheral) and some carbohydrates (externally); forms a selectively permeable boundary of the cell	Acts as a physical barrier to enclose cell contents; regulates material movement into and out of the cell; establishes and maintains an electrical charge difference across the plasma membrane; functions in cell communication	Plasma membrane
Cilia	Short, numerous membrane extensions supported by microtubules, which occur on exposed membrane surfaces of some cells	Move substances (eg, mucus, and dissolved materials) over the cell surface	Cilia
Flagellum	Long, singular membrane extension supported by microtubules; present on sperm cells	Propels sperm	Flagellum
Microvilli	Numerous thin membrane folds projecting from the free cell surface; supported by microfilaments	Increase membrane surface area for greater absorption	Microvilli
Nucleus	Large structure enclosed within a double membrane; contains chromatin, nucleolus, and nucleoplasm	Houses the DNA that serves as the genetic material for directing protein synthesis	Nucleus
Nuclear envelope	Double membrane boundary between cytoplasm and nuclear contents; continuous with rough endoplasmic reticulum	Separates nucleus from cytoplasm	Nuclear pores, Nuclear envelope, Nucleolus, Chromatin
Nuclear pores	Openings through the nuclear envelope	Allow passage of materials between the cytoplasm and nucleoplasm, including ribonucleic acid (RNA), protein, ions, and small water-soluble molecules	
Nucleolus	Large, prominent structure within the nucleus	Functions in synthesis of ribosomes	
Cytoplasm	Contents of cells between the plasma membrane and nuclear envelope	Responsible for many cellular processes	Cytoplasm, Cytosol, Organelles
Cytosol	Viscous fluid medium with dissolved solutes (eg, ions, proteins, carbohydrates, lipids)	Provides support for organelles; serves as the viscous fluid medium through which diffusion occurs	
Organelles	Membrane-bound and non-membrane-bound structures	Carry out specific metabolic activities of the cell	Inclusions
Rough endoplasmic reticulum (rough ER)	Extensive interconnected membrane network that varies in shape (eg, cisternae, tubules); ribosomes attached on cytoplasmic surface	Modifies, transports, and stores proteins produced by attached ribosomes; these proteins are secreted, become components of the plasma membrane, or serve as enzymes of lysosomes	
Smooth endoplasmic reticulum (smooth ER)	Extensive interconnected membrane network lacking ribosomes	Synthesizes, transports, and stores lipids (eg, steroids); metabolizes carbohydrates; detoxifies drugs, alcohol, and poisons; forms vesicles and peroxisomes	

(Continued)

TABLE **2–6** | Summary of cellular structural components. (Continued)

Component	Structure	Major Function	Appearance
Golgi apparatus	Series of several elongated, flattened saclike membranous structures	Modifies, packages, and sorts materials that arrive from the ER in transport vesicles; forms secretory vesicles and lysosomes	
Vesicles	Spherical-shaped membrane-bound sacs; contain various types of materials to be transported through the cell	Transport cellular material	
Lysosomes	Spherical-shaped membrane-bound organelles formed from the Golgi apparatus; contain digestive enzymes	Digest microbes or materials (eg, ingested by the cell, worn-out cellular components, or the entire cell)	
Peroxisomes	Smaller, spherical-shaped membrane-bound organelles formed from the ER or through fission; contain oxidative enzymes	Detoxify specific harmful substances either produced by the cell or taken into the cell; engage in beta oxidation of fatty acids to acetyl CoA	
Mitochondria	Double membrane-bound organelles containing a circular strand of DNA (genes for producing mitochondrial proteins)	Synthesize most ATP during aerobic cellular respiration by digestion of fuel molecules (eg, glucose) in the presence of oxygen	
Ribosomes	Organelles composed of both protein and ribosomal RNA (rRNA) that are organized into both a large and small subunit; may be bound to a membrane or free in cytosol	Engage in protein synthesis: Bound ribosomes produce proteins that are secreted, incorporated into plasma membrane, and within lysosomes; free ribosomes produce proteins used within the cell	Bound ribosomes Free ribosomes
Cytoskeleton	Organized network of protein filaments and hollow tubules, including microfilaments, intermediate filaments, and microtubules	Maintains intracellular structural support and organization of cells; participates in cell division; facilitates movement	Cytoskeleton Intermediate filament Microtubule Microfilament
Microfilaments	Actin protein monomers organized into two thin, intertwined protein filaments (actin filaments)	Maintain cell shape; support microvilli; separate two cells during cytokinesis (a process of cell division); facilitate change in cell shape; participate in muscle contraction	
Intermediate filaments	Various protein components	Provide structural support; stabilize junctions between cells	
Microtubules	Hollow cylinders composed of tubulin protein	Maintain cell shape and rigidity; organize and move organelles; support cilia and flagella; participate in vesicular transport; separate chromosomes during the process of cell division	
Centrosome	Amorphous region adjacent to nucleus; contains a pair of centrioles	Organizes microtubules; participates in mitotic spindle formation during cell division	Centriole Centrosome
Proteasomes	Large, barrel-shaped protein complexes located in both the cytosol and nucleus	Degrade and digest damaged or unneeded proteins; ensure quality of exported proteins	
Inclusions	Aggregates of specific types of molecules (eg, melanin protein, glycogen, or lipid)	Serve as temporary storage for these molecules	Variable appearance

The Cytoplasm SUMMARY OF KEY POINTS

- **Cell differentiation** is the process by which cells of an embryo become specialized structurally to augment specific cytoplasmic activities for functions at the level of tissues and organs.
- **Organelles** are metabolically active structures or complexes, with or without membranes, in the cytoplasm of eukaryotic cells.

Plasma Membrane

- The **plasma membrane (cell membrane** or **plasmalemma)** is the lipid bilayer with embedded proteins that surrounds a cell and is seen only with the TEM.
- The **lipid bilayer** forms from amphipathic **phospholipids,** stabilized by **cholesterol,** and contains many **embedded (integral) proteins** and many **peripheral proteins** on its cytoplasmic surface.
- Membrane proteins move laterally within the lipid bilayer, with less movement in areas referred to as **lipid rafts,** which have higher concentrations of cholesterol and saturated fatty acids.
- Integral membrane proteins include **receptors** for external ligands, **channels** for passive or active movement of molecules across the membrane, and **pumps** for active membrane transport.
- **Endocytosis** is cellular uptake of macromolecules or fluid by plasma membrane engulfment or invagination, followed by the "pinching off" of a filled membranous vesicle in the cytoplasm.
- Major types of endocytosis include **phagocytosis** (uptake of particulate material), **pinocytosis** (uptake of dissolved substances), and **receptor-mediated endocytosis** (uptake of specific molecules bound to integral membrane receptor proteins).
- **Exocytosis** is a type of cellular secretion in which cytoplasmic membrane vesicles fuse with the plasma membrane and release their contents to the extracellular space.
- All types of **cell signaling** use membrane receptor proteins that are often linked to enzymes such as kinases or adenylyl cyclase whose activities initiate intracellular signaling pathways.

Ribosomes

- The two **ribosomal subunits,** each a complex of rRNA and many proteins, attach to mRNA and translate that message into protein.
- Multiple ribosomes on the same mRNA make up a **polyribosome (polysome),** and an abundance of these produces basophilic cytoplasm after H&E staining.

Endoplasmic Reticulum

- The ER is a convoluted network of membrane enclosing continuous spaces called **cisternae** and extending from the nucleus to the plasma membrane.
- **Rough ER** has a **granular, basophilic cytoplasmic surface** due to the presence of polysomes making most membrane proteins, proteins in certain other organelles, or for exocytosis; RER is always well developed in cells actively secreting proteins.
- Proteins to be processed through the RER contain initial **signal peptides** which bind receptors in the ER membrane, localizing them to that organelle.
- After **translocation** across the membrane into the cisterna, the proteins undergo **posttranslational modification and folding** in a process monitored by RER molecular chaperones and enzymes.
- **Smooth ER (SER)** lacks ribosomes, but includes enzymes for **lipid and glycogen metabolism,** for **detoxification reactions,** and for temporary **Ca^{2+} sequestration.**

Golgi Apparatus

- The **Golgi apparatus** is a dynamic organelle consisting of stacked membranous cisternae in which proteins made in RER are **processed** further and **packaged** for secretion or other roles.

- Proteins in **transport vesicles** enter the *cis* or receiving face of the Golgi, move through medical cisternae of the Golgi network for enzymatic modifications, and are released in other vesicles at the *trans* face.
- Vesicle movement through the Golgi apparatus is guided by specific **coat proteins** such as COPII and COPI.
- Important protein modifications in the Golgi apparatus include **sulfation** and many **glycosylation** reactions.
- Modified proteins leave the Golgi apparatus after packaging in vesicles with coat proteins that direct movement to lysosomes, the plasma membrane, or secretion by exocytosis.

Lysosomes

- **Primary lysosomes** emerge from the Golgi apparatus containing inactive acid hydrolases specific for degrading a wide variety of cellular macromolecules.
- **Secondary lysosomes** are more heterogeneous, having fused with vesicles produced by endocytosis that contain material to be digested by the hydrolytic enzymes.
- During **autophagy,** lysosomes digest unneeded or nonfunctional organelles after these are surrounded by membrane that then fuses with a lysosome.
- Products of digestion in secondary lysosomes are released to the cytoplasm for reuse; final condensed vesicles containing any indigestible molecules are called **residual bodies.**

Proteasomes

- Proteasomes are small cytoplasmic protein complexes which degrade improperly folded proteins after they are tagged with the polypeptide **ubiquitin.**

Mitochondria

- **Mitochondria** are the major sites of **ATP synthesis** and are abundant in cells or cytoplasmic regions where large amounts of energy are expended.
- Mitochondria are usually **elongated organelles** and form by fission of preexisting mitochondria.
- Mitochondria have two membranes: a **porous outer membrane** encloses the intermembrane space and an **inner membrane with many folds (cristae)** enclosing a gel-like matrix.
- The **mitochondrial matrix** contains enzymes for β-oxidation of fatty acids and the citric acid (Krebs) cycle.
- The inner membrane includes enzyme assemblies of the **electron-transport system and ATP synthase.**
- Mitochondria of stressed cells may release **cytochrome c** from the inner membrane, triggering a regulated series of events culminating in cell death (**apoptosis**).

Peroxisomes

- Peroxisomes are small spherical organelles containing enzymes for various metabolic reactions, notably **for oxidation and detoxification,** and **catalase** that breaks down the H$_2$O$_2$ resulting from those reactions.

Cytoskeleton

- The cytoskeleton contains three types of polymers: (1) **microtubules** 25 nm in diameter; (2) actin filaments or **microfilaments** (5-7 nm); and (3) **intermediate filaments** (8-10 nm).
- Microtubules are semirigid tubular structures with walls composed of **polymerized tubulin** heterodimers; their structure is often very dynamic, with steady addition and dissociation of tubulin.
- Microtubules are important in **maintaining cell shape** and as **tracks for transport** of vesicles and organelles by the **motor proteins kinesin** and **dynein.**

- Microfilaments are short, flexible, highly dynamic filaments of **actin subunits**, in which changes in length and interactions with binding proteins regulate cytoplasmic viscosity and movement.
- **Myosins** are **motor proteins** that bind and move along actin filaments, carrying vesicles or producing cytoplasmic movement.
- Movements of cytoplasm produced by actin filaments and myosins are important for endocytosis, cell cleavage after mitosis, and cell locomotion on substrates.
- Intermediate filaments are the **most stable** cytoskeletal component, conferring strong mechanical stability to cells.

- Intermediate filaments are composed of various protein subunits in different cells; they include **vimentin**; nuclear **lamins**; **neurofilament proteins**; and **keratins**, which are especially important in epithelial cells.

Inclusions

- Unlike organelles, inclusions are **not metabolically active** and are primarily **storage sites**, such as lipid droplets, glycogen granules, pigment granules, or residual bodies (also called lipofuscin).

3 The Nucleus

Containing the code for all of a cell's enzymes and other proteins, the **nucleus** is the command center of the cell. The nucleus also contains the molecular machinery to replicate the DNA and to synthesize and process all types of RNA. During interphase pore complexes in the membrane enclosing the nucleus regulate macromolecular transfer between the nuclear and cytoplasmic compartments. Mature RNA molecules pass into the cytoplasm for their roles in protein synthesis, while proteins needed for nuclear activities are imported from the cytoplasm. Restricting protein synthesis to the cytoplasm helps ensure that newly made RNA molecules do not become involved in translation before processing is complete.

❯ COMPONENTS OF THE NUCLEUS

The nucleus frequently appears as a large rounded or oval structure, often near the center of the cell (Figure 3–1). Consisting of a **nuclear envelope**, a mass of DNA and associated proteins called **chromatin**, and a specialized subdomain called the **nucleolus**, the nucleus is typically the largest structure within a cell. In specific tissues the size and morphologic features of nuclei normally tend to be uniform.

Nuclear Envelope

The **nuclear envelope** forms a selectively permeable barrier between the nuclear and cytoplasmic compartments. Electron microscopy reveals that the envelope has two concentric membranes separated by a narrow (30-50 nm) **perinuclear space** (Figure 3–2). This space and the outer nuclear membrane are continuous with the extensive cytoplasmic network of the rough endoplasmic reticulum (RER). Closely associated with the inner nuclear membrane is a highly organized meshwork of proteins called the **nuclear lamina** (Figure 3–4), which stabilizes the nuclear envelope. Major components of

this layer are the class of intermediate filament proteins called **lamins** that bind to membrane proteins and associate with chromatin in nondividing cells.

The inner and outer nuclear membranes are bridged at **nuclear pore complexes** (Figures 3–2 through 3–6). Various core proteins of a nuclear pore complex, called **nucleoporins**, display eightfold symmetry around the lumen. Although ions and small solutes pass through the channels by simple diffusion, the pore complexes regulate movement of macromolecules between the nucleus and cytoplasm. A growing cell has 3000-4000 such channels, each providing passage for up to 1000 macromolecules per second. Individual pores permit molecular transfer in both directions simultaneously. Macromolecules shipped out of the nucleus include ribosomal subunits and other RNAs associated with proteins, while inbound traffic consists of chromatin proteins, ribosomal proteins, transcription factors, and enzymes. Using mechanisms similar to that by which specific proteins are recognized and translocated across the RER membrane, proteins of complexes destined for the cytoplasm have specific nuclear export sequences and proteins to be imported have nuclear localization sequences. Such sequences bind specifically to transport proteins (importins, exportins, etc) that in turn interact with proteins of the pore complexes for transfer across the nuclear envelope. Energy for the transport is derived from guanosine 5′-triphosphate (GTP), with specific GTPases helping provide directionality to the transfer.

Chromatin

In nondividing nuclei, chromatin consists of the DNA and its attendant proteins in a largely uncoiled state. Two types of chromatin can be distinguished with both the light and electron microscopes (Figures 3–2). **Heterochromatin** (Gr. *heteros*, other + *chroma*, color) appears as coarse, electron-dense material in the electron microscope and as intensely basophilic clumps in the light microscope. **Euchromatin** is visible as finely dispersed

FIGURE **3–1** Nuclei of large, active cells.

Liver cells have large, central nuclei. One or more highly basophilic nucleoli are visible within each nucleus, indicating intense protein synthesis by these cells. Most of the chromatin is light staining or euchromatic, with small areas of more darkly stained heterochromatin scattered throughout the nucleus and just inside the nuclear envelope. This superficial heterochromatin allows the boundary of the organelle to be seen more easily by light microscopy. One cell here has two nuclei, which is fairly common in the liver. X500. Pararosaniline–toluidine blue.

granular material in the electron microscope and as lightly stained basophilic areas in the light microscope. The dispersed euchromatin contains regions of the DNA undergoing active transcription and is more prominent in metabolically active cells.

The chromatin pattern of a nucleus is a guide to the cell's activity. Generally cells with lightly stained nuclei are more active in protein synthesis than those with condensed, dark nuclei. In light-stained nuclei with much euchromatin and few heterochromatic clumps, more DNA surface is available for the transcription of RNA. In dark-stained nuclei rich in

highly condensed heterochromatin, the tightly coiled DNA is less accessible for transcription.

Although heterochromatin tends to be concentrated near the nuclear lamina, evidence for spatial organization of chromatin is not normally seen. Recent in situ hybridization studies of cultured human fibroblast nuclei, using a differently labeled fluorescent probes for sequences on each individual chromosome, have revealed that these structures occupy discrete chromosomal territories within dispersed chromatin (Figure 3–7). Such studies show further that chromosomal domains with few genes form a layer beneath the nuclear envelope, while domains with many active genes are located deeper in the nucleus.

Routine microscopy of mammalian cell nuclei reveals a small, dense mass of heterochromatin present in females but not males. This "sex chromatin" (or **Barr body**) is one of the two X chromosomes present in females. This X chromosome represents *facultative* heterochromatin and remains tightly coiled between mitoses, while the other X chromosome is uncoiled, transcriptionally active, and not visible. The male cell has one X chromosome and one Y chromosome; like the other chromosomes, the interphase X chromosome is uncoiled and therefore no sex chromatin is visible in males.

Formation of facultative heterochromatin involves specific chemical modifications of chromatin proteins and usually occurs only within specific regions of a chromosome, with variability in cells of different tissues. *Constitutive* heterochromatin on the other hand is also specifically modified but is always located at the same sites, such as the centromere region of every chromosome.

DNA in chromatin is extensively packaged by associating with basic proteins called **histones** and with various nonhistone proteins. The structural unit of DNA and histones is the **nucleosome** (Figure 3–8), which has a core of eight small histones (two copies each of histones H2A, H2B, H3, and H4), around which is wrapped DNA with about 150 base pairs. Each nucleosome also has a larger histone (H1) associated with both the wrapped DNA and the surface of the core. The series of nucleosomes in chromatin interacts with many nonhistone proteins having a wide variety of enzymatic functions.

DNA bound to nucleosomes undergoes additional folding and packing to form the 30-nm fiber (Figure 3–9), although the folding mechanism and structures of this and the larger structures are not well understood. Higher orders of chromatin coiling include the formation of transcriptionally active DNA (euchromatin) into loops that are tethered to a central scaffold of proteins that include the condensins. Each long DNA double helix with its associated proteins is a **chromatid**; after DNA replication two chromatids held together by complexes of cohesin proteins make up each **chromosome**. Further packaging during the early phase of cell division causes chromosomes to become visible by light microscopy after staining (Figure 3–9).

FIGURE **3–2** Relationship of nuclear envelope to the rough ER (RER).

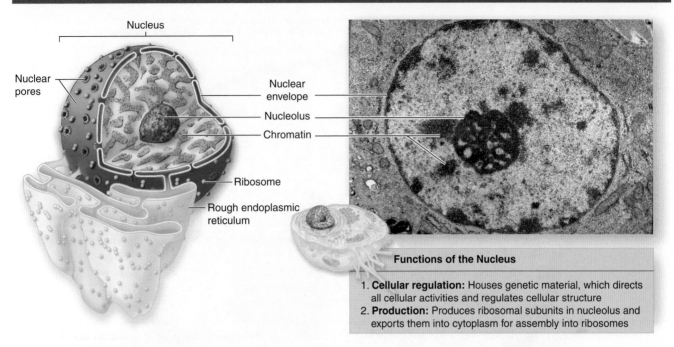

Functions of the Nucleus

1. **Cellular regulation:** Houses genetic material, which directs all cellular activities and regulates cellular structure
2. **Production:** Produces ribosomal subunits in nucleolus and exports them into cytoplasm for assembly into ribosomes

Three-dimensional representation of a cell nucleus shows a single large nucleolus and the distribution of the nuclear pores in the nuclear envelope. The outer membrane of the nuclear envelope is continuous with the RER. TEM X20,000.

Barr bodies or gender chromatin permit gender to be determined microscopically in patients whose external sex organs do not permit that determination, as in hermaphroditism and pseudohermaphroditism. Sex chromatin analysis also helps reveal other anomalies involving the sex chromosomes, such as the presence of XXY chromosomes (Klinefelter syndrome), which causes testicular abnormalities and azoospermia (absence of sperm).

The X and Y sex chromosomes contain genes determining whether an individual will develop as a female or a male. In addition to the pair of sex chromosomes, cells contain pairs of autosomes. Each of these pairs of chromosomes contains one chromosome originally derived from the mother and one derived from the father. The members of each chromosomal pair are called **homologous** because, although from different parents, they contain forms (alleles) of the same genes. Cells of most tissues (somatic cells) are considered **diploid** because they contain pairs of chromosomes. Geneticists refer to diploid cells as 2*n*, where *n* is the number of unique chromosomes in a species, 23 in humans. Sperm cells and mature oocytes

(germ cells) are **haploid**, with half the diploid number of chromosomes, each pair having been separated during meiosis (described below).

Microscopic analysis of chromosomes usually begins with cultured cells arrested in mitotic metaphase by colchicine or other compounds that disrupt microtubules. After processing and staining the cells, the condensed chromosomes of one nucleus are photographed by light microscopy and rearranged to produce a **karyotype** in which stained chromosomal regions (bands) can be analyzed (Figure 3–10).

Karyotyping is important for many prenatal diagnoses, in which chromosomal analysis of cultured cells from the fetus or amnion can detect certain genetic anomalies. As with karyotypes of adults, missing or extra chromosomes and chromosomal deletions or translocations are readily seen. New methods of chromosomal staining and molecular techniques such as fluorescence in situ hybridization (FISH) are continuously being developed and used for cytogenetic diagnosis.

FIGURE 3–3   Ultrastructure of a nucleus.

Regions of euchromatin and heterochromatin display variable electron densities with the transmission electron microscope (TEM). An active nucleus typically has much diffuse, light-staining euchromatin and smaller subdomains of electron-dense heterochromatin (**H**), with many of these associated at the periphery associated with the nuclear lamina. The more heterogeneous electron-dense subdomain is the nucleolus (**N**), the site of rRNA synthesis and ribosomal subunit assembly. X25,000.

Nucleolus

The **nucleolus** is a generally spherical, highly basophilic subdomain of nuclei in cells, actively making proteins (Figures 3–1 through 3–3). The intense basophilia of nucleoli is due not to heterochromatin but to the presence of densely concentrated ribosomal RNA (rRNA) that is transcribed, processed, and complexed into ribosomal subunits in nucleoli. Chromosomal regions with the genes for rRNA organize one or more nucleoli in cells requiring intense ribosome production for synthesis of proteins during growth or secretion. Ultrastructural analysis of an active nucleolus reveals fibrillar and granular subregions with different staining characteristics that reflect stages of rRNA maturation (Figure 3–11). Molecules of rRNA are processed in the nucleolus and very quickly associate with the ribosomal proteins imported from the cytoplasm via nuclear pore complexes. The newly organized small and large ribosomal subunits are then exported back to the cytoplasm through those same nuclear pores.

›› MEDICAL APPLICATION

Tissues with either stable or rapidly renewing cell populations can include cells that become transformed to grow at a higher rate and in an uncoordinated manner. Such **neoplastic proliferation** typically follows damage to the DNA of proto-oncogenes and failure of the cells to be eliminated. Neoplastic growth can be either benign (with slow growth and no invasiveness to neighboring organs) or malignant (with rapid growth and great capacity to invade other organs). **Cancer** is the common term for all malignant tumors.

FIGURE **3–4** The nuclear envelope, nuclear lamina, and nuclear pore complexes.

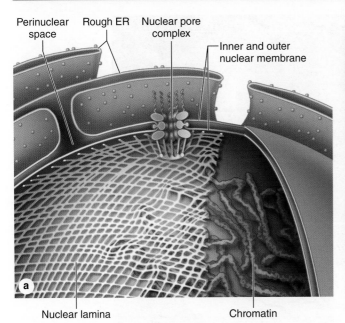

Perinuclear space • Rough ER • Nuclear pore complex • Inner and outer nuclear membrane

Nuclear lamina • Chromatin

(a) Bound to the inner membrane of the nuclear envelope is the **nuclear lamina**, a meshwork assembled from lamins (class V intermediate filament proteins). **Nuclear pore complexes** contain more than 30 core proteins (nucleoporins), span both membranes of the nuclear envelope, and regulate the bidirectional transfer of macromolecular complexes between the nucleus and cytoplasm.

(b) Scanning EM of the inner nuclear membrane (nucleoplasmic face) showing portions of the nuclear lamina (**NL**)

meshwork with many embedded nuclear pore complexes (**NPC**). The preparation is from an actively growing amphibian oocyte. Nuclei of these very large cells can be isolated manually, facilitating ultrastructural studies of the nuclear envelope. X100,000.

(Used, with permission, of Dr M.W. Goldberg, Department of Biological and Biomedical Sciences, Durham University, UK.)

FIGURE **3–5** Nuclear pores.

(a) A TEM section through the nuclear envelope between nucleus (**N**) and cytoplasm (**C**) shows its two-membrane structure. The electron-dense nuclear pore complexes bridging the nuclear envelope can also be seen (arrows). Electron-dense heterochromatin is adjacent to the envelope, except at the nuclear pores. **(b)** A tangential section through a nuclear

envelope shows the nuclear pore complexes (arrows) and the electron-lucent patches in the peripheral heterochromatin, which represent the areas just inside pores. X80,000.

FIGURE **3–6** Cryofracture of nuclear envelope showing nuclear pores.

An electron micrograph obtained by freeze-fractured cell shows the two layers of the nuclear envelope and nuclear pores. The fracture plane occurs partly *between* the two nuclear envelope membranes (left) but mostly just *inside* the envelope with the chromatin removed. The size and distribution of the nuclear pore complexes are clearly seen. X60,000.

>> MEDICAL APPLICATION

Certain mutations in the gene coding for lamin A are associated with a subtype of the disorder progeria, which causes premature aging. In this and other rare "laminopathies," the nuclear envelope is abnormal, but how this is linked to the disorder is unclear. Laminopathies affect some tissues much more than others, although the lamins involved are in all the body's cells.

> THE CELL CYCLE

Before differentiation, most cells undergo repeated cycles of macromolecular synthesis (growth) and division (mitosis). The regular sequence of events that result in new cells is termed the **cell cycle**. Improved knowledge about how each phase of the cell cycle is controlled and how the quality of molecular synthesis, particularly DNA replication, is monitored has led to understanding the causes of many types of cancer, in which cells proliferate without those controls.

The cell cycle has four distinct phases: **mitosis** and periods termed G_1 (the time gap between mitosis and DNA replication), **S** (the period of DNA synthesis), and G_2 (the gap between DNA duplication and the next mitosis). The approximate durations of these phases in rapidly dividing human cells are illustrated in Figure 3–12. G_1 is usually the longest and most variable phase of the cycle and is a period of active RNA and protein synthesis, including proteins controlling progress through the cell cycle. Also in G_1, the cell volume, reduced by half during mitosis, returns to its previous size. The S phase is characterized by DNA replication, histone synthesis, and the beginning of centrosome duplication. In the relatively short G_2 phase, proteins required for mitosis accumulate. As postmitotic cells begin to specialize and differentiate, cell cycle activities may be temporarily or permanently suspended, with the cells sometimes referred to as being in the G_0 phase. Some differentiated cells, such as those of the liver, renew cycling under certain conditions; others, including most muscle and nerve cells, are *terminally differentiated*.

FIGURE **3–7** Chromosome territories of a human fibroblast nucleus.

Fluorescence in situ hybridization (FISH) can be used with a combination of labeled probes, each specific for sequences on different chromosomes. A nucleus of a cultured human fibroblast was processed by 24-color FISH, photographed by confocal microscopy in appropriate channels, and the results superimposed to form an RGB (red-green-blue) image **(a)** of the 24 differently labeled chromosome types (1-22, X, and Y). Individual chromosome territories in the image were identified and false-colored after classification by software developed for such analyses **(b)**.

(*Used, with permission, of Dr Thomas Cremer, Department of Biology II, Anthropology and Human Genetics, Ludwig Maximilian University, Munich, Germany.*)

Cycling is activated in postmitotic G_0 cells by protein signals from the extracellular environment called **mitogens** or **growth factors** binding to cell surface receptors and triggering a cascade of kinase signaling in the cells. The cells are then

FIGURE **3–8** Components of a nucleosome.

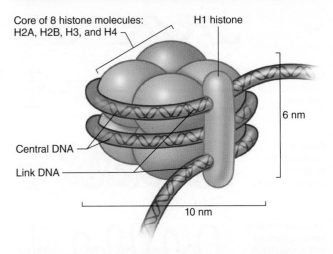

Nucleosome is a structure that produces the initial organization of free double-stranded DNA into chromatin. Each nucleosome has an octomeric core complex made up of four types of **histones**, two copies each of H2A, H2B, H3, and H4. Around this core is wound DNA approximately 150 base pairs in length. One H1 histone is located outside the DNA on the surface of each nucleosome. DNA associated with nucleosomes in vivo thus resembles a long string of beads. Nucleosomes are very dynamic structures, with H1 loosening and DNA unwrapping at least once every second to allow other proteins, including transcription factors and enzymes, access to the DNA.

maintained at the *restriction point* at the G_1/S "boundary" until sufficient nutrients and enzymes required for DNA replication have accumulated and when all ready DNA replication begins (S phase).

As shown in Figure 3–13, entry or progression through other phase of the cycle is also monitored at other specific *checkpoints*, where certain conditions must be met before the cell continues cycling. Overall cycling is regulated by a family of cytoplasmic proteins called **cyclins**. With different cyclins present during different cell cycle phases, each complex activates one or more specific **cyclin-dependent kinases (CDKs)**. Each activated CDK then phosphorylates specific proteins, including enzymes, transcription factors for specific sets of genes, and cytoskeletal subunits, triggering the activities that characterize the next phase of the cycle. When each successive set of activities is complete, the cyclin controlling that cell cycle phase is removed rapidly by proteasomes and a new cyclin that promotes activities for the next phase takes over. In this way diverse cellular activities are coordinated with specific phases of the cell cycle. The major cyclins, CDKs, and important target proteins are summarized in Table 3–1.

FIGURE **3–9** From DNA to chromatin.

Several orders of DNA packing occur in chromatin and during chromatin condensation of mitotic prophase. The top drawing shows the 2-nm DNA double helix, followed by the association of DNA with histones to form 11-nm filaments of **nucleosomes** connected by the DNA ("beads on a string"). Nucleosomes on the DNA then interact in a manner not well understood to form a more compact **30-nm** fiber. For transcription, DNA forms loops that remain tethered to and stabilized by interactions with **protein scaffolds** that eventually make up a central framework at the long axis of each chromosome. **Heterochromatin** is not transcribed and remains more highly condensed. The bottom drawing shows a metaphase chromosome, with maximum packing of DNA. The **chromosome** consists of two **chromatids** held together at a constriction called the **centromere**.

›› MEDICAL APPLICATION

Many mitogenic growth factors for research are produced commercially from microorganisms or cells with recombinant DNA, and some have important medical uses.

FIGURE **3–10** Human karyotype.

Karyotypes provide light microscopic information regarding the number and morphology of chromosomes in an organism. Such preparations are made by staining and photographing the chromosomes of a cultured cell arrested with colchicine during mitosis, when chromosomes are maximally condensed. From the image individual chromosomes are typically placed together in pairs. With certain stains each chromosome has a particular pattern of banding that facilitates its identification and shows the relationship of the banding pattern to genetic anomalies. Hybridization with fluorescent probes specific for each chromosome (FISH) followed by karyotyping yields an image like that shown here. Note that the 22 pairs of autosomes, as well as the X and Y chromosomes, differ in size, morphology, and location of the centromere.

Important examples include analogs of granulocyte colony-stimulating factor (G-CSF), which stimulates neutrophil production in immunocompromised patients, and erythropoietin, which can stimulate red blood cell formation in patients with anemia.

Progression through the cell cycle is halted by a variety of adverse conditions such as inadequate nutrition (nutrient stress), inappropriate cellular microenvironments, or DNA damage. Nuclear DNA is monitored very closely, and damage here can arrest the cell cycle not only at the G_1 **restriction point** but also during S or at a checkpoint in G_2 (Figure 3–13). G_1 arrest may permit repair of the damage before the cell enters S phase, so that the damaged DNA does not reproduce gene defects during replication. If the problem encountered at

FIGURE **3–11** Regions within a nucleolus.

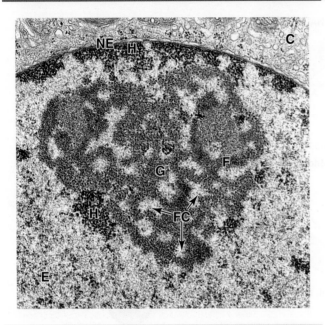

TEM reveals morphologically distinct regions within a nucleolus. Small, light-staining areas are fibrillar centers (**FC**), containing the DNA sequences for the *rRNA* genes (the nucleolar organizers). The darker fibrillar material (**F**) surrounding the fibrillar centers consists of accumulating rRNA transcripts. More granular material (**G**) of the nucleolus contains mainly the large and small ribosomal subunits being assembled from rRNA and ribosomal proteins synthesized in the cytoplasm. Various amounts of heterochromatin (**H**) are also typically found near the nucleolus, scattered in the euchromatin (**E**), and adjacent to the nuclear envelope (**NE**) that separates chromatin from cytoplasm (**C**). X35,000.

any checkpoint cannot be corrected fairly quickly while cycling is halted, proteins encoded by tumor suppressor genes are activated and that cell's activity is redirected toward cell suicide or apoptosis.

Many genes coding for proteins important in the control of cell proliferation and differentiation are often called **proto-oncogenes**; changes in the structure or expression of these can convert them to **oncogenes** causing uncontrolled cell growth and a potential for cancer. Altered proto-oncogenes are associated with many types of tumors and hematologic cancers. Proto-oncogenes can encode almost any protein involved in the control of mitotic activity, including various specific growth factors, the receptors for growth factors, and various kinases and other proteins involved in intracellular signaling of growth factors.

Retinoblastoma is a type of cancer occurring in the eyes, usually in young children. One form of the disease is inherited or familial. Research on the genetic basis of this disease led to the discovery of Rb, a gene coding for a key protein active at the G_1 restriction point that blocks cell cycle progression until a mitogenic stimulus arrives. A kinase activated by a growth factor receptor phosphorylates the Rb protein, causing it to release the E2F transcription factor. This factor then activates genes needed for DNA replication.

DNA changes (mutations) resulting from damage are not always detected and corrected (or eliminated). If such a change occurs in a gene important for cell cycle activities, such as genes for certain growth factors, their receptors or signaling kinases, normal controls on the cell cycle may be affected and growth may occur in a less-regulated manner that is usually detected by the tumor suppressor proteins such as p53. Failure to detect unregulated cell cycling can lead to additional defects and the cellular changes found in the various types of cancer. In many forms of human cancer, the gene for the key tumor suppressor p53 is itself mutated, thus reducing the ability to eliminate cells with damaged DNA and facilitating proliferation of cells with new genetic defects.

▶ MITOSIS

The period of cell division, or **mitosis** (Gr. *mitos*, a thread), is the only cell cycle phase that can be routinely observed with the light microscope. During mitosis, a parent cell divides and each of the two daughter cells receives a chromosomal set identical to that of the parent cell. The chromosomes replicated during the preceding S phase are distributed to the daughter cells. The long growth period between mitoses is also commonly called **interphase**. The events of mitosis can be subdivided into four phases (Figure 3–12). Important details of each mitotic phase are included in Figure 3–14 and summarized here. During the relatively long **prophase**, several changes occur:

- The nucleolus disappears and the replicated chromatin condenses into discrete threadlike chromosomes, each consisting of duplicate sister chromatids joined by cohesins.
- At the centromere region of each chromosome, a large protein complex called the **kinetochore** serves as a site for attachment to microtubules.
- The centrosomes with their now-duplicated centrioles separate and migrate to opposite poles of the cell.

FIGURE **3–12** The cell cycle.

The ability to recognize microscopically cells during both mitosis and DNA replication (by autoradiography after administering radiolabeled thymidine) led to the concept of the cell "cycle" with the phases occurring as shown here. In rapidly dividing cells, **G₁** is a period in which cells accumulate the enzymes and nucleotides required for DNA replication, **S** is the period devoted primarily to DNA replication, **G₂** is a usually short period of preparation for mitosis, and **M** includes all phases of mitosis itself. In rapidly growing human tissues the cell cycle varies from 24 to 36 hours. The length of G₁ depends on many factors and is usually the longest and most variable period; the length of S is largely a function of the genome size. G₂ and mitosis together normally last only 2-3 hours. Differentiating cells in growing tissues may have very long G₁ periods and such cells are often said to be in the **G₀** phase of the cell cycle.

- The microtubules of the mitotic spindle polymerize between the two centrosomes.
- Late in prophase, lamins and inner nuclear membrane are phosphorylated, causing the nuclear lamina and nuclear pore complexes to disassemble and disperse in cytoplasmic membrane vesicles.

During **metaphase**, chromosomes condense further and attach to the mitotic spindle at large electron-dense protein complexes called **kinetochores** (Gr. *kinetos*, moving) at each centromere (Figure 3–15). The cell is now more spherical and the chromosomes are moved to align at its equatorial plane.

In **anaphase** sister chromatids (now called **chromosomes** themselves) separate and move toward opposite spindle poles by a combination of microtubule motor proteins and dynamic changes in the lengths of the microtubules as the spindle poles move farther apart.

At **telophase** the following occur:

- The two sets of chromosomes are at the spindle poles and begin reverting to their decondensed state.

- The spindle depolymerizes and the nuclear envelope begins to reassemble around each set of daughter chromosomes.
- A belt-like contractile ring of actin filaments associated with myosins develops in the peripheral cytoplasm at the cell's equator. During **cytokinesis** at the end of telophase, constriction of this ring produces a cleavage furrow and progresses until the cytoplasm and its organelles are divided into two daughter cells, each with one nucleus.

Most tissues undergo cell turnover with slow cell division and cell death. Nerve tissue and cardiac muscle are exceptions because their differentiated cells cannot undergo mitosis. As discussed in later chapters, a capacity for mitosis within a tissue, either by differentiated cells or by reserve cells, largely determines that tissue's potential to regeneration. The cell turnover rate is rapid in the epithelium lining the digestive tract and uterus or covering the skin. Mitotic cells are usually difficult to identify conclusively in sections of adult organs but may often be detected in rapidly growing tissues by their condensed chromatin (Figure 3–16).

FIGURE **3–13** Controls at cell cycle checkpoints.

Start (G₁/S) checkpoint:
- Are cell nutrition, size, and environment favorable?
- Is all DNA intact?

Prepare for DNA replication and enter S phase

Progress driven by shifts in active kinases, each targeting different sets of proteins

Metaphase/anaphase checkpoint:
- Is all DNA intact?
- Are all chromosomes attached to the mitotic spindle?

Begin chromatid separation and prepare for cytokinesis

G₂/M checkpoint:
- Is DNA completely replicated?

Enter mitosis

Each phase of the cell cycle has one or more checkpoints where the quality of specific cell activities is checked. Progression to the next phase of the cycle does not occur until all activities of the preceding phase are completed satisfactorily. Three important checkpoints are shown here, including

- The *start or restriction checkpoint* just before the start of S
- The *G₂/M checkpoint* that ensures that DNA replication is complete

- The metaphase *spindle checkpoint* that ensures that all chromosomes will be segregated

Overall progression in the cycle is regulated by proteins called **cyclins** and **cyclin-dependent kinases (CDKs)** that phosphorylate/activate enzymes and other proteins needed for phase-specific functions. Major cyclins, their CDKs, and important protein targets are summarized in Table 3–1.

❯ STEM CELLS & TISSUE RENEWAL

Throughout an individual's lifetime, many tissues and organs contain a small population of undifferentiated **stem cells** whose cycling serves to renew the differentiated cells of tissues as needed. Many stem cells divide infrequently and the divisions are asymmetric; that is, one daughter cell remains as a stem cell while the other becomes committed to a path that leads to differentiation (Figure 3–17). Stem cells of many tissues are found

in specific locations or niches where the microenvironment helps maintain their uniquely undifferentiated properties; they are often rare and inconspicuous by routine histologic methods.

Stem cells are best studied in tissues with *rapidly renewing cell populations*, including blood cells, skin cells, and cells lining the digestive tract. Most mitotic cells here are not stem cells but the more rapidly dividing progeny of the cells committed to differentiation (Figure 3–17). They are commonly called **progenitor cells** or **transit amplifying cells** because they

TABLE **3–1** Major cyclin and cyclin-dependent kinase complexes regulating the human cell cycle and important target proteins.

Cycle Phase or Checkpoint	Active Cyclin-CDK Complex	Examples of Target Proteins
Early G₁	Cyclin D-CDK4 or 6	Phosphorylates Rb protein, releasing E2F, a transcription factor that activates genes for many G₁ activities and for cyclin A
Late G₁/entry of S	Cyclin E-CDK2	Further activation E2F-mediated gene transcription; protein p53; other kinases
Progression through S	Cyclin A-CDK2	DNA polymerase and other proteins for DNA replication
G₂/entry of M	Cyclin A-CDK1	Specific phosphatases and cyclin B
Progression through M	Cyclin B-CDK1	Nuclear lamins; histone H1; chromatin- and centrosome-associated proteins

FIGURE **3–14** Stages of mitosis in cultured cells. (Opposite)

The phases of mitosis are shown well in these images of cultured cells obtained with a confocal laser scanning microscope, with chromosomes stained orange and microtubules, green. **(a)** Prophase: The chromosomes have undergone DNA replication and each consists of two very close sister chromatids. Two microtubule-organizing centers, the centrosomes, have moved apart and each is associated with microtubules forming the mitotic spindle. **(b)** Prometaphase: Chromosomes attach to spindle microtubules at their kinetochores and begin to be moved. **(c)** Metaphase: Chromosomes have become aligned at the middle of the spindle, near the cell equator. Kinetochore microtubules attach to each sister chromatid and to opposite poles of the spindle. **(d)** Anaphase: Sister chromatids separate from each other to become individual chromosomes that are pulled toward the spindle poles. The poles move apart and the kinetochore microtubules get shorter. **(e)** Telophase: The two sets of daughter chromosomes arrive at the spindle poles. **(f)** Late telophase and cytokinesis: A contractile ring of myosin-associated actin filaments forms a cleavage furrow that pinches the cell into two daughter cells, each with one nucleus and a complete set of chromosomes ready to undergo another round of DNA replication. a, d, e, and f: X1500; b and c: X3000.

(With permission, from Drs Julie C. Canman and Ted Salmon, Department of Biology, University of North Carolina, Chapel Hill.)

FIGURE **3–15** Mitotic spindle and metaphase chromosomes.

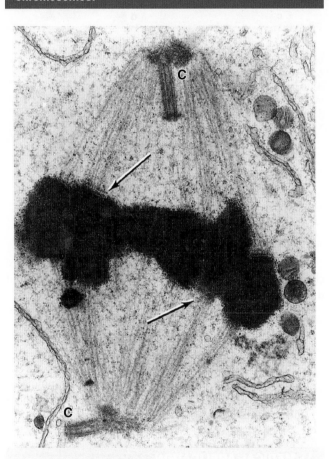

TEM of a sectioned metaphase cell shows several features of the mitotic apparatus, including the very electron-dense chromosomes bound at kinetochores (arrows) to the microtubules of the spindle. The microtubules converge on the centrosomes (**C**), each containing a pair of centrioles. The flattened membrane vesicles near the mitotic spindle may represent fragments of the nuclear envelope, which begin to reassemble during late telophase. X19,000.

(With permission, from Richard McIntosh, Department of Molecular, Cellular and Developmental Biology, University of Colorado, Boulder.)

are in transit along the path from the stem cell niche to a differentiated state, while still amplifying by mitosis the number of new cells available for the differentiated tissue. Cells formed by progenitor cells may often become *terminally differentiated*, meaning that renewed cycling cannot occur and the specialized cells exist for only a short time.

In tissues with *stable cell populations*, such as most connective tissues, smooth muscle, and the cells lining blood vessels, stem cells are not readily apparent and differentiated cells appear to undergo slow and episodic division to maintain tissue integrity.

❯ MEIOSIS

Meiosis is a specialized process involving *two* unique and closely associated cell divisions that occurs only in the cells that will form sperm and egg cells. Differentiation of these two forms of "germ cells" or **gametes** is discussed fully in Chapters 21 and 22 , but the chromosomal aspects of meiosis are described here for comparison with the events of mitosis (Figure 3–18).

Two key features characterize meiosis. (1) Early in the process the homologous chromosomes of each pair (one from the mother, one from the father) come together in an activity termed **synapsis**. During synapsis double-stranded breaks and repairs occur in the DNA, some of which result in reciprocal DNA exchanges called **crossovers** between the aligned maternal and paternal chromosomes. Crossing over produces new combinations of genes in the chromosomes in the germ cells so that few if any chromosomes are exactly the same as those in the mother and father. (2) The cells produced are **haploid**, having just one chromosome from each pair present in the body's somatic cells. The union of haploid eggs and sperm at fertilization forms a new diploid cell (the zygote) that can develop into a new individual.

As shown in Figure 3–18, the important events of meiosis unfold as follows:

■ A cell approaching the first meiotic division has just completed a typical S phase and replicated its DNA; each chromosome contains the two identical DNA molecules called *sister chromatids*.

FIGURE **3–16** Mitotic cells in adult tissues.

Dividing cells in recognizable stages of mitosis are rarely observed in adult tissues because they are rare and the cells are small, with variable shapes and orientations. However, *mitotic figures*, nuclei with clumped, darkly stained chromatin, can sometimes be identified, as shown here in various rapidly renewing tissues.

(a) In the lining of the small intestine, many mitotic *transit amplifying cells* can be found in the area above the most

basal region of the intestinal crypts. Condensed chromosomes of cells in late anaphase and prophase phase can be distinguished here. **(b)** Metaphase cell in a gland of proliferating uterine endometrium. **(c)** Telophase cell in the esophagus lining. **(d)** Metaphase in the basal layer of epidermis. X400. H&E.

- During a greatly elongated prophase of the first meiotic division (prophase I), the partially condensed chromatin of homologous chromosomes begins to come together and physically associate along their lengths during synapsis. Because each of the paired chromosomes has two chromatids, geneticists refer to synaptic chromosomes as *tetrads* to emphasize that four copies of each genetic sequence are present. During synapsis recombination or crossing over occurs among the four chromatids, which mixes up the genes inherited from each parent and yields a new and different set of genes to be passed on to the next generation. In human spermatogenesis prophase I normally lasts for 3 weeks; oocytes arrest in this meiotic phase from the time of their formation in the fetal ovary through the woman's reproductive maturity, that is, for about 12 years to nearly five decades!
- When synapsis and crossing over are completed, the chromosomes become fully condensed and undergo metaphase, anaphase, and telophase as the cell divides. This first meiotic division separates the homologous chromosomes that paired during synapsis; each of the separated chromosomes still contains two chromatids held together at the centromere.
- The two new cells now each divide again, much more rapidly and without an intervening S phase. In the second meiotic division the chromatids separate to

opposite poles as individual chromosomes. In each new cell a nuclear envelope forms around this new haploid set of chromosomes.

In summary, meiosis and mitosis share many aspects of chromatin condensation and separation (Figure 3–18), but differ in key ways:

- Mitosis is a cell division that produces *two diploid cells*. Meiosis involves two cell divisions and produces *four haploid cells*.
- During meiotic crossing over, new combinations of genes are produced and every haploid cell is genetically unique. Lacking synapsis and the opportunity for DNA recombination, mitosis yields two cells that are the same genetically.

›› MEDICAL APPLICATION

In humans chromosome 21 is a very small chromosome and the one most likely to be "overlooked" at the metaphase/anaphase checkpoint. Failure of these homologous chromosomes to separate (nondisjunction) in the first meiotic division also occurs with greater frequency in older oocytes (or sperm progenitor cells). A gamete retaining this chromosome pair forms a viable zygote after fertilization, but the developing **trisomy 21** individual has morphologic and cognitive impairments associated with Down syndrome.

FIGURE **3–17** Stem cells.

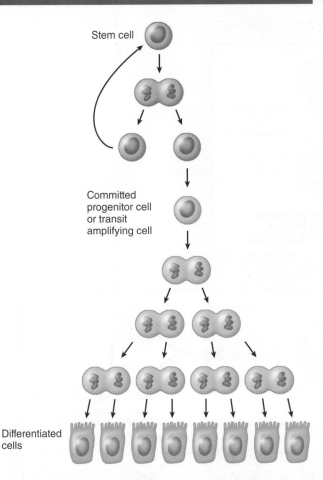

Stem cell

Committed
progenitor cell
or transit
amplifying cell

Differentiated
cells

In rapidly growing adult tissues and perhaps in other tissues there are slowly dividing populations of **stem cells**. Stem cells divide asymmetrically, producing one cell that remains as a stem cell and another that becomes committed to a differentiative pathway but divides a few more times at a more rapid rate. Such cells have been termed **progenitor cells**, or "transit amplifying cells," each of which eventually stops dividing and becomes fully differentiated.

❯ APOPTOSIS

Less evident, but no less important than cell proliferation for body functions, is the process of cell suicide called **apoptosis** (Gr. *apo*, off + *ptosis*, a falling). Apoptosis is a rapid, highly regulated cellular activity that shrinks and eliminates defective and unneeded cells (Figure 3–19). It results in small membrane-enclosed *apoptotic bodies*, which quickly undergo phagocytosis by neighboring cells or cells specialized for debris removal. Apoptotic cells do not rupture and release none of their contents, unlike damaged cells that undergo *necrosis* as a result of injury. This difference is highly significant because release of cellular components triggers a local inflammatory reaction and

immigration of leukocytes. Such a response is avoided when cells are routinely and rapidly eliminated following DNA damage or as part of normal organ development by apoptosis.

❯❯ MEDICAL APPLICATION

Cancer cells often deactivate the genes that control the apoptotic process, thus preventing their elimination in this type of cell death and allowing progression toward a more malignant state. The Bcl-2 family of proteins that controls the onset of apoptosis was first identified by a genetic mutation in a specific B-cell lymphoma, which provided the name for the original protein.

Apoptosis is controlled by cytoplasmic proteins in the **Bcl-2 family**, which regulate the release of death-promoting factors from mitochondria. Activated by either external signals or irreversible internal damage, specific Bcl-2 proteins induce a process with the following features:

- **Loss of mitochondrial function and caspase activation:** Bcl-2 proteins associated with the outer mitochondrial membrane compromise membrane integrity, stopping normal activity and releasing cytochrome c into the cytoplasm where it activates proteolytic enzymes called **caspases**. The initial caspases activate a cascade of other caspases, resulting in protein degradation throughout the cell.
- **Fragmentation of DNA: Endonucleases** are activated, which cleave DNA between nucleosomes into small fragments. (The new ends produced in the fragmented DNA allow specific histochemical staining of apoptotic cells using an appropriate enzyme that adds labeled nucleotides at these sites.)
- **Shrinkage of nuclear and cell volumes:** Destruction of the cytoskeleton and chromatin causes the cell to shrink quickly, producing small structures with dense, darkly stained **pyknotic nuclei** that may be identifiable with the light microscope (see Figure 3–19).
- **Cell membrane changes:** The plasma membrane of the shrinking cell undergoes dramatic shape changes, such as "blebbing," as membrane proteins are degraded and lipid mobility increases.
- **Formation and phagocytic removal:** Membrane-bound remnants of cytoplasm and nucleus separate as very small **apoptotic bodies** (Figure 3–20). Newly exposed phospholipids on these bodies induce their phagocytosis by neighboring cells or white blood cells.

❯❯ MEDICAL APPLICATION

Nuclei of cells in malignant tumors are often enlarged, abnormally shaped, and extremely dark staining, with abnormal nucleoli, in comparison with nuclei of normal cells. Such changes are useful to pathologists looking for evidence of cancer during microscopic examinations of biopsies.

FIGURE **3–18** Mitosis and meiosis.

MITOSIS

Interphase

Prophase
Chromosomes
condense.

Metaphase
Chromosomes
line up single file.

Anaphase/Telophase
Genetically identical
daughter cells produced.

Mitosis adds
and replaces
identical cells.

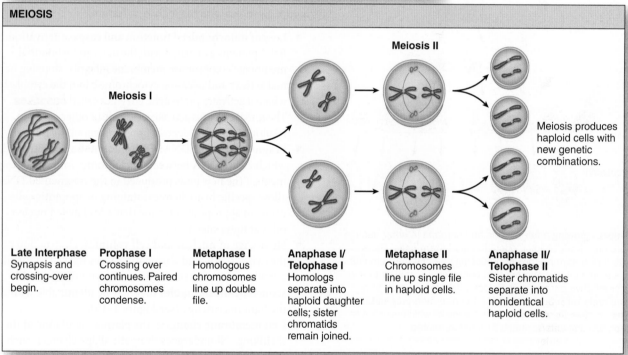

MEIOSIS

Meiosis I

Meiosis II

Meiosis produces
haploid cells with
new genetic
combinations.

Late Interphase
Synapsis and
crossing-over
begin.

Prophase I
Crossing over
continues. Paired
chromosomes
condense.

Metaphase I
Homologous
chromosomes
line up double
file.

**Anaphase I/
Telophase I**
Homologs
separate into
haploid daughter
cells; sister
chromatids
remain joined.

Metaphase II
Chromosomes
line up single file
in haploid cells.

**Anaphase II/
Telophase II**
Sister chromatids
separate into
nonidentical
haploid cells.

Mitosis and meiosis share many aspects of chromatin conden-sation and separation but differ in key ways. Mitosis produces *two diploid cells* that are the same genetically. In meiosis, the two homologous maternal and paternal chromosomes physically align in **synapsis** and regions are exchanged during *crossing over* or genetic recombination. This is followed by **two meiotic divisions** with no intervening S phase, producing *four haploid cells*.

A few examples of apoptosis emphasize the significance of this process. In the thymus, T lymphocytes with the poten-tial to react against self-antigens receive signals that activate the apoptotic program and die without leaving the thymus. In the ovary, apoptosis is the mechanism for both the monthly loss of luteal cells and the removal of excess oocytes and their follicles. Apoptosis was first discovered as programmed cell death in embryos, where it plays an essential part in shaping various developing organs or body regions, such as the free spaces between embryonic fingers and toes. Apoptosis also plays an important role in the final development of the central nervous system.

Triggered by p53 and other tumor suppressor proteins, apoptosis is also an important means of eliminating cells whose survival is blocked by lack of nutrients or by damage caused by free radicals or radiation. In all these examples apoptosis occurs very rapidly, in less time than required for mitosis, and the affected cells are removed without a trace.

FIGURE **3–19** Apoptotic cells.

Apoptotic cells in adult tissues are rare because the process is completed very rapidly. Moreover, with their highly condensed chromatin in pyknotic nuclei and rounded shape, cells early in apoptosis may superficially resemble some mitotic cells. Shown here are apoptotic cells (**A**) in the epithelium covering an intestinal villus (**a**), in a corpus luteum beginning to undergo involution (**b**), in the epithelium of a uterine endometrial gland at the onset of menstruation (**c**), and in the liver (**d**). X400. H&E.

FIGURE **3–20** Late apoptosis—apoptotic bodies.

TEM of a cell in late apoptosis shows radical changes in cell shape, with membrane blebbing and the formation of many membrane-bound cytoplasmic regions. These apoptotic bodies may separate from one another but remain enclosed by plasma membrane so that no contents are released into the extracellular space. The membrane changes are recognized by neighboring cells, and macrophages and apoptotic bodies are very rapidly phagocytosed. X10,000.

The Nucleus SUMMARY OF KEY POINTS

Nuclear Envelope

- Cytoplasm is separated from nucleoplasm by the **nuclear envelope**, a double set of membranes with a narrow perinuclear space; the outer membrane binds ribosomes and is continuous with the RER.
- The nuclear envelope is penetrated by **nuclear pore complexes**, large assemblies of nucleoporins with eightfold symmetry through which proteins and protein-RNA complexes move in both directions.
- The nuclear envelope is supported internally by a meshwork, the nuclear lamina, composed of intermediate filament subunits called **lamins**.

Chromatin

- Chromatin is the combination of DNA and its associated proteins.
- Chromatin with DNA that is active in transcription stains lightly and is called **euchromatin**; inactive chromatin stains more darkly and is called **heterochromatin**.
- The DNA molecule initially wraps around complexes of basic proteins called **histones** to form **nucleosomes**, producing a structure resembling beads on a string.
- Additional levels of chromatin fiber condensation are less well understood and involve nonhistone proteins, including complexes of condensins.

- The extra X chromosome in cells of female mammals forms facultative heterochromatin and can be seen as the Barr body.

Nucleolus

- The **nucleolus** is a very basophilic or electron-dense area of chromatin localized where **rRNA transcription and ribosomal subunits assembly** occur.
- By TEM, an active nucleolus is seen to have **fibrous and granular parts** where rRNA forms and ribosomal subunits are assembled, respectively.

The Cell Cycle

- The **cell cycle** is the sequence of events that controls cell growth and division.
- The G_1 phase, the longest part of the cycle, begins immediately after mitosis and includes all preparations for DNA replication.
- The period of DNA (and histone) synthesis is the **S phase**.
- In a short G_2 phase the cell prepares for division during **mitosis (M)**.
- Cell cycling is controlled by the sequential appearance of key cytoplasmic proteins, the **cyclins**, which bind **cyclin-dependent kinases (CDKs)**.
- CDKs phosphorylate and activate the enzymes and transcription factors whose functions characterize each phase of the cell cycle.
- Progress through the cell cycle stages is monitored at checkpoints, including the G_1 **restriction point**; only when each phase's activities are completed are the cyclins changed to trigger those of the next phase.

Mitosis

- Stages of mitotic cell divisions include **prophase**, when chromosomes condense, the nuclear envelope disassembles, and the microtubular spindle forms; **metaphase**, when chromosomes are aligned; **anaphase**, when they begin to separate toward the two centrosomes; and **telophase**, when nuclear envelope re-forms around the separated chromosomes.
- Telophase ends with **cytokinesis** or cell cleavage into two daughter cells by a contractile ring of actin filaments and myosin.

Stem Cells & Tissue Renewal

- **Stem cells** occur in all tissues with rapid cell turnover; they divide slowly in an **asymmetric** manner, with one daughter cell remaining a stem cell and one becoming committed toward differentiation.

- Cells committed to differentiate (**transit amplifying or progenitor cells**) typically divide more rapidly than stem cells before slowing or stopping division to differentiate.

Meiosis

- **Meiosis** is the process by which two successive cell divisions produce cells called **gametes** containing half the number of chromosomes found in somatic cells.
- Prophase of the first meiotic division is a unique, extended period in which homologous chromosomes pair and undergo genetic recombination during the process called **synapsis**.
- Synaptic pairs separate toward two daughter cells at the first meiotic division.
- The second meiotic division occurs with no intervening S phase and separates the sister chromatids into two final cells that are **haploid**.

Apoptosis

- **Apoptosis** is the process by which redundant or defective cells are rapidly eliminated in a manner that does not provoke a local inflammatory reaction in the tissue.
- Apoptosis involves a cascade of events controlled by the **Bcl-2 family of proteins** regulating the release of death-promoting factors from mitochondria.
- Cytochrome c from mitochondria activates cytoplasmic proteases called **caspases**, which degrade proteins of the cytosol, cytoskeleton, and cell membrane.
- **Endonucleases** are activated, which degrade all nuclear DNA.
- Cell and nuclear volumes shrink rapidly, and the cell membrane changes produce extensive blebbing of the cell surface.
- Late in apoptosis, the cell breaks into many small **apoptotic bodies** that undergo **phagocytosis** by neighboring cells.
- Apoptosis occurs rapidly, with little or no release of proteins that would trigger inflammation, unlike the **death of injured cells by necrosis** that typically induces local inflammation.

4 Epithelial Tissue

D espite its complexity, the human body is composed of only **four basic types of tissue:** epithelial, connective, muscular, and nervous. These tissues, which all contain cells and molecules of the extracellular matrix (ECM), exist in association with one another and in variable proportions and morphologies, forming the different organs of the body. The main characteristics of these basic types of tissue are shown in Table 4–1. Also of great functional importance are the free cells found in body fluids such as blood and lymph.

Connective tissue is characterized by the abundant ECM produced by its cells; muscle tissue is composed of elongated cells specialized for contraction and movement; and nervous tissue is composed of cells with long, fine processes specialized to receive, generate, and transmit nerve impulses. Most organs can be divided into **parenchyma**, which is composed of the cells responsible for the organ's specialized functions, and **stroma**, the cells of which have a supporting role in the organ. Except in the brain and spinal cord, the stroma is always connective tissue.

Epithelial tissues are composed of closely aggregated polyhedral cells with strong adhesion to one another and attached to a thin layer of ECM. Epithelia are cellular sheets that line the cavities of organs and cover the body surface.

The principal functions of epithelial (Gr. *epi*, upon + *thele*, nipple) tissues include the following:

- Covering, lining, and protecting surfaces (eg, epidermis)
- Absorption (eg, the intestinal lining)
- Secretion (eg, parenchymal cells of glands)

Specific cells of certain epithelia may be contractile (myoepithelial cells) or specialized sensory cells, such as those of taste buds or the olfactory epithelium. Because epithelial cells line all external and internal surfaces of the body, all substances that enter or leave tissues and organs must cross an epithelium.

> CHARACTERISTIC FEATURES OF EPITHELIAL CELLS

The shapes and dimensions of epithelial cells are quite variable, ranging from tall **columnar** to **cuboidal** to low **squamous** cells. The cells' size and morphology are generally dictated by their function. Epithelial cell nuclei vary in shape and may be elliptic (oval), spherical, or flattened. Nuclear shape corresponds roughly to cell shape; tall cells have elongated nuclei and squamous cells have flattened nuclei. Cuboidal or pyramidal cells usually have more spherical nuclei (Figure 4–1).

Because the lipid-rich membranes of epithelial cells are frequently indistinguishable with the light microscope, the number and shape of the stained nuclei can indicate cell density and shape. The nuclei also allow one to determine the number of cell layers in an epithelium, a primary morphologic criterion for classifying epithelia.

Most epithelia rest on connective tissue that contains the microvasculature bringing nutrients and O_2 to both tissues. Even thick epithelia do not themselves normally contain blood vessels. The connective tissue that underlies the epithelia lining the organs of the digestive, respiratory, and urinary systems is called the **lamina propria**. The area of contact between the epithelium and connective tissue may be increased by irregularities at the interface in the form of small evaginations called **papillae** (L. diminutive of *papula*, nipple; singular papilla). Papillae occur most frequently in epithelial tissues subject to friction, such as the covering of the skin or tongue.

TABLE **4–1**	Main characteristics of the four basic types of tissues.		
Tissue	**Cells**	**Extracellular Matrix**	**Main Functions**
Nervous	Elongated cells with extremely fine processes	Very small amount	Transmission of nerve impulses
Epithelial	Aggregated polyhedral cells	Small amount	Lining of surface or body cavities; glandular secretion
Muscle	Elongated contractile cells	Moderate amount	Strong contraction; body movements
Connective	Several types of fixed and wandering cells	Abundant amount	Support and protection of tissues/organs

Epithelial cells generally show **polarity**, with organelles and membrane proteins distributed unevenly within the cell. The region of the cell contacting the connective tissue is called the **basal pole** and the opposite end, usually facing a space, is the **apical pole**. The two poles of epithelial cells differ in both structure and function. Regions of cuboidal or columnar cells that adjoin the neighboring cells are the **lateral surfaces**; cell membranes here often have numerous infoldings to increase the area of that surface, increasing its functional capacity.

Basement Membranes

All epithelial cells in contact with subjacent connective tissue have at their basal surfaces a specialized, feltlike sheet of extracellular material referred to as the **basement membrane** (Figure 4–1). Glycoproteins and other components in this structure can be stained and make it visible beneath epithelia with the light microscope (Figure 4–2).

With the transmission electron microscope (TEM) the basement membrane may be resolved into two structures. Nearest the epithelial basal poles is an electron-dense layer, 20-100 nm thick, consisting of a network of fine fibrils that comprise the **basal lamina** (Figure 4–3). Beneath this layer is often a more diffuse and fibrous **reticular lamina**.

FIGURE **4–2** Basement membranes.

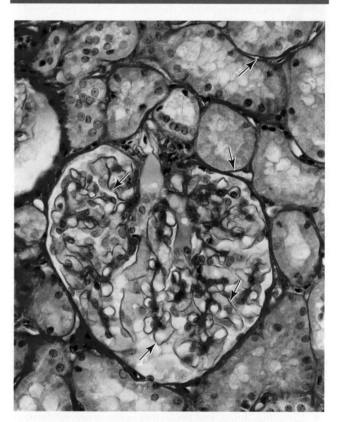

This section of kidney shows the well-stained basement membranes (arrows) of epithelia forming structures within the large, round renal glomerulus and its surrounding tubules. In kidney glomeruli the basement membrane, besides having a supporting function, has a highly developed role as a filter that is key to renal function. X100. Picrosirius-hematoxylin (PSH).

FIGURE **4–1** Epithelia and adjacent connective tissue.

Cuboidal or pyramidal cells of epithelia generally have spherical nuclei, while nuclei of squamous epithelial cells are flattened. An extracellular **basement membrane** (red) always lies at the interface of epithelial cells and connective tissue. Nutrients for epithelial cells must diffuse across the basement membrane. Nerve fibers normally penetrate this structure, but small blood capillaries (being epithelial themselves) normally never enter epithelia.

FIGURE **4–3** Basal and reticular laminae.

The ultrastructural components of the basement membrane are revealed by TEM. The dense **basal lamina (BL)** may appear with thin clear zones on each side and is anchored to a thicker, more diffuse **reticular lamina (RL)** containing collagen III reticular fibers. **Hemidesmosomes (H)** bind the basal surface of the epithelial cell (**C**) to the basal lamina. X54,000.

The terms "basement membrane" and "basal lamina" are often used indiscriminately, causing confusion. Most authors use "basal lamina" to denote the extracellular epithelial layer seen ultrastructurally and "basement membrane" for the entire structure below an epithelium visible with the light microscope.

The macromolecules of the basal lamina are secreted at the basal poles of the epithelial cells and form three-dimensional arrays. ECM components are described more fully in Chapter 5, but those of basal laminae include the following:

- **Laminin:** These are large glycoproteins that self-assemble as a lacelike network immediately below the cells' basal poles where they are held in place by the transmembrane integrins.
- **Type IV collagen:** Monomers of type IV collagen contain three polypeptide chains and self-assemble further to form a feltlike layer.
- The laminin and type IV collagen networks are held together by the adhesive glycoprotein **entactin/ nidogen**, and by **perlecan**, a proteoglycan.

These components of basal laminae are also produced by other cells besides those of epithelia, including muscle cells, adipocytes (fat-storing cells), and the cells supporting peripheral neurons. Surrounding these cells, this *external lamina* binds factors important for interactions with other

cells and serves as semipermeable barriers further regulating macromolecular exchanges between the enclosed cells and connective tissue.

The more diffuse meshwork of reticular laminae contains **type III collagen** and is bound to the basal laminae by anchoring fibrils of **type VII collagen**. These components of the basement membrane are produced by cells of the connective tissue and are also visible by TEM (Figure 4–3).

Basement membranes have many functions. They provide structural support and polarity to epithelial cells and attach epithelia to underlying connective tissue. Proteins of the layered meshwork help filter substances entering the epithelium from below, concentrate mitogenic growth factors, and form a scaffold for epithelial repair and regeneration. Basal lamina components help organize proteins in the plasma membrane of epithelial cells, affecting endocytosis, signal transduction, and other activities. Basement membrane proteins also mediate many cell-to-cell interactions involving epithelia and mark routes for certain cell migrations along epithelia.

Intercellular Adhesion & Other Junctions

Several membrane-associated structures provide adhesion and communication between cells. Some are present in other tissues but all are particularly numerous and prominent in epithelia. Epithelial cells adhere strongly to neighboring cells and basal laminae, particularly in epithelia subject to friction or other mechanical forces.

As shown in Figure 4–4 and summarized in Table 4–2, lateral surfaces of epithelial cells exhibit several specialized intercellular junctions, which serve different functions:

- **Tight** or **occluding junctions** form a seal between adjacent cells.
- **Adherent** or **anchoring junctions** are sites of string cell adhesion.
- **Gap junctions** are channels for communication between adjacent cells.

In many epithelia these junctions are present in a definite order at the apical end of the cells. **Tight junctions**, or **zonulae occludens**, are the most apical of the junctions. The term "zonula" indicates that the junction forms a band completely encircling each cell. In TEM the adjacent membranes at these junctions appear fused or very tightly apposed (Figures 4–5). The seal between the membranes is due to interactions between the transmembrane proteins **claudin** and **occludin** of each cell. Zonulae occludens are clearly seen after cryofracture (Figure 4–6), where they appear as a band of branching strands in the membrane around each cell's apical end. The intercellular seal of this junctional type ensures that molecules crossing an epithelium in either direction do so by going *through* the cells (transcellular path) rather than *between* them (paracellular pathway). Epithelia with one or very few fused sealing strands (eg, proximal renal tubule) are more permeable to water and solutes than are epithelia with numerous fusion sites (eg, the lining of the urinary bladder).

FIGURE **4–4** Junctional complexes of epithelial cells.

Microvilli

Tight junction
(occluding junction)

Adherens junction
(anchoring junction)

Desmosome
(anchoring junction)

Intermediate
filament

Gap junction
(communicating junction)

Hemidesmosome
(anchoring junction)

Basal lamina

Most cuboidal or columnar epithelial cells have four major types of intercellular junctional complexes, as shown schematically here. At the apical end, **tight junctions** (zonulae occludens) and **adherent junctions** (zonulae adherens) are typically close together and each forms a continuous ribbon around the cell. Multiple ridges of the tight junction prevent passive flow of material between the cells but are not very strong; the adhering junctions immediately below them serve to stabilize and strengthen the circular occluding bands and help hold the cells together.

Both **desmosomes** and **gap junctions** are spot-like, not circular, structures between two cells. Bound to intermediate filaments inside the cells, desmosomes form very strong attachment points that supplement the zonulae adherens and play a major role to maintain the integrity of an epithelium. Gap junctions, each a patch of many **connexons** in the adjacent cell membranes, have little strength but serve as intercellular channels for flow of molecules. All of these junctional types are also found in certain other cell types besides epithelia. **Hemidesmosomes** bind epithelial cells to the underlying basal lamina.

TABLE **4–2**	Epithelial cell junctions, their major structural features and functions, and medical significance.				
Junction	**Tight Junction (Zonula Occludens)**	**Adherent Junction (Zonula Adherens)**	**Desmosome (Macula Adherens)**	**Hemidesmosome**	**Gap Junction (Nexus)**
Major transmembrane link proteins	Occludins, claudins, ZO proteins	E-cadherin, catenin complexes	Cadherin family proteins (desmogleins, desmocollin)	Integrins	Connexin
Cytoskeletal components	Actin filaments	Actin filaments	Intermediate filaments (keratins)	Intermediate filaments	None
Major functions	Seals adjacent cells to one another, controlling passage of molecules between them; separates apical and basolateral membrane domains	Provides points linking the cytoskeletons of adjacent cells; strengthens and stabilizes nearby tight junctions	Provides points of strong intermediate filament coupling between adjacent cells, strengthening the tissue	Anchors cytoskeleton to the basal lamina	Allows direct transfer of small molecules and ions from one cell to another
Medical significance	Defects in occludins may compromise the fetal blood-brain barrier, leading to severe neurologic disorders	Loss of E-cadherin in epithelial cell tumors (carcinomas) promotes tumor invasion and the shift to malignancy	Autoimmunity against desmoglein I leads to dyshesive skin disorders characterized by reduced cohesion of epidermal cells	Mutations in the integrin-β4 gene are linked to some types of epidermolysis bullosa, a skin blistering disorder	Mutations in various connexin genes have been linked to certain types of deafness and peripheral neuropathy

Tight junctions also serve a related purpose in epithelia. These continuous zones around epithelial cells prevent membrane proteins at the apical cell surface from moving in the membrane to the basal and lateral surfaces, and vice versa. This produces two membrane domains (apical and basolateral) with different protein populations, which allows the two sides of the epithelium to maintain different receptors and to function differently. Apical cell membranes of epithelia are part of the luminal compartment of a tissue or organ, while the basolateral domains of the epithelial cells are part of a basal compartment that also encompasses the underlying connective tissue.

The second type of junction is the **zonula adherens** (Figures 4–4 and 4–5), which also encircles the epithelial cell, usually immediately below the zonula occludens. This is an adherent junction, firmly anchoring a cell to its neighbors. Cell adhesion here is mediated by **cadherins**, transmembrane glycoproteins of each cell that interact in the presence of Ca^{2+}. At their cytoplasmic ends, cadherins bind **catenin** that is linked via actin-binding proteins to actin filaments. The actin filaments linked to the zonula adherens form part of the terminal web, a cytoskeletal feature at the apical pole in many epithelial cells with a role in cytoplasmic motility and other functions. Together, the tight and adherent junctions encircling the apical ends of epithelial cells function like the plastic form that holds a six-pack of canned drinks together.

A related adherent junction is the **desmosome** or **macula adherens** (L. *macula*, spot). As the latter name implies, this junction resembles a single "spot-weld" and does not form a belt around the cell. Maculae adherens or desmosomes are disc-shaped structures at the surface of one cell that are matched with identical structures at an adjacent cell surface (Figures 4–4 and 4–5). Desmosomes contain larger members of the cadherin family called **desmoglein** and **desmocollin**. On the cytoplasmic side of each cell membrane, these proteins inset into a dense attachment plaque of anchoring proteins (**plakoglobin** and **desmoplakin**) that bind intermediate filaments rather than actin filaments. Cable-like filaments of cytokeratin are most common in desmosomes of epithelia. Because intermediate filaments of the cytoskeleton are very strong, desmosomes provide firm adhesion among the cells. In nonepithelial cells, the intermediate filaments attached to desmosomes are composed of other proteins, such as desmin or vimentin.

>> **MEDICAL APPLICATION**

Various **blistering (bullous) diseases**, such as pemphigus vulgaris, involving the epidermis or stratified squamous epithelia of the oral mucosa, are due to abnormal desmosome function caused by autoimmune reactions against specific desmogleins that reduce cell-to-cell adhesion. Similar disorders arise with genetic mutations for various junctional proteins.

Gap junctions mediate communication rather than adhesion or occlusion between cells (Figure 4–7). Abundant in many epithelia, gap junctions are also functionally important in nearly all mammalian tissues. Cryofracture preparations

FIGURE **4–5** Epithelial cell junctional complex.

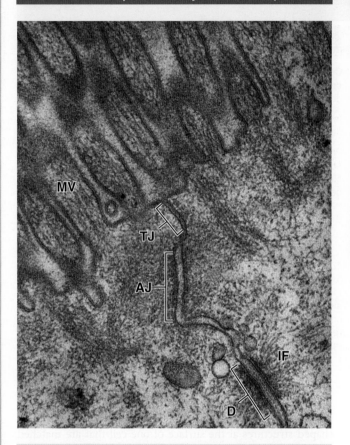

Ultrastructural view of the apical region near microvilli (**MV**) of two epithelial cells, revealing a junctional complex with a tight junction (**TJ**) or zonula occludens, an adherent junction (**AJ**) or zonula adherens, and a desmosome (**D**) associated with intermediate filaments (**IF**). The functions and major protein components of these junction types are summarized in Table 4–2. X195,000.

FIGURE **4–6** View of a tight junction after cryofracture.

Just below the apical microvilli (**MV**) of this epithelial cell, a cryofracture plane splitting fused cell membranes reveals the fused strands of transmembrane proteins forming the tight junction (zonula occludens). X100,000.

show that gap junctions consist of aggregated transmembrane protein complexes that form circular patches in the plasma membrane (Figure 4–7b).

The gap junction proteins, called **connexins**, form hexameric complexes called **connexons**, each of which has a central hydrophilic pore about 1.5 nm in diameter. When two cells attach, connexins in the adjacent cell membranes move laterally and align to form connexons between the two cells (Figure 4–4), with each junction having dozens or hundreds of aligned connexon pairs. Gap junctions permit intercellular exchange of molecules with small (<1.5 nm) diameters. Some molecules mediating signal transduction, such as cyclic nucleotides and ions, move rapidly through gap junctions, allowing cells in many tissues to act in a coordinated manner rather than as independent units. For example, in heart and visceral muscles gap junctions help produce rhythmic contractions.

The basal domain of an epithelial cell (Figure 4–4) attaches to the subjacent basal lamina by junctions called

hemidesmosomes (Gr. *hemi*, half + *desmos* + *soma*), which can be observed by TEM (Figure 4–3). These adhesive structures resemble a half-desmosome ultrastructurally, but, unlike desmosomes, they contain abundant **integrins** rather than cadherins. The transmembrane integrin proteins bind the extracellular macromolecules laminin and collagen type IV.

> **›› MEDICAL APPLICATION**
>
> Proteins of the **zonula occludens** provide the targets for certain common bacteria of medical importance. The enterotoxin secreted by *Clostridium perfringens*, which causes "food poisoning," binds claudin molecules of intestinal cells, prevents insertion of these proteins during maintenance of tight junctions, and causes loss of tissue fluid into the intestinal lumen via the paracellular pathway.
>
> Similarly, *Helicobacter pylori*, which is important in the etiology of **gastric ulcers**, binds the extracellular domains of tight-junction proteins in cells of the stomach and inserts a protein into these cells, which targets ZO-1 and disrupts signaling from the junction.

› SPECIALIZATIONS OF THE APICAL CELL SURFACE

The apical ends of many tall or cuboidal epithelial cells face an organ's lumen and often have specialized projecting structures.

FIGURE **4–7** Gap junctions.

(a) A diagram of a gap junction shows the structural elements that allow the exchange of nutrients and signal molecules between cells without loss of material into the intercellular space. The communicating channels are formed by pairs of abutting particles **(connexons)**, which are in turn each composed of six protein subunits (connexins) that span the lipid bilayer of each cell membrane. The channel formed by paired connexons (arrow) is about 1.5 nm in diameter, limiting the size of transmitted molecules. **(b)** A cryofracture preparation of a gap junction, showing the patch of aggregated transmembrane protein complexes, the connexons. X150,000.

These function either to increase the apical surface area for absorption or to move substances along the epithelial surface.

Microvilli

Many cells are seen to have cytoplasmic projections visible with the electron microscope. Such extensions usually reflect cytoplasmic movements and activity of actin filaments and are both temporary and variable in their length, shape, and number. However, in epithelial cells specialized for absorption, the apical surfaces present an array of projections called **microvilli** (L. *villus*, tuft). In cells such as those lining the small intestine, apical surfaces are densely covered with uniform microvilli, which are visible as a **brush** or **striated border** on these cells (Figure 4–8). The average microvillus is about 1 μm long and 0.1 μm wide, but with hundreds or thousands present on the end of each absorptive cell, the total surface area can be increased by 20- or 30-fold. Glycocalyx covering intestinal microvilli is thick and includes enzymes for digestion of certain macromolecules.

Each microvillus contains many bundles of actin filaments capped and cross-linked to each other and to the surrounding plasma membrane by many different actin-binding proteins (Figure 4–8). Although microvilli are often relatively stable, the microfilament arrays are dynamic and undergo various myosin-based movements, which help maintain optimal conditions for absorption via numerous channels, receptors, and other proteins in the plasmalemma. The actin filaments insert into the terminal web of similar filaments at the base of the microvilli.

›› MEDICAL APPLICATION

Celiac disease, also called **gluten-sensitive enteropathy** or **sprue**, is a disorder of the small intestine in which one of the first pathologic changes is loss of the microvilli brush border of the absorptive cells. This is caused by an immune reaction against the wheat protein gluten during its digestion, which produces diffuse enteritis (intestinal inflammation), changes to the epithelial cells leading to malabsorption, and eventually to pathologic changes in the intestinal wall. The malabsorption problems and structural changes are reversible when gluten is removed from the diet.

FIGURE **4–8** Microvilli.

Formin and
other proteins for
F-actin capping

Fimbrin, villin
(cross-linking
F-actin)

Myosin I
(anchoring
F-actin to
membrane)

Actin filaments
(microfilaments)

Myosin II

d   Intermediate filaments (keratins)

Absorptive cells lining the small intestine demonstrate the highly uniform microvilli of a striated or brush border particularly well. **(a)** A high-magnification light microscope shows many parallel microvilli and their connections to the terminal web (**TW**) in the underlying cytoplasm. X6500. **(b)** SEM of a sectioned epithelial cell shows both the internal and surface structure of individual microvilli and the association with actin filaments and intermediate filaments of the terminal web (**TW**). X7000. **(c)** TEM of microvilli sectioned longitudinally and transversely (inset) reveals the microfilament arrays that form the core of these projections. The terminal web (**TW**) of the cytoskeleton is also seen. The glycocalyx (**G**) extending from glycoproteins and glycolipids of the microvilli plasmalemma contains certain enzymes for late stages of macromolecule digestion. X15,000.

(d) The diagram shows a few microfilaments in a microvillus, with various actin-binding proteins important for F-actin assembly, capping, cross-linking, and movement. Like microfilaments in other regions of the cytoskeleton, those

of microvilli are highly dynamic, with treadmilling and various myosin-based interactions. Myosin motors import various microvilli components along the actin filaments. (*Figure 4–8b, with permission, from Dr John Heuser, Washington University School of Medicine, St. Louis, MO.*)

FIGURE **4–9** Stereocilia.

At the apical ends of the tall epithelial cells lining organs such as the epididymis (shown here) are numerous very long stereocilia, which increase the surface area available for absorption. Stereocilia are much longer than microvilli and often have distal branching. X400. H&E.

Stereocilia

Stereocilia are a much less common type of apical process, restricted to absorptive epithelial cells lining the epididymis (Figure 4–9) and the proximal part of ductus deferens in the male reproductive system. Like microvilli, stereocilia increase the cells' surface area, facilitating absorption. More specialized stereocilia with a motion-detecting function are important components of inner ear sensory cells.

Stereocilia resemble microvilli in containing arrays of actin filaments and various actin-binding proteins, with similar diameters, and with similar connections to the cell's terminal web. However, stereocilia are typically much longer and much less motile than microvilli, and may show distal branching along their length.

Cilia

Cilia are long projecting structures, larger than microvilli, which contain internal arrays of microtubules (Figure 4–10). Most (if not all) cell types have at least one cilium of variable length, usually called a *primary cilium*, which is not motile but is enriched with receptors and signal transduction complexes for detection of light, odors, motion, and flow of liquid past the cells. Primary cilia are also important in the early embryo.

Motile cilia are found only in epithelia, where they are abundant on the apical domains of many cuboidal or columnar cells. Typical cilia are 5-10 μm long and 0.2 μm in diameter, which is much longer and two times wider than a typical microvillus. As shown in Figure 4–11, each cilium has a core structure consisting of nine peripheral microtubular doublets in which a few tubulin protofilaments are shared. The nine doublets form an array around two central microtubules; the **9 + 2 assembly** of microtubules is called an **axoneme** (Gr. *axon*, axis + *nema*, thread). As with other microtubules, kinesin and cytoplasmic dynein *motors* move along the peripheral microtubules for the transport of molecular components into and out of these structures.

Axonemes are continuous with **basal bodies**, which are apical cytoplasmic structures just below the cell membrane (Figures 4–10 and 4–11). Basal bodies have a structure similar to that of centrioles, with triplets of microtubules and dynamic tubulin protofilaments forming rootlets anchoring the entire structure to the cytoskeleton.

Epithelial cilia exhibit rapid beating patterns of movement that propel a current of fluid and suspended matter in one direction over the epithelium. Ciliary motion occurs through successive changes in the conformation of the axoneme, in which a large variety of accessory proteins make each cilium relatively stiff, but elastic. Complexes with **axonemal dyneins** bound to a microtubule in each doublet extend as "arms" toward a microtubule of the next doublet. With energy from adenosine triphosphate (ATP), dynein-powered sliding of adjacent doublets relative to each other bends the axoneme and a rapid series of these sliding movements produces the beating motion of epithelial cilia. The long flagellum that extends from each fully differentiated sperm cell has an axonemal structure like that of cilia and moves with a similar mechanism.

> **>> MEDICAL APPLICATION**
>
> Several mutations have been described in the proteins of the cilia and flagella. They are responsible for the **immotile cilia syndrome** (Kartagener syndrome), whose symptoms are chronic respiratory infections caused by the lack of the cleansing action of cilia in the respiratory tract and immotile spermatozoa, causing male infertility.

› TYPES OF EPITHELIA

Epithelia can be divided into two main groups: **covering** (or **lining) epithelia** and **secretory (glandular) epithelia**. This is an arbitrary division, for there are lining epithelia in which all the cells also secrete (eg, the lining of the stomach) or in which glandular cells are distributed among the lining cells (eg, mucous cells in the small intestine or trachea).

Covering or Lining Epithelia

Cells of covering epithelia are organized into one or more layers that cover the external surface or line the cavities of

FIGURE **4–10** Cilia.

Epithelial cells lining the respiratory tract have many very well-developed cilia. **(a)** By light microscopy cilia (**C**) on the columnar cells appear as a wave of long projections, interrupted by nonciliated, mucus-secreting goblet cells (**G**). X400. Toluidine blue. **(b)** SEM of the apical surfaces of this epithelium shows the density of the cilia (**C**) and the scattered goblet cells (**G**). X300.

(c) TEM of cilia (**C**) sectioned longitudinally reveals the central and peripheral microtubules of the axonemes, with cross sections (inset) clearly showing the 9 + 2 array of the microtubule doublets. At the base of each cilium is a basal body (**B**) anchoring the axoneme to the apical cytoplasm. Much shorter microvilli (**MV**) can be seen between the cilia. X59,000. Inset: X80,000.

an organ. Such epithelia are classified according to the number of cell layers and the cell morphology in the surface layer (Table 4–3). **Simple epithelia** contain one cell layer and **stratified epithelia** contain two or more layers.

Based on cell shape, simple epithelia are classified as **squamous** (thin cells), **cuboidal** (cell width and thickness roughly similar) or **columnar** (cells taller than they are wide) Examples of these epithelial types are shown in Figures 4–12 through 4–14.

Most stratified epithelia (Figure 4–15) are classified according to the cell shape of the *superficial* layer(s): **squamous**, **cuboidal**, or **columnar**.

The very thin surface cells of stratified squamous epithelia can be "keratinized" (filled with keratin intermediate filaments) or "nonkeratinized" (with relatively sparse amounts of keratin). **Stratified squamous keratinized epithelium** is found mainly in the epidermis of skin, where it helps prevent dehydration from the tissue (Figure 4–15). Its cells form many layers, with the less differentiated cuboidal cells near the underlying connective tissue. These cells become more

irregular in shape and flatten as they accumulate keratin in the process of **keratinization** and are moved progressively closer to the skin surface, where they become thin, metabolically inactive packets (squames) of keratin lacking nuclei. As discussed with skin, this surface layer of cells helps protect against water loss across this epithelium. **Stratified squamous nonkeratinized epithelium** (Figure 4–15) lines wet cavities (eg, mouth, esophagus, and vagina) where water loss is not a problem. Here the flattened cells of the surface layer contain much less keratin, retaining their nuclei and metabolic function.

Stratified cuboidal and **stratified columnar epithelia** are both relatively rare. Stratified cuboidal epithelium is restricted to excretory ducts of salivary and sweat glands (Figure 4–15). Stratified columnar epithelium can be found in the conjunctiva lining the eyelids, where it is both protective and mucus secreting.

Transitional epithelium or **urothelium** lines much of the urinary tract, extending from the kidneys to the proximal part of the urethra, and is characterized by a superficial layer of

FIGURE **4–11** Ciliary axoneme.

Microtubule protofilament

Dynein "arms"

Radial spoke to central microtubule

Nexin-link protein to next doublet

Central microtubules

Microtubule doublet

Inner sheath

Microtubule triplet

Distal tips of cilia contain dynamic pools of tubulin, other ciliary precursor proteins, and motor proteins

Pair of dynein arms

Nexin cross-links between doublets

b

Transport of proteins upward through cilia involves kinesin II motors moving along microtubules of peripheral doublets

Plasma membrane

Transport of proteins back to base of cilium involves cytoplasmic dynein motors moving along microtubules of peripheral doublets

Basal body

Rootlet

a

(a) A diagram of a cilium with the **axoneme** consisting of **two central microtubules** surrounded by **nine peripheral microtubular doublets** associated with other proteins. In the doublets, microtubule A is complete, consisting of 13 protofilaments, whereas microtubule B shares some of A's protofilament heterodimers. The axoneme is elastic but relatively stiff, with its structure maintained by nexins linking the peripheral doublets and other protein complexes forming a sheath and radial spokes between the doublets and the central microtubules.

The axoneme is continuous with a **basal body** located in the apical cytoplasm. Basal bodies are structurally very similar to centrioles, consisting of nine relatively short **microtubular triplets** linked together in a pinwheel-like arrangement. A dynamic pool of tubulin and other proteins exists distally in cilia, and proteins are transported into and out of the structure by **kinesin** and **cytoplasmic dynein** motors moving along the peripheral doublets of microtubules.

(b) Ciliary movement involves a rapid series of changes in the shape of the axoneme. Along the length of each doublet, a series of paired "arms" with **axonemal dynein** is bound to microtubule A, with each pair extended toward microtubule B of the next doublet. When activated by ATP, the dynein arms briefly bind the neighboring microtubule and the doublets slide past each other slightly. The sliding motion is restricted by nexin cross-links between the doublets, causing the axoneme to bend. A rapid succession of this movement along the axoneme produces ciliary motion.

TABLE **4–3**	Common types of covering epithelia.		

Major Feature	Cell Form	Examples of Distribution	Main Function
Simple (one layer of cells)	Squamous	Lining of vessels (endothelium); Serous lining of cavities: pericardium, pleura, peritoneum (mesothelium)	Facilitates the movement of the viscera (mesothelium), active transport by pinocytosis (mesothelium and endothelium), secretion of biologically active molecules (mesothelium)
	Cuboidal	Covering the ovary, thyroid	Covering, secretion
	Columnar	Lining of intestine, gallbladder	Protection, lubrication, absorption, secretion
Pseudostratified (layers of cells with nuclei at different levels; not all cells reach surface but all adhere to basal lamina)		Lining of trachea, bronchi, nasal cavity	Protection, secretion; cilia-mediated transport of particles trapped in mucus out of the air passages
Stratified (two or more layers of cells)	Squamous keratinized (dry)	Epidermis	Protection; prevents water loss
	Squamous nonkeratinized (moist)	Mouth, esophagus, larynx, vagina, anal canal	Protection, secretion; prevents water loss
	Cuboidal	Sweat glands, developing ovarian follicles	Protection, secretion
	Transitional	Bladder, ureters, renal calyces	Protection, distensibility
	Columnar	Conjunctiva	Protection

FIGURE **4–12** Simple squamous epithelium.

This is a single layer of thin cells, in which the **cell nuclei** (arrows) are the thickest and most visible structures. Simple epithelia are typically specialized as lining of vessels and cavities, where they regulate passage of substances into the underlying tissue. The thin cells often exhibit transcytosis. Examples shown here are those lining the thin renal loops of Henle **(a)**, covering the outer wall of the intestine **(b)**, and lining the inner surface of the cornea **(c)**. a, c X400; b X600. H&E.

FIGURE **4–13** Simple cuboidal epithelium.

Epithelium
Basement membrane
Lamina propria
Capillaries

a

b

c

Cells here are roughly as tall as they are wide. Their greater thickness allows cytoplasm to be rich in mitochondria and other organelles for a high level of active transport across the epithelium and other functions. Examples shown here are from a renal collecting tubule **(a)**, a large thyroid follicle **(b)**, and the thick mesothelium covering an ovary **(c)**. All X400. H&E.

FIGURE **4–14** Simple columnar epithelium.

Cilia
Terminal bars
Epithelium
Basement membrane
Lamina propria
Capillary

a

b

c

Cells here are always taller than they are wide, with apical cilia or microvilli, and are often specialized for absorption. Complexes of tight and adherent junctions, sometimes called "terminal bars" in light microscopic images, are present at the apical ends of cells. The examples shown here are from a renal collecting duct **(a)**, the oviduct lining, with both secretory and ciliated cells **(b)**, and the lining of the gall bladder **(c)**. All X400. H&E.

FIGURE **4–15** Stratified epithelium.

Stratified squamous epithelia usually have protective functions: protection against easy invasion of underlying tissue by microorganisms and protection against water loss. These functions are particularly important in the epidermis **(a)** in which differentiating cells become **keratinized**, ie, filled with keratin and other substances, eventually lose their nuclei and organelles, and form superficial layers flattened squames that impede water loss. Keratinized cells are sloughed off and replaced by new cells from more basal layers, which are discussed fully with the skin in Chapter 18.

Nonkeratinized epithelia occur in many organs, such as the esophageal lining **(b)** or outer covering of the cornea **(c)**. Here cells accumulate much less keratin and retain their nuclei but still provide protection against microorganisms.

Stratified cuboidal or columnar epithelia are fairly rare but occur in excretory ducts of certain glands, such as sweat glands **(d)** where the double layer of cells allows additional functions. All X400; (b) PT, (a, c, and d) H&E.

large, dome-like cells sometimes called umbrella cells (Figure 4–16). These cells are specialized to protect underlying tissues from the hypertonic and potentially cytotoxic effects of urine. Importantly, unique morphological features of the cells allow *distension* of transitional epithelium as the urinary bladder fills. Transitional epithelium is discussed further with the urinary system.

In addition to the simple and stratified epithelial classifications, there is another type called **pseudostratified columnar epithelium** (Figure 4–17). Here tall, irregular cells all are attached to the basement membrane but their nuclei are at different levels and not all cells extend to the free surface, giving a stratified appearance. A good example of pseudostratified columnar epithelium is that lining the upper respiratory tract, where the cells are also heavily ciliated.

>> MEDICAL APPLICATION

In **chronic bronchitis**, common among habitual smokers, the number of goblet cells in the lining of airways in the lungs often increases greatly. This leads to excessive mucus production in areas where there are too few ciliated cells for its rapid removal and contributes to obstruction of the airways. The ciliated pseudostratified epithelium lining the bronchi of smokers can also be transformed into stratified squamous epithelium by metaplasia.

Secretory Epithelia & Glands

Epithelial cells that function mainly to produce and secrete various macromolecules may occur in epithelia with other

FIGURE **4–16** Transitional epithelium or urothelium.

Surface epithelium (umbrella cells)

Basal epithelium

Basement membrane

Lamina propria

Urothelium is stratified and lines much of the urinary tract. The superficial cells are rounded or dome-shaped, and have specialized membrane features enabling them to withstand the hypertonic effects of urine and protect underlying cells from this toxic solution. Cells of this epithelium are also able to adjust their relationships with one another and undergo a transition in their appearance as the urinary bladder fills and the wall is distended. These unique features of transitional epithelium are discussed more extensively in Chapter 19. X400. H&E.

FIGURE **4–17** Pseudostratified epithelium.

Mucus   Cilia

Terminal bars

Epithelial cell
Goblet cells

Basal cell

Basement membrane

Lamina propria

Cells of pseudostratified epithelia appear to be in several layers, but their basal ends all rest on the basement membrane. The pseudostratified columnar epithelium of the upper respiratory tract shown here contains many ciliated cells, as well as other cells with their nuclei at different levels. X400. H&E.

major functions or comprise specialized organs called **glands**. Products to be secreted are generally stored in the cells within small membrane-bound vesicles called **secretory granules**.

Secretory epithelial cells may synthesize, store, and release proteins (eg, in the pancreas), lipids (eg, adrenal, sebaceous glands), or complexes of carbohydrates and proteins (eg, salivary glands). Epithelia of mammary glands secrete all three substances. The cells of some glands (eg, sweat glands) have little synthetic activity and secrete mostly water and electrolytes (ions) transferred from the blood.

Scattered secretory cells, sometimes called **unicellular glands**, are common in simple cuboidal, simple columnar, and pseudostratified epithelia of many organs. An important, easily seen example is the **goblet cell** abundant in the lin-

ing of the small intestine (Figure 4–18) and respiratory tract, which secretes lubricating mucus that aids the function of these organs.

Glands develop from covering epithelia during fetal life by means of cell proliferation and growth into the underlying connective tissue, followed by further differentiation (Figure 4–19). **Exocrine glands** retain their connection with the surface epithelium, the connection forming the tubular ducts lined with epithelium by which secreted material leaves the gland. **Endocrine glands** lose the connection to their original epithelium and therefore lack ducts. Thin-walled blood vessels (capillaries) adjacent to the endocrine cells absorb their secreted hormone products for transport in blood to target cells throughout the body.

As shown in Figure 4–20, epithelia of exocrine glands are organized as a continuous system composed of many small **secretory portions** and **ducts** that transport the secretion out of the gland. In both exocrine and endocrine glands the secretory units are supported by a stroma of connective

FIGURE **4–18** Goblet cells: unicellular glands.

The simple columnar epithelium lining the large intestine shows many isolated goblet cells secreting mucus into the lumen. **(a)** With a stain for the oligosaccharide components of mucin glycoproteins, the cytoplasmic secretory granules of two goblet cells and secreted mucus are stained purple. X600. PAS-PT. **(b)** As shown ultrastructurally, goblet cells always have basal nuclei surrounded by RER (**R**), a large Golgi complex (**G**), and abundant apical cytoplasm filled with large secretory granules (**SG**). After exocytosis mucin components are hydrated and become mucus. A brush border of microvilli (**M**) is seen on neighboring columnar cells. X17,000.

tissue. A layer of connective tissue also encloses the gland as its *capsule*, surrounds the larger ducts, and forms partitions or *septa* that separate the gland into lobules, each containing secretory units connected to a small part of the duct system (Figure 4–20).

The structure of the secretory portions and ducts allows exocrine glands to be classified as shown schematically in Table 4–4. Although the three-dimensional morphology is often not prominent in histologic sections, the key points are summarized as follows:

- Glands can be **simple** (ducts not branched) or **compound** (ducts with two or more branches).
- Secretory portions can be **tubular** (either short or long and **coiled**) or **acinar** (rounded and saclike); either type of secretory unit may be **branched**, even if the duct is not branched.
- **Compound** glands can have branching ducts and can have multiple tubular, acinar, or tubuloacinar secretory portions.

Epithelial cells in multicellular glands have three basic mechanisms for releasing their product (Figure 4–21), and cells involved in each type of secretion are easily recognized histologically:

1. **Merocrine secretion:** This is the most common method of protein secretion and involves typical exocytosis of proteins or glycoproteins from membrane-bound vesicles.

2. **Holocrine secretion:** In this process cells accumulate product as they mature and undergo terminal cell differentiation, culminating in complete cell disruption with release of the product and cell debris into the gland's lumen. This is best seen in the sebaceous glands of skin (Figure 4–22).

3. **Apocrine secretion:** Here product accumulates at the cells' apical ends, portions of which are then extruded to release the product together with a bit of cytoplasm and plasma membrane. This is the mechanism by which droplets of lipid are secreted in the mammary gland (Figure 4–23).

▶▶ MEDICAL APPLICATION

The holocrine sebaceous glands are the primary structure involved in the common form of **acne**, acne vulgaris. Excessive holocrine secretion of sebum and keratin triggered by the surge of the steroid hormone testosterone that occurs in both genders at puberty frequently leads to blocked ducts within the gland. Activity of the normal commensal skin bacterium *Propionibacterium acnes* within the blocked duct commonly produces localized inflammation.

Exocrine glands with merocrine secretion can be further categorized as either **serous** or **mucous** according to the nature of their secretory products, which give distinct staining properties to the cells. Serous cells synthesize proteins that are mostly nonglycosylated, such as digestive enzymes. The cells have well-developed RER and Golgi complexes and are filled apically with secretory granules in different stages of maturation

FIGURE 4–19 Formation of glands from covering epithelia.

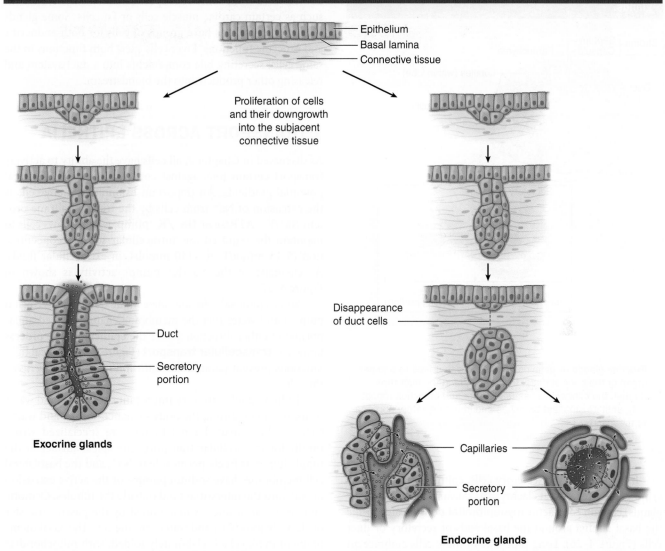

Epithelium
Basal lamina
Connective tissue

Proliferation of cells and their downgrowth into the subjacent connective tissue

Duct

Secretory portion

Exocrine glands

Disappearance of duct cells

Capillaries

Secretory portion

Endocrine glands

During fetal development epithelial cells proliferate and penetrate the underlying connective tissue. These cells may—or may not—maintain a connection with the surface epithelium. The connection is maintained to form a duct in exocrine glands; it is lost as endocrine glands develop. Exocrine glands secrete substances to specific organs via duct systems. Endocrine glands produce hormones and are always rich in capillaries. Hormones are released outside the cells and picked up by these blood vessels for distribution throughout the body, where specific target cells are identified by receptors for the hormones. Endocrine glands can have secretory cells arranged as irregular cords (left) or as rounded follicles (right) with lumens for temporary storage of the secretory product.

(Figure 4–24). Serous cells therefore stain intensely with basophilic or acidophilic stains. Acini of the pancreas and parotid salivary glands are composed of serous cells.

Mucous cells, such as goblet cells, also have RER and Golgi complexes and are filled apically with secretory granules, but these contain heavily glycosylated proteins called **mucins**. When mucins are released from the cell, they become hydrated and form mucus. Most of the hydrophilic mucins are washed from cells during routine histological preparations, causing the mucinogen granules to stain poorly with eosin (Figure 4–25). Sufficient oligosaccharides usually remain, however, to allow mucous cells to be stained by the periodic acid-Schiff (PAS) method (see Figure 4–18a).

Some salivary glands are mixed **seromucous glands**, with both serous acini and mucous tubules capped by groups of serous cells (see Figure 16–6). The product of such glands is a mixture of digestive enzymes and watery mucus.

FIGURE **4–20** General structure of exocrine glands.

Stroma ⎡ Septum
      ⎣ Capsule
Parenchyma
Lobules (within lobe)
Duct
Secretory acini
Lobe

Secretory vesicles

Acinus   Duct
(secretory portion)   (conducting portion)

Exocrine glands by definition have ducts that lead to another organ or the body surface. Inside the gland the duct runs through the connective tissue of septa and branches repeatedly, until its smallest branches end in the secretory portions of the gland.

In addition to the secretory cells, epithelia of many exocrine glands (eg, sweat, lachrymal, salivary, and mammary glands) contain contractile **myoepithelial cells** located *inside* the basal lamina around the basal ends of secretory or duct cells (Figure 4–26). Long processes of these cells embrace an acinus as an octopus might embrace a rounded boulder. Along ducts, they are more longitudinally arranged. Connected to each other and to the other epithelial cells by both gap junctions and desmosomes, myoepithelial cells are rich in actin filaments and myosins. Their contractions serve to help propel secretory products into and up the duct system.

Hormone-producing cells of endocrine glands are usually specialized for either protein or steroid synthesis, with cytoplasmic staining characteristic of RER or SER, respectively. The proteins are released by exocytosis and the lipophilic steroids by diffusion through the cell membrane for uptake by binding proteins outside the cell. As mentioned earlier, **endocrine signaling** involves hormone transport in the blood to target cells throughout the body, often within other endocrine glands. The receptors may also be on cells very close to the hormone-secreting cell or on the secreting cell itself; in these cases the signaling is termed **paracrine** or **autocrine**, respectively.

Important but inconspicuous endocrine or paracrine cells also occur singly or in small groups in epithelia of the

digestive, respiratory, and other organ systems. Hormones are also secreted from some cells specialized for other functions, such as certain cardiac muscle cells or fat cells. Some glands such as the pancreas have groups of cells for both endocrine and exocrine functions. Liver cells exert both functions in the same cells, secreting bile components into a duct system and releasing other products into the bloodstream.

› TRANSPORT ACROSS EPITHELIA

As discussed in Chapter 2, all cells have the ability to actively transport certain ions against concentration and electrical potential gradients. An important example in many cells is the extrusion of Na^+ from cells by the transmembrane protein Na^+/K^+-ATPase or **Na^+/K^+ pump**, which allows cells to maintain the required low intracellular sodium concentration (5-15 mmol/L vs ~140 mmol/L in extracellular fluid). A schematic of the Na^+/K^+ pump's activity is shown in Figure 4–27.

Some epithelial cells specialize in the transfer ions (by ion pumps) and water (via the membrane channels called aquaporins) in either direction across the epithelium, the process known as **transcellular transport** (Figure 4–28). Apical tight junctions prevent paracellular diffusion or backflow *between* the cells.

Kidney tubules are very important sites of ion and water transport, maintaining the body's balance of salts and water. Cells of the proximal renal tubules are specialized structurally for transcellular transport. The apical surface at the tubule lumen is freely permeable to Na^+, and the basolateral cell membranes have sodium pumps for the active extrusion of Na^+ into the interstitial fluid outside the tubules. Osmotic and electrical balance is maintained by the passive transfer of chloride ions (Cl^-) and water into the cell. The basal membrane of these cells is elaborately folded, with mitochondria located between the folds to supply ATP for Na^+/K^+ pumps (Figure 4–29). Lateral membrane interdigitations between cells further increase the surface area for transport. Regulated transfer of ions and water by various epithelial cells along the renal tubules maintains the ionic balance within the body and allows excretion of excess water and salts in the urine.

As discussed in Chapter 2 with the cell membrane, all cells can also internalize extracellular molecules and fluid using endocytosis and formation of cytoplasmic, membrane-bound vesicles. This activity is clearly observed in the simple squamous epithelial cells lining blood and lymphatic capillaries (endothelia) or body cavities (mesothelia). These thin cells have few organelles other than the abundant pinocytotic vesicles, which cross the thin cells in both directions and release their contents on the opposite side by exocytosis. This process of **transcytosis** also occurs between the apical and basolateral membranes domains in cells of simple cuboidal and columnar epithelia and is important in many physiologic processes.

TABLE **4–4**	Structural classes of exocrine glands, features of each class, and examples.

SIMPLE Glands (Ducts Do Not Branch)

Class	Simple Tubular	Branched Tubular	Coiled Tubular	Acinar (or Alveolar)	Branched Acinar
Features	Elongated secretory portion; duct usually short or absent	Several long secretory parts joining to drain into 1 duct	Secretory portion is very long and coiled	Rounded, saclike secretory portion	Multiple saclike secretory parts entering the same duct
Examples	Mucous glands of colon; intestinal glands or crypts (of Lieberkühn)	Glands in the uterus and stomach	Sweat glands	Small mucous glands along the urethra	Sebaceous glands of the skin

COMPOUND Glands (Ducts from Several Secretory Units Converge into Larger Ducts)

Class	Tubular	Acinar (Alveolar)	Tubuloacinar
Features	Several *elongated*, coiled secretory units and their ducts converge to form larger ducts	Several *saclike* secretory units with small ducts converge at a larger duct	Ducts of both tubular and acinar secretory units converge at larger ducts
Examples	Submucosal mucous glands (of Brunner) in the duodenum	Exocrine pancreas	Salivary glands

❯ RENEWAL OF EPITHELIAL CELLS

Epithelial tissues are relatively labile structures whose cells are renewed continuously by mitotic activity and stem cell populations. The rate of renewal varies widely; it can be fast in tissues such as the intestinal epithelium, which is replaced every week, or slow, as in the large glands. In stratified epithelial tissues, stem cells and mitosis occur only within the basal layer in contact with the basal lamina. In some functionally complex epithelia, stem cells are located only in restricted niches some distance from the transit amplifying cells and differentiating cells. For example, the epithelium lining the small intestine is derived completely from stem cells found in the simple glands between the intestinal villi. In the epidermis, stem cells are located at a characteristic position along the wall of hair follicles.

FIGURE **4–21** Mechanisms of exocrine gland secretion.

Secretory contents

Secretory vesicle

Nucleus

Secretory vesicles releasing their contents via exocytosis

(a) **Merocrine gland**

Disintegrating cells with contents becoming the secretion

Cells dividing

(b) **Holocrine gland**

Secretions

Nucleus of secretory cell

Pinching off of apical portion of secretory cell

(c) **Apocrine gland**

Three basic types of secretion are used by cells of exocrine glands, depending on what substance is being secreted.

(a) Merocrine secretion releases products, usually containing proteins, by means of exocytosis at the apical end of the secretory cells. Most exocrine glands are merocrine.

(b) Holocrine secretion is produced by the disintegration of the secretory cells themselves as they complete their terminal differentiation, which involves becoming filled with product. Sebaceous glands of hair follicles are the best examples of holocrine glands.

(c) Apocrine secretion involves loss of membrane-enclosed apical cytoplasm, usually containing one or more lipid droplets. Apocrine secretion, along with merocrine secretion, is seen in mammary glands.

>> **MEDICAL APPLICATION**

Both benign and malignant tumors can arise from most types of epithelial cells. Malignant tumors of epithelial origin are called **carcinomas** (Gr. *karkinos*, cancer + *oma*, tumor). Malignant tumors derived from glandular epithelial tissue are called **adenocarcinomas** (Gr. *adenos*, gland + *karkinos*). Adenocarcinomas are by far the most common tumors in adults after age 45.

>> **MEDICAL APPLICATION**

Some epithelial cells are prone to abnormal growth or dysplasia, which can progress to precancerous growth called **neoplasia**. Early neoplastic growth is often reversible and does not always result in cancer.

Under certain abnormal conditions, one type of epithelial tissue may undergo transformation into another type in another reversible process called **metaplasia**. In heavy cigarette smokers, the ciliated pseudostratified epithelium lining the bronchi can be transformed into stratified squamous epithelium.

>> **MEDICAL APPLICATION**

In individuals with chronic vitamin A deficiency, epithelial tissues of the type found in the bronchi and urinary bladder are gradually replaced by stratified squamous epithelium.

Epithelia are normally capable of rapid repair and replacement of apoptotic or damaged cells. In some large glands, most notably the liver, mitotic activity is normally rare but is actively renewed following major damage to the organ. When a portion of liver tissue is removed surgically or lost by the acute effects of toxic substances, cells of undamaged regions quickly begin active proliferation and a mass of liver tissue with normal function is regenerated.

FIGURE **4–22** Holocrine secretion in a sebaceous gland.

In holocrine secretion, best seen in the sebaceous gland adjacent to hair follicles, entire cells fill with a lipid-rich product as they differentiate. Mature (terminally differentiated) cells separate and completely disintegrate, releasing the lipid that serves to protect and lubricate adjacent skin and hair. Sebaceous glands lack myoepithelial cells; cell proliferation inside a dense, inelastic connective tissue capsule continuously forces product into the duct. X200. H&E.

FIGURE **4–23** Apocrine secretion in the mammary gland.

The secretory portions of a mammary gland demonstrate apocrine secretion, characterized by extrusion of the secretion product along with a bit of apical cytoplasm (**arrows**). The released portion of cell contains lipid droplet(s). Merocrine secretion also occurs from the same and other cells of the gland. X400. PSH.

Epithelial Tissue SUMMARY OF KEY POINTS

- An **epithelium** is a tissue in which cells are bound tightly together structurally and functionally to form a sheetlike or tubular structure with little extracellular material between the cells.
- Cells in epithelia each have an **apical side** facing the sheet's free surface and a **basal side** facing a basement membrane and underlying connective tissue.
- Epithelia are often specialized for absorption or **transcytosis**, pinocytosis of material at the apical side and exocytosis at the basolateral side (or vice versa).
- Cells of most epithelia exhibit **continuous renewal**, with the locations of stem cells and rates of cell turnover variable in various specialized epithelia.

Basement Membrane

- The **basement membrane** of all epithelia is a thin extracellular layer of specialized proteins, usually having two parts: a basal lamina and a more fibrous reticular lamina.
- The **basal lamina** is a thin meshwork of type IV collagen and laminin produced by the epithelial cells.
- The **reticular lamina** contains type III collagen and anchoring fibrils of VII collagen, all secreted by cells of the immediately adjacent connective tissue.
- Together, these components **attach** epithelia to connective tissue, regulate (**filter**) substances passing from connective tissue into epithelia, provide a guide or **scaffold** during tissue regeneration after injury, and **compartmentalize** epithelial cells from other tissues.

FIGURE **4–24** Serous cells.

The small serous acini of the exocrine pancreas each have 5-10 cells facing a very small central lumen. Each acinar cell is roughly pyramidal, with its apex at the lumen. **(a)** As seen by light microscopy, the apical ends are very eosinophilic due to the abundant secretory granules present there. The cells' basal ends contain the nuclei and an abundance of RER, making this area basophilic. A small duct (**D**) is seen, but lumens of acini are too small to be readily visible. The enclosed area is comparable to that shown in part **b**. X300. H&E. **(b)** A portion of one acinar cell is shown ultrastructurally, indicating the abundant RER (**R**), a Golgi complex (**G**), apical secretory granules (**SG**) and the small acinar lumen (**L**). X13,000.

Intercellular Junctions

- Intercellular junctions are well developed in epithelia and consist of three major types, with different functions.
- **Tight or occluding junctions** are formed by interacting transmembrane proteins such as **claudin** and **occludin**; linear arrangements of these linked proteins surround the apical ends of the cells and **prevent paracellular passage** of substances (between the cells.)
- **Adherent or anchoring junctions**, formed by interacting proteins of the **cadherin** family, are points of strong **attachment** holding together cells of the epithelium.
- Adherent junctions may form **zonula adherens** that encircle epithelial cells just below their tight junctions or scattered, spot-like attachment sites called **desmosomes** or **maculae adherens**, both of which are attached to cytoplasmic **keratins**.
- **Hemidesmosomes** composed of transmembrane **integrins** attach cells to proteins of the basal lamina.
- **Gap or communicating junctions** are points of cell contact where both plasma membranes have numerous hexameric complexes of transmembrane **connexons**, each forming a channel allowing passage of small molecules from one cell to the other.

Apical Structures of Epithelial Cells

- **Microvilli** are small membrane projections with cores of **actin filaments** that generally function to increase epithelial cells' apical surface area for **absorption**.

- **Stereocilia** are long microvilli with specialized mechanosensory function in cells of the inner ear and for absorption in tissues of the male reproductive tract.
- **Cilia** are larger projecting structures with a well-organized core of **microtubules** (in a 9 + 2 arrangement called the **axoneme**) in which restricted, dynein-based sliding of microtubules causes ciliary movement that propel material along an epithelial surface.

Morphological Types of Epithelia

- An epithelium in which the basement membrane has one cell layer is **simple**; the cells of different simple epithelia range widely in height, from very thin or **squamous**, to roughly **cuboidal**, to very tall or **columnar**.
- Epithelia with two or more layers of cells are **stratified** and almost all such epithelia are stratified squamous, in which the outer cell layers are thin and flattened.
- Cells of stratified squamous epithelia move gradually from the basal to the surface layers, changing shape and becoming filled with **keratin** intermediate filaments.
- Stratified squamous epithelia such as the epidermis cover the body surface, **protecting** underlying tissues from excess water loss (dehydration) and microbial invasion.
- **Pseudostratified epithelia** are thick and appear to have several cell layers; all cells attach to the basal lamina but not all extend to the free epithelial surface.

FIGURE **4–25** Mucous cells.

Mucous cells of salivary glands are typically larger than serous cells, with flattened basal nuclei. Most of the cytoplasm is filled with secretory granules containing mucinogen like that of goblet cells. The RER and Golgi complexes of mucous cells produce heavily glycosylated glycoproteins with water-binding properties. The lumens (arrows) of mucous tubules are larger than those of serous acini. Much connective tissue surrounds the mucous tubules and ducts (**D**). X200. PT.

FIGURE **4–26** Myoepithelial cells.

(a) The TEM shows two salivary gland cells containing secretory granules, with an associated myoepithelial cell (**M**). X20,000. **(b)** A myoepithelial cell immunostained brown with antibodies against actin shows its association with cells of an acinus stained by H&E. Contraction of the myoepithelial cell compresses the acinus and aids in the expulsion of secretory products into the duct. X200.

- **Transitional epithelium or urothelium,** found only in the lining of the urinary system, is stratified, with large rounded surface cells protective against urine.

Epithelial Secretion/Glands

- The major function in many epithelial cells is synthesis and secretion of specialized products; organs composed primarily of such epithelia are called **glands.**
- **Exocrine glands** have epithelial ducts carrying secretions to specific sites; the ducts of **simple glands** are unbranched and those of **compound glands** are branched.
- The secretory portions of exocrine glands may form round, saclike **acini** (also called **alveoli**) or elongated **tubules**; both types of secretory units may themselves branch.

- **Endocrine glands** lack ducts; secreted substances are hormones carried throughout the body by the interstitial fluid and blood, with specificity produced by the hormone receptors of target cells.
- Glands have three basic secretory mechanisms: **merocrine,** which uses exocytosis; **holocrine,** in which terminally differentiated cells filled with lipid product are released; and **apocrine,** in which apical, product-filled areas of cells are extruded.
- Exocrine glands producing mucus, or similar individual cells called **goblet cells,** are called **mucous glands;** oligosaccharide components of mucus stain poorly with routine dyes but stain well with PAS stain.
- Exocrine glands producing largely enzymes (proteins) are called **serous glands** and stain darkly with H&E due to the cells' content of RER and secretory granules.

FIGURE **4–27** Na⁺/K⁺ pump.

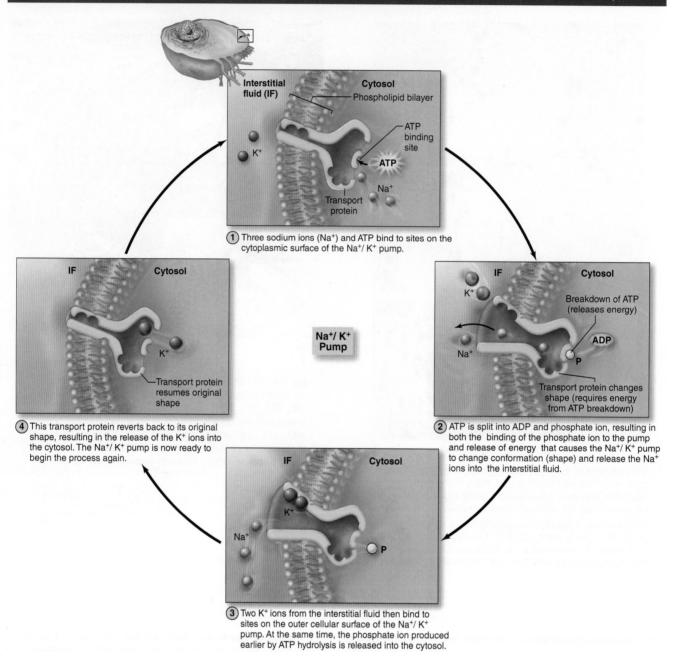

① Three sodium ions (Na⁺) and ATP bind to sites on the cytoplasmic surface of the Na⁺/ K⁺ pump.

② ATP is split into ADP and phosphate ion, resulting in both the binding of the phosphate ion to the pump and release of energy that causes the Na⁺/ K⁺ pump to change conformation (shape) and release the Na⁺ ions into the interstitial fluid.

③ Two K⁺ ions from the interstitial fluid then bind to sites on the outer cellular surface of the Na⁺/ K⁺ pump. At the same time, the phosphate ion produced earlier by ATP hydrolysis is released into the cytosol.

④ This transport protein reverts back to its original shape, resulting in the release of the K⁺ ions into the cytosol. The Na⁺/ K⁺ pump is now ready to begin the process again.

A Na⁺/K⁺-ATPase located in the plasma membrane of many cells uses ATP to transport or pump the cations Na⁺ and K⁺ through the membrane in opposite directions, against their concentrations gradients.

FIGURE **4–28** Ion and water absorption and secretion.

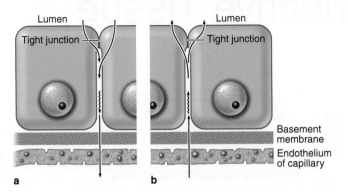

Ion and water transport across epithelia can occur in either direction, depending on which tissue is involved. **(a)** The direction of transport is from the lumen to the blood vessel, as in the gallbladder and intestine. This process is called **absorption**, and serves to concentrate bile and obtain water and ions in these organs.

(b) Transport of water in the other direction from the capillaries into a lumen, as in the choroid plexus and sweat glands, is often part of **secretion** and serves to expel water from the interstitial fluid into specialized aqueous fluids in these tissues. No matter whether an epithelium is absorbing or secreting water, apical occluding junctions are necessary to maintain tight compartmentalization.

FIGURE **4–29** Absorptive cells.

A diagram and TEM of epithelial cells highly specialized for absorption: cells of proximal convoluted tubule of the kidney. Typically, long invaginations of the basal cell membrane outline regions with mitochondria (**M**). Interdigitations from neighboring cells are also present laterally. Immediately below the microvilli (**MV**) are many pinocytotic vesicles, which may fuse with lysosomes as shown or mediate transcytosis by secreting their contents at the basolateral membrane. Junctional complexes between individual cells separate the apical and basolateral compartments. Sodium ions diffuse passively through the apical membranes of renal epithelial cells and are actively transported out of the cells by Na^+/K^+-ATPase located in the basolateral membrane. Immediately below the basal lamina is a capillary (**C**) that removes water absorbed across the epithelium. X9600.

CHAPTER

5 Connective Tissue

CELLS OF CONNECTIVE TISSUE

CHAPTER

5 Connective Tissue

The different types of connective tissue maintain the form of organs throughout the body. Connective tissues provide a matrix that supports and physically connects other tissues and cells together in organs. The interstitial fluid of connective tissue gives metabolic support to cells as the medium for diffusion of nutrients and waste products.

Unlike the other tissue types (epithelium, muscle, and nerve), which consist mainly of cells, the major constituent of connective tissue is the **extracellular matrix (ECM)**. Extracellular matrices consist of different combinations of **protein fibers** (such as collagens and elastic fibers) and **ground substance**. Ground substance is a complex of anionic, hydrophilic proteoglycans, glycosaminoglycans (GAGs), and multiadhesive glycoproteins (laminin, fibronectin, and others). As described briefly in Chapter 4 with the basal lamina, such glycoproteins help stabilize the ECM by binding to other matrix components and to **integrins** in cell membranes. The hydrated nature of connective tissue ground substance provides the medium for the exchange of nutrients and metabolic wastes between cells and the blood supply.

The variety of connective tissue types in the body reflects differences in composition and amount of the cells, fibers, and ground substance which together are responsible for the remarkable structural, functional, and pathologic diversity of connective tissue.

Connective tissues originate from embryonic **mesenchyme**, a tissue developing mainly from the middle layer of the embryo, the mesoderm (Figure 5–1). Mesenchyme consists largely of viscous ground substance with few collagen fibers. **Mesenchymal cells** are undifferentiated and have large nuclei, with prominent nucleoli and fine chromatin. They are often said to be "spindle-shaped," with their scant cytoplasm extended as two or more thin cytoplasmic processes. Mesodermal cells migrate from their site of origin in the embryo, surrounding and penetrating developing organs. In addition to producing all types of connective tissue proper and the specialized connective tissues bone and cartilage, the embryonic mesenchyme includes stem cells for other tissues such as blood, the vascular endothelium, and muscle. This chapter focuses on connective tissue proper.

>> MEDICAL APPLICATION

Some cells in mesenchyme are **multipotent stem cells** potentially useful in **regenerative medicine** after grafting to replace damaged tissue in certain patients. Mesenchyme-like cells remain present in some adult connective tissues, including that of tooth pulp and some adipose tissue, and are being investigated as possible sources of stem cells for therapeutic repair and organ regeneration.

> CELLS OF CONNECTIVE TISSUE

Fibroblasts and certain other cells are typically present in connective tissue proper (Figure 5–2 and Table 5–1). Fibroblasts originate locally from mesenchymal cells and are permanent residents of connective tissue; other cells found here, such as **macrophages**, **plasma cells**, and **mast cells**, originate from hematopoietic stem cells in bone marrow, circulate in the blood, and then move into connective tissue where they function. White blood cells (leukocytes) are transient cells of most connective tissues; they also originate in the bone

FIGURE 5–1 Embryonic mesenchyme.

Mesenchyme consists of a population of undifferentiated cells, generally elongated but with many shapes, having large euchromatic nuclei and prominent nucleoli that indicate high levels of synthetic activity. These cells are called **mesenchymal cells**. Mesenchymal cells are surrounded by an ECM that they produced and that consists largely of a simple ground substance rich in hyaluronan (hyaluronic acid), but with very little collagen. X200. Mallory trichrome.

marrow and move to the connective tissue where they function for a few days, then die by apoptosis.

Fibroblasts

Fibroblasts (Figure 5–3), the most common cells in connective tissue, produce and maintain most of the tissue's extracellular components. Fibroblasts synthesize and secrete collagen (the most abundant protein of the body) and elastin, which form large fibers, as well as the GAGs, proteoglycans, and multiadhesive glycoproteins that comprise the ground substance. As described later, most of the secreted ECM components undergo further modification outside the cell before assembling as a matrix.

Two levels of fibroblast activity can be observed histologically (Figure 5–3b). Cells with intense synthetic activity are morphologically distinct from the quiescent fibroblasts that are scattered within the matrix they have already synthesized. Some histologists reserve the term "fibroblast" to denote the active cell and "fibrocyte" to denote the quiescent cell. The active fibroblast has more abundant and irregularly branched cytoplasm. Its nucleus is large, ovoid, euchromatic, and has a prominent nucleolus. The cytoplasm has much rough endoplasmic reticulum (RER) and a well-developed Golgi apparatus. The quiescent cell is smaller than the active

fibroblast, is usually spindle-shaped with fewer processes and much less RER, and contains a darker, more heterochromatic nucleus.

Fibroblasts are targets of many families of proteins called **growth factors** that influence cell growth and differentiation. In adults, connective tissue fibroblasts rarely undergo division. However, stimulated by locally released growth factors, cell cycling and mitotic activity resume when the tissue requires additional fibroblasts, for example, to repair a damaged organ. Fibroblasts involved in wound healing, sometimes called **myofibroblasts**, have a well-developed contractile function and are enriched with a form of actin also found in smooth muscle cells.

›› MEDICAL APPLICATION

The regenerative capacity of connective tissue is clearly observed in organs damaged by ischemia, inflammation, or traumatic injury. Spaces left after such injuries, especially in tissues whose cells divide poorly or not at all (eg, cardiac muscle), are filled by connective tissue, forming dense irregular **scar tissue**. The healing of surgical incisions and other wounds depends on the reparative capacity of connective tissue, particularly on activity and growth of fibroblasts.

In some rapidly closing wounds, a cell called the myofibroblast, with features of both fibroblasts and smooth muscle cells, is also observed. These cells have most of the morphologic characteristics of fibroblasts but contain increased amounts of actin microfilaments and myosin and behave much like smooth muscle cells. Their activity is important for the phase of tissue repair called **wound contraction**.

Adipocytes

Adipocytes (L. *adeps*, fat + Gr. *kytos*, cell), or fat cells, are found in connective tissue of many organs. These large, mesenchymally derived cells are specialized for cytoplasmic storage of lipid as neutral fats, or less commonly for the production of heat. The large deposits of fat in the cells of adipose connective tissue also serve to cushion and insulate the skin and other organs. Adipocytes have major metabolic significance with medical importance and are described and discussed in Chapter 6.

Macrophages & the Mononuclear Phagocyte System

Macrophages are characterized by their well-developed phagocytic ability and specialize in turnover of protein fibers and removal of dead cells, tissue debris, or other particulate material. They have a wide spectrum of morphologic features corresponding to their state of functional activity and to the tissue they inhabit. A typical macrophage measures between 10 and 30 μm in diameter and has an eccentrically located, oval or kidney-shaped nucleus. Macrophages are present in the connective tissue of most organs and are often referred to by pathologists as "histiocytes."

FIGURE 5–2   Cellular and extracellular components of connective tissue.

Blood vessel

Ground substance

Extracellular matrix

Protein fibers

Elastic fiber

Collagen fiber

Reticular fiber

Resident cells

Mesenchymal cell

Macrophage

Adipocyte

Fibroblast

Connective tissue is composed of **fibroblasts** and other cells and an **extracellular matrix (ECM)** of various protein fibers, all of which are surrounded by watery **ground substance**. In all types of connective tissue the extracellular volume exceeds that of the cells.

TABLE 5–1	Functions of cells in connective tissue proper.
Cell Type	**Major Product or Activity**
Fibroblasts (fibrocytes)	Extracellular fibers and ground substance
Plasma cells	Antibodies
Lymphocytes (several types)	Various immune/defense functions
Eosinophilic leukocytes	Modulate allergic/vasoactive reactions and defense against parasites
Neutrophilic leukocytes	Phagocytosis of bacteria
Macrophages	Phagocytosis of ECM components and debris; antigen processing and presentation to immune cells; secretion of growth factors, cytokines, and other agents
Mast cells and basophilic leukocytes	Pharmacologically active molecules (eg, histamine)
Adipocytes	Storage of neutral fats

›› MEDICAL APPLICATION

Besides their function in turnover of ECM fibers, macrophages are key components of an organism's innate immune defense system, removing cell debris, neoplastic cells, bacteria, and other invaders. Macrophages are also important antigen-presenting cells required for the activation and specification of lymphocytes.

When macrophages are stimulated (by injection of foreign substances or by infection), they change their morphologic characteristics and properties, becoming **activated macrophages**. In addition to showing an increase in their capacity for phagocytosis and intracellular digestion, activated macrophages exhibit enhanced metabolic and lysosomal enzyme activity. Macrophages are also secretory cells producing an array of substances, including various enzymes for ECM breakdown and various growth factors or cytokines that help regulate immune cells and reparative functions.

When adequately stimulated, macrophages may increase in size and fuse to form **multinuclear giant cells**, usually found only in pathologic conditions.

FIGURE 5–3 Fibroblasts.

(a) Fibroblasts typically have large active nuclei and eosinophilic cytoplasm that tapers off in both directions along the axis of the nucleus, a morphology often referred to as "spindle-shaped." Nuclei (**arrows**) are clearly seen, but the eosinophilic cytoplasmic processes resemble the collagen bundles (**C**) that fill the ECM and are difficult to distinguish in H&E-stained sections.

(b) Both active and quiescent fibroblasts may sometimes be distinguished, as in this section of dermis. Active fibroblasts have large, euchromatic nuclei and basophilic cytoplasm, while inactive fibroblasts (or fibrocytes) are smaller with more heterochromatic nuclei (**arrows**). The round, very basophilic round cells are in leukocytes. Both X400. H&E.

In the TEM, macrophages are shown to have a characteristic irregular surface with pleats, protrusions, and indentations, a morphologic expression of their active pinocytotic and phagocytic activities (Figure 5–4). They generally have a well-developed Golgi apparatus and many lysosomes.

Macrophages derive from bone marrow precursor cells that divide, producing **monocytes** that circulate in the blood. These cells cross the epithelial wall of venules to penetrate connective tissue, where they differentiate further, mature, and acquire the morphologic features of phagocytic cells. Therefore, monocytes and macrophages are the same cell at different stages of maturation. Macrophages play an important role in the early stages of repair after tissue damage, and under such conditions of inflammation these cells accumulate in connective tissue by local proliferation of macrophages in addition to monocyte recruitment from the blood. Macrophages are distributed throughout the body and are present in most organs. Along with other monocyte-derived cells, they comprise a family of cells called the **mononuclear phagocyte system**

(Table 5–2). The macrophage-like cells have been given different names in different organs, for example Kupffer cells in the liver, microglial cells in the central nervous system, Langerhans cells in the skin, and osteoclasts in bone tissue. However, all are derived from monocytes. All are long-living cells and may survive for months in the tissues. In addition to debris removal, these cells are highly important for the uptake, processing, and presentation of antigens for lymphocyte activation, a function discussed later with the immune system. The transformation from monocytes to macrophages in connective tissue involves increases in cell size, increased protein synthesis, and increases in the number of Golgi complexes and lysosomes.

Mast Cells

Mast cells are oval or irregularly shaped connective tissue cells, between 7 and 20 μm in diameter, whose cytoplasm is filled with basophilic secretory granules. The nucleus is centrally situated

FIGURE **5–4** Macrophage ultrastructure.

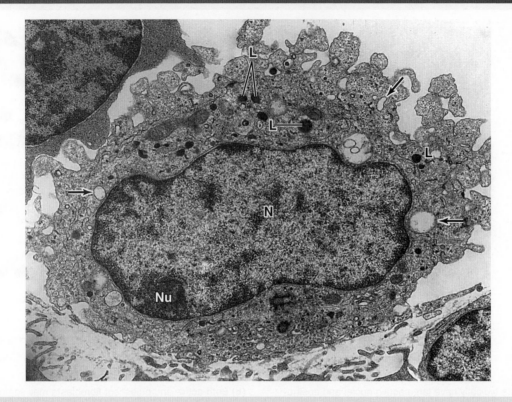

Characteristic features of macrophages seen in this TEM of one such cell are the prominent nucleus (**N**) and the nucleolus (**Nu**) and the numerous secondary lysosomes (**L**). The arrows indicate phagocytic vacuoles near the protrusions and indentations of the cell surface. X10,000.

and often obscured by abundant secretory granules (Figure 5–5). These granules are electron-dense and heterogeneous (ranging from 0.3 to 2.0 μm in diameter.) Because of their high content of acidic radicals in their sulfated GAGs, mast cell granules display **metachromasia**, which means that they can change the color of some basic dyes (eg, toluidine blue) from blue to purple or red. The granules are poorly preserved by common fixatives, so that mast cells are frequently difficult to identify.

TABLE **5–2** Distribution and main functions of the cells of the mononuclear phagocyte system.

Cell Type	Major Locations	Main Function
Monocyte	Blood	Precursor of macrophages
Macrophage	Connective tissue, lymphoid organs, lungs, bone marrow, pleural and peritoneal cavities	Production of cytokines, chemotactic factors, and several other molecules that participate in inflammation (defense), antigen processing, and presentation
Kupffer cell	Liver (perisinusoidal)	Same as macrophages
Microglial cell	Central nervous system	Same as macrophages
Langerhans cell	Epidermis of skin	Antigen processing and presentation
Dendritic cell	Lymph nodes, spleen	Antigen processing and presentation
Osteoclast (from fusion of several macrophages)	Bone	Localized digestion of bone matrix
Multinuclear giant cell (several fused macrophages)	In connective tissue under various pathological conditions	Segregation and digestion of foreign bodies

FIGURE **5–5** Mast cells.

Mast cells are components of loose connective tissues, often located near small blood vessels (**BV**). **(a)** They are typically oval shaped, with cytoplasm filled with strongly basophilic granules. X400. PT.

(b) Ultrastructurally mast cells show little else around the nucleus (**N**) besides these cytoplasmic granules (**G**), except

for occasional mitochondria (**M**). The granule staining in the TEM is heterogeneous and variable in mast cells from different tissues; at higher magnifications some granules may show a characteristic scroll-like substructure (inset) that contains pre-formed mediators such as histamine and proteoglycans. The ECM near this mast cell includes elastic fibers (**E**) and bundles of collagen fibers (**C**).

Mast cells function in the localized release of many bioactive substances with roles in the local inflammatory response, innate immunity, and tissue repair. A partial list of important molecules released from these cells' secretory granules includes the following:

- **Heparin**, a sulfated GAG that acts locally as an anticoagulant
- **Histamine**, which promotes increased vascular permeability and smooth muscle contraction
- **Serine proteases**, which activate various mediators of inflammation
- **Eosinophil** and **neutrophil chemotactic factors**, which attract those leukocytes
- **Cytokines**, polypeptides directing activities of leukocytes and other cells of the immune system
- **Phospholipid** precursors for conversion to prostaglandins, leukotrienes, and other important lipid mediators of the inflammatory response.

Occurring in connective tissue of many organs, mast cells are especially numerous near small blood vessels in skin and mesenteries (*perivascular* mast cells) and in the tissue that lines digestive and respiratory tracts (*mucosal* mast cells); the granule content of the two populations differs somewhat. These major locations suggest that mast cells place themselves strategically to function as sentinels detecting invasion by microorganisms.

Mast cells originate from progenitor cells in the bone marrow. The progenitor cells circulate in the blood, cross the wall of venules and capillaries, and penetrate connective tissues, where they differentiate. Although they are in many respects similar to basophilic leukocytes, they appear to have a different lineage at least in humans.

Release of certain chemical mediators stored in mast cells also promotes the allergic reactions, also known as **immediate hypersensitivity reactions** because they occur within a few minutes after the appearance of an antigen in an individual previously sensitized to the same or a very similar antigen. There are many examples of immediate hypersensitivity reaction; a dramatic one is anaphylactic shock, a potentially fatal condition. The process of anaphylaxis consists of the following sequential events. The first exposure to an antigen (allergen), such as bee venom, results in production of the immunoglobulin E (IgE) class of immunoglobulins (antibodies) by plasma cells. IgE is avidly bound to the surface of mast cells. A second exposure to the antigen results in binding of the antigen to IgE on the mast cells. This event triggers release of the mast cell granules, liberating histamine, leukotrienes, chemokines, and heparin (Figure 5–6). Degranulation of mast cells also occurs as a result of the action of the complement molecules that participate in the immunologic reactions described in Chapter 14.

FIGURE **5–6** Mast cell secretion.

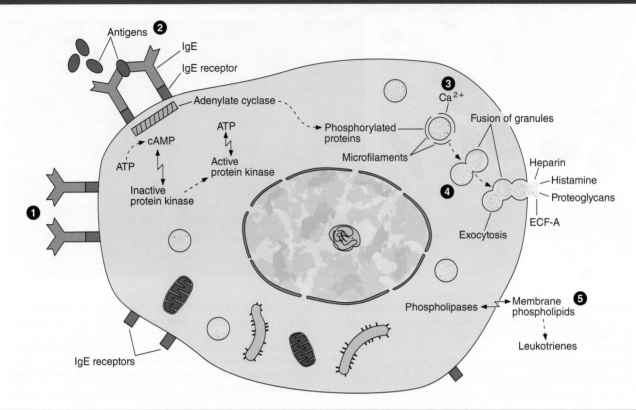

Mast cell secretion is triggered by reexposure to certain antigens and allergens. Molecules of IgE antibody produced in an initial response to an allergen such as pollen or bee venom are bound to surface receptors for IgE (**1**), of which 300,000 are present per mast cell.

When a second exposure to the allergen occurs, IgE molecules bind this antigen and a few IgE receptors very rapidly become cross-linked (**2**). This activates adenylate cyclase, leading to phosphorylation of specific proteins (**3**), entry of

Ca^{2+} and rapid exocytosis of some granules (**4**). In addition, phospholipases act on specific membrane phospholipids, leading to production and release of leukotrienes (**5**).

The components released from granules, as well as the leukotrienes, are immediately active in the local microenvironment and promote a variety of controlled local reactions that together normally comprise part of the inflammatory process called the **immediate hypersensitivity reaction**. "ECF-A" is the eosinophil chemotactic factor of anaphylaxis.

Plasma Cells

Plasma cells are B-lymphocyte–derived, antibody-producing cells. These large, ovoid cells have basophilic cytoplasm due to their richness in RER (Figure 5–7). Next to the nucleus, the Golgi apparatus and centrioles occupy a region that may appear pale in routine histologic preparations (Figure 5–7b).

The nucleus of the plasma cell is generally spherical but eccentrically placed. Many of these nuclei contain compact, peripheral regions of heterochromatin alternating with lighter areas of euchromatin, a configuration that can give the nucleus of a plasma cell the appearance of a clock face. There are at least a few plasma cells in most connective tissues. Their average lifespan is only 10-20 days.

►► MEDICAL APPLICATION

Plasma cells are derived from B lymphocytes and are responsible for the synthesis of immunoglobulin antibodies. Each antibody is specific for the one antigen that stimulated the clone of B cells and reacts only with that antigen or molecules resembling it (see Chapter 14). The results of the antibody-antigen reaction are variable, but they usually neutralize harmful effects caused by antigens. An antigen that is a toxin (eg, tetanus, diphtheria) may lose its capacity to do harm when it binds to its specific antibody. Bound antigen-antibody complexes are quickly removed from tissues by phagocytosis.

FIGURE **5–7** Plasma cells.

Antibody-secreting plasma cells are present in variable numbers in the connective tissue of many organs.

(a) Plasma cells are large, ovoid cells, with basophilic cytoplasm. The round nuclei frequently show peripheral clumps of heterochromatin, giving the structure a "clock-face" appearance. X640. H&E.

(b) Plasma are often more abundant in infected tissues, as in the inflamed lamina propria shown here. A large pale

Golgi apparatus (arrows) at a juxtanuclear site in each cell is actively involved in the terminal glycosylation of the antibodies (glycoproteins). Plasma cells leave their sites of origin in lymphoid tissues, move to connective tissue, and produce antibodies that mediate immunity. X400 PT.

Leukocytes

Besides macrophages and plasma cells, connective tissue normally contains other leukocytes derived from cells circulating in the blood. Leukocytes, or white blood cells, make up a population of wandering cells in connective tissue. They leave blood by migrating between the endothelial cells lining venules to enter connective tissue by a process called **diapedesis**. This process increases greatly during inflammation, which is a vascular and cellular defensive response to injury or foreign substances, including pathogenic bacteria or irritating chemical substances.

Classically, the major signs of inflamed tissues include "redness and swelling with heat and pain" (*rubor et tumor cum calore et dolore*). Inflammation begins with the local release of chemical mediators from various cells, the ECM, and blood plasma proteins. These substances act on the local microvasculature, mast cells, macrophages, and other cells to induce events characteristic of inflammation, for example increased blood flow and vascular permeability, diapedesis and migration of leukocytes, and activation of macrophages for phagocytosis.

Most leukocytes function for a few hours or days in connective tissue and then die. However, as discussed with the immune system, some lymphocytes and phagocytic antigen-presenting cells normally leave the interstitial fluid of connective tissue, enter blood or lymph, and move to selected lymphoid organs.

⟩⟩ MEDICAL APPLICATION

Increased vascular permeability is caused by the action of vasoactive substances such as histamine released from mast cells during **inflammation**. Increased blood flow and vascular permeability produce local swelling (edema), redness, and heat. **Pain** is due mainly to the action of the chemical mediators on nerve endings. All these activities help protect and repair the inflamed tissue. **Chemotaxis** (Gr. *chemeia*, alchemy + *taxis*, orderly arrangement), the phenomenon by which specific cell types are attracted by specific molecules, draws much larger numbers of leukocytes into inflamed tissues.

⟩ FIBERS

The fibrous components of connective tissue are elongated structures formed from proteins that polymerize after secretion from fibroblasts (Figure 5–2). The three main types of fibers include **collagen**, **reticular**, and **elastic fibers**. Collagen and reticular fibers are both formed by proteins of the collagen family, and elastic fibers are composed mainly of the protein **elastin**. These fibers are distributed unequally among the different types of connective tissue, with the predominant fiber type usually responsible for conferring specific tissue properties.

Collagen

The **collagens** constitute a family of proteins selected during evolution for their ability to form a variety of extracellular structures. The various fibers, sheets, and networks made of collagens are all extremely strong and resistant to normal shearing and tearing forces. Collagen is a key element of all connective tissues, as well as epithelial basement membranes and the external laminae of muscle and nerve cells.

Collagen is the most abundant protein in the human body, representing 30% of its dry weight. A major product of fibroblasts, collagens are secreted by several other cell types and are distinguishable by their molecular compositions, morphologic characteristics, distribution, functions, and pathologies. A family of 28 collagens exists in vertebrates, the most important of which are listed in Table 5–3. They can be grouped into the following categories according to the structures formed by their interacting subunits:

- **Fibrillar collagens**, notably **collagen types I**, **II**, and **III**, have subunits that aggregate to form large fibrils clearly visible in the electron or light microscope (Figure 5–8). Collagen type I, the most abundant and widely distributed collagen, forms large, eosinophilic bundles usually called **collagen fibers**. These often densely fill the connective tissue, forming structures such as tendons, organ capsules, and dermis.
- **Sheet-forming collagens** such as **type IV collagen** have subunits produced by epithelial cells and are the major structural proteins of external laminae and the basal lamina in all epithelia.
- **Linking/anchoring collagens** are short collagens that link fibrillar collagens to one another (forming larger fibers) and to other components of the ECM. **Type VII collagen** binds type IV collagen and anchors the basal lamina to the underlying reticular lamina in basement membranes (see Figure 4–3).

TABLE **5–3**	Collagen types.				
Type	**Molecule Composition**	**Structure**	**Optical Microscopy**	**Major Locations**	**Main Function**
Fibril-Forming Collagens					
I	$[\alpha1\,(I)]_2[\alpha2\,(I)]$	300-nm molecule, 67-nm banded fibrils	Thick, highly picrosirius birefringent, fibers	Skin, tendon, bone, dentin	Resistance to tension
II	$[\alpha1\,(II)]_3$	300-nm molecule, 67-nm banded fibrils	Loose aggregates of fibrils, birefringent	Cartilage, vitreous body	Resistance to pressure
III	$[\alpha1\,(III)]_3$	67-nm banded fibrils	Thin, weakly birefringent, argyrophilic (silver-binding) fibers	Skin, muscle, blood vessels, frequently together with type I	Structural maintenance in expansible organs
V	$[\alpha1\,(V)]_3$	390-nm molecule, N-terminal globular domain	Frequently forms fiber together with type I	Fetal tissues, skin, bone, placenta, most interstitial tissues	Participates in type I collagen function
XI	$[\alpha1\,(XI)]\,[\alpha2\,(XI)]$ $[\alpha3\,(XI)]$	300-nm molecule	Small fibers	Cartilage	Participates in type II collagen function
Sheet-Forming Collagens					
IV	$[\alpha1\,(VII)]_2\,[\alpha1\,(IV)]$	2-dimensional cross-linked network	Detected by immunocytochemistry	All basal and external laminae	Support of epithelial cells; filtration
Linking/Anchoring Collagens					
VII	$[\alpha1\,(VII)]_3$	450 nm, globular domain at each end	Detected by immunocytochemistry	Epithelial basement membranes	Anchors basal laminae to underlying reticular lamina
IX	$[\alpha1\,(IX)]\,[\alpha2\,(IX)]$ $[\alpha3\,(IX)]$	200-nm molecule	Detected by immunocytochemistry	Cartilage, vitreous body	Binds various proteoglycans; associated with type II collagen
XII	$[\alpha1\,(XII)]_3$	Large N-terminal domain	Detected by immunocytochemistry	Placenta, skin, tendons	Interacts with type I collagen
XIV	$[\alpha1\,(XIV)]_3$	Large N-terminal domain; cross-shaped molecule	Detected by immunocytochemistry	Placenta, bone	Binds type I collagen fibrils, with types V and XII, strengthening fiber formation

FIGURE **5–8** Type I collagen.

Subunits of type I collagen, the most abundant collagen, assemble to form extremely strong fibrils, which are then bundled together further by other collagens into much larger structures called **collagen fibers**.

(a) TEM shows fibrils cut longitudinally and transversely. In longitudinal sections fibrils display alternating dark and light bands; in cross section the cut ends of individual collagen molecules appear as dots. Ground substance completely surrounds the fibrils. X100,000.

(b) The large bundles of type I collagen fibrils (**C**) appear as acidophilic collagen fibers in connective tissues, where they

may fill the extracellular space. Subunits for these fibers were secreted by the fibroblasts (**arrows**) associated with them. X400. H&E.

Collagen synthesis occurs in many cell types but is a specialty of cells that produce the various kinds of connective tissue. The initial **procollagen α chains** are made in the cells' abundant RER. The collagen gene family is very large, and many different α chains have been identified, varying in length and sequence. In the ER three α chains are selected, aligned, and stabilized by disulfide bonds at their carboxyl terminals, and folded as a **triple helix**, which is the defining feature of

collagens. The triple helix undergoes exocytosis and is cleaved to a rodlike **procollagen molecule** (Figure 5–9) that is the basic subunit from which the fibers or sheets are assembled. These subunits may be homotrimeric, with all three chains identical, or heterotrimeric, with two or all three chains having different sequences. Different combinations of procollagen α chains produce the various types of collagen with different structures and functional properties.

FIGURE **5–9** The collagen subunit.

← 8.6 nm →

In the most abundant form of collagen, type I, each procollagen molecule or subunit has two α1- and one α2-peptide chains, each with a molecular mass of approximately 100 kDa, intertwined in a right-handed helix and held together by hydrogen

bonds and hydrophobic interactions. The length of each molecule (sometimes called tropocollagen) is 300 nm, and its width is 1.5 nm. Each complete turn of the helix spans a distance of 8.6 nm.

An unusually large number of posttranslational processing steps are required to prepare collagen for its final assembly in the ECM. These steps have been studied most thoroughly for type I collagen, which accounts for 90% of all the body's collagen. The most important parts of this process are summarized in Figure 5–10 and here:

1. The procollagen α chains are produced on polyribosomes of the RER and translocated into the cisternae, where the signal peptide is clipped off. Collagens typically have long central domains rich in proline and lysine; in type I collagen every third amino acid is glycine.

2. **Hydroxylase** enzymes in the ER cisternae add hydroxyl groups to some prolines and lysines in important reactions that require O_2, Fe^{2+}, and ascorbic acid (vitamin C) as cofactors.

3. Glycosylation of some hydroxylysine residues also occurs, with the various collagen types having different amounts of bound galactose.

4. Both the amino- and carboxyl-terminal sequences of α chains have globular structures that lack the gly-X-Y repeats. In the RER the C-terminal regions of three selected α chains (α1, α2) are stabilized by cysteine disulfide bonds, which align the three polypeptides and facilitates their central domains folding as the triple helix. With its globular terminal sequences intact, the trimeric procollagen molecule is transported through the Golgi apparatus, packaged in vesicles and secreted.

5. Outside the cell, specific proteases called **procollagen peptidases** remove the terminal globular peptides, converting the procollagen molecules to collagen molecules. These now self-assemble (an entropy-driven process) into polymeric collagen fibrils, usually in specialized niches near the cell surface.

6. Certain proteoglycans and collagens (types V and XII) associate with the new collagen fibrils, stabilize these assemblies, and promote the formation of larger fibers from the fibrils.

7. Fibrillar structure is reinforced and disassembly is prevented by the formation of covalent cross-links between the collagen molecules, a process catalyzed by the enzyme **lysyl oxidase**.

The other fibrillar and sheetlike collagens are formed in processes similar to that described for collagen type I and stabilized by linking or anchoring collagens. Because there are so many steps in collagen biosynthesis, there are many points at which the process can be interrupted or changed by defective enzymes or by disease processes (Table 5–4).

Type I collagen fibrils have diameters ranging from 20 to 90 nm and can be several micrometers in length. Adjacent rodlike collagen subunits of the fibrils are staggered by 67 nm, with small gaps (lacunar regions) between their ends (Figure 5–11). This structure produces a characteristic feature of type I collagen visible by EM: transverse striations with a regular periodicity (Figure 5–11). Type I collagen fibrils assemble further to form large, extremely strong collagen fibers that are bundled by linking collagens and proteoglycans. Collagen type II (present in cartilage) occurs as fibrils but does not form fibers or bundles. Sheet-forming collagen type IV subunits assemble as a lattice-like network in epithelial basal laminae.

When present in large numbers (eg, in tendons or the eye's sclera region), bundles of collagen appear white. The highly regular orientation of subunits makes collagen fibers birefringent under the polarizing microscope (see Figure 1–7). In the light microscope, collagen fibers are acidophilic; they stain pink with eosin and blue with Mallory trichrome stain, and red with Sirius red. Because of the long and tortuous course of collagen bundles, their length and diameter are better studied in spread preparations than in histologic sections (see Figure 1–7). Mesentery is frequently used for this purpose; when spread on a slide, this structure is sufficiently thin to let the light pass through; it can be stained and examined directly under the microscope.

Collagen turnover and renewal in normal connective tissue is generally a very slow but ongoing process. In some organs, such as tendons and ligaments, the collagen is very stable, whereas in others, as in the periodontal ligament surrounding teeth, the collagen turnover rate is high. To be renewed, the collagen must first be degraded. Degradation is initiated by specific enzymes called **collagenases**, which are members of an enzyme class called **matrix metalloproteinases (MMPs)**. Collagenases clip collagen fibrils or sheets in such a way that they are then susceptible to further degradation by nonspecific proteases. Various MMPs are secreted by macrophages and play an important role in remodeling the ECM during tissue repair.

Reticular Fibers

Found in delicate connective tissue of many organs, **reticular fibers** consist mainly of collagen type III. This collagen forms an extensive network (reticulum) of extremely thin (diameter

FIGURE **5–10** Collagen synthesis.

Hydroxylation and glycosylation of procollagen α chains and their assembly into triple helices occur in the RER, and further assembly into fibrils occurs in the ECM after secretion of procollagen. Because there are many slightly different genes for procollagen α chains and collagen production depends on several posttranslational events involving several other enzymes, many diseases involving defective collagen synthesis have been described.

TABLE **5–4**	Examples of clinical disorders resulting from defects in collagen synthesis.	
Disorder	**Defect**	**Symptoms**
Ehlers-Danlos type IV	Faulty transcription or translation of collagen type III	Aortic and/or intestinal rupture
Ehlers-Danlos type VI	Faulty lysine hydroxylation	Increased skin elasticity, rupture of eyeball
Ehlers-Danlos type VII	Decrease in procollagen peptidase activity	Increased articular mobility, frequent luxation
Scurvy	Lack of vitamin C, a required cofactor for prolyl hydroxylase	Ulceration of gums, hemorrhages
Osteogenesis imperfecta	Change of 1 nucleotide in genes for collagen type I	Spontaneous fractures, cardiac insufficiency

FIGURE **5–11** Assembly of type I collagen.

Shown here are the relationships among type I collagen molecules, fibrils, fibers, and bundles.

1. Rodlike triple-helix collagen molecules, each 300 nm long, self-assemble in a highly organized, lengthwise arrangement of overlapping regions.

2. The regular, overlapping arrangement of subunits continues as large collagen fibrils are assembled.

3. This structure causes fibrils to have characteristic cross striations with alternating dark and light bands when observed in the EM.

4. Fibrils assemble further and are linked together in larger collagen fibers visible by light microscopy.

5. Type I fibers often form into still larger aggregates bundled and linked together by other collagens.

The photo shows an SEM view of type I collagen fibrils closely aggregated as part of a collagen fiber. Striations are visible on the surface of the fibrils.

FIGURE **5–12** Reticular fibers.

In these silver-stained sections of adrenal cortex **(a)** and lymph node **(b)**, networks of delicate, black **reticular fibers** are prominent. These fibers serve as a supportive stroma in most lymphoid and hematopoietic organs and many endocrine glands. The fibers consist of type III collagen that is heavily glycosylated, producing the black argyrophilia. Cell nuclei are also dark, but cytoplasm is unstained. X100.

0.5-2 μm), heavily glycosylated fibers. Reticular fibers are seldom visible in hematoxylin and eosin (H&E) preparations but are characteristically stained black by impregnation with silver salts (Figure 5–12) and are termed **argyrophilic** (Gr. *argyros*, silver). Reticular fibers are also periodic acid-Schiff (PAS) positive, which, like argyrophilia, is due to the high content of sugar chains bound to type III collagen. Reticular fibers contain up to 10% carbohydrate as opposed to 1% in most other collagen fibers.

Reticular fibers produced by fibroblasts occur in the reticular lamina of basement membranes and typically also surround adipocytes, smooth muscle and nerve fibers, and small blood vessels. Delicate reticular networks serve as the supportive stroma for the parenchymal secretory cells and rich microvasculature of the liver and endocrine glands. Abundant reticular fibers also characterize the stroma of hemopoietic tissue (bone marrow) and some lymphoid organs (eg, spleen and lymph nodes) where they support rapidly changing populations of proliferating cells and phagocytic cells.

Elastic Fibers

Elastic fibers are also thinner than the type I collagen fibers and form sparse networks interspersed with collagen bundles in many organs, particularly those subject to much bending or stretching. As the name implies, elastic fibers have physical properties similar to those of rubber, allowing tissues to be stretched or distended and return to their original shape. In the wall of large blood vessels, especially arteries, elastin also occurs as fenestrated sheets called **elastic lamellae**. Elastic fibers and lamellae are not strongly acidophilic and stain poorly with H&E; they are stained more darkly than collagen in other stains such as orcein and aldehyde fuchsin (Figure 5–13).

Elastic fibers (and lamellae) are a composite of **fibrillin microfibrils** embedded in a larger mass of cross-linked **elastin**. Both components are secreted from fibroblasts (and smooth muscle cells in vascular walls) and produce elastic fibers in a stepwise manner. Initially, microfibrils with diameters of 10 nm form from the protein **fibrillin** (350 kDa) and from several other glycoproteins. The microfibrils act as scaffolding upon which elastin is deposited in the second step of elastic fiber formation. Elastin accumulates between the microfibrils, surrounding most of these, and eventually comprises most of the elastic fiber. Stages of elastic fiber formation are shown in Figure 5–14.

The properties of elastic fibers and lamellae result from the structure of the 60 kDa elastin subunits and the unique cross-links holding them together. Elastin molecules are rich

FIGURE **5–13** Elastic fibers.

Elastic fibers or lamellae (sheets) add resiliency to connective tissue. Such fibers may be difficult to discern in H&E-stained tissue, but elastin has a distinct, darker-staining appearance with other staining procedures.

(a) The length, diameter, distribution, and density of dark **elastic fibers** are easily seen in this spread preparation of nonstretched connective tissue in a mesentery. X200. Hematoxylin and orcein.

(b) In sectioned tissue at higher magnification, **elastic fibers** can be seen among the acidophilic collagen bundles of dermis. X400. Aldehyde fuchsin.

(c) Elastic lamellae in the wall of the aorta are more darkly stained, incomplete sheets of elastin between the layers of eosinophilic smooth muscle. X80. H&E.

FIGURE **5–14** Formation of elastic fibers.

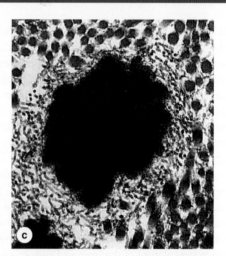

Stages in the formation of elastic fibers can be seen by TEM.

(a) Initially, a developing fiber consists of many 10-nm-diameter **fibrillin microfibrils** composed of molecular subunits secreted by fibroblasts and smooth muscle cells.

(b) Elastin is deposited on the scaffold of microfibrils, forming growing, amorphous composite structures. The elastin molecules are also secreted by the fibroblasts and quickly become cross-linked into larger assemblies.

(c) Elastin accumulates and ultimately occupies most of the electron-dense center of the single elastic fiber shown here. Fibrillin microfibrils typically remain at the fiber surface. Collagen fibrils, seen in cross section, are also present surrounding the elastic fiber. All X50,000.

FIGURE **5–15** Molecular basis of elastic fiber elasticity.

Stretched

Cross-link

Relaxed

Single elastin molecule

The diagram shows a small piece of an elastic fiber, in two conformations. Elastin polypeptides, the major components of elastic fibers, have multiple random-coil domains that straighten or stretch under force, and then relax. Most of the cross-links between elastin subunits consist of the covalent, cyclic structure **desmosine**, each of which involves four converted lysines in two elastin molecules. This unusual type of protein cross-link holds the aggregate together with little steric hindrance to elastin movements. These properties give the entire network its elastic quality.

in glycine, proline, and lysine, giving much of the protein a random-coil conformation (like that of natural rubber). Many lysines are present as pairs. During deposition on microfibrils the enzyme lysyl oxidase converts the paired lysines' amino groups to aldehydes. Oxidized lysines on two different elastin molecules then condense as a **desmosine** ring that acts as a covalent cross-link between the polypeptides, which maintain their rubberlike properties (Figure 5–15). Elastin resists digestion by most proteases, but it is hydrolyzed by pancreatic **elastase**.

≫ MEDICAL APPLICATION

Fibrillins comprise a family of proteins involved in making the scaffolding necessary for the deposition of elastin. Mutations in the fibrillin genes result in **Marfan syndrome**, a disease characterized by a lack of resistance in tissues rich in elastic fibers. Because the walls of large arteries are rich in elastic components and because the blood pressure is high in the aorta, patients with this disease often experience aortic swellings called **aneurysms**, which are life-threatening conditions.

≫ GROUND SUBSTANCE

The **ground substance** of the ECM is a highly hydrated (with much bound water), transparent, complex mixture of macromolecules, principally of three classes: **glycosaminoglycans (GAGs)**, **proteoglycans**, and **multiadhesive glycoproteins**. It fills the space between cells and fibers in connective tissue and, because it is viscous, acts as both a lubricant and a barrier to the penetration of invaders. Many macromolecules and physical properties of ground substance profoundly influence a variety of cellular activities. When adequately fixed for histologic analysis, its components aggregate and precipitate in the tissues as granular material that is observed in TEM preparations as electron-dense filaments or granules (Figure 5–16).

GAGs (also called **mucopolysaccharides**) are long polysaccharides consisting of repeating disaccharide units, usually a uronic acid and a hexosamine. The hexosamine can be **glucosamine** or **galactosamine**, and the uronic acid can be **glucuronic** or **iduronic acid**. The largest, almost unique, and most ubiquitous GAG is **hyaluronic acid** (HA or hyaluronan). With a molecular weight from 100s to 1000s kDa, hyaluronic acid is a long polymer of the disaccharide glucosamine-glucuronate. It is synthesized directly into the ECM by an enzyme complex, **hyaluronate synthase**, located in the cell membrane of many cells. Hyaluronic acid forms a dense, viscous network of polymers, which binds a considerable amount of water, giving it an important role in allowing diffusion of molecules in connective tissue and in lubricating various organs and joints.

All other GAGs are much smaller (10-40 kDa), sulfated, covalently attached to proteins (as parts of proteoglycans), and are synthesized in Golgi complexes. The four major GAGs found in proteoglycans are **dermatan sulfate**, **chondroitin sulfates**, **keratan sulfate**, and **heparan sulfate**, all of which have different disaccharide units and tissue distributions (Table 5–5). Like hyaluronic acid, these GAGs are intensely hydrophilic, contributing to the viscosity of ground substance, and are polyanions, binding a great number of cations (usually sodium) by electrostatic (ionic) bonds.

Proteoglycans are composed of a core protein to which are covalently attached various numbers and combinations of the sulfated GAGs. Like glycoproteins, they are synthesized on RER, mature in the Golgi, where the GAG side chains are added, and secreted from cells by exocytosis. Unlike glycoproteins, some proteoglycans, such as the major cartilage constituent aggrecan, contain a greater mass of polysaccharide chains than polypeptide. These structural differences between a typical glycoprotein and aggrecan are shown in Figure 5–17.

Proteoglycans are distinguished by their diversity, which is generated in part by enzymatic differences in the Golgi complexes. A region of ECM may contain several different core proteins, each with one or many GAGs of different lengths and composition. A small proteoglycan, **decorin**, has few GAG side chains and binds fibrils of type I collagen. Cell surface proteoglycans such as **syndecan** have transmembrane core

FIGURE **5–16** Ultrastructure of the extracellular matrix (ECM).

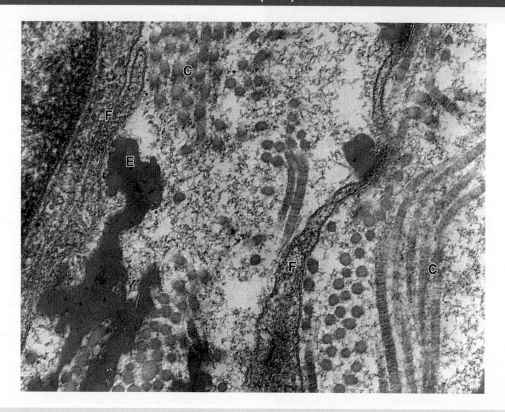

TEM of the connective tissue ECM reveals ground substance as either empty or containing fine granular material that fills spaces between the collagen (**C**) and elastic (**E**) fibers and surrounds fibroblast cells and processes (**F**). The granularity of ground substance is an artifact of the glutaraldehyde–tannic acid fixation procedure. X100,000.

TABLE **5–5** Composition and distribution of glycosaminoglycans in connective tissue and their interactions with collagen fibers.

Glycosaminoglycan	Repeating Disaccharides		Distribution	Electrostatic Interaction with Collagen
	Hexuronic Acid	Hexosamine		
Hyaluronic acid	D-glucuronic acid	D-glucosamine	Umbilical cord, synovial fluid, vitreous humor, cartilage	
Chondroitin 4-sulfate	D-glucuronic acid	D-galactosamine	Cartilage, bone, cornea, skin, notochord, aorta	High levels of interaction, mainly with collagen type II
Chondroitin 6-sulfate	D-glucuronic acid	D-galactosamine	Cartilage, umbilical cord, skin, aorta (media)	High levels of interaction, mainly with collagen type II
Dermatan sulfate	L-iduronic acid or D-glucuronic acid	D-galactosamine	Skin, tendon, aorta (adventitia)	Low levels of interaction, mainly with collagen type I
Heparan sulfate	D-glucuronic acid or L-iduronic acid	D-galactosamine	Aorta, lung, liver, basal laminae	Intermediate levels of interaction, mainly with collagen types III and IV
Keratan sulfate	D-galactose	D-glucosamine	Cartilage, nucleus pulposus, annulus fibrosus	None

FIGURE **5–17** Glycoproteins and proteoglycans.

a A typical glycoprotein

0.5 μm

b Proteoglycans linked to hyaluronan

Both macromolecules have a protein core that is glycosylated to variable degrees in the Golgi apparatus.

(a) Glycoproteins are usually globular proteins with branched oligosaccharide side-chains. Their polypeptide content is generally greater than their polysaccharide content.

(b) Proteoglycans contain a core of protein with one or many side chains of sulfated GAGs as well as branched oligosaccharides, generally having more carbohydrate than do glycoproteins. Shown here is a TEM darkfield image of many proteoglycans linked to an axis of hyaluronan. This large aggregate was purified from cartilage, where the major proteoglycan

is **aggrecan**. The core protein of this extremely large proteoglycan has hydrated chondroitin sulfate and keratan sulfate side chains, and is attached to hyaluronan by link proteins. These features are included in the diagram representing a small portion of the photo. Chemical structures of the repeating disaccharide subunits of hyaluronan, chondroitin sulfate, and keratan sulfate are also indicated.

(*Figure 5-17b, Reproduced, with permission, from Rosenberg L, Hellman W, Kleinschmidt AK: Electron microscopic studies of proteoglycan aggregates from bovine articular cartilage. J Biol Chem 1975;250:1877. © 1975 The American Society for Biochemistry and Molecular Biology.*)

proteins and serve as additional attachments of the cell to the ECM. One of the best known proteoglycans, **aggrecan**, is very large (250 kDa), with a core protein bearing many chondroitin sulfate and keratan sulfate chains. Aggrecan is bound via a link protein to polymer of hyaluronic acid (Figure 5–17). In cartilage aggrecan-hyaluronate, complexes fill the space between collagen fibers and cells and contribute greatly to the physical properties of this tissue.

GAGs bind large amounts of water, which causes the polyanions to swell and occupy a large space in the tissue. Embryonic mesenchyme (Figure 5–1) is very rich in hyaluronate and water, producing the characteristic wide spacing of cells and a matrix ideal for cell migrations and growth. Both matrix-linked

and cell surface proteoglycans also bind and sequester certain signaling proteins, for example fibroblast growth factor (FGF). Degradation of proteoglycans during the early phase of tissue repair releases these stored growth factors that then stimulate new cell growth and ECM synthesis.

›› MEDICAL APPLICATION

The degradation of proteoglycans is carried out by several cell types and depends in part on the presence of several lysosomal enzymes. Several disorders have been described, including a deficiency in certain lysosomal enzymes causing degradation of certain GAGs, with the consequent accumulation of these macromolecules in tissues. The lack of specific hydrolases in the lysosomes has been found to be the cause of several disorders, including the **Hurler, Hunter, Sanfilippo,** and **Morquio syndromes.**

Because of their high viscosity, HA and proteoglycans tend to form a barrier against bacterial penetration of tissues. Bacteria that produce hyaluronidase, an enzyme that hydrolyzes hyaluronic acid and disassembles proteoglycans complexes, reduce the viscosity of the connective tissue ground substance and have greater invasive power.

The third class of ground substance components, the **multiadhesive glycoproteins,** all have multiple binding sites for cell surface receptors (integrins) and for other matrix macromolecules. The adhesive glycoproteins are very large molecules with branched oligosaccharide chains and have important roles in the adhesion of cells to their substrate. The large (200-400 kDa), trimeric, cross-shaped glycoprotein **laminin** provides adhesion for epithelial and other cells, with binding sites for integrins, type IV collagen, and specific proteoglycans. As shown in Figure 5–18a, all basal and external laminae are rich in laminin, which is essential for the assembly and maintenance of these structures.

Fibronectin (L. *fibra*, fiber + *nexus*, interconnection), synthesized largely by fibroblasts, is a 235-270 kDa dimeric molecule, has binding sites for collagens and certain GAGs, and forms insoluble fibrillar networks throughout connective tissue (Figure 5–18b). The fibronectin substrate provides specific binding sites for integrins and is important both for cell adhesion and cellular migration through the ECM.

The **integrin** family of integral membrane proteins act as matrix receptors for specific sequences on laminin, fibronectin, some collagens, and certain other ECM proteins (Figure 5–19). Integrins bind their ligands in the ECM with relatively low affinity, allowing cells to explore their environment without losing attachment to it or becoming glued to it. They are heterodimers of two transmembrane polypeptides: the α and β chains. Great diversity in the subsets of integrin α and β chain cells express allows the cells to have different specific ligands preferentially.

Cytoplasmic portions of integrins associate with the peripheral membrane proteins talin and vinculin, which together bind actin filaments (Figure 5–19). In this way integrins mediate physical connections between ECM components and the cytoskeleton of cells in connective tissue, which allows the cells to monitor many physical aspects of their microenvironment. These connections between cells and the ECM exert effects in both directions and are important for the physical orientation of both cells and fibers.

Integrins and other proteins associated with intermediate filaments form the hemidesmosomes of epithelia (see Chapter 4); clustered integrin-microfilament complexes in fibroblasts form structures called **focal adhesions** that can be localized by TEM or immunocytochemistry. This type of adhesive junction is typically present at the ends of actin filaments bundled by α-actinin as cytoplasmic stress fibers. Focal adhesion

FIGURE 5–18 Laminin and fibronectin localization by immunohistochemistry.

Both of these glycoproteins (and other similar glycoproteins) are multiadhesive, with binding sites for ECM components and for integrins at cell surfaces, and have important roles in cell migration and maintaining tissue structure.

(a) Laminin is concentrated in the basal lamina of the stratified epithelium (top) and in the external laminae surrounding cross-sectioned nerves and muscle fibers. X200.

(b) A fine network of **fibronectin** is localized more diffusely throughout the ECM. X400.

FIGURE **5–19** Integrin and actin filament interaction.

Extracellular matrix
linking domain

Integrin

α chain   β chain

Extracellular

Cell membrane

Cytosol

Talin

Vinculin

Capping
protein

F actin

By binding to a matrix protein and to the **actin** cytoskeleton (via talin) inside the cell, **integrins** serve as transmembrane links by which cells adhere to components of the ECM. The molecule is a heterodimer, with α and β chains. The head portion extends from the cell surface into the ECM where it interacts with sites on fibronectin, laminin, collagens, or other matrix components.

kinases provide a mechanism by which pulling forces or other physical properties of the ECM can change activities in the cytoplasm.

In addition to the hydrated ground substance of connective tissue, a small quantity of free **interstitial fluid**, with ion composition similar to that of blood plasma, is also present. Interstitial fluid contains plasma proteins of low molecular weight that pass through the thin walls of capillaries, the smallest blood vessels. Although only a small proportion of connective tissue proteins are plasma proteins, it is estimated that as much as one-third of the body's plasma proteins are stored in the matrix of connective tissue because of its volume and wide distribution.

> **›› MEDICAL APPLICATION**
>
> **Edema** is the excessive accumulation of water in the extracellular spaces of connective tissue. This water comes from the blood, passing through the capillary walls that become more permeable during inflammation and normally producing slight swelling.

Capillaries in connective tissue throughout the body bring the various nutrients required by cells and carry away their metabolic waste products to the detoxifying and excretory organs, the liver and kidneys. Interstitial water provides the solvent for these substances.

Two forces act on the water in capillaries (Figure 5–20):

- The **hydrostatic pressure** of the blood caused by the pumping action of the heart, which forces water out across the capillary wall
- The colloid **osmotic pressure** produced by plasma proteins such as albumin, which draws water back into the capillaries

The colloid osmotic pressure exerted by the blood proteins—which are unable to pass through the capillary walls—is not counterbalanced by outside pressure and tends to pull back into the vessel the water forced out by hydrostatic pressure (Figure 5–20). (Because the ions and low-molecular-weight compounds that pass easily through the capillary walls have similar concentrations inside and outside these blood vessels, the osmotic pressures they exert are approximately equal on either side of the capillaries and cancel each other.)

The quantity of water drawn back into capillaries is often less than that which was forced out. Normally this excess fluid does not accumulate in connective tissue but drains continuously into lymphatic capillaries that eventually return it to the blood. Discussed later with the lymphoid system, lymphatic capillaries originate in connective tissue as delicate, open-ended endothelial tubes (Figure 5–20).

› TYPES OF CONNECTIVE TISSUE

Different combinations and densities of the cells, fibers, and extracellular macromolecules just described produce graded variations in histological structure within connective tissue. Descriptive names or classifications used for the various types of connective tissue denote either a major component or a structural characteristic of the tissue. Table 5–6 gives a classification commonly used for the main types of connective tissue. Adipose tissue, an important specialized connective tissue, and two other supporting tissues, cartilage and bone, will be covered in Chapters 6, 7, and 8.

Connective Tissue Proper

In adults there are two general classes of connective tissue proper, loose and dense, terms that refer to amounts of

FIGURE 5–20 Movement of fluid in connective tissue.

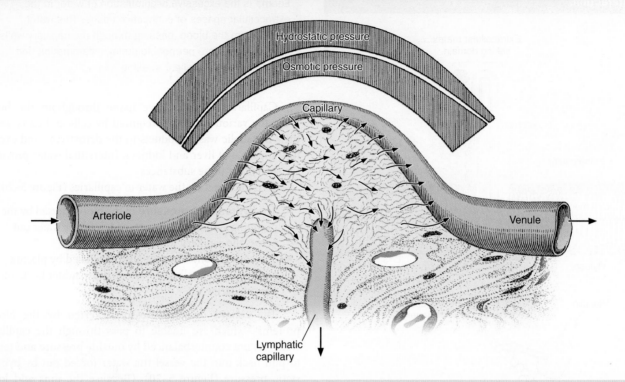

Water normally passes through capillary walls into the ECM of surrounding connective tissues primarily at the arterial end of a capillary, because the **hydrostatic pressure** is greater than the colloid **osmotic pressure**. However, hydrostatic pressure decreases toward the venous end of the capillary, as indicated at the top of the figure. The fall in hydrostatic pressure parallels a rise in osmotic pressure of the capillary blood because the plasma protein concentration increases as water is pushed out across the capillary wall.

As a result of the increased protein concentration and decreased hydrostatic pressure, osmotic pressure at the venous end is greater than hydrostatic pressure and water is drawn back into the capillary. In this way plasma and interstitial fluid constantly mix, nutrients in blood circulate to cells in connective tissue, and cellular wastes are removed.

Not all water that leaves capillaries by hydrostatic pressure is drawn back in by osmotic pressure. This excess tissue fluid is normally drained by the lymphatic capillaries, open-ended vessels that arise in connective tissue and enter the one-way lymphatic system that eventually delivers the fluid (now called **lymph**) back to veins.

collagen present (Figure 5–21). **Loose connective tissue** is very common and generally supports epithelial tissue. It comprises a thick layer (the lamina propria) beneath the epithelial lining of the digestive system and fills the spaces between muscle and nerve fibers (Figure 5–18a). Usually well-vascularized whatever their location, thin layers of loose connective tissue surround most small blood vessels of the body.

Also called **areolar tissue**, the loose connective tissue typically contains cells, fibers, and ground substance in roughly equal parts. The most numerous cells are fibroblasts, but the other types of connective tissue cells are also present, along with nerves and blood vessels. Collagen fibers predominate, but elastic and reticular fibers are also present. With a moderate amount of ground substance, loose connective tissue has a delicate consistency; it is flexible and not very resistant to stress.

Dense connective tissue is adapted to offer stress resistance and protection. It has the same components found in

loose connective tissue, but with fewer cells and a clear predominance of collagen fibers over ground substance. Dense connective tissue is less flexible and far more resistant to stress than loose connective tissue. In **dense irregular connective tissue** bundles of collagen fibers appear randomly interwoven, with no definite orientation. The collagen fibers form a tough three-dimensional network, providing resistance to stress from all directions. Dense irregular connective tissue is often found closely associated with loose connective tissue, with the two types frequently grading into each other and making distinctions between them somewhat arbitrary (Figure 5–21).

The type I collagen bundles of **dense regular connective tissue** are arranged according to a definite pattern, with fibers and fibroblasts aligned in parallel for resistance to prolonged or repeated stresses exerted in the same direction (Figure 5–22).

Common examples of dense regular connective tissue, such as tendons and ligaments, are strong, flexible straps or

	General Organization	Major Functions	Examples
Connective Tissue Proper			
Loose (areolar) connective tissue	Much ground substance; many cells and little collagen, randomly distributed	Supports microvasculature, nerves, and immune defense cells	Lamina propria beneath epithelial lining of digestive tract
Dense irregular connective tissue	Little ground substance; few cells (mostly fibroblasts); much collagen in randomly arranged fibers	Protects and supports organs; resists tearing	Dermis of skin, organ capsules, submucosa layer of digestive tract
Dense regular connective tissue	Almost completely filled with parallel bundles of collagen; few fibroblasts, aligned with collagen	Provide strong connections within musculoskeletal system; strong resistance to force	Ligaments, tendons, aponeuroses, corneal stroma
Embryonic Connective Tissues			
Mesenchyme	Sparse, undifferentiated cells, uniformly distributed in matrix with sparse collagen fibers	Contains stem/progenitor cells for all adult connective tissue cells	Mesodermal layer of early embryo
Mucoid (mucous) connective tissue	Random fibroblasts and collagen fibers in viscous matrix	Supports and cushions large blood vessels	Matrix of the fetal umbilical cord
Specialized Connective Tissues			
Reticular connective tissue (see Chapter 14)	Delicate network of reticulin/collagen III with attached fibroblasts (reticular cells)	Supports blood-forming cells, many secretory cells, and lymphocytes in most lymphoid organs	Bone marrow, liver, pancreas, adrenal glands, all lymphoid organs except the thymus
Adipose Tissue (Chapter 6)			
Cartilage (Chapter 7)			
Bone (Chapter 8)			
Blood (Chapter 12)			

TABLE 5–6 Classification of connective or supporting tissues.

cords that hold together components of the musculoskeletal system. Consisting almost entirely of densely packed collagen fibers, they are white in the fresh state and almost inextensible. The parallel, closely packed bundles of collagen are separated by very little ground substance (Figure 5–22a). The fibrocytes have elongated nuclei lying parallel to the fibers and sparse cytoplasmic folds that envelop portions of the collagen bundles (Figure 5–22b). The cytoplasm of these "tendinocytes" is rarely revealed in H&E stains, not only because it is sparse but also because it stains the same color as the fibers. Some ligaments, such as the yellow ligaments of the vertebral column, also contain abundant parallel elastic fiber bundles.

The collagen bundles of tendons vary in size and are enveloped by small amounts of irregular connective tissue containing small blood vessels and nerves. Overall, however, tendons are poorly vascularized and repair of damaged tendons is very slow. In some tendons, the dense irregular connective tissue sheath is covered by flattened **synovial cells** of mesenchymal origin, which produce lubricant fluid (similar to the fluid of synovial joints, Chapter 8) containing water, proteins, hyaluronate, and other GAGs.

>> **MEDICAL APPLICATION**

Overuse of tendon-muscle units can result in **tendonitis**, characterized by inflammation of the tendons and their attachments to muscle. Common locations are the elbow, the Achilles tendon of the heel, and the shoulder rotator cuff. The swelling and pain produced by the localized inflammation restricts the affected area's normal range of motion and can be relieved by injections of anti-inflammatory agents such as cortisone. Fibroblasts eventually repair damaged collagen bundles of the area.

Reticular Tissue

In **reticular tissue** fibers of type III collagen (see Figure 5–12) form a delicate 3D network that supports various types of cells. The fibrous network of this specialized connective tissue is produced by modified fibroblasts called **reticular cells** that remain associated with and partially covering the fibers (Figure 5–23). The loose disposition of glycosylated reticular

FIGURE 5–21 Loose connective tissue and dense irregular connective tissue.

Examples of these connective tissue types shown here indicate the close association that often occurs between these two types. **(a)** Loose connective tissue (**L**) of a gland contains faintly stained ground substance with fine fibers of collagen and frequently forms a thin layer near epithelia, while dense irregular connective tissue (**D**) forms a thicker layer and is invariably much richer in larger bundles of collagen. Scattered leukocytes can be seen in both connective tissues, along with the large irregular spaces of lymphatic vessels (left). X100. H&E.

(b) Trichrome staining of a section from skin demonstrates the blue staining of collagen with this method and its relative density in loose (**L**) and dense irregular (**D**) connective tissue. X100. Mallory trichrome.

(c) Another example of dense irregular connective tissue, showing the randomly arranged large collagen bundles. The arrangement of collagen strengthens the tissues and resists tearing from all directions. X150. H&E.

(d) Dense irregular connective tissue (**D**) forms a thick, protective capsule around many organs such as the testis shown here. Here the capsule is covered by a simple epithelium of serous mesothelial cells (**S**), which produce a hyaluronate-rich lubricant around such organs. X150. H&E.

FIGURE 5–22 Dense regular connective tissue.

(a) Micrograph shows a longitudinal section of dense regular connective tissue in a tendon. Long, parallel bundles of collagen fibers fill the spaces between the elongated nuclei of fibrocytes. X100. H&E stain.

(b) The electron micrograph shows one fibrocyte in a cross section of tendon, revealing that the sparse cytoplasm of the fibrocytes is divided into numerous thin cytoplasmic processes extending among adjacent collagen fibers. X25,000.

FIGURE 5–23 Reticular tissue.

(a) The diagram shows only the fibers and attached reticular cells (free, transient cells are not represented). Reticular fibers of type III collagen are produced and enveloped by the reticular cells, forming an elaborate network through which interstitial fluid or lymph and wandering cells from blood pass continuously.

(b) The micrograph shows a silver-stained section of lymph node in which reticular fibers are seen as irregular black lines. Reticular cells are also heavily stained and dark. Most of the smaller, more lightly stained cells are lymphocytes passing through the lymph node. X200. Silver.

fibers provides a framework with specialized microenvironments for cells in hemopoietic tissue and some lymphoid organs (bone marrow, lymph nodes, and spleen). The resulting cell-lined system creates a meshwork (see Figure 5–12) for the passage of lymphocytes and lymph. Macrophages and other cells of the mononuclear phagocyte system are also dispersed within these reticular tissues to monitor cells formed there or passing through and to remove debris.

Mucoid Tissue

Mucoid (or mucous) connective tissue is another embryonic type of connective tissue, found mainly in the umbilical cord and fetal organs. With abundant ground substance composed chiefly of hyaluronic acid, mucoid tissue is jellylike with sparse collagen fibers and scattered fibroblasts (Figure 5–24). Mucoid tissue is the principal component of the umbilical cord, where it is referred to as **Wharton's jelly**. A similar form of connective tissue is also found in the pulp cavities of young teeth, which remain as a postnatal source of mesenchymal stem cells.

FIGURE **5–24** Mucoid tissue.

A section of umbilical cord shows large fibroblasts surrounded by a large amount of very loose ECM containing mainly ground substances very rich in hyaluronan, with wisps of collagen. Histologically mucoid (or mucous) connective tissue resembles embryonic mesenchyme in many respects and is rarely found in adult organs. X200. H&E

Connective Tissue SUMMARY OF KEY POINTS

- Connective tissue is specialized to physically **support** and **connect** other tissues and maintain the water required for metabolite diffusion to and from cells.
- Connective tissues all consist primarily of **extracellular** material rather than cells.
- Within most organs connective tissue proper forms the supportive **stroma**, which supports the organ's unique functional components or **parenchyma**.
- The **extracellular matrix (ECM)** of connective tissue proper usually consists of both large protein **fibers** and nonfibrous areas of unstained **ground substance** rich in various GAGs and water.
- All adult connective tissues are derived from an embryonic form of connective tissue called **mesenchyme**, which contains uniformly undifferentiated cells scattered in a gel-like matrix.

Cells of Connective Tissue

- **Fibroblasts** (fibrocytes), the major cells of connective tissue proper, are elongated, irregularly shaped cells with oval nuclei that synthesize and secrete most components of the ECM.
- **Adipocytes** (fat cells) are very large cells specialized for storage of triglycerides; they predominate in a specialized form of connective tissue called **adipose tissue**.
- **Macrophages** are short-lived cells that differentiate in connective tissue from precursor cells called **monocytes** circulating in the blood; they function in ECM turnover, phagocytosis of dead cells and debris, and antigen presentation to lymphocytes.
- **Mast cells** also originate from blood cell precursors and are filled with granules for the release of various vasoactive agents and other substances during inflammatory and allergic reactions.

- **Plasma cells** are short-lived cells that differentiate from B lymphocytes and are specialized for the abundant secretion of specific antibodies (immunoglobulins).
- Besides macrophages and plasma cells, other **leukocytes** normally wander through all types of connective tissue proper, providing surveillance against bacterial invaders and stimulating tissue repair.

Fibers of Connective Tissue

- The most important and abundant fibers of connective tissue are composed of the protein **collagen**, of which there are some 20 related types.
- Synthesis of collagen by fibroblasts and certain other cells involves posttranslational modifications in the RER, notably **hydroxylation** of the numerous prolines and lysines, and formation of helical trimeric subunits of **procollagen**.
- Upon exocytosis, the nonhelical ends of the procollagen subunits are removed, forming trimeric **collagen molecules** that aggregate and become covalently bound together in large **collagen fibrils**.
- The highly regular assembly of collagens in the fibrils produces a characteristic pattern of **crossbanding** visible ultrastructurally along the fibrils of some collagen types.
- Fibrils of type I collagen are bundled together by other forms of nonfibrillar, linking collagens to produce large **collagen bundles**.
- Collagen fibrils are degraded by collagenase enzymes classified as **matrix metalloproteinases (MMPs)**, produced primarily by macrophages.

- Type III collagen produces a network of delicate **reticular fibers**, which stain very dark with silver stains and are abundant in immune and lymphoid tissues.
- **Elastic fibers**, or sheets called **elastic lamellae**, are composed of the proteins **elastin** and **fibrillin**, which exist in a stretchable conformation that provides elastic properties to connective tissues rich in this material.

Ground Substance

- **Ground substance** is the watery, largely unstained extracellular material that is more abundant than fibers in some types of connective tissue proper.
- Ground substance is rich in **hydrated glycosaminoglycans (GAGs)**, **proteoglycans**, and **multiadhesive glycoproteins**.
- The major types of GAGs are **hyaluronic acid** (HA or hyaluronan), which is a very long polymer of the disaccharide glucosamine-glucuronate, and various shorter chains of **sulfated GAGs** composed of other disaccharide polymers.
- Sulfated GAGs such as **chondroitin sulfate** and **keratan sulfate** have various sizes and compositions, but they are all bound to the core proteins of **proteoglycans** and are produced in the Golgi apparatus before secretion.
- Proteoglycans attach to polymers of HA via **linker proteins** to form huge complexes in ground substance that bind water and other substances, including certain polypeptide growth factors that help regulate fibroblast proliferation.
- **Multiadhesive glycoproteins** such as fibronectin and laminin have binding sites for collagens and for integrin proteins in cell membranes, thus allowing temporary attachments between cells and the ECM required for cell migration and positioning.

Types of Connective Tissue

- **Connective tissue proper** is usually classified as loose or dense according to the amount of collagen and ground substance present.
- **Loose connective tissue** (or **areolar tissue**) has relatively more ground substance than collagen, and it typically surrounds small blood vessels and occupies areas adjacent to other types of epithelia.
- **Dense irregular connective tissue** is filled primarily with randomly distributed bundles of type I collagen, with some elastic fibers, providing resistance to tearing from all directions as well as some elasticity.
- **Dense regular connective tissue**, prominent in tendons and ligaments, features bundles of essentially parallel collagen, providing great strength (but little stretch) in binding together components of the musculoskeletal system.
- **Reticular tissue** consists of delicate networks of type III collagen (reticulin) and is most abundant in certain lymphoid organs where the fibers form attachment sites for lymphocytes and other immune cells.
- **Mucoid tissue** is an embryonic form of gel-like connective tissue with few cells, resembling mesenchyme, and is best seen around blood vessels in the umbilical cord.

6 Adipose Tissue

Connective tissue in which **adipocytes** or fat cells predominate is commonly called **adipose tissue**. These large cells are found isolated or in small groups within loose or dense irregular connective tissue but occur in large aggregates as adipose tissue or "fat" in many body regions and organs. Located throughout the body, adipose tissue normally represents 15%-20% of the body weight in men, somewhat more in women. Besides serving as storage depots for neutral fats (chiefly triglycerides, long-chain fatty acyl esters of glycerol), adipocytes function as key regulators of the body's overall energy metabolism. With a growing worldwide epidemic of obesity and its associated health problems, including diabetes and heart disease, adipocytes and adipose tissue now constitute a major area of medical research.

Two properties of triglycerides explain their selection as the preferred form of nutrient storage against fluctuating availability and energy demands. Fats are insoluble in water and can be concentrated with no adverse osmotic effects on cells. Moreover, the caloric density of triglycerides (9.3 kcal/g) is twice that of proteins or carbohydrates, including glycogen, making these simple molecules the most efficient form of nutrient storage. Adipocytes specialize in concentrating triglycerides as lipid droplet(s), with other cells normally accumulating relatively little lipid.

Adipocytes are very active cells metabolically, responding to both nervous and hormonal stimuli. These cells release hormones and various other important substances, and adipose tissue is now recognized as an important endocrine tissue. With its unique physical properties, adipose tissue conducts heat poorly and helps thermally insulate the body. Adipose tissue also fills up spaces between other tissues and helps cushion and keep some organs in place. Subcutaneous layers of adipose tissue help shape the body surface, where pad-like deposits act as shock absorbers, chiefly in the soles and palms.

There are two types of adipose tissue with different locations: structures, colors, and pathologic characteristics. **White adipose tissue**, the more common type, is composed of cells that, when completely developed, contain one very large droplet of whitish-yellow fat in their cytoplasm. **Brown adipose tissue** contains cells with multiple lipid droplets interspersed among abundant mitochondria, which give these cells a darker appearance. Both types of adipose tissue have a rich blood supply.

› WHITE ADIPOSE TISSUE

Specialized for relatively long-term energy storage, adipocytes of white adipose tissue are spherical when isolated but are polyhedral when closely packed in situ. Each cell is very large, between 50 and 150 μm in diameter, and contains a single huge droplet of lipid that fills almost the entire cell. White adipocytes are called **unilocular** because the triglycerides are stored in this single large droplet (Figure 6–1). Because lipid is removed from cells by xylene or other solvents used in routine histological techniques, unilocular adipocytes are often empty in standard light microscope preparations. The cells are sometimes said to have a signet-ring appearance, with the lipid droplet displacing and flattening the nucleus against the cell membrane (Figure 6–1d). This membrane and the thin rim of cytoplasm that remains after removal of the stored triglycerides may shrink, collapse, or rupture, distorting the tissue structure.

›› MEDICAL APPLICATION

Unilocular adipocytes can generate benign tumors called **lipomas** that are relatively common, although malignant adipose tumors (**liposarcomas**) occur infrequently. Fetal lipomas of brown fat are sometimes called **hibernomas**.

Most of the cytoplasm in a white adipocyte surrounds the nucleus and contains mitochondria, a small Golgi apparatus,

FIGURE **6–1** White adipose tissue.

White or unilocular adipose tissue is commonly seen in sections of many human organs. **(a)** Large white adipocytes (**A**) are seen in the connective tissue associated with small blood vessels. The fat cells are empty because lipid was dissolved away in slide preparation. Nuclei at the cell membranes are visible in some of the fat cells. X100. H&E.

(b) Large (empty) adipocytes predominate in this typical white adipose tissue, which shows only a small portion of microvasculature. In a single histologic section, nuclei of most very large adipocytes are not included. X100. H&E.

(c) Tissue was fixed here with osmium tetroxide, which preserves lipid (**L**) and stains it black. Many adipocytes in this slide retain at least part of their large lipid droplets. X440. Osmium tetroxide.

(d) The specimen here was from a young mammal, and the adipocytes marked with asterisks are not yet unilocular, having many small lipid droplets in their cytoplasm, which indicates that their differentiation is not yet complete. The eccentric nuclei of unilocular cells are indicated by arrowheads. X200. PT.

a few cisternae of RER, and free polyribosomes. The thin, submembranous layer of cytoplasm surrounding the lipid droplet contains cisternae of smooth ER (SER) and pinocytotic vesicles. TEM studies reveal that most adipocytes, especially immature cells, contain minute lipid droplets in addition to the single large droplet seen with the light microscope. The lipid droplet-cytoplasm interface is reinforced by intermediate filaments of vimentin. Unlike other connective tissue cells, adipocytes are surrounded by a thin external lamina containing type IV collagen.

White adipose tissue is subdivided into incomplete lobules by partitions of connective tissue containing a vascular bed and nerve network. Fibroblasts, macrophages, and other cells make up about half the total number of cells. Reticular fibers form a fine interwoven network that supports individual fat cells and binds them together. The microvasculature between adipocytes may not always be apparent in tissue sections.

Almost all adipose tissue in adults is unilocular and it is found in and around many organs throughout the body. The distribution of this tissue changes significantly through childhood and adult life and is partly regulated by sex hormones, which control adipose deposition in the breasts and thighs. The color of freshly dissected white adipose tissue depends on the diet, varying from white to yellow with the amount of carotenoids dissolved in the lipid.

Storage & Mobilization of Lipids

Triglycerides stored by cells of white adipose tissue can be derived from dietary fats brought to adipocytes as circulating **chylomicrons**, from triglycerides synthesized in the liver and transported as **very-low-density lipoproteins (VLDLs)**, and by the local synthesis of free fatty acids and glycerol from glucose.

Chylomicrons (Gr. *chylos*, juice + *micros*, small) are small particles of variable size, up to 1200 nm in diameter, formed in intestinal epithelial cells and transported in blood plasma and lymph. They consist of a central core, composed mainly of triglycerides and a small quantity of cholesterol esters, surrounded by a stabilizing monolayer of apolipoproteins, cholesterol, and phospholipids. Lipoproteins are also complexes of lipids and proteins, but are generally smaller than chylomicrons (providing a greater surface-to-volume ratio) and have much higher levels of lipoproteins, cholesterol, and phospholipids in the surface layer. Circulating lipoproteins are routinely measured in clinical tests for blood lipids; varying levels of surface apolipoprotein allow their categorization according to density, from VLDL to high-density lipoprotein (HDL).

In adipose tissue both chylomicrons and VLDL are hydrolyzed at the luminal surfaces of blood capillaries by **lipoprotein lipase**, an enzyme synthesized by the adipocyte and transferred to the capillary cell membrane (Figure 6–2). Free fatty acids enter the adipocyte by both active transport and diffusion. Within the adipocyte, the fatty acids combine with glycerol phosphate, supplied by glucose metabolism, to again form triglycerides, which are then deposited in the growing lipid droplet. Mitochondria and SER participate actively in the process of lipid uptake and storage.

Synthesis by adipocytes of fatty acids from glucose is accelerated by insulin, which also stimulates the uptake of glucose into adipocytes and increases the synthesis of lipoprotein lipase.

When adipocytes are stimulated by nerves or hormones, stored lipids are mobilized and fatty acids and glycerol are released into the blood. Norepinephrine released by postganglionic sympathetic nerves in adipose tissue activates **hormone-sensitive lipase** that breaks down triglycerides at the surface of the stored lipid droplets (Figure 6–2). The free fatty acids diffuse across the membranes of the adipocyte and the capillary endothelium, and bind the carrier protein albumin in blood for transport throughout the body. The more water-soluble glycerol remains free and is taken up by the liver. Insulin inhibits the hormone-sensitive lipase, reducing fatty acid release, and also stimulates enzymes for lipid synthesis. Various other hormones can also regulate lipid synthesis and mobilization in adipocytes. Glucagon and growth hormone promote triglyceride breakdown and release of fatty acids.

White adipose tissue also functions as an important endocrine organ. Adipocytes are the sole source of the 16-kDa polypeptide hormone **leptin** (Gr. *leptos*, thin), a "satiety factor" with target cells in the hypothalamus and other organs. Leptin helps regulate the appetite under normal conditions and participates in regulating the formation of new adipose tissue.

FIGURE 6–2 Lipid storage and mobilization from adipocytes.

Triglycerides are transported by blood and lymph from the intestine and liver in lipoprotein complexes known as **chylomicrons (Chylo)** and **VLDLs**. In the capillary endothelial cells of adipose tissue, these complexes are partly broken down by **lipoprotein lipase**, releasing free fatty acids and glycerol. The free fatty acids diffuse from the capillary into the adipocyte, where they are reesterified to glycerol phosphate, forming triglycerides that are stored in the lipid droplet until needed.

Norepinephrine from nerve endings stimulates the cyclic AMP (cAMP) system, which activates **hormone-sensitive lipase** to hydrolyze the stored triglycerides to free fatty acids and glycerol. These substances diffuse into the capillary, where the fatty acids bind albumin for transport throughout the body for use as an energy source.

Leptin was discovered and is well studied in genetically obese mice, but such studies have not led to new treatments for human obesity. In most obese humans adipocytes produce adequate or excess quantities of leptin, but target cells are not responsive due apparently to insufficient or defective receptors or postreceptor signal transduction.

Although all white adipose tissue appears histologically similar, differences in gene expression have been noted between visceral deposits (in the abdomen) and subcutaneous deposits of white fat. Such differences may be important in the medical risks of obesity; it is well established that increased visceral adipose tissue raises the risk of diabetes and cardiovascular disease whereas increased subcutaneous fat does not. The release of visceral fat products directly to the portal circulation and liver may also influence the medical importance of this form of obesity.

In response to body needs, lipids are mobilized rather uniformly in all parts of the body, although adipose tissue in the palms, soles, and retro-orbital fat pads resists even long periods of starvation. During starvation, most unilocular adipocytes lose nearly all their fat and become polyhedral or spindle-shaped cells with only very small lipid droplets.

Histogenesis of White Adipose Tissue

Like the fiber-producing cells of connective tissue, adipocytes differentiate from embryonic mesenchymal cells. Such differentiation is first seen with the appearance of **preadipocytes** (Figure 6–3). These cells have the appearance of fibroblasts but accumulate lipid droplets in their cytoplasm. Lipid accumulations are isolated from one another at first but soon fuse to form the single large droplet characteristic of cells in unilocular adipose tissue (Figure 6–1d).

In addition to leptin, white adipose tissue secretes numerous other cytokines and other factors with paracrine and autocrine activity, including many proinflammatory cytokines. It is not clear whether these are produced by adipocytes or other cells of the tissue such as macrophages or fibroblasts. With its increased amounts of white adipose tissue, obesity is characterized by a state of chronic mild inflammation. Proinflammatory factors released from visceral fat are being investigated for links to the **inflammation-related disorders associated with obesit**y, such as diabetes and heart disease.

Humans are born with stores of white adipose tissue, which begin to accumulate at week 30 of gestation and are well developed before birth in both the visceral and subcutaneous compartments. Development of new adipocytes continues postnatally around small blood vessels, where undifferentiated mesenchymal cells are fairly abundant.

FIGURE **6–3** **Development of white and brown fat cells.**

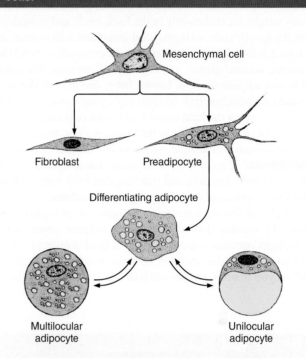

Mesenchymal cell

Fibroblast   Preadipocyte

Differentiating adipocyte

Multilocular   Unilocular
adipocyte   adipocyte

Mesenchymal cells differentiate initially as **preadipocytes** and then develop further as **adipocytes** as they accumulate fat and thus give rise to mature unilocular or multilocular fat cells. The unilocular adipocyte is typically much larger than that shown here in relation to the other cell types. Mesenchymal cells also give rise to a variety of other cell types, including fibroblasts. When large amounts of lipid are mobilized, mature fat cells may return to the lipoblast stage.

Excessive formation of adipose tissue, or obesity, occurs when energy intake exceeds energy expenditure, an increasingly common condition in modern, sedentary lifestyles. Although adipocytes can differentiate from mesenchymal stem cells throughout life, adult-onset obesity mainly involves increased size of existing adipocytes (hypertrophic obesity). Childhood obesity, however, can involve increases in both adipocyte size and numbers due to differentiation of more preadipocytes from mesenchymal stem cells (hyperplastic obesity).

Adult-onset obesity is very often associated with age-related metabolic changes and may involve reduced activity of the hormone-sensitive lipases of adipocytes, causing less effective fat mobilization out of the cells. The increased number of adipocytes produced during **childhood obesity** predisposes an individual to obesity in later life. Despite claims of various fad **diets**, there is no evidence that any particular type of caloric restriction is more effective than others; rather, any intake of calories that is lower than the energy expenditure will result in loss of adipose tissue.

› BROWN ADIPOSE TISSUE

Brown adipose tissue constitutes 2% to 5% of the newborn body weight, located mainly in the back, neck, and shoulders, but it is greatly reduced during childhood and adolescence. In adults it is found only in scattered areas, especially around the kidneys, adrenal glands, aorta, and mediastinum. The color of brown adipose tissue or **brown fat** is due to both the very abundant mitochondria (containing cytochrome pigment) scattered among the lipid droplets of the fat cells and the large number of blood capillaries in this tissue. Adipocytes of brown fat contain many small lipid inclusions and are therefore called **multilocular** (Figure 6–3). The many small lipid droplets, abundant mitochondria, and rich vasculature all help mediate this tissue's principal function of **heat production**.

Cells of brown adipose tissue cells are polygonal and generally smaller than cells of white adipose tissue; their cytoplasm contains a great number of lipid droplets of various sizes and nuclei are often centrally located (Figure 6–4). Adipocytes of brown fat are often closely packed around large

capillaries. The tissue is subdivided by partitions of connective tissue into lobules that are better delineated than the lobules of white adipose tissue. Cells of this tissue receive direct sympathetic innervation.

Function of Brown Adipocytes

The main function of the multilocular adipose cells is to produce heat by nonshivering **thermogenesis**. The physiology of multilocular adipose tissue is best understood from studies of the tissue in hibernating species. In animals ending their hibernation period, or in newborn humans exposed to an environment colder than the uterus, nerve impulses liberate norepinephrine into brown adipose tissue. As in white fat, this neurotransmitter activates the hormone-sensitive lipase of adipocytes, promoting hydrolysis of triglycerides to fatty acids and glycerol. However, unlike the process in white fat, liberated fatty acids of multilocular adipocytes are not released but are quickly metabolized, with a consequent increase in oxygen consumption and heat production. This raises the temperature

---

FIGURE **6–4** Brown adipose tissue.

(a) Brown adipose tissue is shown here around a small blood vessel (**BV**) and adjacent white adipose tissue at the top of the photo. Brown adipocytes are slightly smaller and characteristically contain many small lipid droplets and central spherical nuclei. If the lipid has been dissolved from the cells, as shown here, the many mitochondria among the lipid spaces are retained and can be easily discerned. X200. PT.

(b) A diagram of a single multilocular adipocyte showing the central nucleus, numerous small lipid droplets (yellow), and many mitochondria. Also shown is a sympathetic nerve ending that releases norepinephrine to stimulate mitochondrial production of heat.

within the tissue and warms the locally circulating blood, which then distributes the heat throughout the body.

Heat production is increased in these cells because the mitochondria have in their inner membrane much greater levels of a transmembrane protein called **thermogenin** or **uncoupling protein (UCP-1)**. Thermogenin permits the backflow of protons previously transported to the intermembranous space without passing through the ATP–synthetase complexes. Consequently, the energy generated by proton flow dissipates as heat to warm the blood.

Histogenesis of Brown Adipose Tissue

Brown adipose tissue also develops from embryonic mesenchyme, with cells developing as growing preadipocytes, and emerges earlier than white fat during fetal development. In humans the amount of brown fat is maximal relative to body weight at birth, when thermogenesis is most needed and partially disappears by apoptosis and involution during childhood. In adults the amount and activity of brown fat are higher in lean individuals.

The number of brown adipocytes increases during cold adaptation in adults, usually appearing as clusters of multilocular cells in white adipose tissue. This may represent proliferation and differentiation of new adipocytes from preexisting progenitor cells or a change in the differentiated state of the white adipocytes. Besides stimulating thermogenic activity, autonomic nerves also promote brown adipocyte differentiation and prevent apoptosis in mature brown fat cells.

Adipose Tissue SUMMARY OF KEY POINTS

- The defining cells of adipose tissue (fat), **adipocytes**, are very large cells derived from mesenchyme and specialized for energy storage in lipid droplet(s) with **triglycerides**.
- Adipocytes store lipids from three sources: from dietary fats packaged as **chylomicrons** in the intestine; from triglycerides produced in the liver and circulating as **very-low-density lipoproteins (VLDLs)**; and from fatty acids synthesized locally.
- Lipids are mobilized from adipocytes by **lipases** that are activated by **hormones** (glucagon, growth hormone) and **norepinephrine** released from sympathetic nerves.
- Cells of adipose tissue are supported by reticular fibers, and connective tissue septa divide the tissue into lobules of various sizes.
- There are two types of adipose tissue: white and brown fat.

White Adipose Tissue

- **White adipose tissue** is found in many organs throughout the body, typically forming about 20% of the body weight in adults.
- Adipocytes of white fat are typically very **large cells**, ranging in diameter from 50 to 150 μm.

- These cells each contain primarily **one large lipid droplet** (they are **unilocular**), causing the nucleus and remaining cytoplasm to be pushed against the plasmalemma.
- Fatty acids are released from white adipocytes when nutrients are needed and carried throughout the body on plasma proteins such as albumin.

Brown Adipose Tissue

- **Brown fat** comprises up to 5% of the newborn body weight but smaller amounts in adults.
- Adipocytes of this tissue are typically smaller than those of white fat and contain primarily **many small lipid droplets** (they are **multilocular**) in cytoplasm containing many mitochondria and a central nucleus.
- Fatty acids released in adipocytes of brown fat are metabolized in mitochondria of these cells for **thermogenesis** rather than ATP synthesis, using **uncoupling protein-1** or thermogenin.

7 Cartilage

Cartilage is a tough, flexible form of connective tissue, characterized by an **extracellular matrix** (ECM) with high concentrations of GAGs and proteoglycans, which interact with collagen and elastic fibers. Variations in the composition of these matrix components and cells produce three types of cartilage adapted to local biomechanical needs (Figure 7–1).

The firm consistency of the cartilage ECM allows the tissue to bear mechanical stresses without permanent distortion. In the respiratory tract, ears, and nose, cartilage forms the framework supporting soft tissues. Because of its smooth, lubricated surface and resiliency, cartilage provides shock-absorbing and sliding regions within joints and facilitates bone movements. As described in the next chapter, cartilage also guides development and growth of long bones, both before and after birth.

Cartilage consists of cells called **chondrocytes** (Gr. *chondros*, cartilage + *kytos*, cell) embedded in an extensive ECM. Chondrocytes synthesize and maintain ECM components and are located in matrix cavities called **lacunae**. Collagen, hyaluronic acid, proteoglycans, and various glycoproteins are the principal macromolecules present in all types of cartilage matrix.

The physical properties of cartilage depend on electrostatic bonds between the flexible collagen and elastin fibers and the GAGs on densely packed proteoglycans. Its semi-rigid consistency is attributable to water (solvation water) bound to the negatively charged sulfated GAG chains extending from the proteoglycan core proteins. The high content of bound water allows cartilage to serve as a shock absorber, a role of major functional importance.

Different functional requirements have selected for the three major forms of cartilage, each varying somewhat in matrix composition. In **hyaline cartilage**, the most common form, type II collagen is the principal collagen type (Figure 7–1). The more pliable and distensible **elastic cartilage** possesses abundant elastic fibers in addition to collagen type II. **Fibrocartilage**, present in body regions subjected to pulling forces, is characterized by a matrix containing a dense network of coarse type I collagen fibers.

In all three forms, cartilage is *avascular* and receives nutrients by diffusion from capillaries in adjacent connective tissue (perichondrium). In some instances, large blood vessels traverse cartilage to supply other tissues, but these vessels release few nutrients to the cartilage. As might be expected of cells in an avascular tissue, chondrocytes exhibit low metabolic activity. Cartilage also lacks lymphatic vessels and nerves.

The **perichondrium** (Figure 7–2) is a sheath of dense connective tissue that surrounds cartilage in most places, forming an interface between the cartilage and the tissues supported by the cartilage. The perichondrium harbors the cartilage's vascular supply, as well as nerves and lymphatic vessels. Articular cartilage, which covers the surfaces of bones in movable joints, lacks perichondrium and is sustained by the diffusion of oxygen and nutrients from the synovial fluid.

>> **MEDICAL APPLICATION**

Many genetic conditions in humans or mice that cause defective cartilage, joint deformities, or short limbs are due to recessive mutations in genes for collagen type II, the aggrecan core protein, the sulfate transporter, and other proteins required for normal chondrocyte function.

❭ HYALINE CARTILAGE

Hyaline (Gr. *hyalos*, glassy) cartilage (Figure 7–1), the most common of the three forms, is homogeneous and semitransparent in the fresh state. In adults hyaline cartilage is located in the articular surfaces of movable joints, in the walls of larger respiratory passages (nose, larynx, trachea, bronchi), in the ventral ends of ribs, where they articulate with the sternum, and

FIGURE **7–1** Distribution of cartilage in adults.

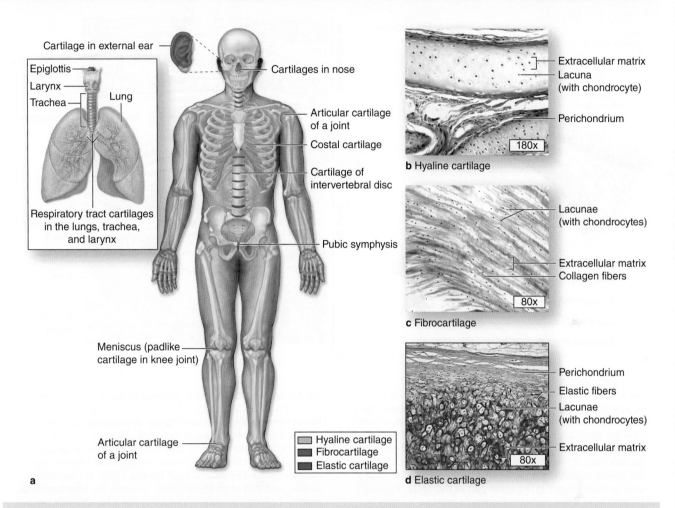

a

Cartilage in external ear

Epiglottis
Larynx
Trachea
Lung

Respiratory tract cartilages in the lungs, trachea, and larynx

Cartilages in nose

Articular cartilage of a joint

Costal cartilage

Cartilage of intervertebral disc

Pubic symphysis

Meniscus (padlike cartilage in knee joint)

Articular cartilage of a joint

☐ Hyaline cartilage
■ Fibrocartilage
■ Elastic cartilage

Extracellular matrix
Lacuna (with chondrocyte)

Perichondrium

180x

b Hyaline cartilage

Lacunae (with chondrocytes)

Extracellular matrix
Collagen fibers

80x

c Fibrocartilage

Perichondrium

Elastic fibers

Lacunae (with chondrocytes)

Extracellular matrix

80x

d Elastic cartilage

(a) There are three types of adult cartilage distributed in many areas of the skeleton, particularly in joints and where pliable support is useful, as in the ribs, ears, and nose. Cartilage support of other tissues throughout the respiratory tract is also prominent. The photomicrographs show the main features of **(b)** hyaline cartilage, **(c)** fibrocartilage, and **(d)** elastic cartilage. Dense connective tissue of perichondrium is shown here with hyaline and elastic cartilage.

in the epiphyseal plates of long bones, where it makes possible longitudinal bone growth. In the embryo, hyaline cartilage forms the temporary skeleton that is gradually replaced by bone.

> **▶▶ MEDICAL APPLICATION**
>
> **Osteoarthritis,** a chronic condition that commonly occurs during aging, involves the gradual loss or changed physical properties of the hyaline cartilage that lines the articular ends of bones in joints. Joints that are weight-bearing (knees, hips) or heavily used (wrist, fingers) are most prone to cartilage degeneration. Fragments released by wear-and-tear to the articular cartilage trigger secretion of matrix metalloproteinases and other factors from macrophages in adjacent tissues, which exacerbate damage and cause pain and inflammation within the joint.

Matrix

The dry weight of hyaline cartilage is 40% collagen embedded in a firm, hydrated gel of proteoglycans and structural glycoproteins. In routine histology preparations, the proteoglycans cause the matrix to be generally basophilic and the thin collagen fibrils are barely discernible. Most of the collagen in hyaline cartilage is **type II collagen**, although small amounts of several minor types are also present.

Aggrecan (250 kD), with approximately 150 GAG side chains of chondroitin sulfate and keratan sulfate, is the most abundant proteoglycan of hyaline cartilage. Hundreds of these proteoglycans are bound noncovalently by link proteins to long polymers of hyaluronic acid, as shown schematically in Figure 7–2a and discussed in Chapter 5. These proteoglycan complexes bind further to the surface of type II collagen fibrils

FIGURE **7–2** The structure of cartilage matrix and cells.

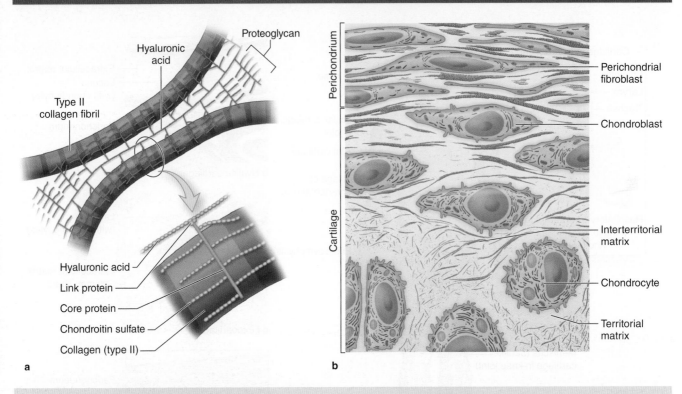

a

b

(a) A schematic representation of the most abundant molecules in cartilage matrix shows the interaction between type II collagen fibrils and proteoglycans linked to hyaluronic acid. Link proteins noncovalently bind the protein core of proteoglycans to the linear hyaluronic acid molecules. The chondroitin sulfate side chains of the proteoglycan electrostatically bind to the collagen fibrils, forming a cross-linked matrix. The circled area is shown larger in the lower part of the figure. Physical properties of these matrix components produce a highly hydrated, pliable material with great strength. Approximately 75% of the wet weight of hyaline cartilage is water.

(b) A diagram of the transitional area between the perichondrium and the cartilage matrix. Fibroblast-like progenitor cells in the perichondrium give rise to larger chondroblasts, which divide and differentiate as chondrocytes. These functional cells produce matrix components and exist in lacunae embedded in the matrix. Staining differences are apparent between the matrix immediately around each lacuna, called the **territorial matrix**, and that more distant from lacunae, the **interterritorial matrix**. Collagen is more abundant in the interterritorial parts of the matrix.

(Figure 7–2a). Water bound to GAGs in the proteoglycans constitutes up 60%-80% of the weight of fresh hyaline cartilage.

Another important component of cartilage matrix is the structural multiadhesive glycoprotein **chondronectin**. Like fibronectin in other connective tissues, chondronectin binds specifically to GAGs, collagen type II, and integrins, mediating the adherence of chondrocytes to the ECM.

Staining variations within the matrix reflect local differences in its molecular composition. Immediately surrounding each chondrocyte, the ECM is relatively richer in GAGs, often causing these areas of **territorial matrix** to stain differently from the intervening areas of interterritorial matrix (Figures 7–2b and 7–3).

Chondrocytes

Cells occupy relatively little of the hyaline cartilage mass. At the periphery of the cartilage, young chondrocytes (or chondroblasts) have an elliptic shape, with the long axis parallel to the surface (Figure 7–3). Deeper in the cartilage, they are round and may appear in groups of up to eight cells that originate from mitotic divisions of a single chondrocyte and are called **isogenous aggregates**. As the chondrocytes become more active in secreting collagens and other ECM components, the aggregated cells are pushed apart and occupy separate lacunae.

Cartilage cells and the matrix often shrink during routine histologic preparation, resulting in both the irregular shape of the chondrocytes and their retraction from the matrix. In living tissue, and in properly prepared sections, the chondrocytes fill the lacunae completely.

Because cartilage is devoid of blood capillaries, chondrocytes respire under low-oxygen tension. Hyaline cartilage cells metabolize glucose mainly by anaerobic glycolysis to produce lactic acid as the end product. Nutrients from the blood diffuse from the perichondrium to reach the deeper

FIGURE **7–3** Hyaline cartilage.

(a) The upper part of the photo shows the more acidophilic perichondrium (**P**), an example of dense connective tissue consisting largely of type I collagen. There is a gradual transition and differentiation of cells from the perichondrium to the cartilage, with elongated fibroblastic cells becoming larger and more rounded chondroblasts and chondrocytes (**C**) located within spaces or lacunae surrounded by the matrix (**M**) secreted by the cells. X200. H&E.

(b) The thin region of hyaline cartilage shown here has perichondrium (**P**) on both sides and shows larger lacunae containing isogenous groups of chondrocytes (**C**) within the matrix (**M**). Such groups of two, four, or more cells are produced by mitosis; the cells will separate into individual lacunae as they begin to secrete matrix. X160. H&E.

chondrocytes. Transport of water and solutes in the matrix is promoted by the pumping action of intermittent cartilage compression and decompression. Because of the limits of diffusion, the maximum thickness of the hyaline cartilage is limited and it usually exists as small, thin plates.

>> **MEDICAL APPLICATION**

The inability of cartilage to regenerate or to be repaired fully may be attributed to the chondrocytes' immobility, low metabolic and mitotic rates, and avascularity. If a cartilage injury involves the perichondrium, new chondroblasts and fibroblasts may be mobilized and limited repair can occur, but most of the new tissue produced is dense connective tissue and normal function of the cartilage is often impaired.

Chondrocyte synthesis of sulfated GAGs and secretion of proteoglycans are accelerated by many hormones and growth factors. A major regulator of hyaline cartilage growth is pituitary-derived growth hormone or **somatotropin**. This hormone acts indirectly, promoting the endocrine release from the liver of insulin-like growth factors, or somatomedins, which directly stimulates proliferation of chondrocytes.

>> **MEDICAL APPLICATION**

Cells of cartilage can give rise to either benign (**chondroma**) or slow-growing, malignant (**chondrosarcoma**) tumors in which cells produce normal matrix components. Chondrosarcomas seldom metastasize and are generally removed surgically.

Perichondrium

Except in the articular cartilage of joints, all hyaline cartilage is covered by a layer of dense connective tissue, the **perichondrium**, which is essential for the growth and maintenance of cartilage (Figures 7–2b and 7–3). The perichondrium consists largely of collagen type I fibers and fibroblasts. Among these fibroblasts in the inner layer of the perichondrium are progenitor cells for chondroblasts that divide and differentiate into chondrocytes.

› ELASTIC CARTILAGE

Elastic cartilage is essentially similar to hyaline cartilage except that it contains an abundant network of elastic fibers in addition to collagen type II (Figure 7–4), which give fresh elastic cartilage a yellowish color. Demonstration of the elastic fibers usually requires stains such as orcein or resorcin fuchsin.

Elastic cartilage is found in the auricle of the ear, the walls of the external auditory canals, the auditory (eustachian) tubes, the epiglottis, and the cuneiform cartilage in the larynx. Elastic cartilage in these locations includes a perichondrium similar to that of most hyaline cartilage.

› FIBROCARTILAGE

Fibrocartilage takes various forms but is essentially a combination of hyaline cartilage and dense connective tissue with gradual transitions between these tissues (Figure 7–1;

Figure 7–5). It is found in intervertebral discs, in attachments of certain ligaments, and in the pubic symphysis.

Chondrocytes of fibrocartilage occur singly and in aligned isogenous aggregates and produce matrix containing type II collagen. In some fibrocartilage this matrix around the chondrocytes is very sparse. Regions with chondrocytes and hyaline matrix are separated by other regions containing bundles of type I collagen and scattered fibroblasts (Figure 7–5). The relative scarcity of proteoglycans makes the matrix of fibrocartilage more acidophilic than that of hyaline or elastic cartilage. There is no distinct surrounding perichondrium in fibrocartilage.

Intervertebral discs of the spinal column are composed primarily of fibrocartilage and act as lubricated cushions and shock absorbers preventing adjacent vertebrae from being damaged by abrasive forces or impacts. Held in place by ligaments, each disc has two major components (see Figure 8–22): the peripheral annulus fibrosus rich in bundles of type I collagen and the central nucleus pulposus with a gel-like matrix

---

FIGURE **7–4** Elastic cartilage.

The chondrocytes (**C**) and overall organization of elastic cartilage are similar to those of hyaline cartilage. Stains for elastin, however, reveal many dark-staining elastic fibers in the matrix (**M**), in addition to the major components found in hyaline matrix. Elastic fibers provide greater flexibility to this form of cartilage. The section in part **b** includes perichondrium (**P**) that is also similar to that of hyaline cartilage. **(a)** X160. Hematoxylin and orcein. **(b)** X100. Weigert resorcin-fuchsin.

FIGURE **7–5** Fibrocartilage.

Fibrocartilage varies in different organs, but is essentially a mixture of hyaline cartilage and dense connective tissue.

(a) A section of pubic symphysis shows lacunae with isolated and grouped chondrocytes (**C**) surrounded by matrix (**M**) and separated in some areas by dense regions (**D**) containing more concentrated acidophilic type I collagen. No separate perichondrium is present on fibrocartilage. X100. H&E.

(b) At higher magnification in a small region of intervertebral disc, the axially arranged aggregates of chondrocytes (**C**) are seen to be surrounded by small amounts of matrix and separated by larger regions with dense collagen (**D**) and a small number of fibroblasts with elongated nuclei (arrows). X250. Picrosirius-hematoxylin.

rich in hyaluronic acid. These structures are discussed further with joints in Chapter 8. Important features of the three major types of cartilage are summarized in Table 7–1.

❯ CARTILAGE FORMATION, GROWTH, & REPAIR

All cartilage forms from embryonic mesenchyme in the process of **chondrogenesis** (Figure 7–6). The first indication of cell differentiation is the rounding up of the mesenchymal cells, which retract their extensions, multiply rapidly, and become more densely packed together. The dividing cells are typically called **chondroblasts** and **chondrocytes** when proliferation has ceased; both have basophilic cytoplasm rich in RER for collagen synthesis (Figure 7–7). Production of the ECM encloses the cells in their lacunae and then gradually separates chondroblasts from one another. During embryonic development, the differentiation of cartilage takes place primarily from the center outward; therefore the more central cells have the characteristics of chondrocytes, whereas the peripheral cells are typical chondroblasts. The superficial mesenchyme forms the perichondrium.

Once initially formed, the cartilage tissue enlarges both by **interstitial growth**, resulting from the mitotic division of preexisting chondroblasts, and by **appositional growth**, which involves differentiation of new chondroblasts from the perichondrium (Figure 7–2b). In both cases, the synthesis of matrix contributes greatly to the growth of the cartilage. Appositional growth of cartilage is more important during postnatal development, although interstitial growth in the articular cartilage and epiphyseal plates of long bones is important in increasing the length of long bones (see Chapter 8). In articular cartilage, cells and matrix near the articulating surface are gradually worn away and must be replaced from within, because there is no perichondrium to add cells by appositional growth.

Except in young children, damaged cartilage undergoes slow and often incomplete **repair**, primarily by activity of cells in the perichondrium, which invade the injured area and produce new cartilage. In extensively damaged areas the perichondrium produces a scar of dense connective tissue instead of forming new cartilage. The poor capacity of cartilage for repair or regeneration is due in part to the avascularity of this tissue.

❯❯ MEDICAL APPLICATION

In contrast to other forms of cartilage and other tissues, hyaline cartilage is susceptible to **calcification** during aging. Calcification of the hyaline matrix, accompanied by degenerative changes in the chondrocytes, is a common part of the aging process and in many respects resembles endochondral ossification by which bone is formed.

FIGURE **7–6** Chondrogenesis.

The diagrams show the major stages by which embryonic cartilage is formed. **(a)** Mesenchyme is the precursor for all types of cartilage. **(b)** Mitosis and early differentiation produces a tissue with condensations of rounded cells called **chondroblasts**. **(c)** Chondroblasts are then separated from one another again by their production of various matrix components, which collectively swell with water and form the very extensive ECM.

(d) Multiplication of chondroblasts within the matrix gives rise to **isogenous cell aggregates** surrounded by a condensation of territorial matrix. In mature cartilage, this interstitial mitotic activity ceases and all chondrocytes typically become more widely separated by their production of matrix.

FIGURE **7–7** Chondrocytes in growing cartilage.

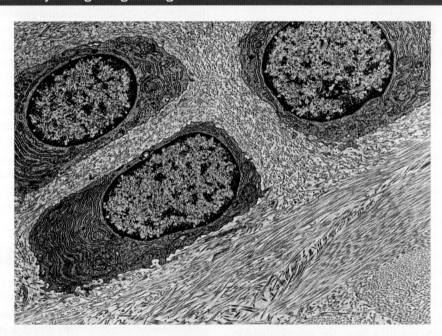

This TEM of **fibrocartilage** shows **chondrocytes** with abundant **RER** actively secreting the collagen-rich matrix. Fine **collagen fibers**, sectioned in several orientations, are prominent around the chondrocytes of fibrocartilage. Chondrocytes in growing hyaline and elastic cartilage have more prominent Golgi complexes and synthesize abundant proteoglycans in addition to collagens. X3750.

TABLE **7–1**	Important features of the major cartilage types.		
	Hyaline Cartilage	**Elastic Cartilage**	**Fibrocartilage**
Main features of the extracellular matrix	Homogeneous, with type II collagen and aggrecan	Type II collagen, aggrecan, and darker elastic fibers	Type II collagen and large areas of dense connective tissue with type I collagen
Major cells	Chondrocytes, chondroblasts	Chondrocytes, chondroblasts	Chondrocytes, fibroblasts
Typical arrangement of chondrocytes	Isolated or in small isogenous groups	Usually in small isogenous groups	Isolated or in isogenous groups arranged axially
Presence of perichondrium	Yes (except at epiphyses and articular cartilage)	Yes	No
Main locations or examples	Many components of upper respiratory tract; articular ends and epiphyseal plates of long bones; fetal skeleton	External ear, external acoustic meatus, auditory tube; epiglottis and certain other laryngeal cartilages	Intervertebral discs, pubic symphysis, meniscus, and certain other joints; insertions of tendons
Main functions	Provides smooth, low-friction surfaces in joints; structural support for respiratory tract	Provides flexible shape and support of soft tissues	Provides cushioning, tensile strength, and resistance to tearing and compression

Cartilage SUMMARY OF KEY POINTS

- Cartilage is a **tough**, **resilient** type of connective tissue that structurally supports certain soft tissues, notably in the respiratory tract, and provides cushioned, low-friction surfaces in joints.
- Cells of cartilage, **chondrocytes**, make up a small percentage of the tissue's mass, which is mainly a flexible mass of **extracellular matrix (ECM)**.
- Chondrocytes are embedded within **lacunae** surrounded by the ECM.
- Cartilage ECM typically includes **collagen** as well as abundant **proteoglycans**, notably **aggrecan**, which bind a large amount of **water**.
- Cartilage always **lacks blood vessels**, lymphatics, and nerves, but it is usually surrounded by a dense connective tissue **perichondrium** that is vascularized.
- There are three major forms of cartilage: (1) **hyaline cartilage**, (2) **elastic cartilage**, and (3) **fibrocartilage**.

Hyaline Cartilage

- The ECM of hyaline cartilage is **homogenous and glassy**, rich in fibrils of type II collagen and aggrecan complexes with bound water.
- The ECM has less collagen and more proteoglycan immediately around the lacunae, producing slight staining differences in this **territorial matrix**.
- Chondrocytes occur **singly** or in small, mitotically derived **isogenous groups**.
- **Perichondrium** is usually present, but not at the hyaline cartilage of articular surfaces or the epiphyses of growing long bones.

Elastic Cartilage

- Elastic cartilage generally resembles hyaline cartilage in its chondrocytes and major ECM components, but its matrix includes **abundant elastic fibers**, visible with special stains, which increase the tissue's flexibility.
- Elastic cartilage provides flexible support for the external ear as well as certain structures of the middle ear and larynx; it is always surrounded by **perichondrium**.

Fibrocartilage

- Fibrocartilage contains varying **combinations of hyaline cartilage** in small amounts of **dense connective tissue**.
- Histologically it consists of small **chondrocytes** in a hyaline matrix, usually layered with larger areas of bundled **type I collagen** with scattered **fibroblasts**.
- Fibrocartilage provides very **tough**, **strong support** at tendon insertions and in **intervertebral discs** and certain other joints.

Cartilage Formation, Growth, & Repair

- All forms of cartilage form from embryonic **mesenchyme**.
- Cartilaginous structures grow by mitosis of existing chondroblasts in lacunae (**interstitial growth**) or formation of new chondroblasts peripherally from progenitor cells in the perichondrium (**appositional growth**).
- Repair or replacement of injured cartilage is very slow and ineffective, due in part to the tissue's **avascularity** and **low metabolic rate**.

8 Bone

As the main constituent of the adult skeleton, bone tissue (Figure 8–1) provides solid support for the body, protects vital organs such as those in the cranial and thoracic cavities, and harbors cavities containing bone marrow where blood cells are formed. Bone (or osseous) tissue also serves as a reservoir of calcium, phosphate, and other ions that can be released or stored in a controlled fashion to maintain constant concentrations in body fluids.

In addition, bones form a system of levers that multiply the forces generated during skeletal muscle contraction and transform them into bodily movements. This mineralized tissue therefore confers mechanical and metabolic functions to the skeleton.

Bone is a specialized connective tissue composed of calcified extracellular material, the **bone matrix**, and three major cell types (Figure 8–2):

- **Osteocytes** (Gr. *osteon*, bone + *kytos*, cell), which are found in cavities (**lacunae**) between bone matrix layers (**lamellae**), with cytoplasmic processes extending into small **canaliculi** (L. *canalis*, canal) between lamellae (Figure 8–1).
- **Osteoblasts** (*osteon* + Gr. *blastos*, germ), which synthesize the organic components of the matrix
- **Osteoclasts** (*osteon* + Gr. *klastos*, broken), which are multinucleated, giant cells involved in the resorption and remodeling of bone tissue.

Because metabolites are unable to diffuse through the calcified matrix of bone, the exchanges between osteocytes and blood capillaries depend on communication through the very thin, cylindrical spaces of the canaliculi.

All bones are lined on both internal and external surfaces by layers of connective tissue containing osteogenic cells—**endosteum** on the internal surface surrounding the marrow cavity and **periosteum** on the external surface.

Because of its hardness, bone cannot be sectioned routinely. Bone matrix is usually softened by immersion in a decalcifying solution before paraffin embedding, or embedded in plastic after fixation and sectioned with a specialized microtome.

› BONE CELLS

Osteoblasts

Osteoblasts synthesize and secrete the organic components of bone matrix, which include type I collagen fibers, proteoglycans, and several glycoproteins such as osteonectin. Deposition of the inorganic components of bone also depends on viable osteoblasts. Mature osteoblasts are located exclusively at the surfaces of bone matrix, usually side by side in a layer somewhat resembling a simple epithelium (Figures 8–2 and 8–3). When actively engaged in matrix synthesis, osteoblasts have a cuboidal to columnar shape and basophilic cytoplasm. When their synthesizing activity declines, they flatten and basophilia is reduced; inactive osteoblasts represent most of the flattened **bone lining cells** in both the endosteum and periosteum.

During matrix synthesis, osteoblasts have the ultrastructure of cells actively synthesizing proteins for secretion. Osteoblasts are polarized cells: matrix components are secreted at the cell surface in contact with existing bone matrix, producing

FIGURE **8–1** Components of bone.

Diaphysis of humerus

Central canal

Osteon

External circumferential lamellae

Perforating fibers

Periosteum

Fibrous layer

Cellular layer

Internal circumferential lamellae

Interstitial lamellae

Inner circumferential lamellae

Trabeculae of spongy bone

Perforating canals

Central canal

(a) Section of humerus

Concentric lamellae

Nerve

Vein

Artery

Collagen fiber orientation

Canaliculi

Central canal

Osteon

Lacuna

Osteocyte

Canaliculi

(b) Compact bone

Space for bone marrow

Trabeculae

Canaliculi opening at surface

Endosteum

Osteoclast

Lamellae

Osteocyte in lacuna

Osteoblasts aligned along trabecula of new bone

Canaliculi opening at surface

(c) Spongy bone

A schematic overview of the basic features of bone, including the three key cell types: **osteocytes**, **osteoblasts**, and **osteoclasts**; their usual locations; and the typical **lamellar organization** of bone. Osteoblasts secrete the matrix that then hardens by calcification, trapping the differentiating cells now called **osteocytes** in individual **lacunae**. Osteocytes maintain the calcified matrix and receive nutrients from microvasculature in the central canals of the osteons via very small channels called

canaliculi that interconnect the lacunae. Osteoclasts are monocyte-derived cells in bone required for bone remodeling.

The **periosteum** consists of dense connective tissue, with a primarily fibrous layer covering a more cellular layer. Bone is vascularized by small vessels that penetrate the matrix from the periosteum. **Endosteum** covers all **trabeculae** around the marrow cavities.

FIGURE 8–2   Osteoblasts, osteocytes, and an osteoclast.

Bone-forming osteoblasts (**Ob**) differentiate from osteoprogenitor cells in the periosteum and endosteum, and cover the surfaces of existing bone matrix. Osteoblasts secrete **osteoid** containing collagen type I, proteoglycans and other molecules, and matrix vesicles. As osteoid undergoes calcification, hardens, and traps the osteoblasts, these cells differentiate further as osteocytes (**Oc**), which occupy lacunae surrounded by bony matrix. The much less numerous large, multinuclear osteoclasts (**Ocl**), produced by the fusion of blood monocytes, reside on bony surfaces and erode the matrix during bone remodeling. 400X. Mallory trichrome.

FIGURE 8–3   Osteoblasts and osteocytes.

(a) Diagram showing the relationship of osteoblasts to osteoid, bone matrix, and osteocytes. Osteoblasts and most of the larger osteoclasts are part of the endosteum covering the bony trabeculae.

(b) The photomicrograph of developing bone shows the location and morphologic differences between active osteoblasts (**Ob**) and osteocytes (**Oc**). Rounded osteoblasts, derived from

cells in the adjacent mesenchyme (**M**), appear as a layer of cells adjacent to a very thin layer of lightly stained osteoid (**Os**) that covers the more heavily stained bony matrix (**B**). Inactive osteoblasts are more flattened and cover the bony surface shown near the top here. Osteocytes are located within lacunae surrounded by matrix. X300. H&E.

a layer of new (but not yet calcified) material called **osteoid** between the osteoblast layer and the preexisting bone surface (Figure 8–2). This process of bone appositional growth is completed by subsequent deposition of calcium salts into the newly formed matrix.

Calcification of the matrix is not completely understood, but basic aspects of the process are shown in Figure 8–4. Prominent among the noncollagen proteins secreted by osteoblasts is the small, vitamin K–dependent polypeptide **osteocalcin**, which together with various glycoproteins binds Ca^{2+} ions and raises their concentration locally. Osteoblasts also release membrane-enclosed **matrix vesicles** rich in alkaline phosphatase and other enzymes whose activity raises the local concentration

>> **MEDICAL APPLICATION**

Cancer originating directly from bone cells (a primary bone tumor) is fairly uncommon (0.5% of all cancer deaths), although a cancer called **osteosarcoma** can arise in osteoprogenitor cells. The skeleton is often the site of secondary, **metastatic tumors**, however, arising when cancer cells move into bones via small blood or lymphatic vessels from malignancies in other organs, most commonly the breast, lung, prostate gland, kidney, or thyroid gland.

FIGURE **8–4** Mineralization in bone matrix.

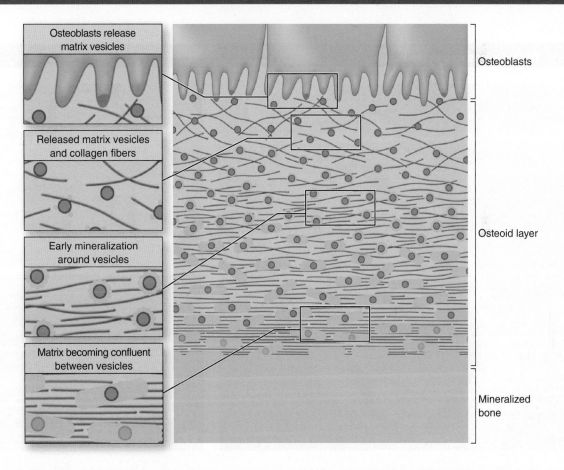

Osteoblasts release matrix vesicles

Released matrix vesicles and collagen fibers

Early mineralization around vesicles

Matrix becoming confluent between vesicles

Osteoblasts

Osteoid layer

Mineralized bone

From their ends adjacent to the matrix, osteoblasts secrete type I collagen, several glycoproteins, and proteoglycans. Some of these factors, notably osteocalcin and certain glycoproteins, bind Ca^{2+} with high affinity, thus raising the local concentration of these ions. Osteoblasts also release very small membrane-enclosed **matrix vesicles** with which alkaline phosphatase and other enzymes are associated. These enzymes hydrolyze PO_4^- ions from various macromolecules,

creating a high concentration of these ions locally. The high ion concentrations cause calcified nanocrystals to form in and around the matrix vesicles. The crystals grow and mineralize further with formation of small growing masses of calcium hydroxyapatite [$Ca_{10}(PO_4)_6(OH)_2$], which surround the collagen fibers and all other macromolecules. Eventually the masses of hydroxyapatite merge as a confluent solid bony matrix as calcification of the matrix is completed.

of PO_4^- ions. With high concentrations of both calcium and phosphate ions, these vesicles serve as foci for the formation of hydroxyapatite $[Ca_{10}(PO_4)_6(OH)_2]$ crystals, the first visible step in calcification. These crystals grow rapidly by accretion of more mineral and eventually produce a confluent mass of calcified material embedding the collagen fibers and proteoglycans.

Osteocytes

Many osteoblasts are gradually surrounded by the material they secreted and differentiate further as **osteocytes** enclosed singly within the **lacunae** that are regularly spaced throughout the mineralized matrix. In the transition from osteoblasts to osteocytes, the cells extend many long dendritic processes, which also become surrounded by calcifying matrix. Osteocytic processes thus come to occupy the many canaliculi, 250-300 nm in diameter, that radiate from each lacuna (Figure 8–5; see Figure 8–1).

Diffusion of metabolites between osteocytes and blood vessels occurs through the small amount of extracellular fluid between the bone matrix and the osteocytes and their processes. Osteocytes also communicate with one another via gap junctions on the dendritic processes in the canaliculi and on osteoblasts and bone lining cells.

When compared with osteoblasts, the flat, almond-shaped osteocytes exhibit significantly less RER, smaller Golgi complexes, and more condensed nuclear chromatin (Figure 8–5a). These cells maintain the bony matrix, and their death is followed by rapid matrix resorption. Osteocytes express a different array of genes compared to osteoblasts, and osteocyte products such as the protein sclerostin and certain cytokines help regulate bone remodeling. The extensive lacunar-canalicular network of osteocytes and their communication with all other bone cells suggest additional roles for osteocytes in calcium homeostasis and as sensors for detection

---

FIGURE **8–5** Osteocytes in lacunae.

(a) TEM showing an osteocyte in a lacuna and two dendritic processes surrounded by matrix. Such processes are extended as osteoid is being secreted, and this material calcifies around the processes, giving rise to canaliculi (**C**) in the bony matrix.

(b) Photomicrograph of bone, not decalcified and sectioned, but ground very thin to demonstrate lacunae and canaliculi. The lacunae and canaliculi (**C**) appear dark and show the

communication between these structures through which nutrients derived from blood vessels diffuse and are passed from cell to cell in living bone. X400. Ground bone.

(c) SEM of non-decalcified, sectioned, and acid-etched bone showing lacunae and canaliculi (**C**). X400.

(*Part c with permission, from Dr Matt Allen, Indiana University School of Medicine, Indianapolis.*)

of mechanical stresses on bone, which is also important in directing bone remodeling.

Osteoclasts

Osteoclasts are very large, motile cells with multiple nuclei (Figure 8–6) and play a major role in matrix resorption during bone growth and remodeling. The large size and multinucleated condition of osteoclasts are due to their origin from the fusion of bone marrow–derived cells. Osteoclast development requires two polypeptides produced by osteoblasts: macrophage-colony–stimulating factor (M-CSF; discussed with hemopoiesis, Chapter 13) and the receptor activator of nuclear factor-κB ligand (RANKL). In areas of bone undergoing resorption, osteoclasts lie within enzymatically etched depressions or cavities in the matrix known as **resorption cavities** (also called **Howship lacunae**).

In active osteoclasts, the surface against the bone matrix is folded into irregular projections, forming a **ruffled border** surrounded by a cytoplasmic zone rich in actin filaments, which is the site of adhesion to the matrix. This circumferential adhesion zone creates a microenvironment between the osteoclast and the matrix in which bone resorption occurs (see Figure 8–6b).

Into this subcellular pocket the osteoclast secretes collagenase, cathepsin K, and other enzymes and pumps protons to produce an acidic environment locally for dissolving hydroxyapatite and promoting the localized digestion of matrix proteins. Osteoclast activity is controlled by local signaling factors and hormones. Osteoclasts have receptors for calcitonin, a thyroid hormone. Osteoblasts activated by parathyroid hormone (PTH) produce M-CSF, RANKL, and other factors that regulate the formation and activity of osteoclasts.

≫ BONE MATRIX

Inorganic material represents about 50% of the dry weight of bone matrix. Calcium hydroxyapatite is most abundant, but bicarbonate, citrate, magnesium, potassium, and sodium ions are also found. Significant quantities of amorphous (noncrystalline) calcium phosphate are also present. The surface ions of hydroxyapatite crystals are hydrated; the layer of water around the crystal facilitates the exchange of ions between the mineral and body fluids.

The organic matter embedded in the calcified matrix includes type I collagen, proteoglycan aggregates, and bone-specific multiadhesive glycoproteins such as **osteonectin**. Calcium-binding glycoproteins, notably osteocalcin, and the phosphatases released in matrix vesicles by osteoblasts promote calcification of the matrix. Other tissues containing type I collagen do not contain osteocalcin or matrix vesicles and are not normally calcified. Because of its high collagen content, decalcified bone matrix is usually acidophilic.

The association of minerals with collagen fibers during calcification is responsible for the hardness and resistance of bone tissue. After a bone is decalcified, its shape is preserved, but it becomes as flexible as a tendon.

≫ PERIOSTEUM & ENDOSTEUM

External and internal surfaces of bone are covered by tissue layers with bone-forming cells, called **periosteum** and **endosteum**, respectively.

The **periosteum** is organized much like the perichondrium (see Figure 7–3a). The outer layer is dense connective tissue, with small blood vessels, collagen bundles, and fibroblasts (see Figure 8–1). Bundles of periosteal collagen fibers, called **perforating (or Sharpey) fibers**, penetrate the bone matrix, binding the periosteum to bone. The inner region of periosteum is a more cellular layer containing bone lining cells, osteoblasts, and mesenchymal stem cells called **osteoprogenitor cells**. With the potential to proliferate and differentiate into osteoblasts, osteoprogenitor cells play a prominent role in bone growth and in bone repair. The principal functions of periosteum are to nourish the osseous tissue and provide a continuous supply of new osteoblasts for **appositional bone growth** or repair.

Internally the very thin **endosteum** covers small **trabeculae** of bony matrix that project into the marrow cavities (Figures 8-1 and 8-3). Although considerably thinner than the periosteum, endosteum also contains osteoprogenitor cells, osteoblasts, and bone lining cells.

FIGURE **8–6** Osteoclasts and their activity.

The osteoclast is a large cell with several nuclei derived by the fusion in bone of several blood-derived monocytes. **(a)** Microscopic section showing two osteoclasts (**Ocl**) digesting or resorbing bone matrix (**B**) in resorption cavities on the matrix surface. A lacuna with an osteocyte (**Oc**) is also shown. X400. H&E.

(b) Diagram showing an osteoclast's circumferential zone where integrins tightly bind the matrix and surround a **ruffled border** of cytoplasmic projections close to this matrix. The sealed space between the cell and the matrix is acidified to ~pH 4.5 by a proton pump located in the osteoclast membrane and receives hydrolytic enzymes secreted from

lysosomes by exocytosis. Acidification of this confined space facilitates the dissolution of calcium apatite from bone and creates the optimal pH for activity of the lysosomal hydrolases. Bone matrix is thus resorbed, with products of matrix digestion released for reuse and calcium, carbonate, and other ions released from uptake by the blood.

(c) SEM showing an active osteoclast cultured on a flat substrate of bone. A trench is formed on the bone surface as the osteoclast crawls along. X5000.

(*Figure 8–6c, with permission, from Alan Boyde, Centre for Oral Growth and Development, University of London.*)

❯ TYPES OF BONE

Gross observation of a bone in cross section (Figure 8–7) shows a dense area near the surface corresponding to **compact (cortical) bone**, which represents 80% of the total bone mass, and deeper areas with numerous interconnecting cavities, called **cancellous (trabecular or spongy) bone**, constituting about 20% of total bone mass. Histological features and important locations of the major types of bone are summarized (Table 8-1) near the end of this chapter.

In long bones, the bulbous ends—called **epiphyses** (Gr. *epiphysis*, an excrescence)—are composed of spongy bone covered by a thin layer of compact bone. The cylindrical part—the **diaphysis** (Gr. *diaphysis*, a growing between)—is almost totally composed of compact bone, with a thin region of spongy bone on the inner surface around the central **marrow cavity** (see Figure 8–1). Short bones such as those of the wrist and ankle usually have cores of spongy bone surrounded completely by compact bone. The flat bones that form the calvaria (skullcap) have two layers of compact bone called **plates**, separated by a thicker layer of spongy bone called the **diploë**.

Microscopic examination of bone tissue shows two types of organization: **lamellar bone** and **woven bone**, which is usually more immature than lamellar bone.

Lamellar Bone

Most bone in adults, compact or cancellous, is organized as **lamellar bone**, characterized by multiple layers or **lamellae** of calcified matrix, each 3-7 μm thick. The lamellae are organized either parallel to each other or concentrically around a central canal. In each lamella, type I collagen fibers are aligned in parallel, with the pitch of the fibers' orientation shifted orthogonally (by about 90 degrees) in successive lamellae. This highly ordered organization of collagen within lamellar bone is visible under the polarizing light microscope as birefringence; alternating bright and dark layers are due to the changing orientation of collagen fibers in the lamellae (Figure 8–8). Like the orientation of wood fibers in plywood, the highly ordered organization of collagen fibers in lamellae adds greatly to the strength of lamellar bone.

An **osteon** (or **Haversian system**) refers to the complex of concentric lamellae surrounding a small central canal that contains blood vessels, nerves, loose connective tissue, and endosteum (see Figures 8–1 and 8–9). Between successive lamellae are lacunae, each with one osteocyte, interconnected by canaliculi containing the cells' dendritic processes (Figure 8–9). Processes of adjacent cells are in contact via gap junctions, and all cells of an osteon receive nutrients and oxygen from the microvasculature in the central canal (see Figure 8–1). The outer boundary of each osteon is a more collagen-rich layer called the **cement line**.

Each osteon is a long, sometimes bifurcated, cylinder generally parallel to the long axis of the diaphysis. It consists of a central canal surrounded by 4-10 concentric lamellae. The central canals communicate with the marrow cavity and the periosteum and with one another through transverse **perforating canals** (or **Volkmann canals**) (Figures 8–1 and 8–10). The transverse canals have few, if any, concentric lamellae. All central osteonic canals and perforating canals come into existence when matrix is laid down around areas with preexisting blood vessels.

Scattered among the intact osteons are numerous irregularly shaped groups of parallel lamellae called **interstitial lamellae**. These structures are lamellae remaining from osteons partially destroyed by osteoclasts during growth and remodeling of bone (Figures 8-10 and 8-11).

In compact bone (eg, the diaphysis of long bones) besides forming osteons, the lamellae also exhibit a typical organization consisting of multiple **external circumferential lamellae** (see Figure 8–1) and often some **inner circumferential lamellae**. Inner circumferential lamellae are located around the marrow cavity, and external circumferential lamellae are located immediately beneath the periosteum.

Bone remodeling is continuous throughout life and involves a process of bone resorption and bone formation. In compact bone, remodeling resorbs parts of old osteons and produces new ones. Resorption involves the actions of osteoclasts, often working in groups to remove old bone in tunnel-like cavities having the approximate diameter of new osteons. Such tunnels are quickly invaded by many osteoprogenitor cells from the endosteum or periosteum and sprouting loops of capillaries. Osteoblasts develop, line the wall of the tunnels, and begin to secrete osteoid in a cyclic manner, forming the concentric lamellae of bone with trapped osteocytes (Figures 8–11 and 8–12). In healthy adults 5%-10% of the bone turns over annually.

FIGURE **8–7** Compact and cancellous bone.

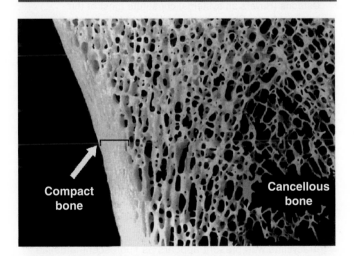

Macroscopic photo of a thick section of bone showing the cortical **compact bone** and the lattice of trabeculae in **cancellous bone** at the bone's interior. In living tissue the compact bone is covered externally with periosteum and all trabecular surfaces of cancellous bone are covered with endosteum. X10.

FIGURE **8–8** Lamellar bone.

FIGURE **8–9** An osteon.

Osteons (Haversian systems) constitute most of the compact bone. Shown here is an osteon with four to five concentric lamellae (**L**) surrounding the central canal (**CC**). Osteocytes (**O**) in lacunae are in communication with each other and with the central canal and periphery of the osteon via through hundreds of dendritic processes located within fine canaliculi (**C**). Also shown are the partial, interstitial lamellae (**I**) of an osteon partially eroded when the intact osteon was formed. Ground bone. X500.

Two photographs of the same area of an unstained section of compact bone, showing osteons with concentric lamellae around central canals. Lamellae are seen only faintly by bright-field microscopy **(a)**, but they appear as alternating bright and dark bands under the polarizing light microscope **(b)**. Bright bands are due to birefringence from the highly ordered collagen fibers in a lamella. Alternating bright and dark bands indicate that fibers in successive lamellae have different orientations, an organization that makes lamellar bone very strong. Both X100.

(With permission, from Dr Matt Allen, Indiana University School of Medicine, Indianapolis.)

❯❯ MEDICAL APPLICATION

The antibiotic **tetracycline** is a fluorescent molecule that binds newly deposited osteoid matrix during mineralization with high affinity and specifically labels new bone under the UV microscope (Figure 8–12). This discovery led to methods for measuring the rate of bone growth, an important parameter in the diagnosis of certain bone disorders. In one technique tetracycline is administered twice to patients, with an intervening interval of 11-14 days. A bone biopsy is then performed, sectioned without decalcification, and examined. Bone formed while tetracycline was present appears as fluorescent lamellae and the distance between the labeled layers is proportional to the rate of bone appositional growth. This procedure is of diagnostic importance in such diseases as **osteomalacia**, in which mineralization is impaired, and **osteitis fibrosa cystica**, in which increased osteoclast activity results in removal of bone matrix and fibrous degeneration.

FIGURE **8–10** Lamellar bone: Perforating canals and interstitial lamellae.

(a) Transverse perforating (Volkmann) canals (**P**) connecting adjacent osteons are shown in this micrograph of compact lamellar bone. Such canals "perforate" lamellae and provide another source of microvasculature for the central canals of osteons. Among the intact osteons are also found remnants of eroded osteons, seen as irregular interstitial lamellae (**I**). Ground bone. X100.

(b) Schematic diagram shows remodeling of compact lamellar bone with three generations of osteons and their successive

contributions to the formation of interstitial lamellae. The shading indicates that successive generations of osteons have different degrees of mineralization, with the most newly formed being the least mineralized. Remodeling is a continuous process that involves the coordinated activity of osteoblasts and osteoclasts, and is responsible for adaptation of bone to changes in stress, especially during the body's growth.

FIGURE **8–11** Development of an osteon.

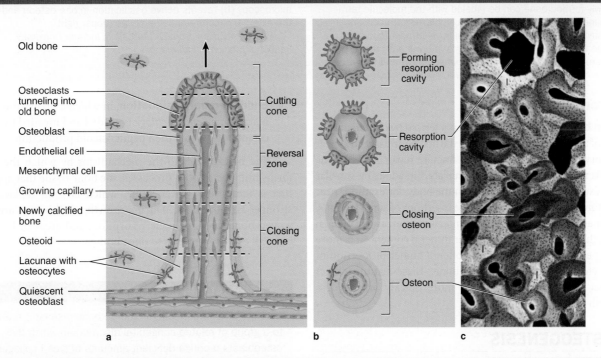

During remodeling of compact bone, osteoclasts act as a cutting cone tunneling into existing bone matrix. Behind the osteoclasts, a population of osteoblasts enters the newly formed tunnel and lines its walls. The osteoblasts secrete osteoid in a cyclic manner, producing layers of new matrix (lamellae) with cells (osteocytes) trapped in lacunae. The

tunnel becomes constricted with multiple concentric layers of new matrix, and its lumen finally exists as only a narrow central canal with small blood vessels. The dashed lines in (a) indicate the levels of the structures shown in cross-section (b). An x-ray image (c) shows the different degrees of mineralization in osteons and in interstitial lamellae (**I**).

FIGURE **8–12**   Tetracycline localization of new bone matrix.

Newly formed bone can be labeled with the molecule tetra-cycline, which forms fluorescent complexes with calcium at ossification sites and provides an in vivo tracer to localize bone formation. A group of osteons in bone after tetracycline incorporation in vivo seen with bright-field **(a)** and fluorescent

microscopy **(b)** reveals active ossification in one osteon and the external circumferential lamellae (upper right).

(*With permission, from Dr Matt Allen, Indiana University School of Medicine, Indianapolis.*)

Woven Bone

Woven bone is nonlamellar and characterized by random dispo-sition of type I collagen fibers and is the first bone tissue to appear in embryonic development and in fracture repair. Woven bone tissue is usually temporary and is replaced in adults by lamellar bone, except in a very few places in the body, for example, near the sutures of the calvaria and in the insertions of some tendons.

In addition to the irregular, interwoven array of collagen fibers, this type of bone has a lower mineral content (it is more easily penetrated by x-rays) and often a higher proportion of osteocytes than mature lamellar bone. These features reflect the fact that woven bone forms more quickly but has less strength than lamellar bone.

› OSTEOGENESIS

Bone development or **osteogenesis** occurs by one of two processes:

- **Intramembranous ossification**, in which osteoblasts differentiate directly from mesenchyme and begin secret-ing osteoid

- **Endochondral ossification**, in which a preexisting matrix of *hyaline cartilage* is eroded and invaded by osteoblasts, which then begin osteoid production.

The names refer to the mechanisms by which the bone forms initially; in both processes, the bone tissue that appears first is temporary woven bone, which is soon replaced by stronger lamellar bone. During growth of all bones, areas of woven bone, areas of bone resorption, and areas of lamellar bone all exist contiguous to one another.

›› MEDICAL APPLICATION

Osteogenesis imperfecta, or "brittle bone disease," refers to a group of related congenital disorders in which the osteoblasts produce deficient amounts of type I collagen or defective type I collagen due to genetic mutations. Such defects lead to a spectrum of disorders, all characterized by significant fragility of the bones. The fragility reflects the deficit in normal collagen, which normally reinforces and adds a degree of resiliency to the mineralized bone matrix.

Intramembranous Ossification

Intramembranous ossification, by which most flat bones begin to form, is so called because it takes place within condensations ("membranes") of embryonic mesenchymal tissue. The frontal and parietal bones of the skull—as well as parts of the occipital and temporal bones and the mandible and maxilla—are produced initially by intramembranous ossification.

Within the condensed layer of mesenchyme, the starting points for bone formation are called **ossification centers**. In these areas mesenchymal cells differentiate into osteoprogenitor cells which proliferate and form incomplete layers of osteoblasts around a network of developing capillaries. From their surfaces facing away from these blood vessels, the polarized osteoblasts secrete the osteoid components that calcify as described earlier and form trabeculae of woven bone (Figure 8-13). Differentiating osteocytes now enclosed within matrix lacunae retain intercellular contacts via their thin cytoplasmic processes within matrix canaliculi. Continued matrix secretion, calcification, and trabecular growth lead slowly to the fusion of neighboring ossification centers and gradually produce layers of compact bone that broadly enclose a region of cancellous bone with marrow and larger blood vessels.

In cranial flat bones, bone formation predominates over bone resorption at both the internal and external surfaces. Thus, two layers of compact bone (internal and external plates) arise, while the central portion (diploë) maintains its cancellous, spongy nature. The fontanelles or "soft spots" on the heads of newborn infants are areas in the skull that correspond to parts of the connective tissue that are not yet ossified. Regions of the connective tissue that do not undergo ossification give rise to the endosteum and the periosteum of the new bone.

Endochondral Ossification

Endochondral (Gr. *endon*, within + *chondros*, cartilage) ossification takes place within a piece of hyaline cartilage whose shape resembles a small version, or model, of the bone to be formed. This type of ossification is principally responsible for initiating most bones of the body and is especially well studied in developing long bones.

Endochondral ossification of a long bone consists of the sequence of events shown schematically in Figure 8–14. The first bone tissue appears as a collar surrounding the diaphysis of the cartilage model. This **bone collar** is produced by activity of osteoblasts that form within the surrounding perichondrium. The collar impedes diffusion of oxygen and nutrients into the underlying cartilage, promoting degenerative changes there. The chondrocytes begin to produce alkaline phosphatase and swell up (hypertrophy), enlarging their lacunae. These changes both compress the matrix into narrow

---

FIGURE 8–13 Intramembranous ossification.

A section of fetal pig mandible developing by intramembranous ossification. **(a)** Areas of typical mesenchyme (**M**) and condensed mesenchyme (**CM**) are adjacent to layers of new osteoblasts (**O**). Some osteoblasts have secreted matrices of bone (**B**), the surfaces of which remain covered by osteoblasts. Between these trabeculae of new woven bone are areas with small blood vessels (**V**). X40. H&E.

(b) At higher magnification another section shows these same structures, along with the developing periosteum (**P**) adjacent to masses of woven bone that will soon merge to form a continuous plate of bone. The larger mesenchyme-filled region at the top is part of the developing marrow cavity. Osteocytes in lacunae can be seen within the eosinophilic bony matrix. X100. H&E.

FIGURE **8–14** Osteogenesis of long bones by endochondral ossification.

This process, by which most bones form initially, begins with embryonic models of the skeletal elements made of hyaline cartilage (**1**). Late in the first trimester, a bone collar develops beneath the perichondrium around the middle of the long bones' cartilage models, causing degeneration of the underlying cartilage (**2**).

This is followed by invasion of the degenerating cartilage by capillaries and osteoprogenitor cells from what is now the periosteum to produce a **primary ossification center** in the diaphysis (**3**). Here osteoid is deposited by the new osteoblasts, undergoes calcification into woven bone, and is remodeled as compact bone.

(**4**) Around the time of birth **secondary ossification centers** begin to develop by a similar process in the epiphyses. During childhood the primary and secondary ossification centers gradually come to be separated only by the **epiphyseal plate** (**5**) that provides for continued bone elongation. The two ossification centers do not merge until the epiphyseal plate disappears (**6**) when full stature is achieved. Osteoblasts of the periosteum provide for growth in the bone's diameter.

trabeculae and lead to calcification in these structures. Death of the chondrocytes creates a porous structure consisting of calcified cartilage remnants which become covered by a layer of osteoblasts (Figure 8–15). Blood vessels from the perichondrium (now the periosteum) penetrate through the bone collar, bringing osteoprogenitor cells to the porous central region. Next, osteoblasts adhere to the remnants of calcified cartilage matrix and produce woven bone. The calcified cartilage at this stage appears basophilic, and the new bone is more acidophilic (Figure 8–15).

This process in the diaphysis forms the **primary ossification center** (Figure 8–14), beginning in many bones as early as the first trimester. **Secondary ossification centers** appear later at the epiphyses of the cartilage model and develop in a similar manner. During their expansion and remodeling, the primary and secondary ossification centers produce cavities that are gradually filled with bone marrow and trabeculae of cancellous bone.

With the primary and secondary ossification centers, two regions of cartilage remain:

▪ The layer of **articular cartilage** within joints (Figure 8–14), which usually persists through adult life and does not contribute to bone growth

FIGURE 8–15 Cells and matrices of a primary ossification center.

A small region of a primary ossification center showing key features of endochondral ossification. Compressed remnants of calcified cartilage matrix (**C**) are basophilic and devoid of chondrocytes. This material becomes enclosed by more lightly stained osteoid and woven bone (**B**) which contains osteocytes in lacunae. The new bone is produced by active osteoblasts (**O**) arranged as a layer on the remnants of old cartilage. X200. Pararosaniline–toluidine blue.

- The specially organized **epiphyseal cartilage** (also called **epiphyseal plate** or growth plate), which connects each epiphysis to the diaphysis (Figures 8–16 and 8–17).

The epiphyseal cartilage is responsible for the growth in length of the bone and disappears at adulthood, causing bone growth to cease. Elimination of these epiphyseal plates ("epiphyseal closure") occurs at different times with different bones and is complete in all bones by about age 20. In forensics or through x-ray examination of the growing skeleton, it is possible to determine the "bone age" of a young person, noting which epiphyses are open and which are closed. Once the

epiphyses have closed, additional growth in length of bones is no longer possible although bone widening may still occur.

An epiphyseal growth plate shows distinct regions of cellular activity and is often discussed in terms of five zones (Figure 8–16), starting from the thin region of normal cartilage:

1. The **resting zone** consists of hyaline cartilage with typical chondrocytes.

2. In the **proliferative zone**, chondrocytes begin to divide rapidly and form columns of stacked cells parallel to the long axis of the bone.

3. The **hypertrophic cartilage zone** contains swollen, degenerative chondrocytes whose cytoplasm has accumulated glycogen. This hypertrophy compresses the matrix into thin septa between the chondrocytes.

4. In the **calcified cartilage zone**, loss of the chondrocytes by apoptosis is accompanied by calcification of the septa of cartilage matrix by the formation of hydroxyapatite crystals (Figure 8–17).

5. In the **ossification zone**, bone tissue first appears. Capillaries and osteoprogenitor cells originally from the periosteum invade the cavities left by the chondrocytes. Many of these cavities will be merged and become the marrow cavity. Osteoblasts settle in a layer over the septa of calcified cartilage matrix and secrete osteoid over these structures, forming woven bone (Figures 8–15, 8–16, and 8–17).

In summary, growth in length of a long bone occurs by proliferation of chondrocytes in the epiphyseal plate. At the same time, chondrocytes in the diaphyseal side of the plate hypertrophy, their matrix becomes calcified, and the cells die. Osteoblasts lay down a layer of new bone on the calcified cartilage matrix. Because the rates of these two opposing events (proliferation and destruction) are approximately equal, the epiphyseal plate does not change thickness. Instead, it is displaced away from the middle of the diaphysis, resulting in growth in length of the bone.

›› MEDICAL APPLICATION

Calcium deficiency in children can lead to **rickets**, a disease in which the bone matrix does not calcify normally and the epiphyseal plate can become distorted by the normal strains of body weight and muscular activity. Ossification processes are consequently impeded, which causes bones to grow more slowly and often become deformed. The deficiency can be due either to insufficient calcium in the diet or a failure to produce the steroid prohormone vitamin D, which is important for the absorption of Ca^{2+} by cells of the small intestine.

In adults calcium deficiency can give rise to **osteomalacia** (osteon + Gr. *malakia*, softness), characterized by deficient calcification of recently formed bone and partial decalcification of already calcified matrix.

FIGURE 8–16 Epiphyseal growth plate: Locations and zones of activity.

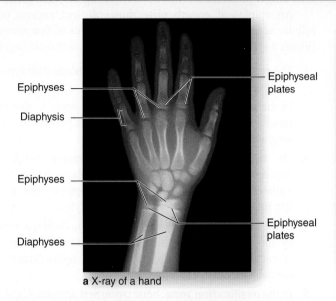

a X-ray of a hand

Zone 1: Zone of resting cartilage

Zone 2: Zone of proliferating cartilage

Zone 3: Zone of hypertrophic cartilage

Zone 4: Zone of calcified cartilage

Zone 5: Zone of ossification

b Epiphyseal plate

The large and growing primary ossification center in long bone diaphyses and the secondary ossification centers in epiphyses are separated in each developing bone by a plate of cartilage called the **epiphyseal plate**.

(a) Epiphyseal plates can be identified in an x-ray of a child's hand as marrow regions of lower density between the denser ossification centers. Cells in epiphyseal growth plates are responsible for continued elongation of bones until the body's full size is reached. Developmental activities in the epiphyseal growth plate occur in overlapping zones with distinct histological appearances.

(b) From the epiphysis to the diaphysis, five general zones have cells specialized for the following: (**1**) a reserve of normal hyaline cartilage, (**2**) cartilage with proliferating chondroblasts aligned as axial aggregates in lacunae, (**3**) degenerating cartilage in which the aligned cells are hypertrophic and the matrix condensed, (**4**) an area in which the chondrocytes have disappeared and the matrix is undergoing calcification, and (**5**) a zone in which blood vessels and osteoblasts invade the lacunae of the old cartilage, producing marrow cavities and osteoid for new bone. X100. H&E.

❯ BONE GROWTH, REMODELING, & REPAIR

Osteogenesis and bone growth involves the partial resorption of bone tissue formed earlier, while simultaneously laying down new bone at a rate exceeding that of bone removal. The sum of osteoblast and osteoclast activities in a growing bone constitutes the process of bone modeling, which maintains each bone's general shape while increasing its mass. The rate of **bone turnover** is very active in young children, where it can be 200 times faster than that of adults. In adults the skeleton is renewed continuously in a process of bone remodeling that also involves coordinated, spatially linked cellular activities for bone resorption and bone formation.

The constant remodeling of bone ensures that, despite its hardness, this tissue remains plastic and capable of adapting its internal structural in the face of changing stresses. A well-known example of bone plasticity is the ability of the positions of teeth in the jawbone to be modified by the lateral pressures produced by orthodontic appliances. Bone forms on the side where traction is applied and is resorbed on the opposite side where pressure is exerted. In this way, teeth are moved within the jaw while the bone is being remodeled.

Cranial bones grow mainly because of the formation of bone tissue by the periosteum between the sutures and on the external bone surface. At the same time, resorption takes place on the internal surface. The plasticity of bone allows it to respond to the growth of the brain and form a skull of adequate size. The skull is small if the brain does not develop completely and larger than normal in a person with hydrocephalus, a disorder characterized by abnormal accumulation of spinal fluid and dilation of the cerebral ventricles.

Because it contains osteoprogenitor stem cells in the periosteum, endosteum, and marrow and is very well vascularized, bone normally has an excellent capacity for **repair**. Repair of bone fractures and other damage efficiently uses cells, signaling molecules, and processes already active in bone remodeling. Surgically created gaps in bone can be filled with new bone, especially when periosteal tissue remains. The major phases that occur typically during bone fracture repair are shown in Figure 8–18.

FIGURE **8–17** Cells and matrices of the epiphyseal growth plate.

(a) At the top of the micrograph the growth plate (**GP**) shows its zones of hyaline cartilage with chondrocytes at rest (**R**), proliferating (**P**), and hypertrophying (**H**). As the chondrocytes swell and degenerate, they release phosphatase, activities that compress the matrix and cause an initial deposition of calcium phosphate. This produces calcified spicules (**C**) in the former cartilage matrix. The tunnel-like lacunae in which the chondrocytes have undergone apoptosis are invaded from the diaphysis by capillaries that begin to convert these spaces into marrow (**M**) cavities. Endosteum with osteoblasts also moves in from the diaphyseal primary ossification center, covering the spicules of calcified cartilage and laying down layers of osteoid to form a matrix of woven bone (**B**). X40. H&E.

(b) Higher magnification shows more detail of the cells and matrix spicules in the zones undergoing hypertrophy (**H**) and ossification. Staining properties of the matrix clearly change as it is compressed and begins to calcify (**C**), and when osteoid and bone (**B**) are laid down. The large spaces between the ossifying matrix spicules become the marrow cavity (**M**), in which pooled masses of eosinophilic red blood cells and aggregates of basophilic white blood cell precursors can be distinguished. Difficult to see at this magnification is the thin endosteum between the calcifying matrices and the marrow. X100. H&E.

❯❯ MEDICAL APPLICATION

Bone fractures are repaired by a developmental process involving fibrocartilage formation and osteogenic activity of the major bone cells (Figure 8–18). Bone fractures disrupt blood vessels, causing bone cells near the break to die. The damaged blood vessels produce a localized hemorrhage or hematoma. Clotted blood is removed along with tissue debris by macrophages and the matrix of damaged, cell-free bone is resorbed by osteoclasts.

The periosteum and the endosteum at the fracture site respond with intense proliferation and produce a soft callus of fibrocartilage-like tissue that surrounds the fracture and covers the extremities of the fractured bone.

The fibrocartilaginous callus is gradually replaced in a process that resembles a combination of endochondral and intramembranous ossification. This produces a hard callus of woven bone around the fractured ends of bone.

Stresses imposed on the bone during repair and during the patient's gradual return to activity serve to remodel the bone callus. The immature, woven bone of the callus is gradually resorbed and replaced by lamellar bone, remodeling and restoring the original bone structure.

FIGURE **8–18** Main features of bone fracture repair.

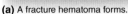

(a) A fracture hematoma forms.

(b) A fibrocartilaginous (soft) callus forms.

(c) A hard (bony) callus forms.

(d) The bone is remodeled.

Repair of a fractured bone occurs through several stages but utilizes mechanisms already in place for bone remodeling. **(a)** Blood vessels torn within the fracture release blood that clots to produce a large fracture hematoma. **(b)** This is gradually removed by macrophages and replaced by a soft fibrocartilage-like mass of procallus tissue rich in collagen and fibroblasts. If broken, the periosteum reestablishes continuity over this tissue. **(c)** This soft procallus is invaded by regrowing blood vessels and osteoblasts. In the next few weeks the fibrocartilage is gradually replaced by trabeculae of woven bone, forming a hard callus throughout the original area of fracture. **(d)** The woven bone is then remodeled as compact and cancellous bone in continuity with the adjacent uninjured areas and fully functional vasculature is reestablished.

❯ METABOLIC ROLE OF BONE

Calcium ions are required for the activity of many enzymes and proteins mediating cell adhesion, cytoskeletal movements, exocytosis, membrane permeability, and other cellular functions. The skeleton serves as the calcium reservoir, containing 99% of the body's total calcium in crystals of hydroxyapatite. The concentration of calcium in the blood (9-10 mg/dL) and tissues is generally quite stable because of a continuous interchange between blood calcium and bone calcium.

The principal mechanism for raising blood calcium levels is the mobilization of ions from hydroxyapatite crystals to interstitial fluid, which occurs primarily in cancellous bone. Ca^{2+} mobilization from hydroxyapatite is regulated mainly by paracrine interactions between bone cells, many of which are not well understood, but two polypeptide hormones also target cells in bone to influence calcium homeostasis:

- **PTH** from the parathyroid glands acts in bone to raise low blood calcium levels by stimulating osteoclasts and osteocytes to resorb matrix and release Ca^{2+}. As discussed earlier the PTH effect on osteoclasts is indirect; PTH receptors occur on *osteoblasts*, which respond by secreting paracrine factors that stimulate osteoclast activity.
- **Calcitonin,** synthesized within the thyroid gland, reduces elevated blood calcium levels by opposing the effects of PTH in bone. This hormone directly targets osteoclasts to slow matrix resorption and bone turnover.

❯❯ MEDICAL APPLICATION

In addition to PTH and calcitonin, several other hormones act on bone. The anterior lobe of the pituitary synthesizes growth hormone (GH or somatotropin), which stimulates the liver to produce insulin-like growth factor-1 (IGF-1 or somatomedin). IGF has an overall growth-promoting effect, especially on the epiphyseal cartilage. Consequently, lack of growth hormone during the growing years causes **pituitary dwarfism**; an excess of growth hormone causes excessive growth of the long bones, resulting in **gigantism**. Adult bones cannot increase in length even with excess IGF because they lack epiphyseal cartilage, but they do increase in width by periosteal growth. In adults, an increase in GH causes **acromegaly**, a disease in which the bones—mainly the long ones—become very thick.

❯❯ MEDICAL APPLICATION

In **rheumatoid arthritis** chronic inflammation of the synovial membrane causes thickening of this connective tissue and stimulates the macrophages to release collagenases and other hydrolytic enzymes. Such enzymes eventually cause destruction of the articular cartilage, allowing direct contact of the bones projecting into the joint.

› JOINTS

Joints are regions where adjacent bones are capped and held together firmly by connective tissues. The type of joint determines the degree of movement between the bones. Joints classified as **synarthroses** (Gr. *syn*, together + *arthrosis*, articulation) allow very limited or no movement. Synarthroses can be subdivided into fibrous and cartilaginous joints, depending on the type of tissue that joins the bones. Major subtypes of synarthroses include the following:

- **Synostoses**, in which bones are united only by bone tissue and no movement takes place. In older adults, synostoses unite the skull bones, which in children and young adults are held together by **sutures**, or thin layers of connective tissue with osteogenic cells.
- **Syndesmoses** join bones by dense connective tissue only. Examples include the interosseous ligament of the inferior tibiofibular joint and the posterior region of the sacroiliac joints.

- **Symphyses** are immobile joints with a pad of fibrocartilage between the articular cartilage covering the ends of the bones. All symphyses, such as the pubic symphysis, occur in the midline of the body.

Joints classified as **diarthroses** permit free bone movement. Diarthroses (Figure 8–19) such as the elbow and knee generally unite long bones and allow great mobility. In a diarthrosis, ligaments and a capsule of dense connective tissue maintain proper alignment of the bones. The capsule encloses a sealed **joint cavity** that contains **synovial fluid**, a clear, viscous liquid. The joint cavity is lined, not by epithelium, but by a specialized connective tissue called the **synovial membrane** that extends folds and villi into the cavity and secretes the lubricant synovial fluid. Synovial fluid is derived from blood plasma, but with a high concentration of hyaluronan produced by cells of the synovial membrane.

In different diarthrotic joints the synovial membrane may have prominent regions with dense connective tissue or fat.

FIGURE **8–19** Diarthroses or synovial joints.

a Typical synovial joint

b

Diarthroses are joints that allow free movement of the attached bones, such as knuckles, knees, and elbows.
(a) Diagram showing major components of a diarthrosis, including the **articular capsule** continuous with a ligament inserting into the periosteum of both bones; the **joint cavity** containing synovial fluid as a lubricant; and the ends of epiphyses covered by **articular cartilage**. The **synovial membrane** lines the capsule and produces the synovial fluid.

(b) Longitudinal section through a diarthrosis with growing bones of a rodent knee, showing the position near the boundaries of the capsule (**C**) of the epiphyseal growth plate (**E**) where endochondral ossification occurs. Also shown are the articular cartilage (**A**) and the folds of synovial membrane (**SM**), which extend prominently into the joint cavity from connective tissue of the capsule for production of synovial fluid. X10. PSH stain.

FIGURE **8–20** Synovial membrane.

The synovial membrane is a specialized connective tissue that lines capsules of synovial joints and contacts the synovial fluid lubricant, which it is primarily responsible for maintaining. **(a)** The synovial membrane projects folds into the joint cavity (**JC**) and these contain many small blood vessels (**V**). The joint cavity surrounds the articular cartilage (**AC**). X100. Mallory trichrome.

(b) Higher magnification of the fold showing a high density of capillaries and two specialized types of cells called **synoviocytes**. Contacting the synovial fluid at the tissue surface are many rounded **macrophage-like synovial cells (type A)** derived from blood monocytes. These cells bind, engulf, and remove tissue debris from synovial fluid. These cells often form a

layer at the tissue surface (**A**) and can superficially resemble an epithelium, but there is no basal lamina and the cells are not joined together by cell junctions. **Fibroblast-like (type B) synovial cells** (**B**) are mesenchymally derived and specialized for synthesis of hyaluronan that enters the synovial fluid, replenishing it. X400.

(c) Schematic representation of synovial membrane histology. Among the macrophage-like and fibroblast-like synovial cells are collagen fibers and other typical components of connective tissue. Surface cells have no basement membrane or junctional complexes denoting an epithelium, despite the superficial resemblance. Blood capillaries are fenestrated, which facilitates exchange of substances between blood and synovial fluid.

However the tissue's surface region is usually well vascularized, with many porous (fenestrated) capillaries. Besides having cells typical of connective tissue proper and a changing population of leukocytes, the synovial membrane in this area is characterized by two specialized cells with distinctly different functions and origins (Figure 8–20):

- **Macrophage-like synovial cells**, also called **type A cells**, are derived from blood monocytes and remove wear-and-tear debris from the synovial fluid. These modified macrophages, which represent approximately 25% of the cells lining the synovium, are important in regulating inflammatory events within diarthrotic joints.
- **Fibroblastic synovial cells**, or **type B cells**, produce abundant hyaluronan and other extracellular components. Much of this material is transported by water from the capillaries into the synovial fluid, which lubricates the joint, reducing friction on all internal surfaces, and supplies nutrients and oxygen to the articular cartilage.

The collagen fibers of the hyaline articular cartilage are disposed as arches with their tops near the exposed surface, which, unlike most cartilage, is not covered by perichondrium (Figure 8–21). This arrangement of collagen helps distribute more evenly the forces generated by pressure on joints. The resilient articular cartilage is also an efficient absorber of the intermittent mechanical pressures to which many joints are subjected.

A similar mechanism is seen in **intervertebral discs** (Figure 8–22) that are thick discs of fibrocartilage between the articular surfaces of successive bony vertebral bodies. These discoid components of the intervertebral joints facilitate movements of the vertebral column. The **annulus fibrosus** of each disc has an external layer of dense connective tissue but is mainly composed of overlapping laminae of fibrocartilage in which collagen bundles are orthogonally arranged in adjacent layers. The multiple lamellae provide the disc with unusual resilience and enable it to withstand pressures generated by the vertebrae.

FIGURE **8–21** Articular cartilage.

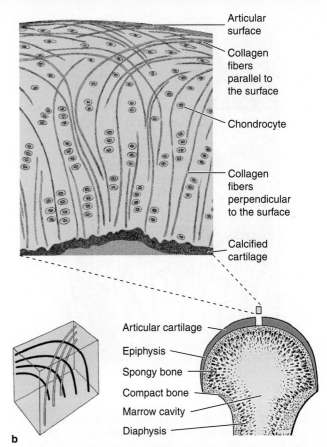

(a) Articular surfaces of a diarthrosis are made of hyaline cartilage that lacks the usual perichondrium covering. X40. H&E. **(b)** The large diagram shows a small region of articular cartilage in which collagen fibers run perpendicular to the tissue surface and then bend gradually, forming a broad arch parallel to that surface. The lower left diagram shows a 3D view of collagen fibers in articular cartilage. Proteoglycan aggregates bound to hyaluronic acid and collagen fill the space among the collagen fibers and bind a large amount of water, functioning as a biomechanical spring in articular cartilage. When pressure is applied, some water is forced out of the cartilage matrix into the synovial fluid. When pressure is released, water is attracted back into the interstices of the matrix. These water movements are brought about constantly by using the joint and are essential for nutrition of the cartilage and for facilitating the interchange of O_2, CO_2, and other molecules between the synovial fluid and the articular cartilage.

TABLE **8–1** | Summary of bone types and their organization.

Type of Bone	Histological Features	Major Locations	Synonyms
Woven bone, newly calcified	Irregular and random arrangement of cells and collagen; lightly calcified	Developing and growing bones; hard callus of bone fractures	Immature bone; primary bone; bundle bone
Lamellar bone, remodeled from woven bone	Parallel bundles of collagen in thin layers (lamellae), with regularly spaced cells between; heavily calcified	All normal regions of adult bone	Mature bone; secondary bone
Compact bone, ~80% of all lamellar bone	Parallel lamellae or densely packed osteons, with interstitial lamellae	Thick, outer region (beneath periosteum) of bones	Cortical bone
Cancellous bone, ~20% of all lamellar bone	Interconnected thin spicules or trabeculae covered by endosteum	Inner region of bones, adjacent to marrow cavities	Spongy bone; trabecular bone; medullary bone

FIGURE 8–22 Intervertebral disc.

Section of a rat tail showing an intervertebral disc and two adjacent vertebrae with bone marrow (**BM**) cavities. The disc consists of concentric layers of fibrocartilage, comprising the annulus fibrosus (**AF**), which surrounds the nucleus pulposus (**NP**). The nucleus pulposus contains scattered residual cells of the embryonic notochord embedded in abundant gel-like matrix. The intervertebral discs function primarily as shock absorbers within the spinal column and allow greater mobility within the spinal column. X40. PSH.

The **nucleus pulposus** is situated in the center of the annulus fibrosus and allows each disc to function as a shock absorber within the vertebral column. It typically contains scattered, vacuolated cells (the only cells derived from the embryonic notochord), but it is largely composed of water in a gel-like matrix rich in hyaluronan and fibers of type II collagen. The nucleus pulposus is large in children, but these structures gradually become smaller with age and are partially replaced by fibrocartilage.

›› MEDICAL APPLICATION

Within an intervertebral disc, collagen loss or other degenerative changes in the annulus fibrosus are often accompanied by displacement of the nucleus pulposus, a condition variously called a **slipped or herniated disc**. This occurs most frequently on the posterior region of the intervertebral disc where there are fewer collagen bundles. The affected disc frequently dislocates or shifts slightly from its normal position. If it moves toward nerve plexuses, it can compress the nerves and result in severe pain and other neurologic disturbances. The pain accompanying a slipped disc may be perceived in areas innervated by the compressed nerve fibers—usually the lower lumbar region.

Bone SUMMARY OF KEY POINTS

- Bone is a type of connective tissue with a **calcified** extracellular matrix (ECM), specialized to **support** the body, **protect** many internal organs, and act as the body's **Ca²⁺ reservoir**.

Major Cells & Matrix Components of Bone

- **Osteoblasts** differentiate from (stem) osteoprogenitor cells and secrete components of the initial matrix, called **osteoid**, that allow matrix mineralization to occur.
- Important components of osteoid include type I collagen, the protein **osteocalcin**, which binds Ca^{2+} and **matrix vesicles** with enzymes generating PO_4^-.
- High concentrations of Ca^{2+} and PO_4^- ions cause formation of **hydroxyapatite** crystals, whose growth gradually calcifies the entire matrix.
- **Osteocytes** differentiate further from osteoblasts when they become enclosed within matrix **lacunae** and act to maintain the matrix and detect mechanical stresses on bone.

- Osteocytes maintain communication with adjacent cells via a network of long **dendritic processes** that extend through the matrix via narrow **canaliculi** radiating from each lacuna.
- **Osteoclasts** are very large cells, formed by fusion of several blood monocytes, which locally erode bone matrix during osteogenesis and bone remodeling.

Periosteum & Endosteum

- **Periosteum** is a layer of dense connective tissue on the outer surface of bone, bound to bone matrix by bundles of type I collagen called **perforating** (or **Sharpey**) **fibers**.
- Regions of periosteum adjacent to bone are rich in **osteoprogenitor cells** and **osteoblasts** that mediate increases in bone thickness by **appositional growth**.
- The **endosteum** is a thin layer of active and inactive osteoblasts, which lines all the internal surfaces within bone; osteoblasts here are also required for bone growth.

Types & Organization of Bone (Table 8-1)

- Dense bone immediately beneath the periosteum is called **compact bone**; deep to the compact bone are small bony trabeculae or spicules of **cancellous (or spongy) bone**.
- In long bones of the limbs these two types of mature bone tissue occur in both the knobby, bulbous ends, called **epiphyses**, and in the intervening shaft or **diaphysis**.
- Immature bone, called **woven bone**, is formed during osteogenesis or repair and has a calcified matrix with randomly arranged collagen fibers.
- By the action of osteoclasts and osteoblasts, woven bone undergoes rapid turnover and is remodeled into **lamellar bone** with new matrix deposited in distinct layers with parallel collagen bundles; both compact and cancellous bone is lamellar bone.
- Most lamellar bone consists of lamellae organized concentrically around small **central canals** containing blood vessels and nerves; this organization is called an **osteon or haversian system**.
- Within each osteon osteocytic lacunae occur between the lamellae, with **canaliculi** radiating through the lamellae, which allow all cells to communicate with the central canal.

Osteogenesis

- Bones of the skull and jaws form initially by **intramembranous ossification**, with osteoblasts differentiating directly from progenitor cells in condensed **"membranes" of mesenchyme**.
- All other bones form by **endochondral ossification**, in which osteoprogenitor cells surround and then invade hyaline **cartilage models** of the skeletal elements in the embryo.
- **Primary ossification centers** in diaphyses of fetal long bones form when chondrocytes die after enclosure of the cartilage within a collar of woven bone, creating an initial cavity that is entered by periosteal osteoblasts and vasculature.
- Later, **secondary ossification centers** develop similarly within the epiphyses, with cartilage of the **epiphyseal growth plate** between the primary and secondary ossification sites.
- The growth plates are the key to **bone elongation** during childhood and are organized as an interrelated series of developing zones.
- Most distally is a **"resting" or reserve zone** of typical hyaline cartilage.
- In an adjacent **proliferative zone**, chondrocytes undergo mitosis and appear stacked within elongated lacunae.
- The most mature chondrocytes in these lacunae swell up, compress the matrix, and undergo apoptosis in a **zone of hypertrophic cartilage** closer to the large primary ossification center.
- Spaces created in the matrix by these events characterize the **zone of cartilage calcification** when they are invaded by osteoblasts, osteoclasts, and vasculature from the primary center.
- In the **ossification zone**, woven bone is laid down initially by osteoblasts and remodeled into lamellae bone.

Bone Growth, Remodeling, & Repair

- **Growth** of bones occurs throughout life, with cells and matrix turning over continuously through activities of osteoblasts and osteoclasts.
- Lamellae and osteons are temporary structures and are replaced and rebuilt continuously in a process of **bone remodeling** by which bones change size and shape according to changes in mechanical stress.
- **Bone repair** after fracture or other injury involves the activation of periosteal fibroblasts to produce an initial **soft, fibrocartilage-like callus**.
- The soft callus is gradually replaced by a **hard callus of woven bone** that is soon remodeled to produce stronger lamellar bone.

Metabolic Role of Bone

- Ca^{2+}, a key ion for all cells, is **stored** in bone when dietary calcium is adequate and **mobilized** from bone when dietary calcium is deficient.
- Maintenance of proper **blood calcium levels** involves activity of all three major bone cells and is largely regulated by subtle paracrine interaction among these and other cells.
- Hormones affecting calcium deposition and removal from bone include **parathyroid hormone (PTH)**, which indirectly stimulates osteoclasts to elevate levels of calcium in blood, and **calcitonin**, which can inhibit osteoclast activity, lowering blood calcium levels.

Joints

- **Joints** are places where bones meet, or articulate, allowing at least the potential for bending or movement in that portion of the skeleton.
- Joints with very limited or no movement are classified collectively as **synarthroses** and freely mobile joints are called **diarthroses**.
- Diarthroses have a **joint cavity** filled with lubricant **synovial fluid**, enclosed within a tough, fibrous **articular capsule**; ends of the bones involved are covered with hyaline **articular cartilage**.
- Specialized connective tissue of the **synovial membrane** lines the capsule, with folds extended into some areas of the joint cavity.
- **Macrophage-like synovial cells** remove wear-and-tear debris from synovial fluid.
- **Fibroblast-like synovial cells** produce hyaluronate that is moved in the synovial fluid with water from local capillaries, forming the synovial fluid that nourishes and lubricates the articular cartilage.
- **Intervertebral discs** allow limited vertebral mobility and consist of large pads of **fibrocartilage** that cushion adjacent vertebrae.
- Each intervertebral disc consists mainly of a thick outer layer of fibrocartilage forming a tough **annulus fibrosus**, and a shock-absorbing inner, gel-like core, the **nucleus pulposus**.

9 Nerve Tissue & the Nervous System

The human nervous system, by far the most complex system in the body, is formed by a network of many billion nerve cells (**neurons**), all assisted by many more supporting cells called **glial cells**. Each neuron has hundreds of interconnections with other neurons, forming a very complex system for processing information and generating responses.

Nerve tissue is distributed throughout the body as an integrated communications network. Anatomically, the general organization of the nervous system (Figure 9–1) has two major divisions:

- **Central nervous system (CNS)**, consisting of the brain and spinal cord
- **Peripheral nervous system (PNS)**, composed of the cranial, spinal, and peripheral nerves conducting impulses to and from the CNS (sensory and motor nerves, respectively) and **ganglia** that are small groups of nerve cells outside the CNS.

Cells in both central and peripheral nerve tissue are of two kinds: **nerve cells**, or **neurons**, which usually show numerous long processes; and various **glial cells** (Gr. *glia*, glue), which have short processes, support and protect neurons, and participate in many neural activities, neural nutrition, and defense of cells in the CNS.

Neurons respond to environmental changes (**stimuli**) by altering the ionic gradient that exists across their plasma membranes. All cells maintain such a gradient, also called an electrical potential, but cells that can rapidly change this potential in response to stimuli (eg, neurons, muscle cells, some gland cells)

are said to be **excitable** or irritable. Neurons react promptly to stimuli with a reversal of the ionic gradient (**membrane depolarization**) that generally spreads from the place that received the stimulus and is propagated across the neuron's entire plasma membrane. This propagation, called the **action potential**, the **depolarization wave**, or the **nerve impulse**, is capable of traveling long distances along neuronal processes, transmitting such signals to other neurons, muscles, and glands.

By collecting, analyzing, and integrating information in such signals, the nervous system continuously stabilizes the intrinsic conditions of the body (eg, blood pressure, O_2 and CO_2 content, pH, blood glucose levels, and hormone levels) within normal ranges and maintains behavioral patterns (eg, feeding, reproduction, defense, interaction with other living creatures).

› DEVELOPMENT OF NERVE TISSUE

The nervous system develops from the outermost of the three early embryonic layers, the ectoderm, beginning in the third week of development (Figure 9–2). With signals from the underlying axial structure, the notochord, ectoderm on the mid-dorsal side of the embryo thickens to form the epithelial **neural plate**. The lateral sides of this plate fold upward, bend and grow toward each other medially, and within a few days fuse to form the **neural tube**. Cells of this tube give rise to the entire CNS, including neurons and most glial cells.

FIGURE **9–1** The general organization of the nervous system.

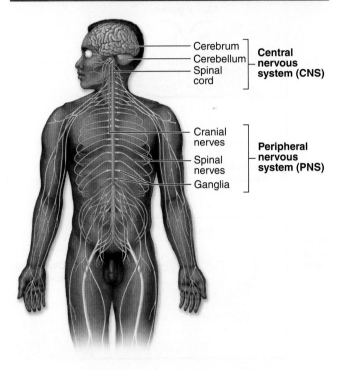

Cerebrum
Cerebellum
Spinal cord

Central nervous system (CNS)

Cranial nerves
Spinal nerves
Ganglia

Peripheral nervous system (PNS)

Components of the nervous system are subdivided both structurally and functionally. Major structural divisions (shown here) are the **CNS**, which includes the brain and spinal cord, and the **PNS**, which is composed of nerves and ganglia. Functional categories are the **sensory (afferent)** and **motor (efferent)** divisions. Sensory nerves are further subdivided into voluntary **somatic** and involuntary or **visceral** components. Motor nerves are subdivided into **voluntary (somatic)** and **involuntary (autonomic)** components. The array of autonomic motor nerves is often called the **autonomic nervous system**.

As the folds fuse and the neural tube separates from the now overlying surface ectoderm that will form epidermis, a large population of developmentally important cells, the **neural crest**, separates from the neuroepithelium and becomes mesenchymal. Neural crest cells migrate extensively and differentiate as all the cells of the PNS, as well as a number of other nonneuronal cell types.

❯ NEURONS

The functional unit in both the CNS and PNS is the **neuron** or nerve cell. Some neuronal components have special names, such as "neurolemma" for the cell membrane. Most neurons consist of three main parts (Figure 9–3):

- The **cell body**, or **perikaryon**, which contains the nucleus and most of the cell's organelles and serves as the synthetic or trophic center for the entire neuron.

- The **dendrites**, which are the numerous elongated processes extending from the perikaryon and specialized to receive stimuli from other neurons at unique sites called **synapses**.
- The **axon** (Gr. *axon*, axis), which is a single long process ending at synapses specialized to generate and conduct nerve impulses to other cells (nerve, muscle, and gland cells). Axons may also receive information from other neurons, information that mainly modifies the transmission of action potentials to those neurons.

Neurons and their processes are extremely variable in size and shape. Cell bodies can be very large, measuring up to 150 μm in diameter. Other neurons, such as the cerebellar granule cells, are among the body's smallest cells.

Neurons can be classified according to the number of processes extending from the cell body (Figure 9–4):

- **Multipolar neurons**, which have one axon and two or more dendrites
- **Bipolar neurons**, with one dendrite and one axon
- **Unipolar** or **pseudounipolar neurons**, which have a single process that bifurcates close to the perikaryon, with the longer branch extending to a peripheral ending and the other toward the CNS.
- **Anaxonic neurons**, with many dendrites but no true axon, do not produce action potentials, but regulate electrical changes of adjacent neurons.

Most neurons are multipolar. Bipolar neurons are found in the retina, olfactory mucosa, and the (inner ear) cochlear and vestibular ganglia, where they serve the senses of sight, smell, and balance, respectively. Pseudounipolar neurons are found in the spinal ganglia (the sensory ganglia found with the spinal nerves) and in most cranial ganglia. Because the fine processes emerging from perikarya are seldom seen in sections of nervous tissue, it is difficult to classify neurons structurally by microscopic inspection.

Nervous components can also be subdivided functionally (Figure 9–1). **Sensory neurons** are **afferent** and receive stimuli from the receptors throughout the body. **Motor neurons** are **efferent**, sending impulses to effector organs such as muscle fibers and glands. **Somatic** motor nerves are under voluntary control and typically innervate most skeletal muscle; **autonomic** motor nerves control the "involuntary" activities of glands, cardiac muscle, and most smooth muscle.

Interneurons establish relationships among other neurons, forming complex functional networks or **circuits** (as in the CNS and retina). Interneurons are generally multipolar or anaxonic and are estimated to include 99% of the neurons in the human CNS.

In the CNS most neuronal perikarya occur in the **gray matter**, with axons concentrated in the **white matter**. These terms refer to the general appearance of unstained CNS tissue caused in part by the different densities of nerve cell bodies. In the PNS cell bodies are found in ganglia and in some sensory regions, such as the olfactory mucosa, and axons are bundled in **nerves**.

FIGURE 9–2 Neurulation in the early embryo.

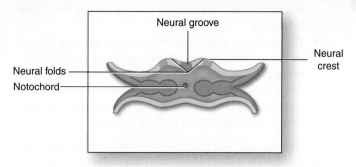

(a) Neural folds and neural groove form from the neural plate.

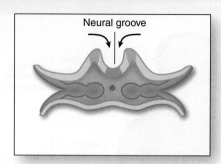

(b) Neural folds elevate and approach one another.

(c) As neural folds prepare to fuse and form the neural tube and dorsal epidermis, neural crest cells loosen and become mesenchymal.

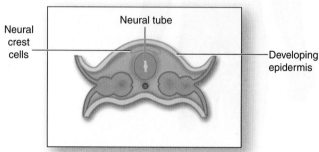

(d) The mass of neural crest cells initially lies atop the newly formed neural tube.

Cross sections through the human embryo during the fourth week of development show stages in the process of **neurulation**, the embryonic process by which cells of the CNS and PNS are initially produced. Part (a) shows a cross section of a 21-day human embryo, when it is approximately 1 mm in length, with the surrounding amniotic membrane and yolk sac removed. Under an inductive influence from the axial notochord, the overlying layer of ectodermal cells thickens to become the **neural plate**. All other ectoderm will become epidermis. The neural plate forms two lateral **folds**, separated by the **neural groove (b)**.

These folds rise and fuse at the midline **(c)**, converting the neural groove into the **neural tube (d)**. The neural tube, which

is large at the cranial end of the embryo and much narrower caudally, will give rise to the CNS. As the neural folds fuse and the resulting tube detaches from the now overlying ectoderm **(d)**, a population of neural cells separates and becomes a mass of mesenchymal cells called the **neural crest**.

Located initially between the neural tube and the epidermis, neural crest cells represent an important population of embryonic mesenchymal cells which immediately begin migrating laterally. Neural crest cells form the sensory ganglia and all other cells of the PNS, as well as contributing to many other developing structures, including certain non-neural tissues.

›› MEDICAL APPLICATION

Parkinson disease is a slowly progressing disorder affecting muscular activity characterized by tremors, reduced activity of the facial muscles, loss of balance, and postural stiffness. It is caused by gradual loss by apoptosis of dopamine-producing neurons whose cell bodies lie within the nuclei of the CNS substantia nigra. Parkinson disease is treated with ʟ-dopa (L-3,4-dihydroxyphenylalanine), a precursor of dopamine which augments the declining production of this neurotransmitter.

Cell Body (Perikaryon)

The **cell body** is the neuronal region that contains the nucleus and surrounding cytoplasm, exclusive of the cell processes (Figure 9–3). It acts as a trophic center, producing cytoplasm for movement into the processes, although most cell bodies also receive a great number of nerve endings conveying excitatory or inhibitory stimuli generated in other nerve cells. Most nerve cells have a generally spherical, unusually large, euchromatic (pale-staining) nucleus with a prominent nucleolus. The chromatin is finely dispersed, reflecting the intense synthetic activity of these cells.

FIGURE **9–3** Structures of neuron.

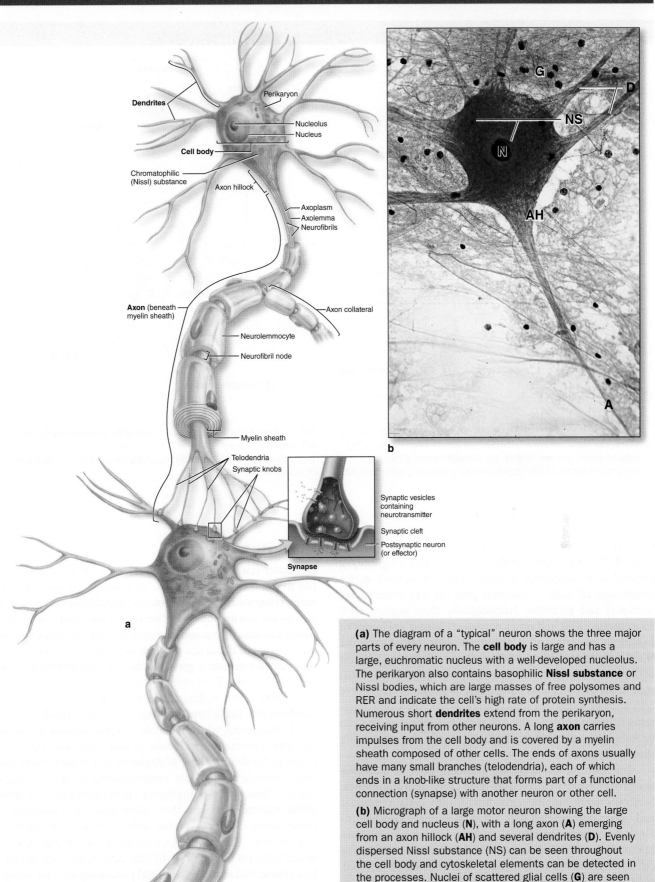

Dendrites

Perikaryon

Nucleolus

Nucleus

Cell body

Chromatophilic (Nissl) substance

Axon hillock

Axoplasm
Axolemma
Neurofibrils

Axon (beneath myelin sheath)

Axon collateral

Neurolemmocyte

Neurofibril node

Myelin sheath

Telodendria
Synaptic knobs

Synaptic vesicles containing neurotransmitter

Synaptic cleft

Postsynaptic neuron (or effector)

Synapse

a

b

G

D

NS

N

AH

A

(a) The diagram of a "typical" neuron shows the three major parts of every neuron. The **cell body** is large and has a large, euchromatic nucleus with a well-developed nucleolus. The perikaryon also contains basophilic **Nissl substance** or Nissl bodies, which are large masses of free polysomes and RER and indicate the cell's high rate of protein synthesis. Numerous short **dendrites** extend from the perikaryon, receiving input from other neurons. A long **axon** carries impulses from the cell body and is covered by a myelin sheath composed of other cells. The ends of axons usually have many small branches (telodendria), each of which ends in a knob-like structure that forms part of a functional connection (synapse) with another neuron or other cell.

(b) Micrograph of a large motor neuron showing the large cell body and nucleus (**N**), with a long axon (**A**) emerging from an axon hillock (**AH**) and several dendrites (**D**). Evenly dispersed Nissl substance (NS) can be seen throughout the cell body and cytoskeletal elements can be detected in the processes. Nuclei of scattered glial cells (**G**) are seen among the surrounding tissue. X100. H&E.

FIGURE **9–4** Structural classes of neurons.

(a) Multipolar neuron

(b) Bipolar neuron

(c) Unipolar neuron

(d) Anaxonic neuron

Shown are the three main types of neurons, with descriptions. (a) Most neurons, including all motor neurons and CNS interneurons, are **multipolar**. (b) **Bipolar** neurons include sensory neurons of the retina, olfactory mucosa, and inner ear.

(c) All other sensory neurons are **unipolar** or **pseudounipolar**.
(d) **Anaxonic** neurons of the CNS lack true axons and do not produce action potentials, but regulate local electrical changes of adjacent neurons.

Cytoplasm of perikarya often contains a highly developed RER with many parallel cisternae and neighboring regions with numerous polyribosomes, indicating active production of both cytoskeletal proteins and proteins for transport and secretion. Histologically these regions with concentrated RER and other polysomes appear as clumps of basophilic material called **chromatophilic substance** (or **Nissl substance**, **Nissl bodies**) (Figure 9–3). The amount of this basophilic material varies with the type and functional state of the neuron and is particularly abundant in large nerve cells such as motor neurons (Figure 9–3b). The Golgi apparatus is located only in the cell body, but mitochondria can be found throughout the cell and are usually abundant in the axon terminals.

Intermediate filaments are abundant both in perikarya and processes and in this cell are often called **neurofilaments**. Neurofilaments become cross-linked with certain fixatives and, when impregnated with silver stains, they form neurofibrils visible with the light microscope. Neurons also contain microtubules identical to those found in other cells. Nerve cells occasionally contain inclusions of pigmented material, such as lipofuscin, consisting of residual bodies left from lysosomal digestion.

Dendrites

Dendrites (Gr. *dendron*, tree) are usually short and divided like tree branches (Figure 9–3). They are usually covered with many synapses and are the principal signal reception and processing sites on neurons. Most nerve cells have many dendrites, which increase the receptive area of the cell considerably. The arborization of dendrites makes it possible for one neuron to receive and integrate a great number of axon terminals from other nerve cells. For example, it has been estimated that up to 200,000 axonal endings make functional contact with the dendrites of a single large Purkinje cell of the cerebellum.

Unlike axons, which maintain a nearly constant diameter, dendrites become much thinner as they subdivide. The cytoplasm of the dendrite base is similar to that of the perikaryon, with cytoskeletal elements predominating in the branched regions. Most synapses impinging on neurons occur on **dendritic spines**, which are short blunt structures projecting at points along dendrites, visible with silver staining methods (Figure 9–5). Dendritic spines occur in vast numbers, estimated to be on the order of 10^{14} for cells of the human cerebral cortex, and serve as the initial processing sites for synaptic signals. The morphology of these spines depends on actin filaments and can be highly plastic; dendritic spines are of key

FIGURE **9–5** Dendrites and dendritic spines.

The large Purkinje neuron in this silver-impregnated section of cerebellum has many dendrites (**D**) emerging from its cell body (**CB**) and forming branches. The small dendritic branches have many short projecting dendritic spines (**DS**) spaced closely along their length, each of which is a site of a synapse with another neuron. X650. Silver stain.

importance in the constant changes of the **neural plasticity** underlying adaptation, learning, and memory.

Axons

Most neurons have only one axon, a fine cylindrical process that varies in length and diameter according to the type of neuron. Axons are usually very long processes. For example, axons of the motor neurons of the spinal cord that innervate the foot muscles may have a length of nearly 100 cm and require large cell bodies for their maintenance. Axons originate from a pyramid-shaped region of the perikaryon called the **axon hillock** (Figure 9–3). The plasma membrane of the axon is often called the **axolemma** and its contents are known as **axoplasm**.

Just beyond the axon hillock, at an area called the initial segment, is the site where various excitatory and inhibitory stimuli impinging on the neuron are algebraically summed, resulting in the decision to propagate—or not to propagate—a nerve impulse. The axolemma of the initial segment contains various ion channels important in generating the action potential.

In contrast to dendrites, the typical axon is much longer, has a constant diameter, and branches less profusely. As shown in Figure 9–3, however, the distal end of an axon forms a **terminal arborization**, and axons of interneurons and some motor neurons have branches called **collaterals** that end at synapses influencing the activity of many other neurons. Each branch ends with a dilation called a **terminal bouton** (Fr. *bouton*, button) that contacts another neuron or

non-nerve cell at a synapse to initiate an impulse in that cell. Axoplasm contains mitochondria, microtubules, neurofilaments, and some cisternae of smooth ER, but essentially no polyribosomes or RER, emphasizing its dependence on the perikaryon for maintenance. If an axon is severed, its peripheral part quickly degenerates.

There is a lively bidirectional transport of small and large molecules along the axon. Organelles and macromolecules synthesized in the cell body move by **anterograde transport** along the axon from the perikaryon to the synaptic terminals. **Retrograde transport** in the opposite direction carries certain other macromolecules, such as material taken up by endocytosis (including viruses and toxins), from the periphery to the cell body. Retrograde transport can be used to study the pathways of neurons: if peroxidase or another marker is injected into regions with axon terminals, its distribution along the entire axon after a period of time can be determined histochemically.

Axonal transport in both directions uses motor proteins on microtubules, as discussed in Chapter 2. **Kinesin**, a microtubule-activated ATPase, mediates anterograde vesicular transport, and the similar ATPase called cytoplasmic **dynein** provides retrograde transport. Anterograde and retrograde transports both occur fairly rapidly, at rates of 50-400 mm/d. A much slower anterograde stream (only a few millimeters per day) involves movement of the axonal cytoskeleton itself. This slow axonal transport system corresponds roughly to the rate of axon growth.

Nerve Impulses

A **nerve impulse**, or **action potential**, travels along an axon like a spark moves along an explosive's fuse. It is an electrochemical process initiated at the axon hillock when other impulses received at the cell body or dendrites meet a certain threshold. The action potential is propagated along the axon as a wave of membrane depolarization produced by **voltage-gated Na^+ and K^+ channels** in the axolemma that allow diffusion of these ions into and out of the axoplasm. The extracellular compartment around all regions of the neuron is a very thin zone immediately outside the cell that is formed by enclosing glial cells that regulate its ionic contents.

In unstimulated neurons, ATP-dependent Na-K pumps and other membrane proteins maintain an axoplasmic Na^+ concentration only one-tenth that outside the cell and a K^+ level many times greater than the extracellular concentration. This produces a potential electrical difference across the axolemma of about −65 mV, with the inside negative to the outside. This difference is the axon's **resting potential**.

⟩⟩ MEDICAL APPLICATION

Most **local anesthetics** are low-molecular-weight molecules that bind to the voltage-gated sodium channels of the axolemma, interfering with sodium ion influx and, consequently, inhibiting the action potential responsible for the nerve impulse.

When the threshold triggering an impulse is met, channels at the axon's initial segment open and allow a very rapid influx of extracellular Na⁺ that makes the axoplasm positive in relation to the extracellular environment and shifts (depolarizes) the resting potential from negative to positive, to +30 mV. Immediately after the membrane depolarization, the voltage-gated Na⁺ channels close and those for K⁺ open, and this rapidly returns the membrane to its resting potential. This cycle of events occurs in less than 1 millisecond.

Depolarization stimulates adjacent portions of the axolemma to depolarize and return immediately to the resting potential, causing the nerve impulse, or wave of depolarization, to move rapidly along the axon. After a refractory period also measured in milliseconds, the neuron is ready to repeat the process and generate another action potential. Impulses arriving at the synaptic nerve endings promote the discharge of stored neurotransmitter that stimulates or inhibits action potentials in another neuron or a non-neural cell.

Synaptic Communication

Synapses (Gr. *synapsis*, union) are sites where nerve impulses are transmitted from one neuron to another or from neurons and other effector cells. The structure of a synapse (Figure 9–6) ensures that transmission is unidirectional. Synapses convert an electrical signal (nerve impulse) from the **presynaptic cell** into a chemical signal that affects the **postsynaptic cell**. Most synapses act by releasing **neurotransmitters**, which are usually small molecules that bind specific receptor proteins to either open or close ion channels or initiate

---

FIGURE 9–6 Major components of a synapse.

(a) Diagram showing a synapse releasing neurotransmitters by exocytosis from the terminal bouton. Presynaptic terminals always contain a large number of **synaptic vesicles** containing neurotransmitters, numerous **mitochondria**, and smooth ER as a source of new membrane. Some neurotransmitters are synthesized in the cell body and then transported in vesicles to the presynaptic terminal. Upon arrival of a nerve impulse, voltage-regulated Ca²⁺ channels permit Ca²⁺ entry, which triggers neurotransmitter release into the synaptic cleft. Excess membrane accumulating at the presynaptic region as a result of exocytosis is recycled by clathrin-mediated endocytosis, which is not depicted here.

(b) The TEM shows a large presynaptic terminal (**T₁**) filled with synaptic vesicles and asymmetric electron-dense regions around 20- to 30-nm-wide synaptic clefts (**arrows**). The postsynaptic membrane contains the neurotransmitter receptors and mechanisms to initiate an impulse at the postsynaptic neuron. The postsynaptic membrane on the right is part of a dendrite (**D**), associated with fewer vesicles of any kind, showing this to be an axodendritic synapse. On the left is another presynaptic terminal (**T₂**), suggesting an axoaxonic synapse with a role in modulating activity of the other terminal. X35,000.

second-messenger cascades. A synapse (Figure 9–6a) has the following components:

- Presynaptic axon terminal (**terminal bouton**) from which neurotransmitter is released by exocytosis from **synaptic vesicles.**
- **Postsynaptic cell membrane** with receptors for the transmitter and ion channels or other mechanisms to initiate a new impulse.
- A 20- to 30-nm-wide intercellular space called the **synaptic cleft** separating the presynaptic and postsynaptic membranes.

At the presynaptic region the nerve impulse briefly opens calcium channels, promoting a Ca^{2+} influx that triggers neurotransmitter release by exocytosis or similar mechanisms. Released neurotransmitter molecules diffuse immediately across the synaptic cleft and bind receptors at the postsynaptic region, producing either an excitatory or an inhibitory effect at the postsynaptic membrane.

- Neurotransmitters from **excitatory synapses** cause postsynaptic Na^+ channels to open, and the resulting influx of this ion initiates a depolarization wave in that neuron or effector cell as described previously.
- At **inhibitory synapses** neurotransmitters open Cl^- or other anion channels, causing influx of anions and **hyperpolarization** of the postsynaptic cell, making its membrane potential more negative and more resistant to depolarization.

Interplay between excitatory and inhibitory effects on postsynaptic cells allows synapses to process neuronal input and fine-tune the reaction of the effector cell. Impulses passing from presynaptic neurons to postsynaptic cells are usually modified at the synapse by similar connections there from other neurons (see Figure 9–6b). Activity of postsynaptic neurons is determined by the summation of activity at hundreds of synapses on that cell.

Once released, neurotransmitters are removed quickly by enzymatic breakdown, diffusion, or endocytosis (recycling) mediated by specific receptors on the presynaptic membrane. Removal of neurotransmitters prevents sustained stimulation of the postsynaptic cell.

Morphologically, various types of synapses are seen between neurons (Figure 9–7). If an axon forms a synapse with a cell body, it is called an **axosomatic synapse**; with a dendrite, **axodendritic**; or with another axon, **axoaxonic**. Axoaxonic synapses modulate activity of the other two types. Synaptic structure cannot be resolved by light microscopy, although components such as dendritic spines may be shown by methods such as silver precipitation (see Figure 9–5).

The chemical transmitter used at neuromuscular junctions is acetylcholine. Within the CNS major categories of neurotransmitters include the following:

- Catecholamines, such as epinephrine (adrenalin), norepinephrine, and dopamine;

- Amino acids (often modified), such as glutamate, glycine, serotonin (5-hydroxytryptamine or 5-HT), and γ-aminobutyrate (GABA); and
- Small peptides, such as endorphins and substance P.

The actions of these and other common neurotransmitters are summarized in Table 9–1.

> **>> MEDICAL APPLICATION**
>
> Levels of neurotransmitters in the synaptic cleft and available for binding postsynaptic receptors are normally regulated by several local mechanisms. **Selective serotonin reuptake inhibitors (SSRIs)**, a widely used class of drugs for treatment of depression and anxiety disorders, were designed to augment levels of this neurotransmitter at the postsynaptic membrane of serotonergic CNS synapses by specifically inhibiting its reuptake at the presynaptic membrane.

> GLIAL CELLS & NEURONAL ACTIVITY

Glial cells support neuronal survival and activities, and are ten times more abundant in the mammalian brain than the neurons. Like neurons, most glial cells develop from progenitor cells of the embryonic neural plate. In the CNS glial cells surround both the neuronal cell bodies, which are often larger than glial cells, and the processes of axons and dendrites occupying the spaces between neurons. Except around the larger blood vessels, the CNS has only a very small amount of connective tissue and collagen. Glial cells substitute for cells of connective tissue in some respects, supporting neurons and creating a microenvironment immediately around those cells that is optimal for neuronal activity. The fibrous intercellular network surrounding cells of the CNS may superficially resemble collagen with light microscopy, but it is actually the network of cellular processes emerging from neurons and glial cells. Such processes are collectively called the **neuropil** (Figure 9–8).

There are six kinds of glial cells; these are shown schematically in Figure 9–9 and basic features are summarized in Table 9–2.

Oligodendrocytes

Oligodendrocytes (Gr. *oligos*, small, few + *dendron*, tree + *kytos*, cell) produce the myelin sheaths around axons that provide the electrical insulation for neurons in the CNS. Oligodendrocytes extend sheetlike processes that wrap around parts of several axons, producing myelin sheaths as shown in Figure 9–9a. These are the predominant glial cells in CNS white matter, which is white because of the lipid concentrated in the wrapped membrane sheaths. The processes and sheaths are not visible by routine light microscope

FIGURE **9–7** Types of synapses.

Axosomatic synapse

- Axon

Cell body

Axodendritic synapse

- Axon

Dendrite

Dendritic spine

Axoaxonic synapse

Axons

Dendrites

Axodendritic synapse

Axosomatic synapse

Cell body

Axon hillock

Axon

Axoaxonic synapse

Terminal arborizations

Axon terminals usually transmit the nerve impulse to another neuron's cell body (or soma) or to its dendrites (or a dendritic spine). Less frequently, axon terminals form synapses with another axon terminal, an arrangement that helps modulate synaptic activity. Features of these three common morphologic types of synapses are shown at the top of the figure.

TABLE **9–1**	Common neurotransmitters and their actions.

Neurotransmitter	Description/Action
ACETYLCHOLINE (ACh)	
	Chemical structure significantly different from that of other neurotransmitters; active in CNS and in both somatic and autonomic parts of PNS; binds to ACH receptors (cholinergic receptors) in PNS to open ion channels in postsymaptic membrane and stimulate muscle contraction
AMINO ACIDS	
	Molecules with both carboxyl (—COOH) and amine (—NH$_2$) groups and various R groups; act as important transmitters in the CNS
Glutamate	Excites activity in neurons to promote cognitive function in the brain (learning and memory); most common neurotransmitter in the brain; opens Na$^+$ channels
Gamma-aminobutyric acid (GABA)	Synthesized from glutamate; primary inhibitory neurotransmitter in the brain; also influences muscle tone; opens or closes various ion channels
Glycine	Inhibits activity between neurons in the CNS, including retina; opens Cl$^-$ channels
MONOAMINES	
	Molecules synthesized from an amino acid by removing the carboxyl group and retaining the single amine group; also called biogenic amines
Serotonin or 5-hydroxytryptamine (5-HT)	Has various functions in the brain related to sleep, appetite, cognition (learning, memory), and mood; modulates actions of other neurotransmitters
Catecholamines	A distinct group of monoamines
Dopamine	Produces inhibitory activity in the brain; important roles in cognition (learning, memory), motivation, behavior, and mood; opens K$^+$ channels, closes Ca^{2+} channels
Norepinephrine (noradrenaline)	Neurotransmitter of PNS (sympathetic division of autonomic nervous system) and specific CNS regions
Epinephrine (adrenaline)	Has various effects in the CNS, especially the spinal cord, thalamus, and hypothalamus
NEUROPEPTIDES	
	Small polypeptides act as signals to assist in and modulate communication among neurons in the CNS
Enkephalin	Helps regulate response to noxious and potentially harmful stimuli
Neuropeptide Y	Involved in memory regulation and energy balance (increased food intake and decreased physical activity)
Somatostatin	Inhibits activities of neurons in specific brain areas
Substance P	Assists with pain information transmission into the brain
Cholecystokinin (CCK)	Stimulates neurons in the brain to help mediate satiation (fullness) and repress hunger
Beta-endorphin	Prevents release of pain signals from neurons and fosters a feeling of well-being
Neurotensin	Helps control and moderate the effects of dopamine
OTHERS	
Adenosine	Also part of a nucleotide, inhibits activities in certain CNS neurons
Nitric oxide	Involved in learning and memory; relaxes muscle in the digestive tract; important for relaxation of smooth muscle in blood vessels (vasodilation)

FIGURE 9–8 Neurons, neuropil, and the common glial cells of the CNS.

(a) Most neuronal cell bodies (**N**) in the CNS are larger than the much more numerous glial cells (**G**) that surround them. The various types of glial cells and their relationships with neurons are difficult to distinguish by most routine light microscopic methods. However, **oligodendrocytes** have condensed, rounded nuclei and unstained cytoplasm due to very abundant Golgi complexes, which stain poorly and are very likely represented by the

cells with those properties seen here. The other glial cells seen here similar in overall size, but with very little cytoplasm and more elongated or oval nuclei, are mostly **astrocytes**. Routine H&E staining does not allow neuropill to stand out well. X200. H&E. **(b)** With the use of gold staining for neurofibrils, **neuropil (Np)** is more apparent. X200. Gold chloride and hematoxylin.

staining, in which oligodendrocytes usually appear as small cells with rounded, condensed nuclei and unstained cytoplasm (Figure 9–8a).

Astrocytes

Astrocytes (Gr. *astron*, star + *kytos*) have a large number of radiating processes (Figures 9–9b and 9–10) and are also unique to the CNS. Astrocytes are by far the most numerous glial cells of the CNS, as well as the most diverse structurally

and functionally. Those with relatively few, long processes are called **fibrous astrocytes** and are typical in white matter; those with many shorter, branched processes are called **protoplasmic astrocytes** and predominate in the gray matter. Terminal branching of astrocytic processes is very extensive, allowing a single astrocyte to associate with over a million synaptic sites. The larger processes of all astrocytes are reinforced with bundles of intermediate filaments made of **glial fibrillary acid protein (GFAP)**, which serves as a unique marker for astrocytes, the most common source of brain tumors.

TABLE 9–2 │ Origin, location and principal functions of neuroglial cells.

Glial Cell Type	Origin	Location	Main Functions
Oligodendrocyte	Neural tube	CNS	Myelin production, electrical insulation
Schwann cell (Neurolemmocyte)	Neural crest	Peripheral nerves	Myelin production, electrical insulation
Astrocyte	Neural tube	CNS	Structural and metabolic support of neurons; BBB; repair processes
Satellite cells (of ganglia)	Neural crest	Peripheral ganglia	Structural and metabolic support for neuronal cell bodies
Ependymal cell	Neural tube	Line ventricles and central canal of CNS	Aid production and movement of CSF
Microglia	Bone marrow (monocytes)	CNS	Defense and immune-related activities

FIGURE **9–9** Glial cells of the CNS and PNS.

CNS Glial Cells

a Oligodendrocyte

b Astrocyte

c Ependymal cells

d Microglial cell

PNS Glial Cells

e Schwann cells

f Satellite cells

There are four major glia in the CNS. **(a) Oligodendrocytes** myelinate parts of several axons. **(b) Astrocytes** have multiple processes and form perivascular feet that completely enclose all capillaries (only a few such feet are shown here to allow their morphology to be seen). **(c) Ependymal cells** are epithelial-like cells that line the ventricles and central canal.

(d) Microglial cells have a protective, phagocytic, immune-related function. Two glial cells occur in the PNS. **(e) Schwann cells**, also called **neurolemmocytes**, form a series ensheathing axons. **(f) Satellite cells** are restricted to ganglia where they cover and support the large neuronal cell bodies.

FIGURE **9–10** Astrocytes.

(a) Astrocytes are the most abundant glial cells of the CNS and are characterized by numerous cytoplasmic processes (**P**) radiating from the glial cell body or soma (**S**). Astrocytic processes are not seen with routine light microscope staining but are easily seen after gold staining. Morphology of the processes allows astrocytes to be classified as fibrous (relatively few and straight processes) or protoplasmic (numerous branching processes), but functional differences between these types are not clear. X500. Gold chloride.

(b) All astrocytic processes contain intermediate filaments of GFAP, and antibodies against this protein provide a simple method to stain these cells, as seen here in a fibrous

astrocyte (**A**) and its processes. The small pieces of other GFAP-positive processes in the neuropil around this cell give an idea of the density of this glial cell and its processes in the CNS. Astrocytes are an important part of the blood-brain barrier (BBB), regulating entry of molecules and ions from blood into CNS tissue. Capillaries at the extreme upper right and lower left corners are enclosed by GFAP-positive perivascular feet (**PF**) at the ends of numerous astrocytic processes. X500. Anti-GFAP immunoperoxidase and hematoxylin counterstain.

(c) A length of capillary (**C**) is shown here completely covered by silver-stained terminal processes extending from astrocytes (**A**). X400. Rio Hortega silver.

›› MEDICAL APPLICATION

Most brain tumors are **astrocytomas** derived from those glial cells and characterized pathologically by their expression of GFAP.

Functions associated with various astrocytes include the following:

- Regulating the extracellular ionic concentrations around neurons, with particular importance in buffering extracellular K^+ levels.
- Guiding and physically supporting movements and locations of differentiating neurons in the developing CNS.
- Extending processes with expanded **perivascular feet** that cover capillary endothelial cells and contribute to the BBB.
- Regulating vasodilation within the CNS and moving nutrients, wastes, and other metabolites between neurons and capillaries.
- Extending processes that associate with or cover synapses in the CNS, affecting the formation, function, and plasticity of these structures.
- Forming a barrier layer of expanded processes, called the **glial limiting membrane**, lining the meninges at the external CNS surface.

Finally, astrocytes communicate directly with one another via gap junctions, forming a very large cellular network for the coordinated regulation of their various activities in different brain regions.

›› MEDICAL APPLICATION

Alzheimer disease, a common type of dementia in the elderly, affects both neuronal perikarya and synapses within the cerebrum. Functional defects are due to **neurofibrillary tangles,** which are accumulations of tau protein associated with microtubules of the neuronal perikaryon and axon hillock regions, and **neuritic plaques,** which are dense aggregates of β-amyloid protein that form around the outside of these neuronal regions.

Ependymal Cells

Ependymal cells are columnar or cuboidal cells that line the ventricles of the brain and central canal of the spinal cord (Figures 9–9c and 9–11). In some CNS locations, the apical ends of ependymal cells have cilia, which facilitate the

FIGURE **9–11** Ependymal cells.

Ependymal cells are epithelial-like cells that form a single layer lining the fluid-filled ventricles and central canal of the CNS. **(a)** Lining the ventricles of the cerebrum, columnar ependymal cells (**E**) extend cilia and microvilli from the apical surfaces into the ventricle (**V**). These modifications help circulate the CSF and monitor its contents. Ependymal cells have junctional complexes at their apical ends like those of epithelial cells but lack a basal lamina. The cells' basal ends are tapered, extending processes that branch and penetrate some distance into the adjacent neuropil (**N**). Other areas of ependyma are responsible for production of CSF. X100. H&E. **(b)** Ependymal cells (**E**) lining the central canal (**C**) of the spinal cord help move CSF in that CNS region. X200. H&E.

movement of cerebrospinal fluid (CSF), and long microvilli, which are likely involved in absorption.

Ependymal cells are joined apically by junctional complexes similar to those of epithelial cells. However, unlike a true epithelium there is no basal lamina. Instead, the basal ends of ependymal cells are elongated and extend branching processes into the adjacent neuropil.

Microglia

Less numerous than oligodendrocytes or astrocytes but nearly as common as neurons, **microglia** are small cells with short irregular processes evenly distributed throughout gray and white matter (Figures 9–9d and 9–12). Unlike other glial cells, microglia migrate through the neuropil, scanning the tissue for damaged cells and invading microorganisms. They secrete a number of immunoregulatory cytokines and constitute the major mechanism of immune defense in the CNS. Microglia do not originate from neural progenitor cells like other glia, but from circulating blood monocytes, belonging to the same family as macrophages and other antigen-presenting cells.

Nuclei of microglial cells can be recognized in routine hematoxylin and eosin (H&E) preparations by their small, dense, elongated structure, which contrasts with the larger, spherical, more lightly stained nuclei of other glial cells. Immunohistochemistry using antibodies against cell surface antigens of immune cells demonstrates microglial processes. When activated by damage or invaders, microglia retract their processes, proliferate, and

FIGURE **9–12** Microglial cells.

Microglia are monocyte-derived, antigen-presenting cells of the CNS, less numerous than astrocytes but nearly as common as neurons and evenly distributed in both gray and white matter. By immunohistochemistry, here using a monoclonal antibody against human leukocyte antigens (HLA) of immune-related cells, the short branching processes of microglia can be seen. Routine staining demonstrates only the small dark nuclei of the cells. Unlike other glia of the CNS, microglia are not interconnected; they are motile cells, constantly used in immune surveillance of CNS tissues. When activated by products of cell damage or by invading microorganisms, the cells retract their processes, begin phagocytosing the damage- or danger-related material, and behave as antigen-presenting cells. X500. Antibody against HLA-DR and peroxidase.

(*Used, with permission, from Wolfgang Streit, Department of Neuroscience, University of Florida College of Medicine, Gainesville.*)

assume the morphologic characteristics and functions of antigen-presenting cells (see Chapter 14).

Schwann Cells

Schwann cells (named for 19th century German histologist Theodor Schwann), sometimes called **neurolemmocytes**, are found only in the PNS and differentiate from precursors in the neural crest. Schwann cells have trophic interactions with axons and importantly allow for their myelination, like the oligodendrocytes of the CNS. As discussed with peripheral nerves, one Schwann cell forms myelin around a segment of one axon, in contrast to the ability of oligodendrocytes to branch and ensheath parts of more than one axon. Figure 9–9e shows how a series of Schwann cells covers the full length of an axon.

Satellite Cells of Ganglia

Also derived from the embryonic neural crest, small **satellite cells** form an intimate covering layer over the large neuronal cell bodies in the ganglia of the PNS (Figures 9–9f and 9–13). Satellite cells exert a trophic or supportive effect on these neurons, insulating, nourishing, and regulating their microenvironments.

› CENTRAL NERVOUS SYSTEM

The major regions of the central nervous system (CNS) are the **cerebrum**, **cerebellum**, and **spinal cord** (see Figure 9–1). The CNS is covered by three connective tissue layers, the meninges, but contains very little collagen or fibrous tissue throughout its substance, making it relatively soft and easily damaged by injuries affecting its protective cranium or vertebral bones. Most neurons of the CNS and their functional organization are more appropriately covered in neuroscience rather than histology courses, but certain important cells and basic topics are described here. Many structural features of CNS tissues can be seen in unstained, freshly dissected specimens.

The entire CNS displays organized areas of **white matter** and **gray matter**, differences caused by the differential distribution of myelin. The main components of white matter are myelinated axons (Figure 9–14), often grouped together as **tracts**, and the myelin-producing oligodendrocytes.

FIGURE 9–13 Satellite cells around neurons of ganglia in the PNS.

Satellite cells are very closely associated with cell bodies of sensory nerves and support these cells in various ways. **(a)** Nuclei of the many satellite cells (**S**) surrounding the perikarya of neurons (**N**) in a dorsal root ganglion can be seen by light microscopy, but the cytoplasmic extensions from the cells are not visible. These long-lived neurons commonly accumulate brown lipofuscin (**L**). X560. H&E.

(b) Immunofluorescent staining of satellite cells (**S**) reveals cytoplasmic sheets extending from these cells and surrounding neuronal cell bodies (**N**). Like the effect of Schwann cells on axons, satellite glial cells insulate, nourish, and regulate the microenvironment of the neuronal cell bodies. X600. Rhodamine red-labeled antibody against glutamine synthetase.

(With permission, from Menachem Hanani, laboratory of Experimental Surgery, Hadassah University Hospital, Jerusalem, Israel.)

FIGURE **9–14** White versus gray matter.

A cross section of H&E-stained spinal cord shows the transition between white matter (left region) and gray matter (right). The gray matter has many glial cells (**G**), neuronal cell bodies (**N**), and neuropil; white matter also contains glia (**G**) but consists mainly of axons (**A**) whose myelin sheaths were lost during preparation, leaving the round empty spaces shown. Each such space surrounds a dark-stained spot that is a small section of the axon. X400.

White matter contains very few neuronal cell bodies, but astrocytes and microglia are present. Gray matter contains abundant neuronal cell bodies, dendrites, the initial unmyelinated portions of axons, astrocytes, and microglial cells. Gray matter is where most synapses occur, and it occupies the thick surface or cortex of both the cerebrum and the cerebellum; most white matter is found in deeper regions. Deep regions of the CNS also have darker aggregates called **nuclei** consisting of large numbers of neuronal cell bodies and surrounded by white matter.

Neuroscientists recognize six layers of neurons with different sizes and shapes in the **cerebral cortex**. The most conspicuous of these cells are the efferent **pyramidal neurons** that come in many sizes (Figure 9–15). Neurons of the cerebral cortex function in the integration of sensory information and the initiation of voluntary motor responses.

The **cerebellar cortex**, which coordinates muscular activity throughout the body, also has a layered organization (Figure 9–16): an outer **molecular layer**, a central layer of very large neurons called **Purkinje cells** (named for the 19th century Czech histologist Jan Purkinje), and an inner **granule layer**. The Purkinje cell bodies are conspicuous even in H&E-stained material, and their dendrites extend throughout the molecular layer as a branching basket of nerve fibers (Figure 9–16d). The granule layer is formed by very small neurons (with diameters of only 4-5 μm), which are packed together densely, in contrast to the neuronal cell bodies in the molecular layer which are sparse (Figure 9–16b).

In cross sections of the **spinal cord**, white matter is peripheral and gray matter is internal and has the general shape of the letter H (Figure 9–17). In the center is an opening, the **central canal**, which develops from the lumen of the embryonic neural tube. The canal is continuous with the ventricles of the brain, contains CSF, and is lined by ependy-mal cells. The gray matter forms the **anterior horns**, which contain motor neurons whose axons make up the ventral roots of spinal nerves, and the **posterior horns**, which receive sensory fibers from neurons in the spinal (dorsal root) ganglia. Spinal cord neurons are large and multipolar, especially the motor neurons in the anterior horns (Figure 9–17).

Meninges

The skull and the vertebral column protect the CNS, but between the bone and nervous tissue are membranes of connective tissue called the **meninges**. Three meningeal layers are distinguished: the dura, arachnoid, and pia maters.

Dura Mater

The thick external **dura mater** (L., *dura mater*, tough mother) consists of dense, fibroelastic connective tissue that is continuous with the periosteum of the skull. Around the spinal cord the dura mater is separated from the periosteum of the vertebrae by the epidural space, which contains a plexus of thin-walled veins and areolar connective tissue (Figures 9-18 and 9-19).

The dura mater is always separated from the arachnoid by the thin **subdural space**. The internal surface of all dura mater, as well as its external surface in the spinal cord, is covered by simple squamous epithelium of mesenchymal origin.

Arachnoid

The **arachnoid** (Gr. *arachnoeides*, spiderweblike) has two components: (1) a sheet of connective tissue in contact with the dura mater and (2) a system of loosely arranged trabeculae composed of collagen and fibroblasts, continuous with the underlying pia mater layer. Surrounding the trabeculae is a large, sponge-like cavity, the **subarachnoid space**, filled with CSF.

FIGURE 9–15 Cerebral cortex.

(a) Important neurons of the cerebrum are the pyramidal neurons (**P**), which are arranged vertically and interspersed with numerous smaller glial cells, mostly astrocytes, in the eosinophilic neuropil. X200. H&E.

(b) From the apical ends of pyramidal neurons (**P**), long dendrites extend in the direction of the cortical surface, which can be best seen in thick silver-stained sections in which only a few other protoplasmic astrocytes (**A**) cells are seen. X200. Silver.

This fluid-filled space helps cushion and protect the CNS from minor trauma. The subarachnoid space communicates with the ventricles of the brain where the CSF is produced.

The connective tissue of the arachnoid is said to be avascular because it lacks nutritive capillaries, but larger blood vessels run through it (Figures 9–18 and 9–19). Because the arachnoid has fewer trabeculae in the spinal cord, it can be more clearly distinguished from the pia mater in that area. The arachnoid and the pia mater are intimately associated and are often considered a single membrane called the pia-arachnoid.

In some areas, the arachnoid penetrates the dura mater and protrudes into blood-filled venous sinuses located within that layer (Figure 9–19). These CSF-filled protrusions, which are covered by vascular endothelial cells lining the sinuses, are called **arachnoid villi**, which function as a site for absorption of CSF into the blood of the venous sinuses.

Pia Mater

The innermost **pia mater** (L., *pia mater*, tender mother) consists of flattened, mesenchymally derived cells closely applied to the entire surface of the CNS tissue. The pia does not directly contact nerve cells or fibers, being separated from the neural elements by the very thin superficial layer of astrocytic processes (the glia limitans), which adheres firmly to the pia mater. Together, the pia mater and the layer of astrocytic end feet form a physical barrier separating CNS tissue from CSF in the subarachnoid space (Figure 9–19).

Blood vessels penetrate the CNS through long **perivascular spaces** covered by pia mater, although the pia disappears when the blood vessels branch to form the small capillaries. However, these capillaries remain completely covered by the perivascular limiting layer of astrocytic processes (Figures 9–9b and 9–10c).

FIGURE **9–16** Cerebellum.

(a) The cerebellar cortex is convoluted with many distinctive small folds, each supported at its center by tracts of white matter in the cerebellar medulla (**M**). Each fold has distinct molecular layers (**ML**) and granular layers (**GL**). X6. Cresyl violet.

(b) Higher magnification shows that the granular layer (**GL**) immediately surrounding the medulla (**M**) is densely packed with several different types of very small rounded neuronal cell bodies. The outer molecular layer (**ML**) consists of neuropil with fewer, much more scattered small neurons. At the interface of these two regions a layer of large Purkinje neuron (**P**) perikarya can be seen. X20. H&E.

(c) A single intervening layer contains the very large cell bodies of unique Purkinje neurons (**P**), whose axons pass through the granular layer (**GL**) to join tracts in the medulla and whose multiple branching dendrites ramify throughout the molecular layer (**ML**). Dendrites are not seen well with H&E staining. X40. H&E.

(d) With appropriate silver staining dendrites from each large Purkinje cell (**P**) are shown to have hundreds of small branches, each covered with hundreds of dendritic spines. Axons from the small neurons of the granular layer are unmyelinated and run together into the molecular layer where they form synapses with the dendritic spines of Purkinje cells. X40. Silver.

FIGURE **9–17** Spinal cord.

The spinal cord varies slightly in diameter along its length but in cross section always shows bilateral symmetry around the small, CSF-filled central canal (**C**). Unlike the cerebrum and cerebellum, in the spinal cord the gray matter is internal, forming a roughly H-shaped structure that consists of two posterior (**P**) horns (sensory) and two anterior (**A**) (motor) horns, all joined by the gray commissure around the central canal.

(a) The gray matter contains abundant astrocytes and large neuronal cell bodies, especially those of motor neurons in the ventral horns. **(b)** The white matter surrounds the gray matter and contains primarily oligodendrocytes and tracts of myelinated axons running along the length of the cord. Center X5, a, b X100. All silver-stained.

(c) With H&E staining the large motor neurons (**N**) of the ventral horns show large nuclei, prominent nucleoli, and cytoplasm rich in Nissl substance, all of which indicate extensive protein synthesis to maintain the axons of these cells that extend great distances. **(d)** In the white commissure ventral to the central canal, tracts (**T**) run lengthwise along the cord, seen here in cross section with empty myelin sheaths surrounding axons, as well as small tracts running from one side of the cord to the other. Both X200. H&E.

FIGURE **9–18** Spinal cord and meninges.

Anterior view

(a) A diagram of the spinal cord indicates the relationship of the three meningeal layers of connective tissue: the innermost **pia mater**, the **arachnoid**, and the **dura mater**. Also depicted are the blood vessels coursing through the subarachnoid space and the nerve rootlets that fuse to form the posterior and anterior roots of the spinal nerves. The posterior root ganglia contain the cell bodies of sensory nerve fibers and are located in intervertebral foramina.

(b) Section of an area near the anterior median fissure showing the tough dura mater (**D**). Surrounding the dura, the epidural space (not shown) contains cushioning adipose tissue and vascular plexuses. The subdural space (**SD**) is an artifact created by separation of the dura from underlying tissue.

The middle meningeal layer is the thicker weblike arachnoid mater (**A**) containing the large subarachnoid space (**SA**) and connective tissue trabeculae (**T**). The subarachnoid space is filled with CSF and the arachnoid acts as a shock-absorbing pad between the CNS and bone. Fairly large blood vessels (**BV**) course through the arachnoid. The innermost pia mater (**P**) is thin and is not clearly separate from the arachnoid; together, they are sometimes referred to as the pia-arachnoid or the leptomeninges. The space between the pia and the white matter (**WM**) of the spinal cord here is an artifact created during dissection; normally the pia is very closely applied to a layer of astrocytic processes at the surface of the CNS tissue. X100. H&E.

Blood-Brain Barrier

The **blood-brain barrier** (BBB) is a functional barrier that allows much tighter control than that in most tissues over the passage of substances moving from blood into the CNS tissue. The main structural component of the BBB is the **capillary endothelium**, in which the cells are tightly sealed together with well-developed occluding junctions and with little or no transcytosis activity. The **limiting layer of perivascular astrocytic feet** that completely envelops the basal lamina of the capillaries in most CNS regions (Figure 9–10c) forms another BBB component and further regulates passage of molecules and ions from blood to brain.

The BBB protects neurons and glia from bacterial toxins, infectious agents, and other exogenous substances, and helps maintain the stable composition and constant balance of ions in the interstitial fluid that is required for normal neuronal function. The components of the BBB are not found in the choroid plexus where CSF is produced, in the posterior pituitary which releases hormones, or in regions of the hypothalamus where plasma components are monitored.

Choroid Plexus

The **choroid plexus** consists of highly specialized tissue with elaborate folds and many villi projecting into the four large ventricles of the brain (Figure 9–20a). It is found in the roofs of the third and fourth ventricles and in parts of the two lateral ventricular walls, all regions in which the ependymal lining directly contacts the pia mater.

Each villus of the choroid plexus contains a thin layer of well-vascularized pia mater covered by cuboidal ependymal cells (Figure 9–20b). The function of the choroid plexus is to remove water from blood and release it as the **CSF**. CSF is clear, contains Na^+, K^+, and Cl^- ions but very little protein, and its only cells are normally very sparse lymphocytes. It is produced continuously and it completely fills the ventricles, the central canal of the spinal cord, the subarachnoid and perivascular spaces. It provides the ions required for CNS neuronal activity and in the arachnoid serves to help absorb mechanical shocks. Arachnoid villi (Figure 9–19) provide the main pathway for absorption of CSF back into the venous circulation. There are no lymphatic vessels in CNS tissue.

FIGURE **9–19** Meninges around the brain.

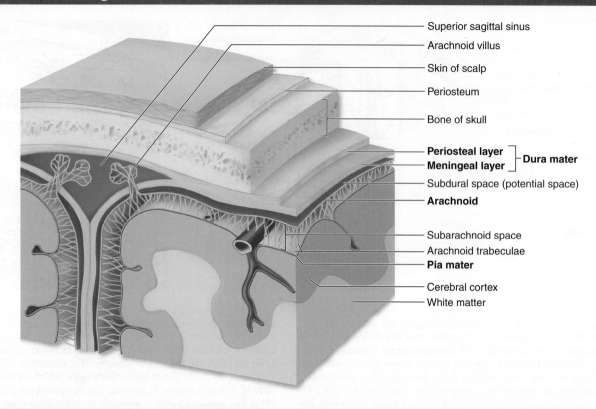

Superior sagittal sinus
Arachnoid villus
Skin of scalp
Periosteum
Bone of skull
Periosteal layer ⎫
Meningeal layer ⎬ **Dura mater**
Subdural space (potential space)
Arachnoid
Subarachnoid space
Arachnoid trabeculae
Pia mater
Cerebral cortex
White matter

The **dura, arachnoid, and pia maters** also surround the brain and as shown here the relationships among the cranial meninges are similar to those of the spinal cord. The diagram includes **arachnoid villi**, which are outpocketings of arachnoid away from the brain, which penetrate the dura mater and enter blood-filled **venous sinuses** located within that layer.

The arachnoid villi function in releasing excess CSF into the blood. Blood vessels from the arachnoid branch into smaller arteries and veins that enter brain tissue carrying oxygen and nutrients. These small vessels are initially covered with pia mater, but as capillaries they are covered only by the perivascular feet of astrocytes.

>> **MEDICAL APPLICATION**

A decrease in the absorption of CSF or a blockage of outflow from the ventricles during fetal or postnatal development results in the condition known as **hydrocephalus** (Gr. *hydro*, water + *kephale*, head), which promotes a progressive enlargement of the head followed by mental impairment.

› PERIPHERAL NERVOUS SYSTEM

The main components of the peripheral nervous system (PNS) are the **nerves**, **ganglia**, and **nerve endings**. Nerves are bundles of nerve fibers (axons) surrounded by Schwann cells and layers of connective tissue.

Nerve Fibers

Nerve fibers are analogous to tracts in the CNS, containing axons enclosed within sheaths of glial cells specialized to facilitate axonal function. In peripheral nerve fibers, axons are sheathed by **Schwann cells**, or neurolemmocytes (Figure 9–9e). The sheath may or may not form myelin around the axons, depending on their diameter.

Myelinated Fibers

As axons of large diameter grow in the PNS, they are engulfed along their length by a series of differentiating neurolemmocytes and become **myelinated nerve fibers**. The plasma membrane of each covering Schwann cell fuses with itself around the axon, and the fused membrane (or mesaxon) becomes wrapped around the axon as the glial cell body moves circumferentially around the axon many times (Figure 9–21). The multiple layers of Schwann cell membrane unite as a thick **myelin sheath**. Composed mainly of lipid bilayers and membrane proteins, myelin is a large lipoprotein complex that, like cell membranes, is partly removed by standard histologic procedures (see Figures 9–14 and 9–17d). Unlike oligodendrocytes of the CNS, a Schwann cell forms myelin around only a portion of one axon.

FIGURE **9–20** Choroid plexus.

Ependymal cells

Capillary

Pia mater

Section of choroid plexus

Cavity of ventricle

CSF forms and enters the ventricle

The choroid plexus consists of ependyma and vascularized pia mater and projects many thin folds from certain walls of the ventricles. **(a)** Section of the bilateral choroid plexus (**CP**) projecting into the fourth ventricle (**V**) near the cerebrum and cerebellum. X12. Kluver-Barrera stain.

(b) At higher magnification each fold of choroid plexus is seen to be well-vascularized with large capillaries (**C**) and covered by a continuous layer of cuboidal ependymal cells (**E**). X150. **(c)** The choroid plexus is specialized for transport of water and ions across the capillary endothelium and ependymal layer and the elaboration of these as CSF.

staining layers are the intraperiod lines that represent the apposed outer bilayers of the Schwann cell membrane.

Membranes of Schwann cells have a higher proportion of lipids than do other cell membranes, and the myelin sheath serves to insulate axons and maintain a constant ionic microenvironment most suitable for action potentials. Between adjacent Schwann cells on an axon the myelin sheath shows small **nodes of Ranvier** (or **nodal gaps**, see Figure 9–9e; Figures 9–23 and 9–24), where the axon is only partially covered by interdigitating Schwann cell processes. At these nodes the axolemma is exposed to ions in the interstitial fluid and has a much higher concentration of voltage-gated Na$^+$ channels, which renew the action potential and produce **saltatory conduction** (L. *saltare*, to jump) of nerve impulses, their rapid movement from node to node. The length of axon ensheathed by one Schwann cell, the **internodal segment**, varies directly with axonal diameter and ranges from 300 to 1500 µm.

Unmyelinated Fibers

Unlike the CNS where many short axons are not myelinated at all but run free among the other neuronal and glial processes, the smallest-diameter axons of peripheral nerves are still

With high-magnification TEM, the myelin sheath appears as a thick electron-dense axonal covering in which the concentric membrane layers may be visible (Figure 9–22). The prominent electron-dense layers visible ultrastructurally in the sheath, the **major dense lines**, represent the fused, protein-rich cytoplasmic surfaces of the Schwann cell membrane. Along the myelin sheath, these surfaces periodically separate slightly to allow transient movement of cytoplasm for membrane maintenance; at these **myelin clefts** (or Schmidt-Lanterman clefts) the major dense lines temporarily disappear (Figure 9–23). Faintly seen ultrastructurally in the light

FIGURE **9–21** Myelination of large-diameter PNS axons.

FIGURE **9–21** Myelination of large-diameter PNS axons.

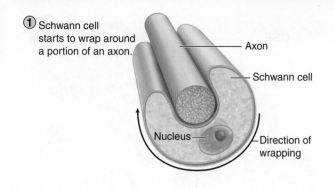

① Schwann cell starts to wrap around a portion of an axon.

Axon

Schwann cell

Nucleus

Direction of wrapping

② Schwann cell cytoplasm and plasma membrane begin to form consecutive layers around axon.

③ The overlapping inner layers of the Schwann cell plasma membrane form the myelin sheath.

Cytoplasm of the Schwann cell

Myelin sheath

④ Eventually, the Schwann cell cytoplasm and nucleus are pushed to the periphery of the cell as the myelin sheath is formed.

Myelin sheath

Schwann cell nucleus

A Schwann cell (neurolemmocyte) engulfs one portion along the length of a large-diameter axon. The Schwann cell membrane fuses around the axon and elongates as it becomes wrapped around the axon while the cell body moves around the axon many times. The Schwann cell membrane wrappings consti-tute the myelin sheath, with the Schwann cell body always on its outer surface. The myelin layers are very rich in lipid, and provide insulation and facilitate formation of action potentials along the axolemma.

enveloped within simple folds of Schwann cells (Figure 9–25). In these **unmyelinated fibers** the glial cell does not form the multiple wrapping of a myelin sheath (Figure 9–22). In unmy-elinated fibers, each Schwann cell can enclose portions of many axons with small diameters. Without the thick myelin sheath, nodes of Ranvier are not seen along unmyelinated nerve fibers. Moreover, these small-diameter axons have evenly distributed voltage-gated ion channels; their impulse conduction is not sal-tatory and is much slower than that of myelinated axons.

Nerve Organization

In the PNS nerve fibers are grouped into bundles to form **nerves**. Except for very thin nerves containing only unmy-elinated fibers, nerves have a whitish, glistening appearance because of their myelin and collagen content.

Axons and Schwann cells are enclosed within layers of connective tissue (Figures 9–24, 9–26, and 9–27). Immedi-ately around the external laminae of the Schwann cells is a thin layer called the **endoneurium**, consisting of reticular fibers, scattered fibroblasts, and capillaries. Groups of axons with Schwann cells and endoneurium are bundled together as **fas-cicles** by a sleeve of **perineurium**, containing flat fibrocytes with their edges sealed together by tight junctions. From two to six layers of these unique connective tissue cells regulate diffusion into the fascicle and make up the **blood-nerve bar-rier** that helps maintain the fibers' microenvironment. Exter-nally, peripheral nerves have a dense, irregular fibrous coat called the **epineurium**, which extends deeply to fill the space between fascicles.

Very small nerves consist of one fascicle (Figure 9–28). Small nerves can be found in sections of many organs and often show a winding disposition in connective tissue.

Peripheral nerves establish communication between cen-ters in the CNS and the sense organs and effectors (muscles, glands, etc). They generally contain both afferent and efferent fibers. **Afferent** fibers carry information from internal body regions and the environment to the CNS. **Efferent** fibers carry

FIGURE **9–22** Ultrastructure of myelinated and unmyelinated fibers.

Cross section of PNS fibers in the TEM reveals differences between myelinated and unmyelinated axons. Large axons (**A**) are wrapped in a thick myelin sheath (**M**) of multiple layers of Schwann cell membrane.

The inset shows a portion of myelin at higher magnification in which the major dense lines of individual membrane layers can be distinguished, as well as the neurofilaments (**NF**) and microtubules (**MT**) in the axoplasm (**A**). At the center of the photo is a Schwann cell showing its active nucleus (**SN**) and Golgi-rich cytoplasm (**SC**). At the right is an axon around which myelin is still forming (**FM**).

Unmyelinated axons (**UM**) are much smaller in diameter, and many such fibers may be engulfed by a single Schwann cell (**SC**). The glial cell does not form myelin wrappings around such small axons but simply encloses them. Whether it forms myelin or not, each Schwann cell is surrounded, as shown, by an external lamina containing type IV collagen and laminin like the basal laminae of epithelial cells. X28,000, inset X70,000.

(Used, with permission, from Dr Mary Bartlett Bunge, The Miami Project to Cure Paralysis, University of Miami Miller School of Medicine, Miami, FL.)

impulses from the CNS to effector organs commanded by these centers. Nerves possessing only sensory fibers are called **sensory nerves**; those composed only of fibers carrying impulses to the effectors are called **motor nerves**. Most nerves have both sensory and motor fibers and are called **mixed nerves**, usually also with both myelinated and unmyelinated axons.

Ganglia

Ganglia are typically ovoid structures containing neuronal cell bodies and their surrounding glial satellite cells supported by delicate connective tissue and surrounded by a denser capsule. Because they serve as relay stations to transmit nerve impulses, at least one nerve enters and another exits from each ganglion. The direction of the nerve impulse determines whether the ganglion will be a **sensory** or an **autonomic** ganglion.

Sensory Ganglia

Sensory ganglia receive afferent impulses that go to the CNS. Sensory ganglia are associated with both cranial nerves (cranial ganglia) and the dorsal roots of the spinal nerves (spinal ganglia). The large neuronal cell bodies of ganglia (Figure 9–29) are associated with thin, sheetlike extensions of small glial **satellite cells** (see Figures 9–9f and 9–13). Sensory ganglia are supported by a distinct connective tissue capsule and an internal framework continuous with the connective tissue layers of the nerves. The neurons of these ganglia are pseudounipolar and relay information from the ganglion's nerve endings to the gray matter of the spinal cord via synapses with local neurons.

Autonomic Ganglia

Autonomic (Gr. *autos*, self + *nomos*, law) nerves effect the activity of smooth muscle, the secretion of some glands, heart rate, and many other involuntary activities by which the body maintains a constant internal environment (**homeostasis**).

Autonomic ganglia are small bulbous dilations in autonomic nerves, usually with multipolar neurons. Some are located within certain organs, especially in the walls of the digestive tract, where they constitute the **intramural ganglia**. The capsules of these ganglia may be poorly defined among the local connective tissue. A layer of satellite cells also envelops the neurons of autonomic ganglia (Figure 9–29), although these may also be inconspicuous in intramural ganglia.

Autonomic nerves use two-neuron circuits. The first neuron of the chain, with the **preganglionic fiber**, is located in the CNS. Its axon forms a synapse with **postganglionic fibers** of the second multipolar neuron in the chain located in a peripheral ganglion system. The chemical mediator present in the synaptic vesicles of all preganglionic axons is acetylcholine.

As indicated earlier autonomic nerves make up the **autonomic nervous system**. This has two parts: the **sympathetic** and the **parasympathetic divisions**. Neuronal cell

Schmidt-Lanterman clefts

Node of Ranvier

Basal lamina

SC   SC

SC

The middle diagram shows schematically a myelinated peripheral nerve fiber as seen under the light microscope. The axon is enveloped by the myelin sheath, which, in addition to membrane, contains some Schwann cell cytoplasm in spaces called **Schmidt-Lanterman or myelin clefts** between the major dense lines of membranes.

The upper diagram shows one set of such clefts ultrastructurally. The clefts contain Schwann cell cytoplasm that was not displaced to the cell body during myelin formation. This cytoplasm moves slowly along the myelin sheath, opening temporary spaces (the clefts) that allow renewal of some membrane components as needed for maintenance of the sheath.

The lower diagram depicts the ultrastructure of a single **node of Ranvier** or nodal gap. Interdigitating processes extending from the outer layers of the **Schwann cells (SC)** partly cover and contact the axolemma at the nodal gap. This contact acts as a partial barrier to the movement of materials in and out of the periaxonal space between the axolemma and the Schwann sheath. The basal or external lamina around Schwann cells is continuous over the nodal gap. The axolemma at nodal gaps has abundant voltage-gated Na^+ channels important for impulse conductance in these axons.

FIGURE **9–24** Node of Ranvier and endoneurium.

A longitudinally oriented nerve shows one node of Ranvier (**N**) with the axon visible. Collagen of the sparse endoneurium (**En**), blue in this trichrome stain, surrounds the Schwann cells and a capillary (**C**). At least one Schwann cell nucleus (**S**) is also clearly seen. X400. Mallory trichome.

FIGURE **9–25** Unmyelinated nerves.

Unmyelinated axons

① Schwann cell starts to envelop multiple axons.

Schwann cell

Axons

② The unmyelinated axons are enveloped by the Schwann cell, but there are *no* myelin sheath wraps around each axon.

Schwann cell nucleus

Unmyelinated axon

Schwann cell

During development, portions of several small-diameter axons are engulfed by one Schwann cell. Subsequently the axons are separated and each typically becomes enclosed within its own fold of Schwann cell surface. No myelin is formed by wrapping. Small-diameter axons utilize action potentials whose formation and maintenance do not depend on the insulation provided by the myelin sheath required by large-diameter axons.

bodies of preganglionic sympathetic nerves are located in the thoracic and lumbar segments of the spinal cord and those of the parasympathetic division are in the medulla and midbrain and in the sacral portion of the spinal cord. Sympathetic second neurons are located in small ganglia along the vertebral column, while second neurons of the parasympathetic series are found in very small ganglia always located near or within the effector organs, for example in the walls of the stomach and intestines. Parasympathetic ganglia may lack distinct capsules altogether, perikarya and associated satellite cells simply forming a loosely organized plexus within the surrounding connective tissue.

› NEURAL PLASTICITY & REGENERATION

Despite its general stability, the nervous system exhibits neuronal differentiation and formation of new synapses even in adults. Embryonic development of the nervous system produces an excess of differentiating neurons, and the cells that do not establish correct synapses with other neurons are eliminated by apoptosis. In adult mammals after an injury, the neuronal circuits may be reorganized by the growth of neuronal processes, forming new synapses to replace ones lost by injury. Thus, new communications are established with some degree of functional recovery. This **neural plasticity** and reformation of processes are controlled by several growth factors produced by both neurons and glial cells in a family of proteins called **neurotrophins**.

Neuronal stem cells are present in the adult CNS, located in part among the cells of the ependyma, which can supply new neurons, astrocytes, and oligodendrocytes.

FIGURE 9–26 Peripheral nerve connective tissue: Epi-, peri-, and endoneurium.

(a) The diagram shows the relationship among these three connective tissue layers in large peripheral nerves. The epineurium (**E**) consists of a dense superficial region and a looser deep region that contains the larger blood vessels. **(b)** The micrograph shows a small vein (**V**) and artery (**A**) in the deep epineurium (**E**). Nerve fibers (**N**) are bundled in fascicles. Each fascicle is surrounded by the perineurium (**P**), consisting of a few layers of unusual squamous fibroblastic cells that are all joined at the peripheries by tight junctions. The resulting blood-nerve barrier helps regulate the microenvironment inside the fascicle. Axons and Schwann cells are in turn surrounded by a thin layer of endoneurium. X140. H&E.

(c) As shown here and in the diagram, septa (**S**) of connective tissue often extend from the perineurium into larger fascicles.

The endoneurium (**En**) and lamellar nature of the perineurium (**P**) are also shown at this magnification, along with some adjacent epineurium (**E**). X200. PT.

(d) SEM of transverse sections of a large peripheral nerve showing several fascicles, each surrounded by perineurium and packed with endoneurium around the individual myelin sheaths. Each fascicle contains at least one capillary. Endothelial cells of these capillaries are tightly joined as part of the blood-nerve barrier and regulate the kinds of plasma substances released to the endoneurium. Larger blood vessels course through the deep epineurium that fills the space around the perineurium and fascicles. X450.

Fully differentiated, interconnected CNS neurons cannot temporarily disengage these connections and divide to replace cells lost by injury or disease; the potential of neural stem cells to allow tissue regeneration and functional recovery within the CNS components is a subject of intense investigation. Astrocytes

do proliferate at injured sites and these growing cells can interfere with successful axonal regeneration in structures such as spinal cord tracts.

In the histologically much simpler peripheral nerves, injured axons have a much greater potential for regeneration

FIGURE **9–27** Peripheral nerve ultrastructure.

This low-magnification TEM shows a fibroblast (**F**) surrounded by collagen (**C**) in the epineurium (**E**) and three layers of flattened cells in the perineurium (**P**) which form another part of the blood-nerve barrier. Inside the perineurium the endoneurium (**En**) is rich in reticulin fibers (**RF**) that surround all Schwann cells. Nuclei of two Schwann cells (**SC**) of myelinated axons (**A**) are visible as well as many unmyelinated axons (**UM**) within Schwann cells. X1200.

and return of function. If the cell bodies are intact, damaged, or severed PNS axons can regenerate as shown in the sequence of diagrams in Figure 9–30. Distal portions of axons, isolated from their source of new proteins and organelles, degenerate; the surrounding Schwann cells dedifferentiate, shed the myelin sheaths, and proliferate within the surrounding layers of connective tissue. Cellular debris including shed myelin is removed by blood-derived macrophages, which also secrete neurotrophins to promote anabolic events of axon regeneration.

The onset of regeneration is signaled by changes in the perikaryon that characterize the process of **chromatolysis**: the cell body swells slightly, Nissl substance is initially diminished, and the nucleus migrates to a peripheral position within the perikaryon. The proximal segment of the axon close to the wound degenerates for a short distance, but begins to grow again distally as new Nissl substance appears and debris is removed. The new Schwann cells align to serve as guides for the regrowing axons and produce polypeptide factors that promote axonal outgrowth. Motor axons reestablish synaptic connections with muscles and function is restored.

›› MEDICAL APPLICATION

Regeneration of peripheral nerves is functionally efficient only when the fibers and the columns of Schwann cells are directed properly. In a mixed nerve, if regenerating sensory fibers grow into columns formerly occupied by motor fibers connected to motor end plates, the function of the muscle will not be reestablished. When there is an extensive gap between the distal and proximal segments of cut or injured peripheral nerves or when the distal segment disappears altogether (as in the case of amputation of a limb), the newly growing axons may form a swelling, or **neuroma**, that can be the source of spontaneous pain.

Nervous System SUMMARY OF KEY POINTS

Development of Nerve Tissue

- Nervous tissue develops in the early embryo when the dorsal ectoderm **neural plate** folds lengthwise to form the **neural tube**, the precursor of the CNS, and releases **neural crest cells**, precursors for much of the PNS.

Neurons

- There are many kinds of **neurons**, but all consist of a **cell body (perikaryon)** containing the nucleus, a long cytoplasmic extension called the **axon**, and one or more shorter processes called **dendrites**.
- Neurons use the common cell property of **excitability** to produce and move an **action potential (nerve impulse)** along the axon to excite another neuron or other effector cell.

- Such nerve communication is transmitted to another neuron or effector cell via a **synapse**, where **neurotransmitter** is released at the **presynaptic membrane** and binds receptors on the **postsynaptic cell**, initiating a new action potential there.

Glial Cells

- Glial cells (glia), required to support neurons in many ways, consist of six major types:
  - **Oligodendrocytes** wrap processes around portions of axons in the CNS, forming **myelin sheaths** that insulate the axons and facilitate nerve impulses.
  - **Astrocytes**, the most numerous cell of the CNS, all produce hundreds of processes to cover and provide regulated microenvironments for neuronal perikarya, synapses, and capillaries.

FIGURE **9–28** Small nerves.

Small nerves can be seen in sections from most organs. **(a)** In cross section an isolated, resin-embedded nerve is seen to have a thin perineurium (**P**), one capillary (**C**), and many large axons (**A**) associated with Schwann cells (**S**). A few nuclei of fibroblasts can be seen in the endoneurium between the myelinated fibers. X400. PT.

(b) In longitudinal sections the flattened nuclei of endoneurial fibroblasts (**F**) and more oval nuclei of Schwann cells (**S**) can be distinguished. Nerve fibers are held rather loosely in the endoneurium and in low-magnification longitudinal section are seen to be wavy rather than straight. This indicates a slack-

ness of fibers within the nerve, which allows nerves to stretch slightly during body movements with no potentially damaging tension on the fibers. X200. H&E.

(c) In sections of mesentery and other tissues, a highly wavy or tortuous disposition of a single small nerve (**N**) will be seen as multiple oblique or transverse pieces as the nerve enters and leaves the area in the section. X200. H&E. **(d)** Often, a section of small nerve will have some fibers cut transversely and others cut obliquely within the same fascicle, again suggesting the relatively unrestrained nature of the fibers within the endoneurium (**E**) and perineurium (**P**). X300. H&E.

- **Ependymal cells** are epithelial-like cells, lacking basement membranes, which line the fluid-filled cerebral ventricles and central canal of the spinal cord.
- **Microglia** differ from all other glial cells in originating from blood monocytes, not from neural tissue precursors; they mediate immune defense activity within the CNS.
- **Schwann cells (neurolemmocytes)** enclose all axons in nerves of the PNS, producing **myelin sheaths** around large-diameter axons, whose impulse conductivity is augmented at the **nodes of Ranvier** between successive Schwann cells.

- **Satellite cells** are located within PNS **ganglia**, aggregated sensory or autonomic neuronal cell bodies, where they enclose each perikaryon and regulate its microenvironment.

Central Nervous System

- Within the brain and spinal cord, regions rich in neuronal perikarya and astrocytes comprise the **gray matter** and regions containing tracts of myelinated axons comprise **white matter**.
- Hundreds of different neurons make up the CNS; large, unique **Purkinje neurons** characterize the cortex of the cerebellum, and layers of small **pyramidal neurons** form the cerebral cortex.

FIGURE **9–29** Ganglia.

(a) A sensory ganglion (**G**) has a distinct connective tissue capsule (**C**) and internal framework continuous with the epineurium and other components of peripheral nerves, except that no perineurium is present and that there is no blood-nerve barrier function. Fascicles of nerve fibers (**F**) enter and leave these ganglia. X56. Kluver-Barrera stain.

(b) Higher magnification shows the small, rounded nuclei of glia cells called satellite cells (**S**) that produce thin, sheetlike

cytoplasmic extensions that completely envelop each large neuronal perikaryon. X400. H&E.

(c) Sympathetic ganglia are smaller than most sensory ganglia but similar in having large neuronal cell bodies (**N**), some containing lipofuscin (**L**). Sheets from satellite cells (**S**) enclose each neuronal cell body with morphology slightly different from that of sensory ganglia. Autonomic ganglia generally have less well-developed connective tissue capsules (**C**) than sensory ganglia. X400. H&E.

- The CNS is completely enclosed by three connective tissue layers called **meninges**: (1) the tough external **dura mater**; (2) the middle **arachnoid layer**; and (3) the delicate **pia mater** that directly contacts neural tissue.
- The **arachnoid layer** contains much CSF, which helps **cushion** the CNS within its bony enclosure.

- The **choroid plexus** consists of elaborate folds of vascularized **pia mater** covered by **ependyma** that project from walls of the cerebral ventricles; there water is removed from capillaries and transferred into the ventricles as **cerebrospinal fluid (CSF)**.
- In most CNS regions, neurons are also protected by the blood-brain barrier, consisting of the **perivascular feet of astrocytic processes** and the nonfenestrated capillary endothelial cells' **tight junctions**.

FIGURE **9–30** Regeneration in peripheral nerves.

| a | b 2 weeks | c 3 weeks | d 3 months |

In an injured or cut peripheral nerve, proximal axon segments can regenerate from their cut ends after a delay. The main changes that take place in an injured nerve fiber are shown here. **(a)** Normal nerve fiber, with its perikaryon, extensive RER (Nissl substance), and effector cell (muscle).

(b) When the axon is injured, the RER is greatly reduced initially and the nerve fiber distal to the injury degenerates along with its myelin sheath. Debris is phagocytosed by macrophages (shown in purple).

(c) In the following weeks after injury, muscle fiber shows denervation atrophy, but Schwann cells proliferate to form a compact cord penetrated by the regrowing axon. The axon grows at the rate of 0.5-3 mm/d.

(d) After some months, the nerve fiber regeneration is successful and functional connections with the muscle fiber are restored.

Peripheral Nervous System

- **Peripheral nerves** consist of axons from motor neurons (in the spinal cord), sensory neurons, and autonomic neurons (in ganglia); all the axons are enclosed within a series of **Schwann cells**, but only large (myelinated) axons have myelin sheaths and nodes of Ranvier.
- **Endoneurium** is a thin connective tissue layer immediately surrounding Schwann cells in peripheral nerves, containing a few nonfenestrated capillaries and much reticulin.
- Groups of axons (with Schwann cells and endoneurium) are surrounded by **perineurium**, consisting of layered, squamous fibroblastic cells joined by **tight junctions** to make a **blood-nerve barrier**.
- In large peripheral nerves, groups of axons are subdivided as **fascicles**, each of which is surrounded by perineurium.
- Surrounding the perineurium is a thick, outermost layer of dense irregular connective tissue, the **epineurium**.

- **Ganglia**, which can be either sensory or autonomic, contain neuronal cell bodies and their **satellite cells** and are surrounded by connective tissue continuous with that of nerves.

Neural Plasticity & Regeneration

- Certain regions of the CNS, such as near the ependyma, retain rare **neural stem and progenitor cells** that allow some replacement of neurons throughout life; **neural plasticity** involving formation and remodeling of synaptic connections is also prevalent throughout life.
- The complexity and distances of the neuronal and glial interconnections with the CNS make regeneration and restoration of function within this tissue after major injury very difficult.
- The more simply organized peripheral nerves have better capacity for **axonal regeneration**, a process involving reactivation of the perikaryon, Schwann cells, and macrophages.

10 Muscle Tissue

Muscle tissue, the fourth basic tissue type with epithelia, connective tissues, and nervous tissue, is composed of cells that optimize the universal cell property of **contractility**. As in all cells, actin microfilaments and associated proteins generate the forces necessary for the muscle contraction, which drives movement within organ systems, of blood, and of the body as a whole. Essentially all muscle cells are of mesodermal origin and differentiate by a gradual process of cell lengthening with abundant synthesis of the myofibrillar proteins actin and myosin.

Three types of muscle tissue can be distinguished on the basis of morphologic and functional characteristics (Figure 10–1), with the structure of each adapted to its physiologic role.

- **Skeletal muscle** contains bundles of very long, multinucleated cells with cross-striations. Their contraction is quick, forceful, and usually under voluntary control.
- **Cardiac muscle** also has cross-striations and is composed of elongated, often branched cells bound to one another at structures called **intercalated discs** that are unique to cardiac muscle. Contraction is involuntary, vigorous, and rhythmic.
- **Smooth muscle** consists of collections of fusiform cells that lack striations and have slow, involuntary contractions.

In all types of muscle, contraction is caused by the sliding interaction of thick myosin filaments along thin actin filaments. The forces necessary for sliding are generated by other proteins affecting the weak interactions in the bridges between actin and myosin.

As with neurons, muscle specialists refer to certain muscle cell organelles with special names. The cytoplasm of muscle cells is often called **sarcoplasm** (Gr. *sarkos*, flesh + *plasma*, thing formed), the smooth ER is the **sarcoplasmic reticulum**, and the muscle cell membrane and its external lamina are the **sarcolemma** (*sarkos* + Gr. *lemma*, husk).

>> **MEDICAL APPLICATION**

The variation in diameter of muscle fibers depends on factors such as the specific muscle, age, gender, nutritional status, and physical training of the individual. Exercise enlarges the skeletal musculature by stimulating formation of new myofibrils and growth in the diameter of individual muscle fibers. This process, characterized by increased cell volume, is called **hypertrophy** (Gr. *hyper*, above + *trophe*, nourishment). Tissue growth by an increase in the number of cells is termed **hyperplasia** (hyper + Gr. *plasis*, molding), which takes place very readily in smooth muscle, whose cells have not lost the capacity to divide by mitosis.

> **SKELETAL MUSCLE**

Skeletal (or **striated**) **muscle** consists of **muscle fibers**, which are long, cylindrical multinucleated cells with diameters of 10 to 100 μm. During embryonic muscle development, mesenchymal myoblasts (L. *myo*, muscle) fuse, forming myotubes with many nuclei. Myotubes then further differentiate to

FIGURE 10-1 The three types of muscle.

Striations ─ Connective
─ Nuclei ─ Muscle fiber │ tissue

a Skeletal muscle

Intercalated disc ─ Glycogen ─
Branching Striations ─ Nucleus ─

b Cardiac muscle

─ Nuclei ─ Muscle cells

c Smooth muscle

Light micrographs of each type, accompanied by labeled drawings. **(a) Skeletal muscle** is composed of large, elongated, multinucleated fibers that show strong, quick, voluntary contractions. **(b) Cardiac muscle** is composed of irregular branched cells bound together longitudinally by intercalated discs and shows strong, involuntary contractions. **(c) Smooth muscle** is composed of grouped, fusiform cells with weak, involuntary contractions. The density of intercellular packing seen reflects the small amount of extracellular connective tissue present. (a, b): X200. (c): X300. All H&E.

form striated muscle fibers (Figure 10–2). Elongated nuclei are found peripherally just under the sarcolemma, a characteristic nuclear location unique to skeletal muscle fibers/cells. A small population of reserve progenitor cells called muscle **satellite cells** remains adjacent to most fibers of differentiated skeletal muscle.

Organization of a Skeletal Muscle

Thin layers of connective tissue surround and organize the contractile fibers in all three types of muscle, and these layers are seen particularly well in skeletal muscle (Figures 10–3 and 10–4). The organization given by these supportive layers resembles that in large peripheral nerves:

- The **epimysium**, an external sheath of dense connective tissue, surrounds the entire muscle. Septa of this tissue extend inward, carrying the larger nerves, blood vessels, and lymphatics of the muscle.
- The **perimysium** is a thin connective tissue layer that immediately surrounds each bundle of muscle fibers

termed a **fascicle** (Figure 10–3). Each fascicle of muscle fibers makes up a functional unit in which the fibers work together. Nerves, blood vessels, and lymphatics penetrate the perimysium to supply each fascicle.

- Within fascicles a very thin, delicate layer of reticular fibers and scattered fibroblasts, the **endomysium**, surrounds the external lamina of individual muscle fibers. In addition to nerve fibers, capillaries form a rich network in the endomysium bringing O_2 to the muscle fibers (Figure 10–5).

Collagen in these connective tissue layers of muscle serve to transmit the mechanical forces generated by the contracting muscle cells/fibers; individual muscle fibers seldom extend from one end of a muscle to the other.

Some skeletal muscles taper at their ends, where the epimysium is continuous with the dense regular connective tissue of a tendon at **myotendinous junctions** (Figure 10–6). Ultrastructural studies show that in these transitional regions, collagen fibers from the tendon insert themselves among muscle fibers and associate directly with complex infoldings of sarcolemma.

FIGURE **10–2** Development of skeletal muscle.

Myoblasts

Satellite cell

Myoblast fusion to form myotubes

Differentiation

Satellite cell

Muscle fiber

Skeletal muscle begins to differentiate when mesenchymal cells, called **myoblasts**, align and fuse together to make longer, multinucleated tubes called **myotubes**. Myotubes synthesize the proteins to make up myofilaments and gradually begin to show cross-striations by light microscopy. Myotubes continue differentiating to form functional myofilaments, and the nuclei are displaced against the sarcolemma.

Part of the myoblast population does not fuse and differentiate but remains as a group of mesenchymal cells called muscle **satellite cells** located on the external surface of muscle fibers inside the developing external lamina. Satellite cells proliferate and produce new muscle fibers following muscle injury.

FIGURE **10–3** Organization of skeletal muscle.

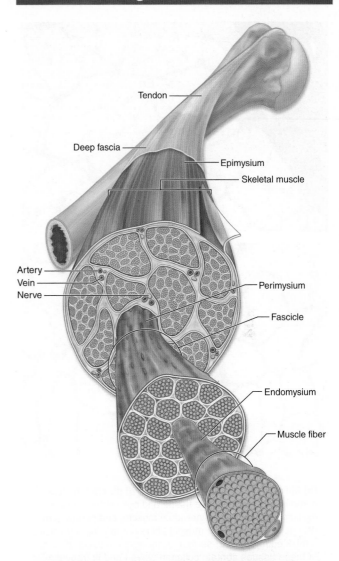

Tendon

Deep fascia

Epimysium

Skeletal muscle

Artery

Vein

Nerve

Perimysium

Fascicle

Endomysium

Muscle fiber

An entire skeletal muscle is enclosed within a thick layer of dense connective tissue called the **epimysium** that is continuous with fascia and the tendon binding muscle to bone. Large muscles contain several **fascicles** of muscle tissue, each wrapped in a thin but dense connective tissue layer called the **perimysium**. Within fascicles individual muscle fibers (elongated multinuclear cells) are surrounded by a delicate connective tissue layer, the **endomysium**.

Organization Within Muscle Fibers

Longitudinally sectioned skeletal muscle fibers show cross-striations of alternating light and dark bands (Figure 10–7). The dark bands are called **A bands** (*an*isotropic or birefringent in polarized light microscopy); the light bands are called **I bands** (*i*sotropic, do not alter polarized light). In the TEM (Figure 10–7c), each I band is seen to be bisected by a dark transverse line, the **Z disc** (Ger. *zwischen*, between). The repetitive functional subunit of the contractile apparatus, the **sarcomere**, extends from Z disc to Z disc (Figure 10–8) and is about 2.5 μm long in resting muscle.

The sarcoplasm has little RER and contains primarily long cylindrical filament bundles, called **myofibrils**, running parallel to the long axis of the fiber (Figure 10–8a). Mitochondria and sarcoplasmic reticulum are found between the myofibrils, which have a diameter of 1 to 2 μm. Myofibrils consist of an end-to-end repetitive arrangement of sarcomeres (Figure 10–8a); the lateral registration of sarcomeres in adjacent myofibrils causes the entire muscle fiber to exhibit a characteristic pattern of transverse striations.

The A and I banding pattern in sarcomeres is due mainly to the regular arrangement of thick and thin **myofilaments**, composed of **myosin** and **F-actin**, respectively, organized within each myofibril in a symmetric pattern containing thousands of each filament type.

The thick myosin filaments are 1.6 μm long and 15 nm wide; they occupy the A band at the middle region of the sarcomere. **Myosin** is a large complex (~500 kDa) with

FIGURE **10–4** Skeletal muscle.

(a) Micrograph shows a cross section of striated muscle demonstrating connective tissue and cell nuclei. The endomysium (**En**) surrounds individual muscle, and perimysium (**P**) encloses a group of muscle fibers comprising a fascicle. A thick epimysium (**E**) surrounds the entire muscle. All three of these tissues contain collagen types I and III (reticulin). X200. H&E.

(b) Adjacent section immunohistochemically stained for laminin, which specifically stains the external laminae of muscle fibers within the endoneurium. X400. Immunoperoxidase.

FIGURE **10–5** Capillaries of skeletal muscle.

The blood vessels were injected with a dark plastic polymer before the muscle was collected and sectioned longitudinally. A rich network of capillaries in endomysium surrounding muscle fibers is revealed by this method. X200. Giemsa with polarized light.

The thin, helical actin filaments are each 1.0 μm long and 8 nm wide and run between the thick filaments. Each G-actin monomer contains a binding site for myosin (Figure 10–9b). Actin filaments are anchored perpendicularly on the Z disc by the actin-binding protein α-**actinin** and exhibit opposite polarity on each side of this disc

FIGURE **10–6** Myotendinous junction.

Tendons develop together with skeletal muscles and join muscles to the periosteum of bones. The collagen fibers of a tendon (**T**) are continuous with those in the connective tissue layers around muscle fibers (**M**), forming a strong unit that allows muscle contraction to move the skeleton. X400. H&E.

two identical heavy chains and two pairs of light chains. Myosin heavy chains are thin, rodlike motor proteins (150 nm long and 2-3 nm thick) twisted together as myosin tails (Figure 10–9). Globular projections containing the four myosin light chains form a head at one end of each heavy chain. The myosin heads bind both actin, forming transient crossbridges between the thick and thin filaments, and ATP, catalyzing energy release (**actomyosin ATPase activity**). Several hundred myosin molecules are arranged within each thick filament with overlapping rodlike portions and the globular heads directed toward either end (Figure 10–9a).

FIGURE **10–7** Striated skeletal muscle in longitudinal section.

Longitudinal sections reveal the striations characteristic of skeletal muscle. **(a)** Parts of three muscle fibers are separated by very small amounts of endomysium. One fibroblast nucleus (**F**) is shown. Muscle nuclei (**N**) are found against the sarcolemma. Along each fiber thousands of dark-staining **A** bands alternate with lighter **I** bands. X200. H&E.
(b) At higher magnification, each fiber can be seen to have three or four myofibrils, here with their striations slightly out of alignment with one another. Myofibrils are cylindrical bundles of thick and thin myofilaments that fill most of each muscle fiber. The middle of each I band can be seen to have a darker Z line (or disc). X500. Giemsa.

(c) TEM showing the more electron-dense **A** bands bisected by a narrow, less electron-dense region called the **H** zone and in the **I** bands the presence of sarcoplasm with mitochondria (**M**), glycogen granules, and small cisternae of SER around the **Z** line. X24,000.

(Figure 10–7c, with permission, from Mikel H. Snow, Department of Cell and Neurobiology, Keck School of Medicine at the University of Southern California, Los Angeles.)

(Figure 10–8c). Thin filaments are also tightly associated with two regulatory proteins (Figure 10–9):

- **Tropomyosin,** a 40-nm-long coil of two polypeptide chains located in the groove between the two twisted actin strands.
- **Troponin,** a complex of three subunits: TnT, which attaches to tropomyosin; TnC, which binds Ca^{2+}; and TnI, which regulates the actin-myosin interaction.

Troponin complexes attach at specific sites regularly spaced along each tropomyosin molecule.

I bands, each bisected by a Z disc, consist of the portions of the thin filaments that do not overlap the thick filaments (which is why I bands stain more lightly). An important accessory protein in I bands is **titin** (3700 kDa), the largest protein in the body, with scaffolding and elastic properties, which supports the thick myofilaments and connects them to the Z disc (Figure 10–8c). Another very large accessory protein, **nebulin** (600-900 kDa), binds each thin myofilament laterally, helps anchor them to α-actinin, and specifies the length of the actin polymers during myogenesis.

The A bands contain both thick filaments and the overlapping portions of thin filaments. Close observation of the A band shows the presence of a lighter zone in its center, the H zone, corresponding to a region with only the rodlike portions of the myosin molecule and no thin filaments (Figure 10–8c). Bisecting the H zone is the M line (Ger. *Mitte*, middle; Figure 10–8c), containing a myosin-binding protein **myomesin** that holds the thick filaments in place, and **creatine kinase**. This enzyme catalyzes transfer of phosphate groups from phosphocreatine, a storage form of high-energy phosphate groups, to ADP, helping to supply ATP for muscle contraction.

Despite the many proteins present in sarcomeres, myosin and actin together represent over half of the total protein in striated muscle. The overlapping arrangement of thin and thick filaments within sarcomeres produces in TEM cross sections hexagonal patterns of structures that were important in determining the functions of the filaments and other proteins in the myofibril (Figures 10–8b and 10–8e).

Sarcoplasmic Reticulum & Transverse Tubule System

In skeletal muscle fibers the smooth ER, or **sarcoplasmic reticulum**, is specialized for Ca^{2+} sequestration. Depolarization of the sarcoplasmic reticulum membrane, which causes release of calcium, is initiated at specialized motor nerve synapses on the sarcolemma. To trigger Ca^{2+} release from sarcoplasmic reticulum throughout the fiber simultaneously and cause uniform contraction of all myofibrils, the sarcolemma is folded into a system of **transverse** or **T tubules** (Figures 10–10a and 10–11). These long fingerlike invaginations of the cell membrane penetrate deeply into the sarcoplasm and encircle every myofibril near the aligned A- and I-band boundaries of sarcomeres (Figures 10–10b and 10–11).

FIGURE **10–8** Structure of a myofibril: A series of sarcomeres.

(a) The diagram shows that each muscle fiber contains several parallel bundles called **myofibrils**.

(b) Each myofibril consists of a long series of sarcomeres, separated by Z discs and containing thick and thin filaments that overlap in certain regions.

(c) Thin filaments are actin filaments with one end bound to α-**actinin** in the Z disc. Thick filaments are bundles of myosin, which span the entire A band and are bound to proteins of the M line and to the Z disc across the I bands by a very large protein called **titin**, which has springlike domains.

(d) The molecular organization of the sarcomeres produces staining differences that cause the dark- and light-staining bands seen by light microscopy and TEM. X28,000.

(e) With the TEM an oblique section of myofibrils includes both **A** and **I** bands and shows hexagonal patterns that indicate the relationships between thin and thick myofilaments and other proteins, as shown in part **b** of this figure. Thin and thick filaments are arranged so that each myosin bundle contacts six actin filaments. Large mitochondria in cross-section and SER cisternae are seen between the myofibrils. X45,000.

FIGURE **10–9** Molecules composing thin and thick filaments.

a Thick filament

b Thin filament

Myofilaments, which include both thick and thin filaments, consist of contractile protein arrays bundled within myofibrils.

(a) A thick myofilament contains 200-500 molecules of **myosin**. **(b)** A thin filament contains **F-actin**, **tropomyosin**, and **troponin**.

Adjacent to each side of every T tubule are expanded **terminal cisterns** of the sarcoplasmic reticulum. In longitudinal TEM sections, this complex of a T tubule with two closely associated small cisterns of sarcoplasmic reticulum on each side is known as a **triad** (Figures 10–10b and 10–11). After depolarization of the sarcoplasmic reticulum membrane, calcium ions concentrated within these cisternae are released through Ca^{2+} channels in the membrane into cytoplasm surrounding the thick and thin filaments. Ca^{2+} binds troponin and allows bridging between actin and myosin molecules. When the membrane depolarization ends, the sarcoplasmic reticulum pumps Ca^{2+} back into the cisternae, ending contractile activity. Together, the triad components make up a signaling apparatus for converting repeated cell membrane depolarizations into spikes of free, cytoplasmic Ca^{2+} that trigger contraction.

Mechanism of Contraction

During contraction, neither the thick nor thin filaments change their length. Contraction results as the overlapping thin and thick filaments of each sarcomere slide past one another.

Contraction is induced when an action potential arrives at a synapse, the neuromuscular junction (NMJ), and is transmitted along the T tubules to the sarcoplasmic reticulum to trigger Ca^{2+} release. Figure 10–11 summarizes the key molecular events in muscle contraction.

In a resting muscle, the myosin heads cannot bind G-actin because the binding sites are blocked by the troponin-tropomyosin complex on the F-actin filaments. Calcium ions released upon neural stimulation bind troponin, changing its shape and moving tropomyosin on the F-actin to expose the myosin-binding active sites and allow crossbridges to form. Binding actin produces a conformational change or pivot in the myosins, which pulls the thin filaments farther into the A band, toward the Z disc. Energy for the pivot and pulling of actin is provided by hydrolysis of ATP bound to the myosin heads, after which myosin binds another ATP and detaches from actin. In the continued presence of Ca^{2+} and ATP, these attach-pivot-detach events occur in a repeating cycle, each lasting about 50 milliseconds, which shortens the sarcomere and contracts the muscle (Figure 10–12). A single muscle contraction results from hundreds of these cycles.

FIGURE **10–10** Transverse tubule system.

Transverse tubules are invaginations of the sarcolemma that penetrate deeply into the muscle fiber around all myofibrils.

(a) TEM cross section of fish muscle shows portions of two fibers and the endomysium (**E**) between them. Several transverse or T tubules (**T**) are shown, perpendicular to the fiber surface, penetrating between myofibrils (**M**). X50,000.

(b) Higher-magnification TEM of skeletal muscle in longitudinal section shows four membranous triads (**Tr**) cut transversely near the **A**-band–**I**-band junctions. Each triad consists of a

central transverse tubule (**T**) and two adjacent terminal cisterns (**TC**) extending from the sarcoplasmic reticulum. Centrally located is the **Z** disc. Besides elements of the triad, sarcoplasm surrounding the myofibril also contains dense glycogen granules (**G**).

Components of the triad are responsible for the cyclic release of Ca^{2+} from the cisternae and its sequestration again that occurs during muscle contraction and relaxation. The association between SR cisternae and T tubules is shown diagrammatically in Figure 10–11. X90,000.

When the neural impulse stops and levels of free calcium diminish, tropomyosin again covers the myosin-binding sites on actin and the filaments passively slide back and sarcomeres return to their relaxed length. In the absence of ATP, the actin-myosin crossbridges become stable, which accounts for the rigidity of skeletal muscles (**rigor mortis**) that occurs as mitochondrial activity stops after death.

Innervation

Myelinated motor nerves branch out within the perimysium connective tissue, where each nerve gives rise to several unmyelinated terminal twigs that pass through endomysium and form synapses with individual muscle fibers. Schwann cells enclose the small axon branches and cover their points of contact with the muscle cells (Figure 10–13); the external lamina of the Schwann cell fuses with that of the sarcolemma. Each axonal branch forms a dilated termination situated within a trough on the muscle cell surface. This synaptic structure is called the **motor end plate (MEP)**, or **NMJ** (Figure 10–13). Within the axon terminal are mitochondria and numerous synaptic vesicles, the latter containing the neurotransmitter **acetylcholine**. Between the axon and the muscle is a space, the **synaptic cleft**. Adjacent to the synaptic cleft, the sarcolemma is

thrown into numerous deep **junctional folds**, which provide for greater postsynaptic surface area and more transmembrane acetylcholine receptors.

When a **nerve action potential** reaches the MEP, acetylcholine is liberated from the axon terminal, diffuses across the cleft, and binds to its receptors in the folded sarcolemma. The **acetylcholine receptor** contains a nonselective cation channel that opens upon neurotransmitter binding, allowing influx of Na^+, depolarizing the sarcolemma, and producing the **muscle action potential**. Acetylcholine quickly dissociates from its receptors, and all free neurotransmitter is removed from the synaptic cleft by the extracellular enzyme **acetylcholinesterase**, preventing prolonged contact of the transmitter with its receptors.

As discussed with Figure 10–11, the action potential initiated at the MEP moves along the surface of the muscle cell and along T tubules that penetrate deeply into sarcoplasm. At triads the depolarization signal triggers the release of Ca^{2+} from terminal cisterns of the sarcoplasmic reticulum, initiating the contraction cycle.

An axon from a single motor neuron can form MEPs with one or many muscle fibers. Innervation of single muscle fibers by single motor neurons provides precise control of muscle activity and occurs, for example, in the extraocular muscles

FIGURE 10–11 Events of muscle contraction.

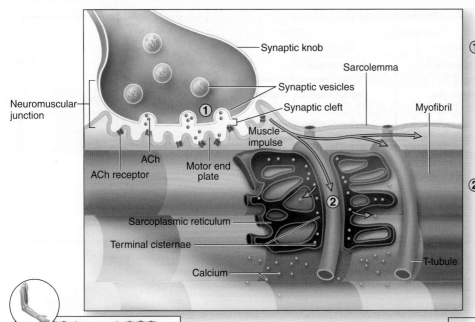

① A nerve impulse triggers release of ACh from the synaptic knob into the synaptic cleft. ACh binds to ACh receptors in the motor end plate of the neuromuscular junction, initiating a muscle impulse in the sarcolemma of the muscle fiber.

② As the muscle impulse spreads quickly from the sarcolemma along T tubules, calcium ions are released from terminal cisternae into the sarcoplasm.

⑤ When the impulse stops, calcium ions are actively transported into the sarcoplasmic reticulum, tropomyosin re-covers active sites, and filaments passively slide back to their relaxed state.

③ Calcium ions bind to troponin. Troponin changes shape, moving tropomyosin on the actin to expose active sites on actin molecules of thin filaments. Myosin heads of thick filaments attach to exposed active sites to form crossbridges.

④ Myosin heads pivot, moving thin filaments toward the sarcomere center. ATP binds myosin heads and is broken down into ADP and P. Myosin heads detach from thin filaments and return to their prepivot position. The repeating cycle of *attach-pivot-detach-return* slides thick and thin filaments past one another. The sarcomere shortens and the muscle contracts. The cycle continues as long as calcium ions remain bound to troponin to keep active sites exposed.

FIGURE 10–12 Sliding filaments and sarcomere shortening in contraction.

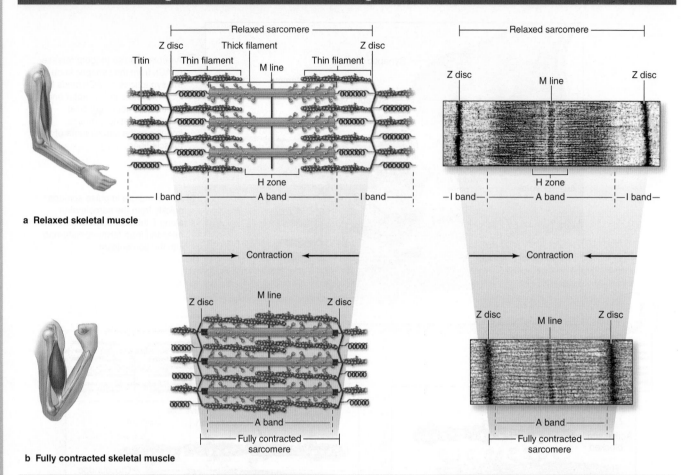

a Relaxed skeletal muscle

b Fully contracted skeletal muscle

Diagrams and TEM micrographs show sarcomere shortening during skeletal muscle contraction. **(a)** In the relaxed state the sarcomere, I band, and H zone are at their expanded length. The springlike action of titin molecules, which span the I band, helps pull thin and thick filaments past one another in relaxed muscle. **(b)** During muscle contraction, the Z discs at the sarcomere boundaries are drawn closer together as they move toward the ends of thick filaments in the A band. Titin molecules are compressed during contraction.

for eye movements. Larger muscles with coarser movements have motor axons that typically branch profusely and innervate 100 or more muscle fibers. In this case the single axon and all the muscle fibers in contact with its branches make up a **motor unit**. Individual striated muscle fibers do not show graded contraction—they contract either all the way or not at all. To vary the force of contraction, the fibers within a muscle fascicle do not all contract at the same time. With large muscles composed of many motor units, the firing of a single motor axon will generate tension proportional to the number of muscle fibers it innervates. Thus, the number of motor units and their variable size control the intensity and precision of a muscle contraction.

Key features of skeletal muscle cells, connective tissue, contraction, and innervation are summarized in Table 10–1.

MEDICAL APPLICATION

Myasthenia gravis is an autoimmune disorder that involves circulating antibodies against proteins of acetylcholine receptors. Antibody binding to the antigenic sites interferes with acetylcholine activation of their receptors, leading to intermittent periods of skeletal muscle weakness. As the body attempts to correct the condition, junctional folds of sarcolemma with affected receptors are internalized, digested by lysosomes, and replaced by newly formed receptors. These receptors, however, are again made unresponsive to acetylcholine by similar antibodies, and the disease follows a progressive course. The extraocular muscles of the eyes are commonly the first affected.

FIGURE **10–13** The neuromuscular junction (NMJ).

Before it terminates in a skeletal muscle, each motor axon bundled in the nerve forms many branches, each of which forms a synapse with a muscle fiber.

(a) Silver staining can reveal the nerve bundle (**NB**), the terminal axonal twigs, and the motor end plates (**MEP**, also called neuromuscular junctions or NMJ) on striated muscle fibers (**S**). X1200.

(b) An SEM shows the branching ends of a motor axon, each covered by an extension of the last Schwann cell and expanded terminally as an MEP embedded in a groove in the external lamina of the muscle fiber.

(c) Diagram of enclosed portion of the SEM indicating key features of a typical MEP: synaptic vesicles of acetylcholine (**ACh**), a synaptic cleft, and a postsynaptic membrane. This membrane, the sarcolemma, is highly folded to increase the number of ACh receptors at the MEP. Receptor binding initiates muscle fiber depolarization, which is carried to the deeper myofibrils by the T tubules.

Muscle Spindles & Tendon Organs

Striated muscles and myotendinous junctions contain sensory receptors acting as proprioceptors (L. *proprius*, one's own + *capio*, to take), providing the central nervous system (CNS) with data from the musculoskeletal system. Among the muscle fascicles are stretch detectors known as **muscle spindles**, approximately 2 mm long and 0.1 mm wide (Figure 10–14a). A muscle spindle is encapsulated by modified perimysium, with concentric layers of flattened cells, containing interstitial fluid and a few thin muscle fibers filled

TABLE 10–1	Important comparisons of the three types of muscle.		
	Skeletal Muscle	**Cardiac Muscle**	**Smooth Muscle**
Fibers	Single multinucleated cells	Aligned cells in branching arrangement	Single small, closely packed fusiform cells
Cell/fiber shape and size	Cylindrical, 10-100 μm diameter, many cm long	Cylindrical, 10-20 μm diameter, 50-100 μm long	Fusiform, diameter 0.2-10 μm, length 50-200 μm
Striations	Present	Present	Absent
Location of nuclei	Peripheral, adjacent to sarcolemma	Central	Central, at widest part of cell
T tubules	Center of triads at A-I junctions	In diads at Z discs	Absent; caveolae may be functionally similar
Sarcoplasmic reticulum (SR)	Well-developed, with two terminal cisterns per sarcomere in triads with T tubule	Less well-developed, one small terminal cistern per sarcomere in diad with T tubule	Irregular smooth ER without distinctive organization
Special structural features	Very well-organized sarcomeres, SR, and transverse tubule system	Intercalated discs joining cell, with many adherent and gap junctions	Gap junctions, caveolae, dense bodies
Control of contraction	Troponin C binds Ca^{2+}, moving tropomyosin and exposing actin for myosin binding	Similar to that of skeletal muscle	Actin-myosin binding occurs with myosin phosphorylation by MLCK triggered when calmodulin binds Ca^{2+}
Connective tissue organization	Endomysium, perimysium, and epimysium	Endomysium; subendocardial and subpericardial CT layers	Endomysium and less-organized CT sheaths
Major locations	Skeletal muscles, tongue, diaphragm, eyes, and upper esophagus	Heart	Blood vessels, digestive and respiratory tracts, uterus, bladder, and other organs
Key function	Voluntary movements	Automatic (involuntary) pumping of blood	Involuntary movements
Efferent innervation	Motor	Autonomic	Autonomic
Contractions	All-or-none, triggered at motor end plates	All-or-none, intrinsic (beginning at nodes of conducting fibers)	Partial, slow, often spontaneous, wavelike and rhythmic
Cell response to increased load	Hypertrophy (increase in fiber size)	Hypertrophy	Hypertrophy and hyperplasia (increase in cell/fiber number)
Capacity for regeneration	Limited, involving satellite cells mainly	Very poor	Good, involving mitotic activity of muscle cells

FIGURE **10–14** Sensory receptors associated with skeletal muscle.

Capsule

Intrafusal muscle fibers

Muscle spindle

Stretch receptor

Afferent nerve fibers

Extrafusal muscle fiber

Golgi tendon organ

Tendon

a

(a) The diagram shows both a **muscle spindle** and a **tendon organ**. Muscle spindles have **afferent sensory** and efferent motor nerve fibers associated with the **intrafusal fibers**, which are modified muscle fibers. The size of the spindle is exaggerated relative to the extrafusal fibers to show better the nuclei packed in the intrafusal fibers. Both types of sensory receptors provide the CNS with information concerning degrees of stretch and tension within the musculoskeletal system.

(b) A TEM cross section near the end of a muscle spindle shows the capsule (**C**), lightly myelinated axons (**MA**) of a sensory nerve, and the intrafusal muscle fibers (**MF**). These thin fibers differ from the ordinary skeletal muscle fibers in having very few myofibrils. Their many nuclei can either be closely aligned (nuclear chain fibers) or piled in a central dilation (nuclear bag fibers). Muscle satellite cells (**SC**) are also present within the external lamina of the intrafusal fibers. X3600.

with nuclei and called **intrafusal fibers** (Figure 10–14). Several sensory nerve axons penetrate each muscle spindle and wrap around individual intrafusal fibers. Changes in length (distension) of the surrounding (extrafusal) muscle fibers caused by body movements are detected by the muscle spindles and the sensory nerves relay this information to the spinal cord. Different types of sensory and intrafusal fibers mediate reflexes of varying complexity to help maintain posture and to regulate the activity of opposing muscle groups involved in motor activities such as walking.

A similar role is played by **Golgi tendon organs**, much smaller encapsulated structures that enclose sensory axons penetrating among the collagen bundles at the myotendinous junction (Figure 10–14a). Tendon organs detect changes in tension within tendons produced by muscle contraction and act to inhibit motor nerve activity if tension becomes excessive. Because both of these proprioceptors detect increases in tension, they help regulate the amount of effort required to perform movements that call for variable amounts of muscular force.

MEDICAL APPLICATION

Dystrophin is a large actin-binding protein located just inside the sarcolemma of skeletal muscle fibers which is involved in the functional organization of myofibrils. Research on **Duchenne muscular dystrophy** revealed that mutations of the dystrophin gene can lead to defective linkages between the cytoskeleton and the extracellular matrix (ECM). Muscle contractions can disrupt these weak linkages, causing the atrophy of muscle fibers typical of this disease.

Muscle Fiber Types

Skeletal muscle cells are highly adapted for the brief, episodic but intense work of contraction. Mitochondria provide muscle fibers energy in the form of ATP and other phosphorylated compounds emerging from the aerobic metabolism of

TABLE **10–2**	Major characteristics of skeletal muscle fiber types.		
	Slow, Oxidative Fibers (Type I)	**Fast, Oxidative-Glycolytic Fibers (Type IIa)**	**Fast, Glycolytic Fibers (Type IIb)**
Mitochondria	Numerous	Numerous	Sparse
Capillaries	Numerous	Numerous	Sparse
Fiber diameter	Small	Intermediate	Large
Size of motor unit	Small	Intermediate	Large
Myoglobin content	High (red fibers)	High (red fibers)	Low (white fibers)
Glycogen content	Low	Intermediate	High
Major source of ATP	Oxidative phosphorylation	Oxidative phosphorylation	Anaerobic glycolysis
Glycolytic enzyme activity	Low	Intermediate	High
Rate of fatigue	Slow	Intermediate	Fast
Myosin-ATPase activity	Low	High	High
Speed of contraction	Slow	Fast	Fast
Typical major locations	Postural muscles of back	Major muscles of legs	Extraocular muscles

fatty acids. Chemical energy is also stored in glycogen granules that are abundant in sarcoplasm (see Figure 10–10b) and constitute about 0.5% to 1% of muscle weight.

Fibers of a given skeletal muscle are grouped physiologically into three types that reflect that muscle's main function (Table 10–2), although a continuum exists among these types. Most muscles contain a mixture of the three types, as can be demonstrated histochemically using myosin ATPase or mitochondrial enzymes (Figure 10–15). Muscles that are often active with slow contractions for long periods tend to have more mitochondria for oxidative phosphorylation and ATP production and to have a higher density of surrounding capillaries. Such fibers have high levels of the cytoplasmic protein **myoglobin**, which contains iron and stores oxygen molecules, giving such fibers a red color in fresh tissue.

Muscles specialized for short-term work and fast contractions are typically larger in diameter and depend more heavily on anaerobic (glycolytic) metabolism of glucose, much of which is derived from stored glycogen. Glycolysis produces lactate that causes rapid muscle fatigue and an oxygen debt that is repaid during the recovery period.

Major cytologic and metabolic features of the three types of skeletal muscle fibers, with examples of muscles rich in each type, are summarized in Table 10–2.

The classification of fiber types in muscle biopsies has clinical significance for the diagnosis of muscle diseases, or myopathies (*myo* + Gr. *pathos*, suffering). Differentiation of muscle into red, white, and intermediate fibers is partly controlled by the frequency of impulses from its motor innervation, and fibers of a single motor unit are of the same type. If nerves to red and

FIGURE **10–15** Skeletal muscle fiber types.

Cross section of skeletal muscle stained histochemically to detect the density of myofibrillar myosin-ATPase can be used to demonstrate the distribution of slow (**S**) type I fibers, intermediate (**I**) type IIa fibers, and fast (**F**) type IIb fibers. X40. Histochemistry.

white fibers are exchanged experimentally, the fibers change their morphologic and physiologic characteristics. Simple denervation of muscle leads to fiber atrophy and local paralysis.

› CARDIAC MUSCLE

During embryonic development, the mesoderm cells of the primitive heart tube align into chainlike arrays. Rather than fusing into multinucleated cells, as in developing skeletal muscle fibers, **cardiac muscle** cells form complex junctions between interdigitating processes (Figure 10–16). Cells within a fiber often branch and bind to cells in adjacent fibers. Consequently, the heart consists of tightly knit bundles of cells, interwoven in a fashion that provides for a characteristic wave of contraction that resembles wringing out of the heart ventricles.

Mature cardiac muscle cells are approximately 15 μm in diameter and from 85 to 100 μm in length. They exhibit a cross-striated banding pattern comparable to that of skeletal muscle. Unlike multinucleated skeletal muscle, however, each cardiac muscle cell possesses only one (or two) centrally located, pale-staining nuclei. Surrounding the muscle cells is a delicate sheath of endomysium with a rich capillary network.

A unique and distinguishing characteristic of cardiac muscle is the presence of dark-staining transverse lines that cross the chains of cardiac cells at irregular intervals where the cells join. These **intercalated discs** represent the interface between adjacent muscle cells and contain many junctional complexes (Figures 10–16 and 10–17). Transverse regions of these steplike discs have many **desmosomes** and **fascia adherentes** (which resemble the zonula adherentes between epithelial cells); together these serve to bind cardiac muscle

FIGURE **10–16** Cardiac muscle.

Desmosome

Intercalated disc

Openings of transverse tubules

Intercalated disc

Gap junction

Cardiac muscle cell

Sarcolemma

Nucleus

Mitochondrion

The diagram of cardiac muscle cells indicates characteristic features of this muscle type. The fibers consist of separate cells in a series with interdigitating processes where they are held together. These regions of contact are called the **intercalated discs**, which cross an entire fiber between two cells. The transverse regions of the steplike intercalated disc have abundant **desmosomes** and other adherent junctions for firm adhesion, while longitudinal regions of the discs contain many physiologically important **gap junctions**.

Cardiac muscle cells have central nuclei and myofibrils that are less dense and less well-organized than those of skeletal muscle. Also, the cells are often branched, allowing the muscle fibers to interweave in a more complicated arrangement within fascicles that produces an efficient contraction mechanism for emptying the heart.

FIGURE **10–17** Cardiac muscle and intercalated discs.

(a) Longitudinal sections of cardiac muscle at the light microscope level show nuclei (**N**) in the center of the muscle fibers and widely spaced intercalated discs (**I**) that cross the fibers. The occasional intercalated discs should not be confused with the repetitive, much more closely spaced striations (**S**), which are similar to those of skeletal muscle but less well-organized. Nuclei of fibroblasts in endomysium are also present. X200. H&E.

(b) TEM of an intercalated disc (arrows) shows a steplike structure representing the short interdigitating processes of the adjacent muscle cells (see Figure 10-16). Transverse regions of the disc have many desmosomes (**D**) and adherent junctions called **fascia adherentes (F)**, similar to the macula adherentes of epithelial cells. Less electron-dense regions of the disc have abundant gap junctions. The sarcoplasm has numerous mitochondria (**M**) and myofibrillar structures similar to those of skeletal muscle but slightly less organized. X31,000.

cells firmly together to prevent their pulling apart under constant contractile activity. The longitudinally oriented portions of each disc have many **gap junctions** providing ionic continuity between cells. These serve as "electrical synapses" and allow cells of cardiac muscle to act like a multinucleated syncytium as in skeletal muscle, with contraction signals passing in a wave from cell to cell.

The structure and function of the contractile proteins in cardiac cells are essentially the same as in skeletal muscle. The T-tubule system and sarcoplasmic reticulum, however, are not as regularly arranged in cardiac fiber. T tubules are more numerous and larger in cardiac muscle, and the sarcoplasmic reticulum is less abundant (Figure 10–18). Cardiac muscle cells contain numerous mitochondria, however, which occupy 40% or more of the cytoplasmic volume, reflecting their need for continuous aerobic metabolism. By comparison, only about 2% of skeletal muscle fiber is occupied by mitochondria. Fatty acids, transported to cardiac muscle cells by lipoproteins, are the major fuel of the heart and are stored as triglycerides in the numerous lipid droplets seen in many cardiac muscle cells. Glycogen granules may also be present. Lipofuscin pigment granules are often found near the nuclei of cardiac muscle cells.

Muscle of the ventricles is much thicker than that of the atria, reflecting its use in pumping systemic blood. Atrial muscle cells are somewhat smaller, with markedly fewer T tubules. Membrane-limited cytoplasmic granules, each about 0.2 to 0.3 μm in diameter, are found near atrial muscle nuclei and are associated with small Golgi complexes (Figure 10–18). These granules release the peptide hormone atrial natriuretic factor (ANF) that acts on target cells in the kidney to affect Na^+ excretion and water balance. The contractile cells of the heart's atria thus also serve an endocrine function.

Cardiac muscle fiber contraction is intrinsic and spontaneous, as evidenced by the continued contraction of the cells in tissue culture. Impulses for the rhythmic contraction or heartbeat are initiated, regulated, and coordinated locally by nodes of unique myocardial fibers specialized for impulse generation and conduction, which are discussed in Chapter 11. As with skeletal muscle, contraction of individual cardiac muscle fibers is all-or-none. The rate of contraction is modified by autonomic innervation of the nodes of conducting cells, with the sympathetic nerve supply accelerating and the parasympathetic supply decreasing the frequency of the impulses.

FIGURE **10–18** Cardiac muscle ultrastructure.

(a) TEM of cardiac muscle shows abundant mitochondria (**M**) and rather sparse sarcoplasmic reticulum (**SR**) in the areas between myofibrils. T tubules are less well-organized and are usually associated with one expanded terminal cistern of SR, forming dyads (**D**) rather than the triads of skeletal muscle. Functionally, these structures are similar in these two muscle types. X30,000.

(b) Muscle cells from the heart atrium show the presence of membrane-bound granules (**G**), mainly aggregated at the nuclear poles. These granules are most abundant in muscle cells of the right atrium (~600 per cell), but smaller quantities

are also found in the left atrium and the ventricles. The atrial granules contain the precursor of a polypeptide hormone, **atrial natriuretic factor (ANF)**. ANF targets cells of the kidneys to bring about sodium and water loss (natriuresis and diuresis). This hormone thus opposes the actions of aldosterone and antidiuretic hormone, whose effects on kidneys result in sodium and water conservation. X10,000.

(*Figure 10–18b, with permission, from Dr J. C. Nogueira, Department of Morphology, Federal University of Minas Gerais, Belo Horizonte, Brazil.*)

Key features of cardiac muscle cells, with comparisons to those of skeletal muscle, are summarized in Table 10–1.

MEDICAL APPLICATION

The most common injury sustained by cardiac muscle is that due to **ischemia**, or tissue damage due to lack of oxygen when coronary arteries are occluded by heart disease. Lacking muscle satellite cells, adult mammalian cardiac muscle has little potential to regenerate after injury. However, certain fish and amphibians, as well as newborn mice, do form new muscle when the heart is partially removed, despite the lack of satellite cells. Research on the possibility of mammalian **heart muscle regeneration** builds on work with the animal models, focusing primarily on the potential of mesenchymal stem cells to form new, site-specific muscle.

❯ SMOOTH MUSCLE

Smooth muscle is specialized for slow, steady contraction and is controlled by a variety of involuntary mechanisms. Fibers of smooth muscle (also called **visceral muscle**) are elongated, tapering, and nonstriated cells, each of which is enclosed by a thin basal lamina and a fine network of reticular fibers, the endomysium (Figure 10–19). The connective tissues serve to combine the forces generated by each smooth muscle fiber into a concerted action, for example peristalsis in the intestine.

Smooth muscle cells may range in length from 20 μm in small blood vessels to 500 μm in the pregnant uterus. Each cell has a single long nucleus located in the center of the cell's central, broadest part. The cells stain uniformly along their lengths, and to achieve the tightest packing the narrow part of one cell lies adjacent to the broad parts of neighboring cells. Such an arrangement viewed in cross section shows a range

FIGURE **10–19** Smooth muscle.

Cells or fibers of smooth muscle are long, tapering structures with elongated nuclei centrally located at the cell's widest part.

(a) In a cross section of smooth muscle in the wall of the small intestine, cells of the inner circular (**IC**) layer are cut lengthwise and cells of the outer longitudinal layer (**OL**) are cut transversely. Only some nuclei (arrows) of the latter cells are in the plane of section, so that many cells appear to be devoid of nuclei. X140. H&E.

(b) Section of smooth muscle in bladder shows fibers in cross section (**XS**) and longitudinal section (**LS**) with the same fascicle. There is much collagen in the branching perimysium (**P**), but very little evidence of endomysium is apparent. X140. Mallory trichrome.

(c) Section stained only for reticulin reveals the thin endomysium around each fiber, with more reticulin in the connective tissue of small arteries (**A**). Reticulin fibers associated with the basal laminae of smooth muscle cells help hold the cells together as a functional unit during the slow, rhythmic contractions of this tissue. X200. Silver.

of cell diameters, with only the largest profiles containing a nucleus (Figures 10–19 and 10–20). All cells are linked by numerous gap junctions. The borders of the cell become scalloped when smooth muscle contracts and the nucleus becomes distorted (Figure 10–21). Concentrated near the nucleus are mitochondria, polyribosomes, RER, and the Golgi apparatus. The short membrane invaginations, called **caveolae**, are often frequent at the smooth muscle cell surface.

The fibers have rudimentary sarcoplasmic reticulum, but lack T tubules; their function is unnecessary in these smaller, tapering cells with many gap junctions. Caveolae of smooth muscle cells contain several pumps and ion channels and may serve to organize proteins signaling calcium release at

myofibrils. The characteristic contractile activity of smooth muscle is generated by myofibrillar arrays of actin and myosin organized differently from those of striated muscles. In smooth muscle cells, bundles of thin and thick myofilaments crisscross obliquely through the cell. Myosin filaments have a less regular arrangement among the thin filaments and fewer crossbridges than in striated muscle, and the actin filaments lack troponin, using instead **calmodulin** and Ca^{2+}-sensitive **myosin light-chain kinase (MLCK)** in the contraction mechanism. Certain other Ca^{2+}-binding regulatory proteins, not used in striated muscle, also occur in these fibers. The sliding filament mechanism of contraction, however, is basically similar to that in striated muscle.

FIGURE **10–20** Smooth muscle ultrastructure.

(a) TEM of a transverse section of smooth muscle showing several cells sectioned at various points along their lengths, yielding profiles of various diameters with only the largest containing a nucleus. Thick and thin filaments are not organized into myofibril bundles, and there are few mitochondria (**M**). There is evidence of a sparse external lamina around each cell, and reticular fibers are abundant in the ECM. A small unmyelinated nerve (**N**) is also seen between the cells. X6650.

(b) Longitudinal section showing several dense bodies (**DB**) in the cytoplasm and at the cell membrane. Thin filaments and intermediate filaments both attach to the dense bodies. In the cytoplasm near the nucleus (**N**) are mitochondria, glycogen granules, and Golgi complexes. In the lower right corner of the photo the cell membrane shows invaginations called caveolae (**C**) that may regulate release of Ca^{2+} from sarcoplasmic reticulum. X9000.

Smooth muscle cells also have an elaborate array of 10-nm intermediate filaments, usually composed of desmin. The intermediate filaments and F-actin filaments both insert into cytoplasmic and plasmalemma-associated **dense bodies** (Figure 10–20). Dense bodies contain α-actinin and are functionally similar to the Z discs of striated and cardiac muscle. The attachments of thin and intermediate filaments to the dense bodies helps transmit contractile force to adjacent smooth muscle cells and their surrounding network of reticular fibers (Figure 10–21).

Smooth muscle is not under voluntary control, and its fibers lack MEPs. Contraction is regulated differently in the smooth muscle of the viscera, the respiratory airways, or large and small blood vessels; the control can involve autonomic nerves, a variety of hormones and similar substances, and local physiologic conditions such as the degree of stretch. Whether smooth muscle fibers contract as small groups or throughout an entire muscle to produce waves of contraction is determined largely by the degree of autonomic innervation and the density of the gap junctions; both conditions vary considerably in different organs.

In smooth muscle, swellings of autonomic nerve axons with synaptic vesicles simply lie in close contact with the sarcolemma, with little or no specialized structure to the junctions. Because smooth muscle is most often spontaneously active without nervous stimuli, its nerve supply serves primarily to modify activity rather than to initiate it. Smooth muscle receives both adrenergic and cholinergic nerve endings that act antagonistically, stimulating or depressing its activity. In some organs, the cholinergic endings activate and the adrenergic nerves depress; in others, the reverse occurs.

In addition to contractile activity, smooth muscle cells also supplement fibroblast activity, synthesizing collagen, elastin, and proteoglycans, with a major influence on the extracellular matrix (ECM) in tissues where these contractile cells are abundant. Active synthesis of ECM by the small cells/fibers of smooth muscle may reflect less specialization for strong contractions than in skeletal and cardiac muscle and is similar to this synthetic function in other contractile cells, such as myofibroblasts and pericytes.

Key histologic and functional features of smooth muscle, with comparisons to those of skeletal and cardiac muscle, are summarized in Table 10–1.

MEDICAL APPLICATION

Benign tumors called **leiomyomas** commonly develop from smooth muscle fibers but are seldom problematic. They most frequently occur in the wall of the uterus, where they are more commonly called **fibroids** and where they can become sufficiently large to produce painful pressure and unexpected bleeding.

FIGURE **10–21** Smooth muscle contraction.

Thick filaments

Thin filaments

Dense body

Adjacent cells physically
coupled at dense bodies

Nucleus

Dense body

a

CT

C

b

Most molecules that allow contraction are similar in the three types of muscle, but the filaments of smooth muscle are arranged differently and appear less organized. **(a)** The diagram shows that thin filaments attach to **dense bodies** located at the cell membrane and deep in the cytoplasm. Dense bodies contain α-actinin for thin filament attachment. Dense bodies at the membrane are also attachment sites for intermediate filaments and for adhesive junctions between cells. This arrangement of both the cytoskeleton and contractile apparatus allows the multicellular tissue to contract as a unit, providing better efficiency and force.

(b) Micrograph showing a contracted (**C**) region of smooth muscle, with contraction decreasing the cell length and deforming the nuclei. The long nuclei of individual fibers assume a cork-screw shape when the fibers contract, reflecting the reduced cell length at contraction. Connective tissue (**CT**) of the perimysium outside the muscle fascicle is stained blue. X240. Mallory trichrome.

❯ REGENERATION OF MUSCLE TISSUE

The three types of adult muscle have different potentials for regeneration after injury and these are also summarized in Table 10–1.

In skeletal muscle, although the multinucleated cells cannot undergo mitosis, the tissue can still display limited regeneration. The source of regenerating cells is the sparse population of mesenchymal **satellite cells** that lies within the external lamina of each mature muscle fiber. Satellite cells are inactive, reserve myoblasts that persist after muscle differentiation. After injury or certain other stimuli, the normally quiescent satellite cells become activated, proliferating and fusing to form new skeletal muscle fibers. A similar activity of satellite cells has been implicated in muscle growth after extensive exercise, a process in which they fuse with their parent fibers to increase muscle mass beyond that which occurs by cell hypertrophy. The regenerative capacity of skeletal muscle is limited, however, occurring less well after major muscle trauma.

Cardiac muscle lacks satellite cells and shows very little regenerative capacity beyond early childhood. Defects or damage (eg, infarcts) to heart muscle are generally replaced by proliferating fibroblasts and growth of connective tissue, forming myocardial scars.

Smooth muscle, composed of simpler, smaller, mononucleated cells, is capable of a more active regenerative response. After injury, viable smooth muscle cells undergo mitosis and replace the damaged tissue. As discussed in Chapter 11, contractile pericytes from the walls of small blood vessels participate in the repair of vascular smooth muscle.

Muscle Tissue SUMMARY OF KEY POINTS

- There are three major types of muscle: (1) **skeletal** or striated muscle, (2) **cardiac** muscle, and (3) **smooth** or visceral muscle.
- **Skeletal muscle cells** are very long, **multinucleated fibers, cylindrically shaped** and with **diameters up to 100 μm.**
- The **sarcolemma** of each fiber is surrounded by an external lamina and thin connective tissue, **endomysium**, containing capillaries.

Organization of Skeletal Muscle Fibers

- Groups of fibers called **fascicles** are surrounded by **perimysium**; all fascicles are enclosed within a dense connective tissue **epimysium.**
- Internally each muscle fiber is filled with myofibrils, composed of thousands of **thick myosin filaments** and **thin actin filaments**, highly organized into contractile units called **sarcomeres.**
- Within sarcomeres thick and thin filaments **interdigitate**; globular myosin heads project from the thick filaments toward the F-actin filaments, which are associated with **tropomyosin** and **troponin.**
- Sarcomeres are separated by **Z discs** that bisect the **light-staining I bands** that contain mainly the thin filaments attached to α-**actinin** in the Z disc.
- Between the two I bands of a sarcomere is the **dark-staining A band** with the thick myosin filaments; alternating light and dark bands appear as microscopic **striations** along the fibers.

Sarcoplasmic Reticulum & Transverse Tubule System

- In the sarcoplasm between parallel myofibrils are **mitochondria** and cisternae of smooth ER, called the **sarcoplasmic reticulum (SR)** specialized for Ca^{2+} sequestration and release.
- At each sarcomere, two **terminal cisterns of SR** contact a deep invagination of the sarcolemma called a **transverse** or **T tubule**, forming a **triad** that triggers Ca^{2+} release when the sarcolemma is depolarized.

Mechanism of Contraction

- Ca^{2+} **binding to troponin** causes **tropomyosin to change shape** and allow the **myosin heads to bind the actin** subunits, forming **crossbridges** between thick and thin filaments.
- The myosin heads then pivot with **ATP hydrolysis**, which pulls the thin filaments along the thick filaments.
- With Ca^{2+} and ATP present, a **contraction cycle** ensues in which **myosin heads repeatedly attach, pivot, detach, and return**, causing the **filaments to slide past one another**, shortening the sarcomere.
- When the membrane **depolarization ends, Ca^{2+} is again sequestered**, ending contraction and allowing the sarcomeres to lengthen again as the **muscle relaxes.**
- Synapses of motor axons with skeletal muscle are called **motor end plates (MEPs), neuromuscular junctions (NMJs)**, or myoneural junctions; the neurotransmitter is **acetylcholine.**

- A motor axon may form many terminal branches, each ending on an MEP of a muscle fiber; all fibers innervated by branches of that axon comprise a **motor unit.**

Muscle Spindles & Tendon Organs

- These are both **sensory proprioceptors** in which sensory **axons wrap around intrafusal fibers** in small specialized fascicles or around **myotendinous collagen bundles**, respectively.

Muscle Fiber Types

- Skeletal muscles contain fibers that can be physiologically classified as the three main types: (1) **slow, oxidative** (type I); (2) **fast, intermediate oxidative-glycolytic** (type IIa); and (3) **fast, glycolytic** (type IIb).

Cardiac Muscle

- **Cardiac muscle fibers** are also **striated**, but they consist of **individual cylindrical cells**, each containing **one (or two) central nuclei** and linked by adherent and gap junctions at prominent **intercalated discs.**
- **Sarcomeres** of cardiac muscle are organized and function similarly to those of skeletal muscle.
- Contraction of cardiac muscle is **intrinsic** at nodes of **impulse-generating pacemaker muscle fibers**; autonomic nerves regulate the rate of contraction.

Smooth Muscle

- **Smooth muscle fibers** are individual **small, fusiform (tapering) cells**, linked by numerous gap junctions.
- **Thin and thick filaments** in smooth muscle fibers do not form sarcomeres, and **no striations** are present.
- Thin actin filaments attach to α-actinin located in **dense bodies** that are located throughout the sarcoplasm and near the sarcolemma; contraction causes cells to shorten individually.
- Sarcoplasmic reticulum is less well-organized in smooth muscle fibers, and there is **no transverse tubule system.**
- Troponin is lacking in smooth muscle; proteins controlling the sliding filaments here include **myosin light-chain kinase (MLCK)** and **calmodulin.**

Regeneration of Muscle Tissue

- Repair and regeneration can occur in **skeletal muscle** because of a population of **reserve muscle satellite cells** that can proliferate, fuse, and form new muscle fibers.
- Cardiac muscle **lacks satellite cells** and has little capacity for regeneration.
- Regeneration is rapid in smooth muscle because the cells/fibers are small and relatively less differentiated, which allow **renewed mitotic activity** after injury.

11 The Circulatory System

The circulatory system pumps and directs blood cells and substances carried in blood to all tissues of the body. It includes both the blood and lymphatic vascular systems, and in an adult the total length of its vessels is estimated at between 100,000 and 150,000 kilometers. The **blood vascular system**, or **cardiovascular system** (Figure 11–1), consists of the following structures:

- The **heart** propels blood through the system.
- **Arteries**, a series of vessels efferent from the heart that become smaller as they branch into the various organs, carry blood to the tissues.
- **Capillaries**, the smallest vessels, are the sites of O_2, CO_2, nutrient, and waste product exchange between blood and tissues. Together with the smallest arterial and venous branches carrying blood to and from them, capillaries in almost every organ form a complex network of thin, anastomosing tubules called the **microvasculature** or microvascular bed.
- **Veins** result from the convergence of venules into a system of larger channels that continue enlarging as they approach the heart, toward which they carry the blood to be pumped again.

As shown in Figure 11–1, two major divisions of arteries, microvasculature, and veins make up the **pulmonary circulation**, where blood is oxygenated in the lungs, and the **systemic circulation**, where blood brings nutrients and removes wastes in tissues throughout the body.

The **lymphatic vascular system**, introduced with the discussion of interstitial fluid in Chapter 5, begins with the **lymphatic capillaries**, which are thin-walled, closed-ended tubules carrying lymph, that merge to form vessels of steadily increasing size. The largest lymph vessels connect with the blood vascular system and empty into the large veins near the heart. This returns fluid from tissue spaces all over the body to the blood.

The internal surface of all components of the blood and lymphatic systems is lined by a single layer of a squamous epithelium, called **endothelium**. As the interface between blood and the organs, cardiovascular endothelial cells have crucial physiologic and medical importance. Not only must endothelial cells maintain a selectively permeable, antithrombogenic (inhibitory to clot formation) barrier, they also determine when and where white blood cells leave the circulation for the interstitial space of tissues and secrete a variety of paracrine factors for vessel dilation, constriction, and growth of adjacent cells.

› HEART

Cardiac muscle in the four chambers of the **heart** wall contracts rhythmically, pumping the blood through the circulatory system (Figure 11–2). The right and left **ventricles** propel blood to the pulmonary and systemic circulation, respectively; right and left **atria** receive blood from the body and the pulmonary veins, respectively. The walls of all four heart chambers consist of three major layers: the internal endocardium; the middle myocardium; and the external epicardium.

- The **endocardium** consists of a very thin inner layer of endothelium and supporting connective tissue, a middle myoelastic layer of smooth muscle fibers and connective tissue, and a deep layer of connective tissue called the **subendocardial layer** that merges with the myocardium Branches of the heart's impulse-conducting system, consisting of modified cardiac muscle fibers, are also located in the subendocardial layer (Figure 11–3).

FIGURE **11–1** Diagram of the cardiovascular system.

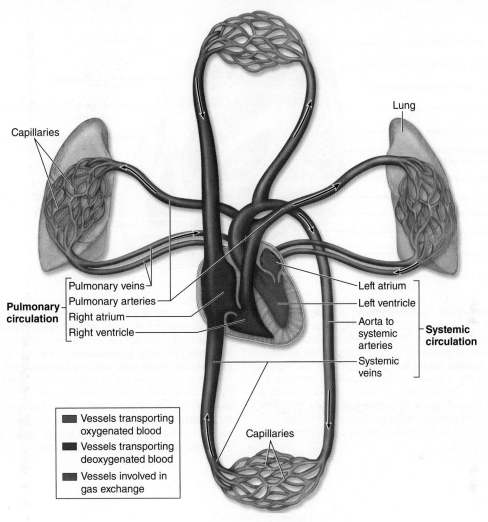

Cardiovascular System

The system consisting of the **heart, arteries, veins,** and **microvascular beds** is organized as the **pulmonary circulation** and the **systemic circulation**. In the pulmonary circulation the right side of the heart pumps blood through pulmonary vessels, through the lungs for oxygenation, and back to the left side of the heart. The larger systemic circulation pumps blood from the left side of the heart through vessels supplying either the head and arms or the lower body, and back to the right side of the heart.

When the body is at rest, approximately 70% of the blood moves through the systemic circulation, about 18% through the pulmonary circulation, and 12% through the heart.

- The thickest layer, the **myocardium**, consists mainly of cardiac muscle with its fibers arranged spirally around each heart chamber. Because strong force is required to pump blood through the systemic and pulmonary circulations, the myocardium is much thicker in the walls of the ventricles, particularly the left, than in the atrial walls (Figure 11–3).
- The **epicardium** is a simple squamous **mesothelium** supported by a layer of loose connective tissue containing blood vessels and nerves (Figure 11–4).

The epicardium corresponds to the **visceral layer of the pericardium**, the membrane surrounding the heart. Where the large vessels enter and leave the heart, the epicardium is reflected back as the **parietal layer** lining the pericardium. During heart movements, underlying structures are cushioned by deposits of adipose tissue in the epicardium and friction within the pericardium is prevented by lubricant fluid produced by both layers of serous mesothelial cells.

FIGURE 11–2 Important features of the heart.

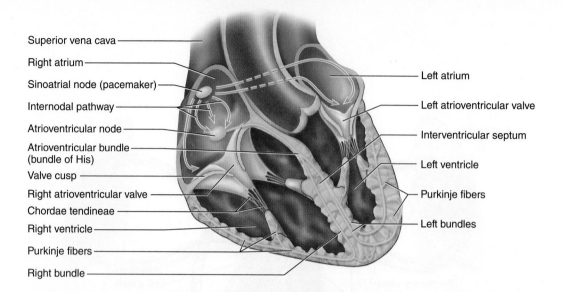

Superior vena cava
Right atrium
Sinoatrial node (pacemaker)
Internodal pathway
Atrioventricular node
Atrioventricular bundle (bundle of His)
Valve cusp
Right atrioventricular valve
Chordae tendineae
Right ventricle
Purkinje fibers
Right bundle

Left atrium
Left atrioventricular valve
Interventricular septum
Left ventricle
Purkinje fibers
Left bundles

As seen in the diagram, the human heart has two **atria** and two **ventricles**. The myocardium of the ventricular walls is thicker than that of the atria. The **valves** are basically flaps of connective tissue anchored in the heart's dense connective tissue, or **cardiac skeleton**, concentrated in the regions shown in white. This fibrous tissue includes the chordae tendineae, cords that extend from the cusps of both atrioventricular valves and attach to papillary muscles, preventing the valves from turning inside-out during ventricular contraction. Valves and cords are covered by the nonthrombogenic endothelium.

Shown in yellow are parts of the cardiac **conducting system**, which initiates the electrical impulse for contraction (heartbeat) and spreads it through the ventricular myocardium. Both the **sinoatrial (SA) node (pacemaker)**, in the right atrial wall, and the **atrioventricular (AV) node**, in the floor of the right atrium, consist of myocardial tissue that is difficult to distinguish histologically from surrounding cardiac muscle. The AV node is continuous with specialized bundles of cardiac muscle fibers, the **AV bundles** (of His) that run along the interventricular septum to the apex of the heart, where they branch further as **conducting (Purkinje) fibers** that extend into myocardium of the ventricles.

Within these major layers the heart contains other structures important for its overall function of moving blood. Dense fibrous connective tissue of the **cardiac skeleton** forms part of the interventricular and interatrial septa, surrounds all valves of the heart, and extends into the valve cusps and the chordae tendineae to which they are attached (Figures 11–2 and 11–5). These regions of dense irregular connective tissue perform the following functions:

- Anchoring and supporting the heart valves
- Providing firm points of insertion for cardiac muscle
- Helping coordinate the heartbeat by acting as electrical insulation between atria and ventricles

Within the subendocardial layer and adjacent myocardium, modified cardiac muscle cells make up the impulse **conducting system of the heart**, which generates and propagates waves of depolarization that spread through the myocardium to stimulate rhythmic contractions. This system (Figure 11–2) consists of two nodes of specialized myocardial tissue in the right atrium: the **sinoatrial (SA) node** (or

pacemaker) and the **atrioventricular (AV) node**, followed by the **AV bundle** (of His) and the **subendocardial conducting network**.

Located in the right atrial wall near the superior vena cava, the SA node is a 6- to 7-mm³ mass of cardiac muscle cells with smaller size, fewer myofibrils, and fewer typical intercalated disks than the neighboring muscle fibers. Impulses initiated by these cells move along the myocardial fibers of both atria, stimulating their contraction. When the impulses reach the slightly smaller AV node, located in the floor of the right atrium near the AV valve and composed of cells similar to those of the SA node, they stimulate depolarization of those cells. Conducting muscle fibers from the AV node form the AV bundle, pass through an opening in the cardiac skeleton into the interventricular septum, and bifurcate into the wall of each ventricle.

At the apex of the heart, the bundles branch further into a subendocardial conducting network of myofibers, usually called **Purkinje fibers**. These are pale-staining fibers, larger than the adjacent contractile muscle fibers, with

FIGURE **11–3** Endocardium, myocardium, and fibers of the subendocardial conducting network.

The **endocardium** consists of the endothelium, a thin layer of connective tissue with smooth muscle cells, and a layer of variable thickness lacking smooth muscle called the **subendocardial layer**.

(a) Below the endothelium (**En**) and myoelastic layer, the subendocardial layer (**SEn**) in the ventricles contains the conducting (Purkinje) fibers (**P**) of the heart's impulse conducting network. These fibers are cardiac muscle cells joined by

intercalated disks but specialized for impulse conduction rather than contraction. With glycogen filling much of the cytoplasm and displacing myofibrils to the periphery, Purkinje fibers typically are more pale staining than contractile cardiac muscle fibers (**M**).

(b) In the atria Purkinje fibers (**P**) are often closer to the endothelium (**En**) and intermingle with the contractile fibers within the myocardium (**M**). Both X200. H&E.

sparse, peripheral myofibrils and much glycogen (Figure 11–3). Purkinje fibers mingle distally with contractile fibers of both ventricles and trigger waves of contraction through both ventricles simultaneously.

Both parasympathetic and sympathetic neural components innervate the heart. Ganglionic nerve cells and nerve fibers are present in the regions close to the SA and AV nodes, where they affect heart rate and rhythm, such as during physical exercise and emotional stress. Stimulation of the parasympathetic division (vagus nerve) slows the heartbeat, whereas stimulation of the sympathetic nerve accelerates activity of the pacemaker. Between fibers of the myocardium are afferent free nerve endings that register pain, such as the discomfort called angina pectoris that occurs when partially occluded coronary arteries cause local oxygen deprivation.

›› MEDICAL APPLICATION

Abnormalities in the structure of heart valves can be produced by developmental defects, scarring after certain infections, or cardiovascular problems such as hypertension. Such abnormal valves may not close tightly, allowing slight regurgitation and backflow of blood. This produces an abnormal heart sound referred to as a **heart murmur**. If the valve defect is severe, the heart will have to work harder to circulate the normal amount of blood, eventually enlarging to accommodate the increased workload. Defective heart valves often may be repaired surgically or replaced by an artificial valve or one from a large animal donor. Because such valve replacements lack a complete endothelial covering, the patients require exogenous anticoagulant agents to prevent thrombus formation at these sites.

FIGURE 11–4 Epicardium or visceral pericardium.

The external tunic of the heart, the epicardium, is the site of the coronary vessels and contains considerable adipose tissue. This section of atrium shows part of the myocardium (**M**) and epicardium (**Ep**). The epicardium consists of loose connective tissue (**CT**) containing autonomic nerves (**N**) and variable amounts of fat (**F**). The epicardium is the visceral layer of the pericardium and is covered by the simple mesothelium (**Mes**) that also lines the pericardial space. The mesothelial cells secrete a lubricant fluid that prevents friction as the beating heart contacts the parietal pericardium on the other side of the pericardial cavity. X100. H&E.

FIGURE 11–5 Valve leaflet and cardiac skeleton.

The fibrous **cardiac skeleton** consists of dense irregular connective tissue, primarily in the endocardium (**En**), which anchors the valves and surrounds the two atrioventricular canals, maintaining their proper shape. The micrograph shows a section through a cusp of an **atrioventricular valve** (arrow) and attached chordae tendineae (**CT**). These structures are largely dense connective tissue (**C**) covered with a thin layer of endothelium. The collagen-rich connective tissue of the valves is stained pale blue here and is continuous with the fibrous ring of connective tissue at the base of the valves, which fills the endocardium between the atrium (**A**) and ventricle (**V**). The thick ventricular myocardium (**M**) is also shown. X20. Masson trichrome.

› TISSUES OF THE VASCULAR WALL

Walls of all blood vessels except capillaries contain smooth muscle and connective tissue in addition to the endothelial lining. The amount and arrangement of these tissues in vessels are influenced by **mechanical factors**, primarily blood pressure, and **metabolic factors** reflecting the local needs of tissues.

The **endothelium** is a specialized epithelium that acts as a semipermeable barrier between two internal compartments: the blood plasma and the interstitial tissue fluid. Vascular endothelial cells are squamous, polygonal, and elongated with the long axis in the direction of blood flow. Endothelium with its basal lamina is highly differentiated to mediate and actively monitor the bidirectional exchange of molecules by simple and active diffusion, receptor-mediated endocytosis, transcytosis, and other mechanisms discussed in Chapter 4.

Besides their key role in metabolite exchanges between blood and tissues, endothelial cells have several other functions:

- The endothelium presents a **nonthrombogenic surface** on which blood will not clot and actively secretes agents that control local clot formation (such as heparin, tissue plasminogen activator, and von Willebrand factor).
- The cells regulate local **vascular tone and blood flow** by secreting various factors that stimulate smooth muscle contraction (such as endothelin 1 and angiotensin-converting enzyme [ACE]) or relaxation (including nitric oxide [NO] and prostacyclin).
- Endothelium has several roles in **inflammation and local immune responses.** In venules endothelial cells induce specific white blood cells to stop and undergo transendothelial migration at sites of injury or infection. Under those conditions **P-selectin** is expressed rapidly on the luminal surface when unique elongated granules, called **Weibel-Palade bodies,** fuse with the cell membrane. As described further in Chapter 12, adhesion to selectins is the first step in the activation of white blood cells specifically where they are needed. Endothelial cells also secrete various factors called **interleukins** that affect the activity of local white blood cells during inflammation.
- Under various conditions endothelial cells secrete various **growth factors**, including proteins promoting proliferation of specific white blood cell lineages and cells that make up the vascular wall.

Growth factors such as vascular endothelial growth factor (VEGF) stimulate formation of the vascular system from embryonic mesenchyme (**vasculogenesis**), help maintain the vasculature in adults, and promote capillary sprouting and outgrowth from small existing vessels (**angiogenesis**) during normal growth, during tissue repair and regeneration, and in tumors and other pathological conditions. In both processes other growth factors, called **angiopoietins**, stimulate endothelial cells to recruit smooth muscle cells and fibroblasts to form the other tissues of the vascular wall.

The normal vascular endothelium is antithrombogenic, allowing adhesion of no blood cells or platelets and preventing blood clot formation. When endothelial cells of the microvasculature are damaged by tissue injury, collagen is exposed in the subendothelial tissues and induces the aggregation of blood platelets. These platelets release factors that initiate a cascade of events that produce fibrin from circulating plasma fibrinogen. An intravascular clot, or **thrombus** (plural, thrombi), with a fibrin framework quickly forms to stop blood loss from the damaged vessels.

From large thrombi, solid masses called **emboli** (singular, embolus) may detach and be carried by the blood to obstruct distant vessels. In both cases vascular flow may be blocked, producing a potentially life-threatening condition. Thus, the integrity of the endothelial layer preventing contact between platelets and the subendothelial connective tissue is an important antithrombogenic mechanism.

Individuals in the initial stages of medical conditions involving thrombus formation, such as myocardial infarct, stroke, or pulmonary embolism, are treated intravenously with tissue plasminogen activator, commonly abbreviated as tPA. This is a serine protease that breaks down fibrin and quickly dissolves the clot.

Smooth muscle fibers occur in the walls of all vessels larger than capillaries and are arranged helically in layers. In arterioles and small arteries, the smooth muscle cells are connected by many more gap junctions and permit vasoconstriction and vasodilation which are of key importance in regulating the overall blood pressure.

Connective tissue components are present in vascular walls in variable amounts and proportions based on local functional requirements. Collagen fibers are found in the subendothelial layer, between the smooth muscle layers, and in the outer covering. Elastic fibers provide the resiliency required for the vascular wall to expand under pressure. Elastin is a major component in large arteries where it forms parallel lamellae, regularly distributed between the muscle layers. Variations in the amount and composition of ground substance components such as proteoglycans and hyaluronate also contribute to the physical and metabolic properties of the wall in different vessels, especially affecting their permeability.

The walls of all blood vessels larger than the microvasculature have many components in common and similar organization. Branching of the vessels helps produce reductions in their size which are accompanied by gradual changes in the composition of the vascular wall. Transitions such as those from "small arteries" to "arterioles" are not clear-cut. However, all of these larger vessels have walls with three concentric layers, or tunics (L. *tunica*, coat), as shown in the diagram of Figure 11–6 and in the micrographs of Figures 11–7 through 11–9.

- The innermost tunica **intima** consists of the endothelium and a thin subendothelial layer of loose connective tissue sometimes containing smooth muscle fibers (Figure 11–7). In arteries and large veins, the intima includes a prominent limiting layer, the **internal elastic lamina**, composed of elastin, with holes allowing better diffusion of substances from blood deeper into the wall.

- The tunica **media**, the middle layer, consists chiefly of concentric layers of helically arranged smooth muscle cells (Figures 11–6 and 11–7). Interposed among the muscle fibers are variable amounts of elastic fibers and elastic lamellae, reticular fibers, and proteoglycans, all of which are produced by the smooth muscle cells. In arteries, the media may have a thin external elastic lamina, separating it from the outermost tunic.

- The outer **adventitia**, or tunica externa, consists principally of type I collagen and elastic fibers (Figures 11–7 and 11–8). The adventitia is continuous with and bound to the stromal connective tissue of the organ through which the blood vessel runs.

Just as the heart wall is supplied with its own coronary vasculature for nutrients and O_2, large vessels usually have **vasa vasorum** ("vessels of the vessel"): arterioles, capillaries, and venules in the adventitia and outer part of the media (Figure 11–8). The vasa vasorum are required to provide metabolites to cells in those tunics in larger vessels because the wall is too thick to be nourished solely by diffusion from the blood in the lumen. Luminal blood alone does provide the needs of cells in the intima. Because they carry deoxygenated blood, large veins commonly have more vasa vasorum than arteries.

The adventitia of larger vessels also contains a network of unmyelinated autonomic nerve fibers, the vasomotor nerves (Figure 11–8), which release the vasoconstrictor norepinephrine. The density of this innervation is greater in arteries than in veins.

> VASCULATURE

Large blood vessels and those of the microvasculature branch frequently and undergo gradual transitions into structures with different histologic features and functions. For didactic purposes vessels can be classified arbitrarily as the types discussed here and listed in Table 11–1.

Elastic Arteries

Elastic arteries are the aorta, the pulmonary artery, and their largest branches; these large vessels are also called **conducting arteries** because their major role is to carry blood to smaller arteries. As shown in Figure 11–7a, the most prominent feature of elastic arteries is the thick media in which elastic lamellae, each about 10 μm thick, alternate with layers of smooth muscle fibers. The adult aorta has about 50 elastic lamellae (more if the individual is hypertensive).

The intima is well developed, with many smooth muscle cells in the subendothelial connective tissue, and often shows folds in cross section as a result of the loss of blood pressure

FIGURE **11–6** Walls of arteries and veins.

Intima

Endothelium

Subendothelial layer

Internal elastic lamina

Media

External elastic lamina

Adventitia

Vasa vasorum

Valves

Small Artery

Small Vein

Walls of both arteries and veins have three tunics called the **intima**, **media**, and the **adventitia** (or externa), which correspond roughly to the heart's endocardium, myocardium, and epicardium. An artery has a thicker media and relatively narrow lumen. A vein has a larger lumen and its adventitia is the thickest layer. The intima of veins is often folded to form **valves**. Capillaries have only an endothelium, with no subendothelial layer or other tunics.

and contraction of the vessel at death (Figure 11–8). The internal elastic lamina is not easily discerned because it is similar to the elastic laminae of the next layer (Figures 11–7a and 11–9). The adventitia is much thinner than the media.

The numerous elastic laminae of these arteries contribute to their important function of making blood flow more uniform. During ventricular contraction (**systole**), blood is moved through the arteries forcefully and the elastin is stretched, distending the wall within the limit set by the wall's collagen. When the ventricles relax (**diastole**), ventricular pressure drops to a low level, but the elastin rebounds passively, helping to maintain arterial pressure. The aortic and pulmonary valves prevent backflow of blood into the heart, so the

rebound continues the blood flow away from the heart. Arterial blood pressure and blood velocity decrease and become less variable as the distance from the heart increases.

>> MEDICAL APPLICATION

Atherosclerosis (Gr. *athero*, gruel or porridge, and *scleros*, hardening) is a disease of elastic arteries and large muscular arteries that may play a role in nearly half of all deaths in developed parts of the world. It is initiated by damaged or dysfunctional endothelial cells oxidizing low-density lipoproteins (LDLs) in the tunica intima, which

FIGURE 11–7 Tunics of the vascular wall.

Comparison of the three major layers or tunics in the largest artery and vein. **(a)** Aorta, **(b)** vena cava. Simple squamous endothelial cells (arrows) line the intima (**I**) that has subendothelial loose connective tissue and is separated from the media by the internal elastic lamina (**IEL**), a sheet of elastin. The media (**M**) contains many elastic lamellae and elastic fibers (**EF**) alternating with layers of smooth muscle.

The media is much thicker in large arteries than veins, with relatively more elastin. Elastic fibers are also present in the outer tunica adventitia (**A**), which is relatively thicker in large veins. Vasa vasorum (**V**) are seen in the adventitia of the aorta. The connective tissue of the adventitia always merges with the less dense connective tissue around it. Both X122. Elastic stain.

induces adhesion and intima entry of monocytes/macrophages to remove the modified LDL. Lipid-filled macrophages (called **foam cells**) accumulate and, along with the free LDL, produce a pathologic sign of early atherosclerosis called **fatty streaks**. During disease progression these develop into **fibro-fatty plaques**, or **atheromas**, consisting of a gruel-like mix of smooth muscle cells, collagen fibers, and lymphocytes with necrotic regions of lipid, debris, and foam cells. Predisposing factors include dyslipidemia (>3:1 ratios of LDL to HDL [high-density lipoprotein]), hyperglycemia of diabetes, hypertension, and the presence of toxins introduced by smoking.

In elastic arteries atheromas produce localized destruction within the wall, weakening it and causing arterial bulges or **aneurysms** that can rupture. In muscular arteries such as the coronary arteries, atheromas can occlude blood flow to downstream vessels, leading to ischemic heart disease.

Arterial Sensory Structures

Carotid sinuses are slight dilations of the bilateral internal carotid arteries where they branch from the (elastic) common carotid arteries; they act as important **baroreceptors**

FIGURE 11–8 Vasa vasorum.

The adventitia of the larger arteries contains a supply of microvasculature to bring O_2 and nutrients to local cells that are too far from the lumen to be nourished by blood there. These arterioles (**A**), capillaries, and venules (**V**) constitute the vasa vasorum (vessels of vessels). The adventitia of large arteries is also supplied more sparsely with small sympathetic nerves (**N**) for control of vasoconstriction. Above the adventitia in this section can be seen muscle fibers (**SM**) and elastic lamellae (**E**) in the media. X100. H&E.

FIGURE 11–9 Elastic artery.

The largest arteries contain considerable elastic material and expand with blood when the heart contracts. A transverse section through part of a large elastic artery shows a thick media (**M**) consisting largely of many well-developed elastic lamellae. Strong pressure of blood pulsating into such arteries during systole expands the arterial wall, reducing the pressure and allowing strong blood flow to continue during diastole. The intima (**I**) of the empty aorta is typically folded, and the dense irregular connective tissue of the adventitia (**A**) is thinner than the media. X200. PT.

monitoring arterial blood pressure. At these sinuses the media is thinner, allowing greater distension when blood pressure rises, and the adventitia contains many sensory nerve endings from cranial nerve IX, the glossopharyngeal nerve. The brain's vasomotor centers process these afferent impulses and adjust vasoconstriction, maintaining normal blood pressure. Functionally similar baroreceptors are also present in the aortic arch.

Histologically more complex **chemoreceptors** that monitor blood levels of CO_2 and O_2, as well as its hydrogen ion concentration (pH), are found in the **carotid bodies** and **aortic bodies**, located in the walls of the carotid sinuses and aortic arch, respectively. These structures are parts of the autonomic nervous system called **paraganglia** with rich capillary networks. The capillaries are closely surrounded by numerous, large, neural crest-derived **glomus (type I) cells**

filled with dense-core vesicles containing dopamine, acetylcholine, and other neurotransmitters, which are supported by smaller satellite (type II) cells (Figure 11–10). Appropriate ion channels in the glomus cell membranes respond to stimuli in the arterial blood, primarily hypoxia (low O_2), hypercapnia (excess CO_2), or acidosis, by activating release of neurotransmitters. Sensory fibers branching from the glossopharyngeal nerve form synapses with the glomus cells and signal brain centers to initiate cardiovascular and respiratory adjustments that correct the condition.

Muscular Arteries

The muscular arteries distribute blood to the organs and help regulate blood pressure by contracting or relaxing the

TABLE **11–1**	Size ranges, major features, and important roles of major blood vessel types.				
Type of Artery	Outer Diameter (Approx. Range)	Intima	Media	Adventitia	Roles in Circulatory System
Elastic arteries	>10 mm	Endothelium; connective tissue with smooth muscle	Many elastic lamellae alternating with smooth muscle	Connective tissue, thinner than media, with vasa vasorum	Conduct blood from heart and with elastic recoil help move blood forward under steady pressure
Muscular arteries	10-1 mm	Endothelium; connective tissue with smooth muscle, internal elastic lamina prominent	Many smooth muscle layers, with much less elastic material	Connective tissue, thinner than media; vasa vasorum may be present	Distribute blood to all organs and maintain steady blood pressure and flow with vasodilation and constriction
Small arteries	1-0.1 mm	Endothelium; connective tissue less smooth muscle	3-10 layers of smooth muscle	Connective tissue, thinner than media; no vasa vasorum	Distribute blood to arterioles, adjusting flow with vasodilation and constriction
Arterioles	100-10 μm	Endothelium; no connective tissue or smooth muscle	1-3 layers of smooth muscle	Very thin connective tissue layer	Resist and control blood flow to capillaries; major determinant of systemic blood pressure
Capillaries	10-4 μm	Endothelium only	Pericytes only	None	Exchange metabolites by diffusion to and from cells
Venules (postcapillary, collecting, and muscular)	10-100 μm	Endothelium; no valves	Scattered smooth muscle cells	None	Drain capillary beds; site of leukocyte exit from vasculature
Small veins	0.1-1 mm	Endothelium; connective tissue with scattered smooth muscle fibers	Thin, 2-3 loose layers of smooth muscle cells	Connective tissue, thicker than media	Collect blood from venules
Medium veins	1-10 mm	Endothelium; connective tissue, with valves	3-5 more distinct layers of smooth muscle	Thicker than media; longitudinal smooth muscle may be present	Carry blood to larger veins, with no backflow
Large veins	>10 mm	Endothelium; connective tissue, smooth muscle cells; prominent valves	>5 layers of smooth muscle, with much collagen	Thickest layer, with bundled longitudinal smooth muscle	Return blood to heart

smooth muscle in the media. The intima has a very thin subendothelial layer and a prominent internal elastic lamina (Figure 11–11). The media may contain up to 40 layers of large smooth muscle cells interspersed with a variable number of elastic lamellae (depending on the size of the vessel). An external elastic lamina, the last component of the media, is present only in the larger muscular arteries. The adventitia consists of connective tissue. Lymphatic capillaries, vasa vasorum, and nerves are also found in the adventitia, and these structures may penetrate to the outer part of the media.

Arterioles

Muscular arteries branch repeatedly into smaller and smaller arteries, until reaching a size with three or four medial layers of smooth muscle. The smallest arteries branch as **arterioles**, which have only one or two smooth muscle layers; these indicate the beginning of an organ's **microvasculature** (Figures 11–12 and 11–13) where exchanges between blood and tissue fluid occur. Arterioles are generally less than 0.1 mm in diameter, with lumens approximately as wide as

FIGURE 11–10 Cells and capillaries in a glomus body.

Specialized regions in the walls of certain elastic arteries contain tissues acting as chemoreceptors that provide information to the brain regarding blood chemistry. The glomus bodies are two small (0.5–5 mm-diameter) ganglion-like structures found near the common carotid arteries. They contain many large capillaries (**C**) intermingled with clusters of large glomus cells (**G**) filled with vesicles of various neurotransmitters. Supportive satellite cells (**S**) with elongated nuclei ensheath each glomus cell. Glomus cells form synaptic connections with sensory fibers. Significant changes in the blood CO_2, O_2, or H^+ concentrations are detected by the chemoreceptive glomus cells, which then release a neurotransmitter that activates the sensory nerve to relay this information to the brain. X400. PT.

FIGURE 11–11 Muscular artery.

With distance from the heart, arteries gradually have relatively less elastin and more smooth muscle in their walls. Most arteries, large enough to have names, are of the muscular type. A transverse section through a muscular (medium-caliber) artery shows a slightly folded intima with only sparse connective tissue between the endothelial cells (**E**) and internal elastic lamina (**IEL**). Multiple layers of smooth muscle (**SM**) in the media (**M**) are thicker than the elastic lamellae and fibers with which they intersperse. Vasa vasorum (**V**) are seen in the adventitia. X100. H&E.

the wall is thick (Figure 11–14). The subendothelial layer is very thin, elastic laminae are absent, and the media consists of the circularly arranged smooth muscle cells. In both small arteries and arterioles, the adventitia is very thin and inconspicuous.

Arterioles almost always branch to form anastomosing networks or beds of capillaries that surround the parenchymal cells of the organ. Smooth muscle fibers act as sphincters closing arterioles and producing periodic blood flow into capillaries (Figure 11–13). Acting as "resistance vessels," muscle tone usually keeps arterioles partially closed and makes these vessels the major determinants of systemic blood pressure.

›› MEDICAL APPLICATION

Blood pressure depends on cardiac output and the total peripheral resistance to blood flow, which is mostly due to the resistance of arterioles. **Hypertension** or elevated blood pressure may occur secondarily to renal or endocrine problems, but is more commonly essential hypertension, due to a wide variety of mechanisms that increase arteriolar constriction.

FIGURE **11–12** Microvasculature.

Arterioles (**A**), capillaries (**C**), and venules (**V**) comprise the microvasculature where, in almost every organ, molecular exchange takes place between blood and the interstitial fluid of the surrounding tissues. Lacking media and adventitia tunics and with diameters of only 4-10 μm, capillaries (**C**) in paraffin sections can be recognized by nuclei adjacent to small lumens or by highly eosinophilic red blood cells in the lumen. As described in Figure 5–20, not all interstitial fluid formed at capillary beds is drained into venules; the excess is called **lymph** and collects in thin-walled, irregularly shaped lymphatic vessels (**L**), such as those seen in connective tissue and smooth muscle here. 200X H&E.

In certain tissues and organs arterioles deviate from this simple path to accommodate various specialized functions (Figure 11–15). For example, thermoregulation by the skin involves arterioles that can bypass capillary networks and connect directly to venules. The media and adventitia are thicker in these **arteriovenous shunts** (or arteriovenous anastomoses) and richly innervated by sympathetic and parasympathetic nerve fibers. The autonomic fibers control the degree of vasoconstriction at the shunts, regulating blood flow through the capillary beds. High capillary blood flow in the skin allows more heat dissipation from the body, while reduced capillary blood flow conserves heat—important functions when the environmental temperature is hot or cold, respectively.

FIGURE **11–13** Microvascular bed structure and perfusion.

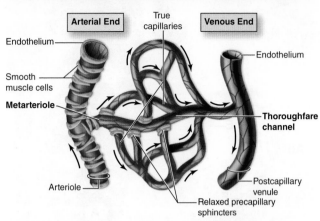

a Sphincters relaxed; capillary bed well perfused

b Sphincters contracted; blood bypasses capillary bed

Arterioles supplying a capillary bed typically form smaller branches called **metarterioles** in which the **smooth muscle cells** are dispersed as bands that act as **precapillary sphincters**. The distal portion of the metarteriole, sometimes called a **thoroughfare channel**, lacks smooth muscle cells and merges with the **postcapillary venule**. Branching from the metarteriole and thoroughfare channel are the smallest vessels, **true capillaries**, which lack smooth muscle cells (although pericytes may be present). The precapillary sphincters regulate blood flow into the true capillaries.

Part **a** shows a well-perfused capillary bed with all the sphincters relaxed and open; part **b** shows a capillary bed with the blood shunted away by contracted sphincters. At any given moment, most sphincters are at least partially closed and blood enters the capillary bed in a pulsatile manner for maximally efficient exchange of nutrients, wastes, O_2, and CO_2 across the endothelium. Except in the pulmonary circulation (see Figure 11–1), blood enters the microvasculature well oxygenated and leaves poorly oxygenated.

Another important alternative microvascular pathway is a venous **portal system** (Figure 11–15), in which blood flows through two successive capillary beds separated by a **portal vein**. This arrangement allows for hormones or

FIGURE 11–14 Arterioles.

(a) Arterioles are microvessels with an intima (I) consisting only of endothelium (E), in which the cells may have rounded nuclei. They have media (M) tunics with only one or two layers of smooth muscle, and usually thin, inconspicuous adventitia (Ad). X350. Masson trichrome. (b) Three arterioles (A) of various sizes and a capillary (C) are shown here. X400. H&E. (c) A large mesenteric arteriole cut obliquely and longitudinally clearly shows the endothelial cells (arrow heads) and one or two layers of smooth muscle cells (M) cut transversely. Adventitia merges imperceptibly with neighboring connective tissue. X300. PT.

FIGURE 11–15 Comparison of the simple microvascular pathway with arteriovenous shunts and portal systems.

Most capillary beds are supplied by arterioles and drain into venules, but alternative pathways are found in certain organs. In skin blood flow can be varied according to external conditions by **arteriovenous (AV) shunts**, or anastomoses, commonly coiled, which directly connect the arterial and venous systems and temporarily bypass capillaries.

In **venous portal systems** one capillary bed drains into a vein that then branches again into another capillary bed. This arrangement allows molecules entering the blood in the first set of capillaries to be delivered quickly and at high concentrations to surrounding tissues at the second capillary bed, which is important in the anterior pituitary gland and liver.

Not shown are **arterial portal system** (afferent arteriole → capillaries → efferent arteriole) which occur in the kidney.

nutrients picked up by the blood in the first capillary network to be delivered most efficiently to cells around the second capillary bed before the blood is returned to the heart for general distribution. The best examples are the hepatic portal system of the liver and the hypothalamic-hypophyseal portal system in the anterior pituitary gland, both of which have major physiologic importance.

Capillary Beds

Capillaries permit and regulate metabolic exchange between blood and surrounding tissues. These smallest blood vessels always function in groups called **capillary beds**, whose size and overall shape conforms to that of the structure supplied (eg, Figure 10–5). The richness of the capillary network is related to the metabolic activity of the tissues. Tissues with

FIGURE **11–16** Capillary with pericytes.

Capillaries consist only of an endothelium rolled as a tube, across which molecular exchange occurs between blood and tissue fluid. **(a)** Capillaries are normally associated with perivascular contractile cells called **pericytes (P)** that have a variety of functions. The more flattened nuclei belong to endothelial cells. X400. H&E of a spread mesentery preparation.

(b) TEM of a capillary cut transversely, showing the nucleus of one thin capillary endothelial cell (**E**). Endothelial cells form the capillary lumen (**L**), are covered by a basal lamina (**BL**), and bound tightly together with junctional complexes (**J**). One pericyte (**P**) is shown, surrounded by its own basal lamina (**BL**) and with cytoplasmic extensions which surround the endothelial cells. X13,000.

high metabolic rates, such as the kidney, liver, and cardiac and skeletal muscle, have an abundant capillary network; the opposite is true of tissues with low metabolic rates, such as smooth muscle and dense connective tissue.

Capillary beds are supplied preferentially by one or more terminal arteriole branches called **metarterioles**, which are continuous with **thoroughfare channels** connected with the **postcapillary venules** (Figure 11–13). True capillaries branch from the metarterioles, which are encircled by scattered smooth muscle cells, and converge into the thoroughfare channels, which lack muscle. At the beginning of each true capillary, muscle fibers act as **precapillary sphincters** that contract or relax to control the entry of blood. These sphincters contract and relax cyclically, with 5 to 10 cycles per minute, causing blood to pass through capillaries in a pulsatile manner. When the sphincters are closed, blood flows directly from the metarterioles and thoroughfare channels into postcapillary venules.

Capillaries are composed of a single layer of **endothelial cells** rolled up as a tube (Figure 11–16). The average diameter of capillaries varies from 4 to 10 μm, which allows transit of blood cells only one at a time, and their individual length is usually not more than 50 μm. These minute vessels make up over 90% of the body's vasculature, with a total length of more than 100,000 km and a total surface area of approximately 5000 m². Because of the cyclical opening and closing of the sphincters, most capillaries are essentially empty at any given time, with only about 5% (~300 mL in an adult) of the total blood volume moving through these structures. Their

thin walls, extensive surface area, and slow, pulsatile blood flow optimize capillaries for the exchange of water and solutes between blood and tissues.

In addition to the endothelial properties mentioned earlier in this chapter, capillary cells have many features specialized for molecular transfer by mechanisms ranging from simple diffusion to transcytosis. The basal lamina helps determine which macromolecules interact with the endothelial cells. The average thickness of the cells is only 0.25 μm and a distinctive feature is often the nucleus curved to accommodate the very small tubular structure (see Figure 11–10). The cytoplasm contains mitochondria and most other organelles, along with a typically large population of membrane vesicles. Along with the basal lamina, junctional complexes between the cells maintain the tubular structure, with variable numbers of tight junctions having an important role in capillary permeability.

Major structural variations in capillaries occur in organs with various functions that permit very different levels of metabolic exchange. Capillaries are generally grouped into three histologic types, depending on the continuity of the endothelial cells and the external lamina (Figure 11–17).

■ **Continuous capillaries** (Figure 11–17a) have many tight, well-developed occluding junctions between slightly overlapping endothelial cells, which provide for continuity along the endothelium and well-regulated metabolic exchange across the cells. This is the most common type of capillary and is found in muscle,

FIGURE **11–17** Types of capillaries.

a Continuous capillary

Basement membrane
Pinocytotic vesicles
Erythrocyte
Intercellular cleft
Lumen
Nucleus of endothelial cell

b Fenestrated capillary

Basement membrane
Nuclei of endothelial cells
Erythrocyte
Intercellular cleft
Lumen
Fenestrations

c Sinusoid

Large fenestrations
Discontinuous basement membrane
Lumen
Intercellular cleft
Nucleus of endothelial cell

The vessels between arterioles and venules can be any of three types. **(a) Continuous capillaries**, the most common type, have tight, occluding junctions sealing the intercellular clefts between all the endothelial cells to produce minimal fluid leakage. All molecules exchanged across the endothelium must cross the cells by diffusion or transcytosis.

(b) Fenestrated capillaries also have tight junctions, but perforations (fenestrations) through the endothelial cells allow greater exchange across the endothelium. The basement membrane is continuous in both these capillary types.

Fenestrated capillaries are found in organs where molecular exchange with the blood is important, such as endocrine organs, intestinal walls, and choroid plexus.

(c) Sinusoids, or discontinuous capillaries, usually have a wider diameter than the other types and have discontinuities between the endothelial cells, large fenestrations through the cells, and a partial, discontinuous basement membrane. Sinusoids are found in organs where exchange of macromolecules and cells occurs readily between tissue and blood, such as in bone marrow, liver, and spleen.

connective tissue, lungs, exocrine glands, and nervous tissue. Ultrastructural studies show numerous vesicles indicating transcytosis of macromolecules in both directions across the endothelial cell cytoplasm.

- **Fenestrated capillaries** (Figure 11–17b) have a sieve-like structure that allows more extensive molecular exchange across the endothelium. The endothelial cells are penetrated by numerous small circular openings or fenestrations (L. *fenestra*, perforation), approximately 80 nm in diameter. Some fenestrations are covered by very thin diaphragms of proteoglycans (Figure 11–18); others may represent membrane invaginations during transcytosis that temporarily involve both sides of the very thin cells. The basal lamina is continuous and covers the fenestrations. Fenestrated capillaries are found in organs with rapid interchange of substances between tissues and the blood, such as the kidneys, intestine, choroid plexus, and endocrine glands.

- **Discontinuous capillaries**, commonly called **sinusoids** (Figure 11–17c), permit maximal exchange of macromolecules as well as allow easier movement of cells between tissues and blood. Individual endothelial cells here have large perforations without diaphragms; collectively they form a discontinuous layer, with wide, irregular spaces between the cells. Sinusoids also differ from other capillaries by having highly discontinuous basal laminae and much larger diameters, often 30 to 40 μm, which slows blood flow. Sinusoidal capillaries

are found in the liver, spleen, some endocrine organs, and bone marrow (Figures 11–19 and 11–20).

At various locations along continuous capillaries and postcapillary venules are mesenchymal cells called **pericytes** (Gr. *peri*, around + *kytos*, cell), with long cytoplasmic processes partly surrounding the endothelial layer. Pericytes produce their own basal lamina, which may fuse with that of the endothelial cells (Figure 11–16). Well-developed networks of myosin, actin, and tropomyosin in pericytes indicate these cells' primary contractile function to facilitate flow of blood cells. After tissue injuries, pericytes proliferate and differentiate to form smooth muscle and other cells in new vessels as the microvasculature is reestablished.

›› MEDICAL APPLICATION

The **hyperglycemia** or excessive blood sugar that occurs with diabetes commonly leads to **diabetic microangiopathy**, a diffuse thickening of capillary basal laminae and concomitant decrease in metabolic exchange at these vessels, particularly in the kidneys, retina, skeletal muscle, and skin.

Venules

The transition from capillaries to venules occurs gradually. The immediate **postcapillary venules** (Figure 11–21a) are

FIGURE **11–18** Continuous capillary.

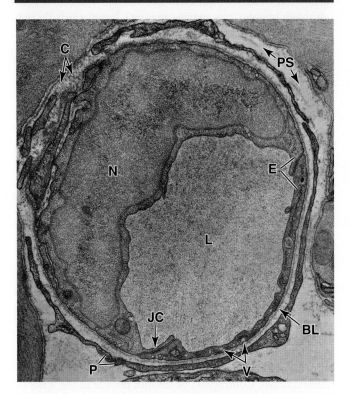

Continuous capillaries exert the tightest control over what molecules leave and enter the capillary lumen (**L**). The TEM shows a continuous capillary in transverse section. An endothelial cell nucleus (**N**) is prominent, and tight or occluding junctions are abundant in the junctional complexes (**JC**) at overlapping folds between the endothelial cells (**E**). Numerous transcytotic vesicles (**V**) are evident. All material that crosses continuous capillary endothelium must pass *through* the cells, usually by diffusion or transcytosis.

Around the capillary are a basal lamina (**BL**) and thin cytoplasmic extensions from pericytes (**P**). Collagen fibers (**C**) and other extracellular material are present in the perivascular space (**PS**). X10,000.

FIGURE **11–19** Fenestrated capillary.

Fenestrated capillaries are specialized for uptake of molecules such as hormones in endocrine glands or for outflow of molecules such as in the kidney's filtration system. TEM of a transversely sectioned fenestrated capillary in the peritubular region of the kidney shows many typical fenestrae closed by diaphragms (arrows), with a continuous basal lamina surrounding the endothelial cell (**BL**). In this cell the Golgi apparatus (**G**), nucleus (**N**), and centrioles (**C**) can also be seen. Fenestrated capillaries allow a freer exchange of molecules than continuous capillaries and are found in the intestinal wall, kidneys, and endocrine glands. X10,000.

(With permission, from Dr Johannes Rhodin, Department of Cell Biology, New York University School of Medicine.)

similar structurally to capillaries with pericytes, but range in diameter from 15 to 20 μm. As described with blood in the Chapter 12, postcapillary venules are the primary site at which white blood cells adhere to endothelium and leave the circulation at sites of infection or tissue damage.

Postcapillary venules converge into larger **collecting venules** that have more contractile cells. With even greater size, the venules become surrounded by a recognizable tunica media with two or three smooth muscle layers and are called **muscular venules**. A characteristic feature of all venules is the large diameter of the lumen compared to the overall thinness of the wall (Figure 11–21).

Veins

Veins carry blood back to the heart from microvasculature all over the body. Blood entering veins is under very low pressure and moves toward the heart by contraction of smooth muscle fibers in the media and by external compressions from surrounding muscles and other organs. Valves project from the tunica intima to prevent backflow of blood. Most veins are **small** or **medium veins** (Figure 11–22), with diameters of 10 mm or less (see Table 11–1). Such veins are usually located close and parallel to corresponding muscular arteries. The intima usually has a thin subendothelial layer, and the media consists of small bundles of smooth muscle cells intermixed with reticular fibers and a delicate network of elastic fibers. The collagenous adventitial layer is well developed.

The big venous trunks, paired with elastic arteries close to the heart, are the **large veins** (see Figure 11–7b). Large veins have a well-developed intima, but the media is relatively thin, with alternating layers of smooth muscle and connective tissue. The adventitial layer is thicker than the media in large veins and frequently contains longitudinal bundles of smooth muscle. Both the media and adventitia contain

FIGURE **11–20** Sinusoidal capillary.

Sinusoidal capillaries or sinusoids generally have much greater diameters than most capillaries and are specialized not only for maximal molecular exchange between blood and surrounding tissue but also for easy movement of blood cells across the endothelium. The sinusoid (**S**) shown here is in bone marrow and is surrounded by tissue containing adipocytes (**A**) and masses of hematopoietic cells (**H**). The endothelial cells are very thin and cell nuclei are more difficult to find than in smaller capillaries. Ultrastructurally sinusoidal capillaries are seen to have large fenestrations through the cells and large discontinuities between the cells and through the basal lamina. X200. H&E.

elastic fibers, but internal and external elastic laminae like those of arteries are not present.

Medium and large veins have valves consisting of paired folds of the intima projecting across the lumen (see Figure 11–6; Figures 11–22 and 11–23). They are rich in elastic fibers and are lined on both sides by endothelium. The valves, which are especially numerous in veins of the legs, help keep the flow of venous blood directed toward the heart.

>> **MEDICAL APPLICATION**

Junctions between endothelial cells of postcapillary venules are the loosest of the microvasculature. This facilitates transendothelial migration of leukocytes at these locations during **inflammation**, as well as a characteristic loss of fluid here during the inflammatory response, leading to tissue **edema**.

› **LYMPHATIC VASCULAR SYSTEM**

In addition to the blood vasculature, the body has a system of very thin-walled channels that collect excess interstitial fluid called **lymph** from the tissue spaces and return it to the blood. In normal tissues lymph does not contain red blood cells (although lymphocytes may be present), but it is usually rich in lightly staining proteins (Figure 11–24a). Most tissues with blood vessels also contain **lymphatic capillaries** (or lymphatics) that originate as closed-ended vessels consisting of a single layer of very thin endothelial cells on an incomplete basal lamina. Openings between these cells are held open by bundles of anchoring filaments containing elastic fibers that also bind the vessels to the surrounding connective tissue. Folds of the endothelial cells across the openings prevent most backflow of lymph out of the vessel (Figure 11–24b).

Lymphatic capillaries converge into larger **lymphatic vessels**. Interposed in the path of these lymphatics are lymph nodes, which are discussed with the immune system in Chapter 14. With exceptions such as the central nervous system (CNS) and the bone marrow, lymphatics are found in almost all organs.

The structure of larger lymphatic vessels resembles that of veins except with thinner walls and no distinct separation among tunics (Figure 11–25). They also have more numerous internal valves than veins. The lymphatic vessels are often dilated with lymph. As in veins, lymphatic circulation is aided by external forces (eg, contraction of surrounding skeletal muscle), with the valves responsible for keeping lymph flow unidirectional. Contraction of smooth muscle in the walls of larger lymphatic vessels also helps propel lymph toward the heart.

Lymphatic vessels ultimately converge as two large trunks: the **thoracic duct** and the **right lymphatic duct**, which empty lymph back into the blood. The thoracic duct enters the cardiovascular system near the junction of the left internal jugular vein with the left subclavian vein, and the lymphatic duct near the confluence of the right subclavian vein and the right internal jugular vein. The structure of these lymphatic ducts is similar to that of large veins, with reinforced smooth muscle in the middle layer arranged both longitudinally and circularly. The adventitia is relatively underdeveloped, but it contains vasa vasorum and a neural network.

Besides gathering interstitial fluid as lymph and returning it to the blood, the lymphatic vascular system is a major distributor of lymphocytes, antibodies, and other immune components which are carried through many organs to and from lymph nodes and other lymphoid tissues.

>> **MEDICAL APPLICATION**

Lymphatics and larger lymphatic vessels are clinically important because (among other reasons) they facilitate the spread of pathogens, parasites, and malignant cells in the body. Surgical removal of lymph nodes, standard procedure to determine the occurrence of cancer metastasis, can disrupt the lymphatic drainage and produce swelling or **lymph edema**, in tissues of the affected region.

FIGURE 11–21 Venules.

A series of increasingly larger and more organized venules lie between capillaries and veins.

(a) Compared to arterioles (**A**), postcapillary venules (**V**) have large lumens and an intima of simple endothelial cells, with occasional pericytes (**P**). X400. Toluidine blue (TB).

(b) Larger collecting venules (**V**) have much greater diameters than arterioles (**A**), but the wall is still very thin, consisting of an endothelium with more numerous pericytes or smooth muscle cells. X200. Toluidine blue.

(c) The muscular venule cut lengthwise here has a better defined tunica media, with as many as three layers of smooth muscle (**M**) in some areas, a very thin intima (**I**) of endothelial

cells (**E**), and a more distinct adventitia (**Ad**). Part of an arteriole (**A**) shows a thicker wall than the venule. X200. Masson trichrome.

As discussed with white blood cells in Chapter 12, postcapillary venules are important as the site in the vasculature where these cells leave the circulation to become functional in the interstitial space of surrounding tissues when such tissues are inflamed or infected.

(d) Postcapillary venule (**V**) from an infected small intestine shows several leukocytes adhering to and migrating across the intima. X200. H&E.

FIGURE 11–22 Veins.

Veins usually travel as companions to arteries and are classified as small, medium, or large based on size and development of the tunics.

(a) Micrograph of small vein (**V**) shows a relatively large lumen compared to the small muscular artery (**A**) with its thick media (**M**) and adventitia (**Ad**). The wall of a small vein is very thin, containing only two or three layers of smooth muscle. X200. H&E.

(b) Micrograph of a convergence between two small veins shows valves (arrow). Valves are thin folds of intima projecting well into the lumen, which act to prevent backflow of blood. X200. H&E.

(c) Micrograph of a medium vein (**MV**) shows a thicker wall but still less prominent than that of the accompanying muscular artery (**MA**). Both the media and adventitia are better developed, but the wall is often folded around the relatively large lumen. X100. H&E.

(d) Micrograph of a medium vein contains blood and shows valve folds (arrows). X200. Masson trichrome.

FIGURE **11–23** Wall of large vein with valve.

Large veins have a muscular media layer (**M**) that is very thin compared to the surrounding adventitia (**A**) of dense irregular connective tissue. The wall is often folded as shown here, with the intima (**I**) projecting into the lumen as a valve (**V**) composed of the subendothelial connective tissue with endothelium on both sides. X100. PT.

FIGURE **11–24** Lymphatic capillary.

Endothelium of
lymphatic capillary

Interstitial fluid

Opening

Lymph

Anchoring filament

Lymphatic capillaries drain interstitial fluid produced when the plasma forced from the microvasculature by hydrostatic pressure does not all return to blood by the action of osmotic pressure. **(a)** Micrograph shows a lymphatic capillary filled with this fluid called lymph (**L**). Lymphatics are blind-ended vessels with a wall of very thin endothelial cells (**E**) and are quite variable in diameter (10-50 μm). Lymph is rich in proteins and other material and often stains somewhat better than the surrounding ground substance, as seen here. X200. Mallory trichrome.

(b) Diagram indicating more details about lymphatics, including the **openings between the endothelial cells**. The openings are held in place by **anchoring filaments** containing elastin and are covered by extensions of the endothelial cells. **Interstitial fluid** enters primarily via these openings, and the endothelial folds prevent backflow of lymph into tissue spaces. Lymphatic endothelial cells are typically larger than those of blood capillaries.

FIGURE **11-25** Lymphatic vessels and valve.

Lymphatic vessels are formed by the merger of lymphatic capillaries, but their walls remain extremely thin. **(a)** Cross section shows a lymphatic vessel (**LV**) near a venule (**V**), whose wall is thick by comparison. Lymphatic vessels normally do not contain red blood cells, which provides another characteristic distinguishing them from venules. X200. Mallory trichrome.

(b) Lymphatic vessel (**LV**) in muscle cut longitudinally shows a valve, the structure responsible for the unidirectional flow of lymph. The solid arrow shows the direction of the lymph flow, and the dotted arrows show how the valves prevent lymph backflow. The lower small lymphatic vessel is a lymphatic capillary with a wall consisting only of endothelium. X200. PT.

The Circulatory System SUMMARY OF KEY POINTS

Heart

- The heart has three major layers: (1) the inner **endocardium** of endothelium and subendothelial connective tissue; (2) the **myocardium** of cardiac muscle; and (3) the **epicardium**, connective tissue with many adipocytes and covered by mesothelium.
- The innate **cardiac conducting system**, which stimulates rhythmic contraction, is made of modified cardiac muscle fibers and consists of the **sinoatrial (SA) and atrioventricular (AV) nodes**, the **atrioventricular bundle (of His)**, and **Purkinje fibers**.
- **Purkinje fibers**, located just beneath the endocardium of both ventricles, are distinguished from contractile fibers by their greater diameter, abundant glycogen, and more sparse bundles of myofibrils.
- Masses of dense irregular connective tissue make up the **cardiac skeleton**, which surrounds the bases of all heart valves, separates the atria from the ventricles, and provides insertions for cardiac muscle.

Vasculature

- Macroscopically visible blood vessels have three major layers or **tunics**: (1) The **intima** includes the endothelium, connective tissue, and an internal elastic lamina in larger vessels; (2) the **media**

contains alternating layers of smooth muscle and collagen or elastic lamellae; and (3) the **adventitia** (or externa) contains connective tissue, small vessels (**vasa vasorum**), and nerves.
- Through the vasculature, **endothelial cells** are not simply heart and vessel liners; they actively produce factors that prevent blood clotting, factors that cause adjacent smooth muscle cells to contract or relax, and factors that initiate inflammation at sites of damage or infection.
- Arteries are grouped by size and wall composition: (1) **large elastic arteries**, with fenestrated elastic laminae in the thick tunica media; (2) **muscular, medium-sized arteries**; and (3) **small arteries**, with fewer than 10 layers of smooth muscle in the media.
- A **microvasculature** too small for surgical manipulation permeates most organs and consists of (1) **arterioles**, with one to three smooth muscle layers; (2) **capillaries**, consisting only of an intima endothelial layer; and (3) **venules**, with large lumens and thin walls, which drain capillaries.
- Terminal arterioles branch into **metarterioles**, in which smooth muscle **sphincters** contract to resist blood flow and relax cyclically to allow pulsatile flow of blood into an anastomosing **capillary bed**, where **metabolic exchange** with surrounding cells occurs.

■ Capillaries are classified as three structural and functional types, with features that allow different degrees of molecular or even cellular exchange: (1) **continuous capillaries** with many tight junctions so that all exchange must occur through the cells; (2) **fenestrated capillaries** with small pores or fenestrations through the cells; and (3) **discontinuous capillaries**, or **sinusoids**, with larger lumens, large spaces between the endothelial cells, and a discontinuous basal lamina.

■ Capillary beds generally drain into **venules**, the last segment of the microvasculature; **postcapillary venules** are the sites at which white blood cells enter damaged or infected tissues.

■ The endothelium of continuous capillaries and postcapillary venules is frequently surrounded by thin cells called **pericytes**, whose contractions facilitate blood flow and which can give rise to smooth muscle and connective tissue during microvascular remodeling or repair.

■ Two alternative microvascular pathways include **arteriovenous anastomoses**, or **AV shunts**, in which arterioles can bypass a capillary bed, and **venous portal systems**, in which venules draining a capillary bed quickly branch again to form another capillary bed.

■ **Small, medium, and large veins**, all with lumen diameters exceeding the thickness of the wall, carry blood back to the heart, with intimal **valves** preventing backflow, and have increasingly well-developed tunics.

Lymphatic Vessels

■ Interstitial fluid that is not pulled into venules by colloidal osmotic pressure drains as **lymph** into blind vessels called **lymphatics**, or **lymphatic capillaries**, which have very thin endothelial cell walls with spaces between the cells.

■ Lymphatics converge into larger, thin-walled **lymphatic vessels** in which lymph is propelled by movements of surrounding muscles and organs, with intimal **valves** keeping the flow unidirectional.

■ The largest lymphatic vessels, the **thoracic duct** and **right lymphatic duct**, both with walls having tunics like those of veins, return lymph to the circulatory system by joining veins near the heart.

12 Blood

Blood is a specialized connective tissue in which cells are suspended in fluid extracellular material called **plasma**. Propelled mainly by rhythmic contractions of the heart, about 5 L of blood in an average adult moves unidirectionally within the closed circulatory system. The so-called **formed elements** circulating in the plasma are **erythrocytes** (red blood cells), **leukocytes** (white blood cells), and **platelets**.

When blood leaves the circulatory system, either in a test tube or in the extracellular matrix (ECM) surrounding blood vessels, plasma proteins react with one another to produce a clot, which includes formed elements and a pale yellow liquid called **serum**. Serum contains growth factors and other proteins released from platelets during clot formation, which confer biological properties very different from those of plasma.

Collected blood in which clotting is prevented by the addition of anticoagulants (eg, heparin or citrate) can be separated by centrifugation into layers that reflect its heterogeneity (Figure 12–1). Erythrocytes make up the sedimented material and their volume, normally about 45% of the total blood volume in healthy adults, is called the **hematocrit**.

The straw-colored, translucent, slightly viscous supernatant comprising 55% at the top half of the centrifugation tube is the plasma. A thin gray-white layer called the **buffy coat** between the plasma and the hematocrit, about 1% of the volume, consists of leukocytes and platelets, both less dense than erythrocytes.

Blood is a distributing vehicle, transporting O_2, CO_2, metabolites, hormones, and other substances to cells throughout the body. O_2 is bound mainly to hemoglobin in erythrocytes and is much more abundant in arterial than venous blood (Figure 12–2), while CO_2 is carried in solution as CO_2 or HCO_3^-, in addition to being hemoglobin-bound. Nutrients are distributed from their sites of synthesis or absorption in the gut, while metabolic residues are collected from cells all over the body and removed from the blood by the excretory organs. Hormone distribution in blood permits the exchange of chemical messages between distant organs regulating normal organ function. Blood also participates in heat distribution, the regulation of body temperature, and the maintenance of acid-base and osmotic balance.

Leukocytes have diversified functions and are one of the body's chief defenses against infection. These cells are generally spherical and inactive while suspended in circulating blood, but, when called to sites of infection or inflammation, they cross the wall of venules, become motile and migrate into the tissues, and display their defensive capabilities.

› COMPOSITION OF PLASMA

Plasma is an aqueous solution, pH 7.4, containing substances of low or high molecular weight that make up 7% of its volume. As summarized in Table 12–1, the dissolved components are mostly plasma proteins, but they also include nutrients, respiratory gases, nitrogenous waste products, hormones, and inorganic ions, collectively called **electrolytes**. Through the capillary walls, the low-molecular-weight components of plasma are in equilibrium with the interstitial fluid of the tissues. The composition of plasma is usually an indicator of the mean composition of the extracellular fluids in tissues.

The major plasma proteins include the following:

- **Albumin**, the most abundant plasma protein, is made in the liver and serves primarily to maintain the osmotic pressure of the blood.
- **α-Globulins and β-globulins**, made by liver and other cells, include transferrin and other transport factors; fibronectin; prothrombin and other coagulation factors; lipoproteins and other proteins entering blood from tissues.
- **γ-Globulins**, which are immunoglobulins (antibodies) secreted by plasma cells in many locations.
- **Fibrinogen**, the largest plasma protein (340 kD), also made in the liver, which, during clotting, polymerizes as insoluble, cross-linked fibers of fibrin that block blood loss from small vessels.
- **Complement proteins**, a system of factors important in inflammation and destruction of microorganisms.

FIGURE **12–1** Composition of whole blood.

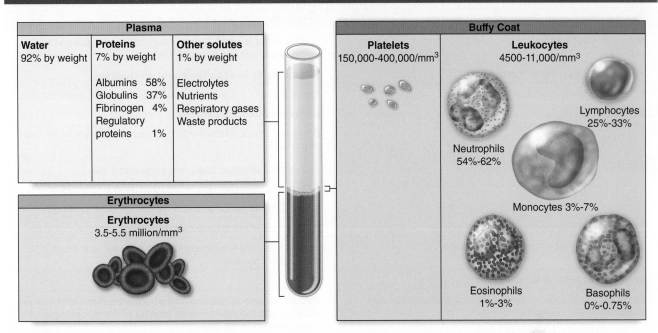

Plasma		
Water 92% by weight	**Proteins** 7% by weight	**Other solutes** 1% by weight
	Albumins 58% Globulins 37% Fibrinogen 4% Regulatory proteins 1%	Electrolytes Nutrients Respiratory gases Waste products

Erythrocytes

Erythrocytes
3.5-5.5 million/mm³

Buffy Coat

Platelets
150,000-400,000/mm³

Leukocytes
4500-11,000/mm³

Lymphocytes
25%-33%

Neutrophils
54%-62%

Monocytes 3%-7%

Eosinophils
1%-3%

Basophils
0%-0.75%

A tube of blood after centrifugation (center) has 36%-53% of its volume represented by erythrocytes in the bottom half of the tube, a volume called the **hematocrit**. Between the sedimented erythrocytes and the supernatant light-colored plasma is a thin layer of leukocytes and platelets called the **buffy coat**. The concentration ranges of erythrocytes, platelets, and leukocytes in normal blood are included here, along with the **differential count** or percent range for each type of leukocyte represented in the buffy coat. A cubic millimeter of blood is equivalent to a microliter (μL). (All complete blood count [CBC] values in this chapter are those used by the US National Board of Medical Examiners.)

FIGURE **12–2** Blood O₂ content in each type of blood vessel.

The amount of O_2 in blood (the O_2 pressure) is highest in arteries and lung capillaries and decreases in tissue capillaries, where exchange of O_2 and CO_2 occurs between blood and tissues.

› BLOOD CELLS

Blood cells can be studied histologically in smears prepared by spreading a drop of blood in a thin layer on a microscope slide (Figure 12–3). In such films the cells are clearly visible and distinct from one another, facilitating observation of their nuclei and cytoplasmic characteristics. Blood smears are routinely stained with special mixtures of acidic (eosin) and basic (methylene blue) dyes. These mixtures may also contain dyes called azures that are more useful in staining cytoplasmic granules containing charged proteins and proteoglycans. Azurophilic granules produce metachromasia in stained leukocytes like that seen with mast cells in connective tissue. Some of these special stains, such as Giemsa and Wright stain, are named after hematologists who introduced their own modifications into the original mixtures.

Erythrocytes

Erythrocytes (red blood cells or RBCs) are terminally differentiated structures lacking nuclei and completely filled with the O_2-carrying protein hemoglobin. RBCs are the only blood cells whose function does not require them to leave the vasculature.

TABLE **12–1**	The composition of blood plasma.

Plasma Component (Percentage of Plasma)	Functions
Water (~92% of plasma)	Is the solvent in which formed elements are suspended and proteins and solutes are dissolved
Plasma Proteins (~7% of Plasma):	**All proteins serve to buffer against pH changes**
Albumin (~58% of plasma proteins)	Exerts osmotic force to retain fluid within the microvasculature Contributes to blood's viscosity Binds and transports some fatty acids, electrolytes, hormones and drugs
Globulins (~37% of plasma proteins)	α-Globulins transport lipids and some metal ions β-Globulins transport iron ions and lipids in bloodstream γ-Globulins are antibodies with various immune functions
Fibrinogen (~4% of plasma proteins)	Participates in blood coagulation (clotting); precursor of fibrin
Regulatory proteins (>1% of plasma proteins)	Consists of enzymes, proenzymes, hormones, and the complement system
Other Solutes (~1% of Blood Plasma)	
Electrolytes (eg, sodium, potassium, calcium, chloride, iron, bicarbonate, and hydrogen)	Help establish and maintain membrane potentials, maintain pH balance, and regulate osmosis (control of the percentages of water and salt in the blood)
Nutrients (eg, amino acids, glucose, cholesterol, vitamins, fatty acids)	Energy source; precursor for synthesizing other molecules
Respiratory gases (eg, oxygen: >2% dissolved in plasma, 98% bound to hemoglobin within erythrocytes; and carbon dioxide: ~7% dissolved in plasma, ~27% bound to hemoglobin within erythrocytes, ~66% converted to HCO_3^-)	Oxygen is needed for aerobic cellular respiration; carbon dioxide is a waste product produced by cells during this process
Wastes (breakdown products of metabolism) (eg, lactic acid, creatinine, urea, bilirubin, ammonia)	Waste products serve no function in the blood plasma; they are merely being transported to the liver and kidneys where they can be removed from the blood

FIGURE **12–3** Preparing a blood smear.

① Prick finger and collect a small amount of blood using a micropipette.

② Place a drop of blood on a slide.

③a Using a second slide, pull the drop of blood across the first slide's surface, leaving a thin layer of blood on the slide.

③b After the blood dries, apply a stain briefly and rinse. Place a coverslip on top.

④ When viewed under the microscope, blood smear reveals the components of the formed elements.

Anemia is the condition of having a concentration of erythrocytes below the normal range. With fewer RBCs per milliliter of blood, tissues are unable to receive adequate O_2. Symptoms of anemia include lethargy, shortness of breath, fatigue, skin pallor, and heart palpitations. Anemia may result from insufficient red cell production, due, for example, to iron deficiency, or from blood loss with a stomach ulcer or excessive menses.

An increased concentration of erythrocytes in blood (**erythrocytosis**, or **polycythemia**) may be a physiologic adaptation found, for example, in individuals who live at high altitudes, where O_2 tension is low. Elevated hematocrit increases blood viscosity, putting strain on the heart, and, if severe, can impair circulation through the capillaries.

Human erythrocytes suspended in an isotonic medium are flexible biconcave discs (Figure 12–4). They are approximately 7.5 μm in diameter, 2.6 μm thick at the rim, but only 0.75 μm thick in the center. Because of their uniform diameters and their presence in most tissue sections, RBCs can often be used by histologists as an internal standard to estimate the size of other cells or structures.

The biconcave shape provides a large surface-to-volume ratio and facilitates gas exchange. The normal concentration of erythrocytes in blood is approximately 3.9 to 5.5 million per microliter (μL, or mm³) in women and 4.1-6.0 million/μL in men.

Erythrocytes are normally quite flexible, which permits them to bend and adapt to the irregular turns and small diameters of capillaries. Observations in vivo show that at the angles of capillary bifurcations, erythrocytes with normal adult hemoglobin frequently assume a cuplike shape. In larger blood vessels RBCs often adhere to one another loosely in stacks called **rouleaux** (Figure 12–4c).

The plasmalemma of the erythrocyte, because of its ready availability, is the best-known membrane of any cell. It consists of about 40% lipid, 10% carbohydrate, and 50% protein. Most of the latter are integral membrane proteins (see Chapter 2), including ion channels, the anion transporter called **band 3 protein**, and **glycophorin A**. The glycosylated extracellular domains of the latter proteins include antigenic sites that form the basis for the ABO blood typing system. Several peripheral proteins are associated with the inner surface of the membrane, including **spectrin**, dimers of which form a lattice bound to underlying actin filaments, and **ankyrin**, which anchors the lattice to the glycophorins and band 3 proteins. This submembranous meshwork stabilizes the membrane, maintains the cell shape, and provides the cell elasticity required for passage through capillaries.

Erythrocyte cytoplasm lacks all organelles but is densely filled with **hemoglobin**, the tetrameric O_2-carrying protein that accounts for the cells' uniform acidophilia. When combined with O_2 or CO_2, hemoglobin forms oxyhemoglobin or carbaminohemoglobin, respectively. The reversibility of these combinations is the basis for the gas-transporting capability of hemoglobin. The combination of hemoglobin with carbon monoxide (CO) is irreversible, however, reducing the cells' capacity to transport O_2.

FIGURE **12–4** Normal human erythrocytes.

(a) Colorized SEM micrograph of normal **erythrocytes** with each side concave. X1800. **(b)** Diagram of an erythrocyte giving the cell's dimensions. The biconcave shape gives the cells a very high surface-to-volume ratio and places most hemoglobin within a short distance from the cell surface, both qualities that provide maximally efficient O_2 transport. Erythrocytes are also quite flexible and can easily bend to pass through small capillaries. **(c)** In small vessels red blood cells also often stack up in aggregates called **rouleaux**. The standard size of RBCs allows one to estimate that the vessel seen is 15 μm in diameter. X250. H&E.

Erythrocyte differentiation (discussed in Chapter 13) includes loss of the nucleus and organelles, shortly before the cells are released by bone marrow into the circulation. Lacking mitochondria, erythrocytes rely on anaerobic glycolysis for their minimal energy needs. Lacking nuclei, they cannot replace defective proteins.

Inherited alterations in hemoglobin molecules are responsible for several pathologic conditions, an example of which is **sickle cell disease**. This disorder is caused by a mutation of one nucleotide (a **point mutation**) in the gene for the hemoglobin β chain. The consequences of this single substitution are profound. When the altered hemoglobin (called **HbS**) is deoxygenated in capillaries, it polymerizes and forms rigid aggregates that cause a characteristic sickle shape (Figure 12-5). The sickled erythrocyte is less flexible and more fragile and has a shortened life span that can lead to anemia. It increases the blood viscosity and can damage the wall of blood vessels, promoting blood coagulation. Sickle cells can block capillaries, restricting O_2 delivery to tissues and leading to varying degrees of ischemia or **anoxia** and organ damage.

FIGURE **12–5** Sickle cell erythrocyte.

A single nucleotide substitute in the hemoglobin gene produces a version of the protein that polymerizes to form rigid aggregates, leading to greatly misshapen cells with reduced flexibility. In individuals homozygous for the mutated *HbS* gene, this can lead to greater blood viscosity, and poor microvascular circulation, both features of sickle cell disease. X6500.

Human erythrocytes normally survive in the circulation for about 120 days. By this time defects in the membrane's cytoskeletal lattice or ion transport systems begin to produce swelling or other shape abnormalities, as well as changes in the cells' surface oligosaccharide complexes. Senescent or worn-out RBCs displaying such changes are removed from the circulation, mainly by macrophages of the spleen, liver, and bone marrow.

Leukocytes

Leukocytes (white blood cells or WBCs) leave the blood and migrate to the tissues where they become functional and perform various activities related to immunity. According to the type of cytoplasmic granules and their nuclear morphology, leukocytes are divided into two groups: **granulocytes** and **agranulocytes** (Table 12-2). Both types are rather spherical while suspended in blood plasma, but they become amoeboid and motile after leaving the blood vessels and invading the tissues. Their estimated sizes mentioned here refer to observations in blood smears in which the cells are spread and appear slightly larger than they are in the circulation.

Granulocytes possess two major types of cytoplasmic granules: lysosomes (often called **azurophilic granules** in blood cells) and **specific granules** that bind neutral, basic, or acidic stains and have specific functions.

Granulocytes have **polymorphic nuclei** with two or more distinct (almost separated) nuclear lobes and include the **neutrophils, eosinophils,** and **basophils** (see Figure 12–1 and Table 12-2). All granulocytes are terminally differentiated cells with a life span of only a few days. Their Golgi complexes and rough ER are poorly developed. They have few mitochondria and depend largely on glycolysis for their low energy needs. Granulocytes normally die by apoptosis in the connective tissue and billions of neutrophils alone die by apoptosis each day in the adult human. The resulting cellular debris is removed by macrophages and, like all apoptotic cell death, does not itself elicit an inflammatory response.

Agranulocytes do not have specific granules, but they do contain azurophilic granules (lysosomes), with affinity for the basic stain azure A. The nucleus is spherical or indented but not lobulated. This group includes **lymphocytes** and **monocytes** (see Figure 12–1 and Table 12–2). The differential count (percentage of all leukocytes) for each type of leukocyte is also presented in Table 12–2.

All leukocytes are key players in the defense against invading microorganisms, and in the repair of injured tissues, specifically leaving the microvasculature in injured or infected tissues. At such sites factors termed **cytokines** are released from various sources and these trigger loosening of intercellular junctions in the endothelial cells of local postcapillary venules (Figure 12–6). Simultaneously the cell adhesion protein **P-selectin** appears on these cells' luminal surfaces produced by exocytosis of Weibel-Palade bodies. Neutrophils and other leukocytes have on their surfaces glycosylated ligands for P-selectin, and their interactions cause cells flowing through the venules to slow down, like rolling tennis balls arriving at a patch of velcro. Other cytokines stimulate the now

TABLE **12–2**	Leukocytes: Numbers, structural features, and major functions.

Eosinophil

Neutrophil

Granulocytes

Agranulocytes

Basophil

Lymphocyte

Monocyte

Type	Nucleus	Specific Granules[a]	Differential Count[b] (%)	Life Span	Major Functions
Granulocytes					
Neutrophils	3-5 lobes	Faint/light pink	57-67	1-4 d	Kill and phagocytose bacteria
Eosinophils	Bilobed	Red/dark pink	1-3	1-2 wk	Kill helminthic and other parasites; modulate local inflammation
Basophils	Bilobed or S-shaped	Dark blue/purple	0-0.75	Several months	Modulate inflammation, release histamine during allergy
Agranulocytes					
Lymphocytes	Rather spherical	(none)	25-33	Hours to many years	Effector and regulatory cells for adaptive immunity
Monocytes	Indented or C-shaped	(none)	3-7	Hours to years	Precursors of macrophages and other mononuclear phagocytic cells

[a]Color with routine blood smear stains. There are typically 4500-11,000 total leukocytes/μL of blood in adults, higher in infants and young children.

[b]The percentage ranges given for each type of leukocyte are those used by the U.S. National Board of Medical Examiners. The value for neutrophils includes 3%-5% circulating, immature band forms.

All micrographs X1600.

FIGURE 12–6 Diagram of events involving leukocytes in a postcapillary venule at sites of inflammation.

Locations in connective tissue with injuries or infection require the rapid immigration of various leukocytes to initiate cellular events for tissue repair and removal of the invading microorganisms. The cytokines and cell binding proteins target various leukocytes and are best known for neutrophils. The major initial events of neutrophil migration during inflammation are summarized here:

1. Local macrophages activated by bacteria or tissue damage release **proinflammatory cytokines** such as interleukin-1 (IL-1) or tumor necrosis factor-α (TNF-α) that signal endothelial cells of nearby postcapillary venules to rapidly insert glycoprotein selectins on the luminal cell surfaces.

2. Passing neutrophils with appropriate cell surface glycoproteins bind the **selectins**, which causes such cells to adhere loosely to the endothelium and "roll" slowly along its surface.

3. Exposure to these and other cytokines causes expression of new **integrins** on the rolling leukocytes and expression of the integrin ligand **ICAM-1** (intercellular adhesion molecule-1) on the endothelial cells. Junctional complexes between the endothelial cells are selectively downregulated, loosening these cells.

4. Integrins and their ligands provide firm endothelial adhesion of neutrophils to the endothelium, allowing the leukocytes to receive further stimulation from the local cytokines.

5. Neutrophils become motile, probe the endothelium with pseudopodia, and, being attracted by other local injury-related factors called chemokines, finally migrate by **diapedesis** between the loosened cells of the venule. Rapid transendothelial migration of neutrophils may be facilitated by the cells' thin, segmented nuclei. All leukocytes first become functional in the ECM after emerging from the circulation by this process.

slowly rolling leukocytes to express integrins and other adhesion factors that produce firm attachment to the endothelium (see Figure 11–21d). In a process called **diapedesis** (Gr. *dia*, through + *pedesis*, to leap), the leukocytes send extensions through the openings between the endothelial cells, migrate out of the venules into the surrounding tissue space, and head directly for the site of injury or invasion. The attraction of neutrophils to bacteria involves chemical mediators in a process of **chemotaxis**, which causes leukocytes to rapidly accumulate where their defensive actions are specifically needed.

The number of leukocytes in the blood varies according to age, sex, and physiologic conditions. Healthy adults have 4500 to 11,000 leukocytes per microliter of blood.

Neutrophils (Polymorphonuclear Leukocytes)

Mature neutrophils constitute 54% to 62% of circulating leukocytes; circulating immature forms raise this value by 3%

to 5%. Neutrophils are 12-15 μm in diameter in blood smears, with nuclei having two to five lobes linked by thin nuclear extensions (see Table 12–2; Figure 12–7). In females, the inactive X chromosome may appear as a drumstick-like appendage on one of the lobes of the nucleus (Figure 12–7c) although this characteristic is not obvious in every neutrophil. Neutrophils are inactive and spherical while circulating but become actively amoeboid during diapedesis and upon adhering to solid substrates such as collagen in the ECM.

Neutrophils are active phagocytes of bacteria and other small particles and are usually the first leukocytes to arrive at sites of infection, where they actively pursue bacterial cells using chemotaxis.

The cytoplasmic granules of neutrophils provide the cells' functional activities and are of two main types (Figure 12–8). **Azurophilic primary granules** resemble lysosomes as large, dense vesicles and have a major role in both killing and

FIGURE 12–7 Neutrophils.

(a) In blood smears neutrophils can be identified by their multilobulated nuclei, with lobules held together by very thin strands. With this feature, the cells are often called **polymorphonuclear leukocytes**, PMNs, or just **polymorphs**. The cells are dynamic and the nuclear shape changes frequently. X1500. Giemsa.

(b) Neutrophils typically have diameters ranging from 12 to 15 μm, approximately twice that of the surrounding erythrocytes. The cytoplasmic granules are relatively sparse and have heterogeneous staining properties, although generally pale and not obscuring the nucleus. X1500. Giemsa.

(c) Micrograph showing a neutrophil from a female in which the condensed X chromosome appears as a drumstick appendage to a nuclear lobe (arrow). X1500. Wright.

degrading engulfed microorganisms. They contain proteases and antibacterial proteins, including the following:

- **Myeloperoxidase** (MPO), which generates hypochlorite and other agents toxic to bacteria
- **Lysozyme**, which degrades components of bacterial cell walls
- **Defensins**, small cysteine-rich proteins that bind and disrupt the cell membranes of many types of bacteria and other microorganisms.

❯❯ MEDICAL APPLICATION

Several kinds of **neutrophil defects**, often genetic in origin, can affect function of these cells, for example, by decreasing adhesion to the wall of venules, by causing the absence of specific granules, or with deficits in certain factors of the azurophilic granules. Individuals with such disorders typically experience more frequent and more persistent bacterial infections, although macrophages and other leukocytes may substitute for certain neutrophil functions.

Specific secondary granules are smaller and less dense, stain faintly pink, and have diverse functions, including secretion of various ECM-degrading enzymes such as collagenases, delivery of additional bactericidal proteins to the phagolysosomes, and insertion of new cell membrane components.

Activated neutrophils at infected or injured sites also have important roles in the inflammatory response that begins the process of restoring the normal tissue microenvironment. They release polypeptide **chemokines** that attract other leukocytes and **cytokines** that direct activities of these and local cells of the tissue. Important **lipid mediators** of inflammation are also released from neutrophils.

Neutrophils contain glycogen, which is broken down into glucose to yield energy via the glycolytic pathway. The citric acid cycle is less important, as might be expected in view of the paucity of mitochondria in these cells. The ability of neutrophils to survive in an anaerobic environment is highly advantageous, because they can kill bacteria and help clean up debris in poorly oxygenated regions, for example, damaged or necrotic tissue lacking normal microvasculature.

Neutrophils are short-lived cells with a half-life of 6 to 8 hours in blood and a life span of 1 to 4 days in connective tissues before dying by apoptosis.

❯❯ MEDICAL APPLICATION

Neutrophils look for bacteria to engulf by pseudopodia and internalize them in vacuoles called **phagosomes**. Immediately thereafter, specific granules fuse with and discharge their contents into the phagosomes which are then acidified by proton pumps. Azurophilic granules then discharge their enzymes into this acidified vesicle, killing and digesting the engulfed microorganisms.

During phagocytosis, a burst of O_2 consumption leads to the formation of superoxide anions (O_2^-) and hydrogen peroxide (H_2O_2). O_2^- is a short-lived, highly reactive free radical that, together with MPO and halide ions, forms a powerful microbial killing system inside the neutrophils. Besides the activity of lysozyme cleaving cell wall peptidoglycans to kill certain bacteria, the protein lactoferrin avidly binds iron, a crucial element in bacterial nutrition whose lack of availability then causes bacteria to die. A combination of these mechanisms will kill most microorganisms, which are then digested by lysosomal enzymes. Apoptotic neutrophils, bacteria, semidigested material, and tissue fluid form a viscous, usually yellow collection of fluid called **pus**.

Several neutrophil hereditary dysfunctions have been described. In one of them, actin does not polymerize normally, reducing neutrophil motility. With a NADPH oxidase deficiency, there is a failure to produce H_2O_2 and hypochlorite, reducing the cells' microbial killing power. Children with such dysfunctions can experience more persistent bacterial infections.

FIGURE **12–8** Neutrophil ultrastructure.

A TEM of a sectioned human neutrophil reveals the two types of cytoplasmic granules: the small, pale, more variably stained specific granules (**S**) and the larger, electron-dense azurophilic granules (**A**). Specific granules undergo exocytosis during and after diapedesis, releasing many factors with various activities, including enzymes to digest ECM components and bactericidal factors. Azurophilic granules are modified lysosomes with components to kill engulfed bacteria. The nucleus (**N**) is lobulated and the central Golgi apparatus (**G**) is small. Rough ER and mitochondria are not abundant, because this cell utilizes glycolysis and is in the terminal stage of its differentiation. X25,000.

Eosinophils

Eosinophils are far less numerous than neutrophils, constituting only 1% to 3% of leukocytes. In blood smears, this cell is about the same size as a neutrophil or slightly larger, but with a characteristic bilobed nucleus (see Table 12-2; Figure 12–9). The main identifying characteristic is the abundance of large, acidophilic specific granules typically staining pink or red.

Ultrastructurally the eosinophilic specific granules are seen to be oval in shape, with flattened crystalloid cores (Figure 12–9c) containing **major basic proteins** (**MBP**), an arginine-rich factor that accounts for the granule's acidophilia and constitutes up to 50% of the total granule protein. MBPs, along with eosinophilic peroxidase, other enzymes and toxins, act to kill parasitic worms or helminths. Eosinophils also modulate inflammatory responses by releasing chemokines, cytokines, and lipid mediators, with an important role in the inflammatory response triggered by allergies. The number of circulating eosinophils increases during helminthic infections and allergic reactions. These leukocytes also remove antigen-antibody complexes from interstitial fluid by phagocytosis.

Eosinophils are particularly abundant in connective tissue of the intestinal lining and at sites of chronic inflammation, such as lung tissues of asthma patients.

>> MEDICAL APPLICATION

An increase in the number of eosinophils in blood (**eosinophilia**) is associated with allergic reactions and helminth parasitic infections. In patients with such conditions, eosinophils are found in the connective tissues underlying epithelia of the bronchi, gastrointestinal tract, uterus, and vagina, and surrounding any parasitic worms present. In addition, these cells produce substances that modulate inflammation by inactivating the leukotrienes and histamine produced by other cells. Corticosteroids (hormones from the adrenal cortex) produce a rapid decrease in the number of blood eosinophils, probably by interfering with their release from the bone marrow into the bloodstream.

Basophils

Basophils are also 12 to 15 μm in diameter but make up less than 1% of blood leukocytes and are therefore difficult to find in normal blood smears. The nucleus is divided into two irregular lobes, but the large specific granules overlying the nucleus usually obscure its shape.

The specific granules (0.5 μm in diameter) typically stain purple with the basic dye of blood smear stains and are fewer, larger, and more irregularly shaped than

FIGURE **12–9** Eosinophils.

Eosinophils are about the same size as neutrophils but have bilobed nuclei and more abundant coarse cytoplasmic granules. The cytoplasm is often filled with brightly eosinophilic specific granules, but it also includes some azurophilic granules. **(a)** Micrograph shows an eosinophil **(E)** next to a neutrophil **(N)** and a small lymphocyte **(L)**. X1500. Wright.

(b) Even with granules filling the cytoplasm, the two nuclear lobes of eosinophils are usually clear. X1500. Giemsa.

(c) Ultrastructurally a sectioned eosinophil clearly shows the unique specific eosinophilic granules **(EG)**, as oval structures with disc-shaped electron-dense, crystalline cores. These granules, along with a few lysosomes and mitochondria **(M)**, fill the cytoplasm around the bilobed nucleus **(N)**. X20,000.

---

the granules of other granulocytes (see Table 12–2; Figure 12–10). The strong basophilia of the granules is due to the presence of heparin and other sulfated GAGs. Basophilic specific granules also contain much histamine and various other mediators of inflammation, including platelet activating factor, eosinophil chemotactic factor, and the enzyme phospholipase A that catalyzes an initial step in producing lipid-derived proinflammatory factors called **leukotrienes**.

By migrating into connective tissues, basophils appear to supplement the functions of mast cells, which are described in Chapter 5. Both basophils and mast cells have metachromatic granules containing heparin and histamine, have surface **receptors for immunoglobulin E (IgE)**, and secrete their granular components in response to certain antigens and allergens.

≫ MEDICAL APPLICATION

In some individuals a second exposure to a strong allergen, such as that delivered in a bee sting, may produce an intense, adverse systemic response. Basophils and mast cells may rapidly degranulate, producing vasodilation in many organs, a sudden drop in blood pressure, and other effects comprising a potentially lethal condition called **anaphylaxis** or **anaphylactic shock**.

Basophils and mast cells also are central to immediate or **type 1 hypersensitivity**. In some individuals substances such as certain pollen proteins or specific proteins in food are allergenic, that is, elicit production of specific IgE antibodies, which then bind to receptors on mast cells and immigrating basophils. Upon subsequent exposure, the allergen combines with the receptor-bound IgE molecules, causing them to cross-link and aggregate on the cell surfaces and triggering rapid exocytosis of the cytoplasmic granules. Release of the inflammatory mediators in this manner can result in **bronchial asthma**, cutaneous **hives**, **rhinitis**, **conjunctivitis**, or **allergic gastroenteritis**.

Lymphocytes

By far the most numerous type of agranulocyte in normal blood smears or CBCs, lymphocytes constitute a family of leukocytes with spherical nuclei (see Table 12–2; Figure 12–11). Lymphocytes are typically the smallest leukocytes and are abundant, constituting up to a third of these cells. Although they are morphologically similar, lymphocytes can be subdivided into functional groups by distinctive surface molecules (called "cluster of differentiation" or

FIGURE **12–10** Basophils.

(a-c) Basophils are also approximately the same size as neutrophils and eosinophils, but they have large, strongly basophilic specific granules that usually obstruct the appearance of the nucleus which usually has two large irregular lobes. a and b: X1500, Wright; c: X1500, Giemsa.

(d) A TEM of a sectioned basophil reveals the single bilobed nucleus (**N**) and the large, electron-dense specific basophilic granules (**B**). Basophils exert many activities modulating the immune response and inflammation and have many functional similarities with mast cells, which are normal, longer-term residents of connective tissue. X25,000.

CD markers) that can be distinguished using antibodies with immunocytochemistry or flow cytometry. Major classes include **B lymphocytes**, helper and cytotoxic **T lymphocytes** (CD4+ and CD8+, respectively), and **natural killer (NK) cells**. These and other types of lymphocytes have diverse roles in immune defenses against invading microorganisms and certain parasites or abnormal cells, and these immune functions are discussed with the immune system in Chapter 14.

Though generally small circulating lymphocytes have a wider range of sizes than most leukocytes. Many have diameters similar to those of RBCs; medium and large lymphocytes are 9 to 18 μm in diameter, with the latter representing activated lymphocytes or NK cells. The small lymphocytes are characterized by spherical nuclei with highly condensed chromatin and only a thin surrounding rim of scant cytoplasm, making them easily distinguishable from granulocytes. Larger lymphocytes have larger, slightly indented nuclei and

more cytoplasm that is slightly basophilic, with a few azurophilic granules (lysosomes), mitochondria, free polysomes, and other organelles (Figure 12–11d).

Lymphocytes vary in life span according to their specific functions; some live only a few days and others survive in the circulating blood or other tissues for many years.

>> MEDICAL APPLICATION

Given their central roles in immunity, lymphocytes are obviously important in many diseases. **Lymphomas** are a group of disorders involving neoplastic proliferation of lymphocytes or the failure of these cells to undergo apoptosis. Although often slow-growing, all lymphomas are considered malignant because they can very easily become widely spread throughout the body.

FIGURE **12–11** Lymphocytes.

Lymphocytes are agranulocytes and lack the specific granules characteristic of granulocytes. Lymphocytes circulating in blood generally range in size from 6 to 15 μm in diameter and are sometimes classified arbitrarily as small, medium, and large. **(a)** The most numerous small lymphocytes shown here are slightly larger than the neighboring erythrocytes and have only a thin rim of cytoplasm surrounding the spherical nucleus. X1500. Giemsa.

(b) Medium lymphocytes are distinctly larger than erythrocytes. X1500. Wright. **(c)** Large lymphocytes, much larger than erythrocytes, may represent activated cells that have returned to the circulation. X1500. Giemsa. **(d)** Ultrastructurally a medium-sized lymphocytes is seen to be mostly filled with a euchromatic nucleus (**N**) surrounded by cytoplasm containing mitochondria (**M**), free polysomes, and a few dark lysosomes (azurophilic granules). X22,000.

Monocytes

Monocytes are agranulocytes that are precursor cells of **macrophages**, osteoclasts, microglia, and other cells of the **mononuclear phagocyte system** in connective tissue (see Chapter 5). All monocyte-derived cells are antigen-presenting cells and have important roles in immune defense of tissues. Circulating monocytes have diameters of 12 to 15 μm, but macrophages are somewhat larger. The monocyte nucleus is large and usually distinctly indented or C-shaped (Figure 12–12). The chromatin is less condensed than in lymphocytes and typically stains lighter than that of large lymphocytes.

The cytoplasm of the monocyte is basophilic and contains many small lysosomes or azurophilic granules, some of which are at the limit of the light microscope's resolution. These granules are distributed through the cytoplasm, giving it a

bluish-gray color in stained smears. Mitochondria and small areas of rough ER are present, along with a Golgi apparatus involved in the formation of lysosomes (Figure 12–12e).

›› MEDICAL APPLICATION

Extravasation or the accumulation of immigrating monocytes occurs in the early phase of inflammation following tissue injury. **Acute inflammation** is usually short-lived as macrophages undergo apoptosis or leave the site, but chronic inflammation usually involves the continued recruitment of monocytes. The resulting continuous presence of macrophages can lead to excessive tissue damage that is typical of chronic inflammation.

FIGURE 12–12 Monocytes.

Monocytes are large agranulocytes with diameters from 12 to 20 μm that circulate as precursors to macrophages and other cells of the mononuclear phagocyte system.
(a-d) Micrographs of monocytes showing their distinctive nuclei which are indented, kidney-shaped, or C-shaped. a: X1500, Giemsa; b-d: X1500, Wright. **(e)** Ultrastructurally the cytoplasm of a monocyte shows a Golgi apparatus (**G**), mitochondria (**M**), and lysosomes or azurophilic granules (**A**). Rough ER is poorly developed and there are some free polysomes (**R**). X22,000.
(Figure 12-12e, with permission, from D.F. Bainton and M.G. Farquhar, Department of Pathology, University of California at San Francisco, CA.)

Platelets

Blood platelets (or **thrombocytes**) are very small non-nucleated, membrane-bound cell fragments only 2 to 4 μm in diameter (Figure 12–13a). As described in Chapter 13, platelets originate by separation from the ends of cytoplasmic processes extending from giant polyploid bone marrow cells called **megakaryocytes**. Platelets promote blood clotting and help repair minor tears or leaks in the walls of small blood vessels, preventing loss of blood from the microvasculature. Normal platelet counts range from 150,000 to 400,000/μL (mm³) of blood. Circulating platelets have a life span of about 10 days.

In stained blood smears, platelets often appear in clumps. Each individual platelet is generally discoid, with a very lightly stained peripheral zone, the **hyalomere**, and a darker-staining central zone containing granules, called the **granulomere**.

A sparse glycocalyx surrounding the platelet plasmalemma is involved in adhesion and activation during blood coagulation. Ultrastructural analysis (Figure 12–13b) reveals a peripheral **marginal bundle** of microtubules and microfilaments, which helps to maintain the platelet's shape. Also in the hyalomere are two systems of membrane channels. An **open**

FIGURE **12–13** Platelets.

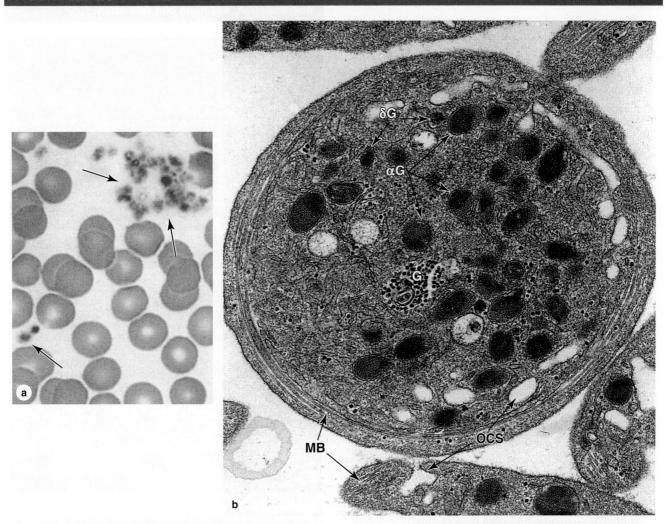

Platelets are cell fragments 2-4 μm in diameter derived from megakaryocytes of bone marrow. Their primary function is to rapidly release the content of their granules upon contact with collagen (or other materials outside of the endothelium) to begin the process of clot formation and reduce blood loss from the vasculature.

(a) In a blood smear, platelets (arrows) are often found as aggregates. Individually they show a lightly stained **hyalomere** region surrounding a more darkly stained central **granulomere** containing membrane-enclosed granules. X1500. Wright.

(b) Ultrastructurally a platelet shows a system of microtubules and actin filaments near the periphery, called the **marginal bundle (MB)**, which is formed as the platelet pinches off from megakaryocyte (Chapter 13), and helps maintain its shape. An open canalicular system (**OCS**) of invaginating membrane vesicles continuous with the plasmalemma facilitates rapid degranulation upon activation and Ca²⁺ release. The central granulomere region contains small dense delta granules (**δG**), larger and more numerous alpha granules (**αG**), and glycogen (**G**). X40,000.

(Figure 12-13b, with permission, from Dr M. J. G. Harrison, Middlesex Hospital and University College London, UK.)

canalicular system of vesicles is connected to invaginations of the plasma membrane, which may facilitate platelets' uptake of factors from plasma. A much less prominent set of irregular tubular vesicles comprising the dense tubular system is derived from the ER and stores Ca²⁺ ions. Together, these two membranous systems facilitate the extremely rapid exocytosis of proteins from platelets (degranulation) upon adhesion to collagen or other substrates outside the vascular endothelium.

Besides specific granules, the central granulomere has a sparse population of mitochondria and glycogen particles (Figure 12–13b). Electron-dense **delta granules** (δG), 250-300 nm in diameter, contain ADP, ATP, and serotonin (5-hydroxytryptamine) taken up from plasma. **Alpha granules** (αG) are larger (300-500 nm in diameter) and contain platelet-derived growth factor (PDGF), platelet factor 4, and several other platelet-specific proteins. Most of the stained granules seen in platelets with the light microscope are alpha granules.

The role of platelets in controlling blood loss (hemorrhage) and in wound healing can be summarized as follows:

- **Primary aggregation:** Disruptions in the microvascular endothelium, which are very common, allow the platelet glycocalyx to adhere to collagen. Thus, a **platelet plug** is formed as a first step to stop bleeding (Figure 12–14).
- **Secondary aggregation:** Platelets in the plug release a specific adhesive glycoprotein and ADP, which induce further platelet aggregation and increase the size of the platelet plug.
- **Blood coagulation:** During platelet aggregation, **fibrinogen** from plasma, **von Willebrand factor** and other proteins released from the damaged endothelium, and **platelet factor 4** from platelet granules promote the sequential interaction (cascade) of plasma proteins, giving rise to a **fibrin** polymer that forms a three-dimensional network of fibers trapping red blood cells and more platelets to form a **blood clot**, or **thrombus** (Figure 12–14). Platelet factor 4 is a chemokine for monocytes, neutrophils, and fibroblasts and proliferation of the fibroblasts is stimulated by PDGF.
- **Clot retraction:** The clot that initially bulges into the blood vessel lumen contracts slightly because of the interaction of platelet actin and myosin.
- **Clot removal:** Protected by the clot, the endothelium and surrounding tunic are restored by new tissue, and the clot is then removed, mainly dissolved by the proteolytic enzyme **plasmin**, formed continuously through the local action of **plasminogen activators** from the endothelium on **plasminogen** from plasma.

≫ MEDICAL APPLICATION

Aspirin and other nonsteroidal anti-inflammatory agents have **an** inhibitory effect on platelet function and blood coagulation because they block the local prostaglandin synthesis that is needed for platelet aggregation, contraction, and exocytosis at sites of injury. **Bleeding disorders** result from abnormally slow blood clotting. One such disease directly related to a defect in the platelets is a rare autosomal recessive **glycoprotein Ib deficiency**, involving a factor on the platelet surface needed to bind subendothelial collagen and begin the cascade of events leading to clot formation.

FIGURE 12–14 Platelet aggregation, degranulation, and fibrin clot formation.

Minor trauma to vessels of the microvasculature is a routine occurrence in active individuals and quickly results in a fibrin clot, shown here by SEM **(a)**. Upon contact with collagen in the vascular basement membrane, platelets (**P**) aggregate, swell, and release factors that trigger formation of a fibrin meshwork (**F**) that traps erythrocytes (**E**) and more degranulating platelets. Platelets in various states of degranulation are shown. Such a clot grows until blood loss from the vasculature stops. After repair of the vessel wall, fibrin clots are removed by proteolysis due primarily to locally generated plasmin, a nonspecific protease. X4100.

(b) Platelets aggregate at the onset of clot formation. This TEM section shows platelets in a platelet plug adhering to collagen (**C**). Upon adhering to collagen, platelets are activated and their granules undergo exocytosis into the open canalicular system, which facilitates extremely rapid release of factors involved in blood coagulation. When their contents are completely released, the swollen degranulated platelets (**arrows**) remain as part of the aggregate until the clot is removed. Several other key proteins for blood coagulation are released locally from adjacent endothelial cell processes (**EP**) and from the plasma. Part of an erythrocyte (**E**) is seen at the right. X7500.

Blood SUMMARY OF KEY POINTS

- The liquid portion of circulating blood is **plasma**, while the cells and platelets comprise the **formed elements**; upon clotting, some proteins are removed from plasma and others are released from platelets, forming a new liquid termed **serum**.
- Important protein components of plasma include **albumin**, diverse **α- and β-globulins**, proteins of the **complement** system, and **fibrinogen**, all of which are secreted within the liver, as well as the **immunoglobulins**.
- **Red blood cells** or **erythrocytes**, which make up the **hematocrit** portion (~45%) of a blood sample, are **enucleated, biconcave discs** 7.5 μm in diameter, filled with **hemoglobin** for the uptake, transport, and release of O_2, and with a normal life span of about **120 days**.
- **White blood cells** or **leukocytes** are broadly grouped as **granulocytes** (neutrophils, eosinophils, basophils) or **agranulocytes** (lymphocytes, monocytes).
- All leukocytes become active outside the circulation, specifically leaving the microvasculature in a process involving cytokines, selective adhesion, changes in the endothelium, and **transendothelial migration** or **diapedesis**.
- All granulocytes have specialized lysosomes called **azurophilic granules** and smaller **specific granules** with proteins for various cell-specific functions.

- **Neutrophils**, the most abundant type of leukocyte, have **polymorphic, multilobed nuclei**, and faint pink cytoplasmic granules that contain many factors for highly efficient phagolysosomal killing and removal of bacteria.
- **Eosinophils** have bilobed nuclei and eosinophilic specific granules containing factors for destruction of helminthic parasites and for modulating inflammation.
- **Basophils**, the rarest type of circulating leukocyte, have irregular bilobed nuclei and resemble mast cells with strongly basophilic specific granules containing factors important in allergies and chronic inflammatory conditions, including **histamine**, **heparin**, **chemokines**, and various **hydrolases**.
- **Lymphocytes**, agranulocytes with many functions as T- and B-cell subtypes in the immune system, range widely in size, depending on their activation state, and have roughly spherical nuclei with little cytoplasm and few organelles.
- **Monocytes** are larger agranulocytes with distinctly indented or C-shaped nuclei that circulate as precursors of macrophages and other cells of the **mononuclear phagocyte system**.
- **Platelets** are small (2-4 μm) cell fragments derived from **megakaryocytes** in bone marrow, with a **marginal bundle** of actin filaments, **alpha granules** and **delta granules**, and an **open canalicular system** of membranous vesicles; rapid degranulation on contact with collagen triggers blood clotting.

13 Hemopoiesis

Mature blood cells have a relatively short life span and must be continuously replaced with new cells from precursors developing during **hemopoiesis** (Gr. *haima*, blood + *poiesis*, a making). In the early embryo these blood cells arise in the **yolk sac** mesoderm. In the second trimester, hemopoiesis (also called **hematopoiesis**) occurs primarily in the developing **liver**, with the spleen playing a more minor role (Figure 13–1). Skeletal elements begin to ossify and **bone marrow** develops in their medullary cavities, so that in the third trimester marrow of specific bones becomes the major hemopoietic organ.

Throughout childhood and adult life, erythrocytes, granulocytes, monocytes, and platelets continue to form from stem cells located in bone marrow. The origin and maturation of these cells are termed, respectively, **erythropoiesis** (Gr. *erythros*, red + *poiesis*), **granulopoiesis**, **monocytopoiesis**, and **thrombocytopoiesis**. As described in Chapter 14 on the immune system, **lymphopoiesis** or lymphocyte development occurs in the marrow and in the lymphoid organs to which precursor cells migrate from marrow.

This chapter describes the stem and progenitor cells of hemopoiesis and their controlling factors, the histology of bone marrow, the major stages of red and white blood cell differentiation, and platelet formation.

› STEM CELLS, GROWTH FACTORS, & DIFFERENTIATION

As discussed in Chapter 3, stem cells are **pluripotent** cells capable of asymmetric division and self-renewal. Some of their daughter cells form specific, irreversibly differentiated cell types, and other daughter cells remain as a small pool of slowly dividing stem cells.

Hemopoietic stem cells can be isolated by using fluorescence-labeled antibodies to mark specific cell surface antigens and passing the cell population through a fluorescence-activated cell-sorting (FACS) instrument. Stem cells are studied using experimental techniques that permit analysis of hemopoiesis in vivo and in vitro.

In vivo techniques include injecting the bone marrow of normal donor mice into irradiated mice whose hematopoietic cells have been destroyed. In these animals, only the transplanted bone marrow cells produce hematopoietic colonies in the bone marrow and spleen, simplifying studies of this process. This work led to the clinical use of bone marrow transplants to treat potentially lethal hemopoietic disorders.

In vitro techniques using semisolid tissue culture media containing substances produced by marrow stromal cells are used to identify and study the cytokines promoting hemopoietic cell growth and differentiation.

Hemopoietic Stem Cells

All blood cells arise from a single major type of **pluripotent stem cell** in the bone marrow that can give rise to all the blood cell types (Figure 13–2). These pluripotent stem cells are rare, but they proliferate and form two major lineages of **progenitor cells** with restricted potentials (committed to produce specific blood cells): one for **lymphoid cells** (lymphocytes) and another for **myeloid cells** (Gr. *myelos*, marrow) that develop in bone marrow. Myeloid cells include granulocytes, monocytes, erythrocytes, and megakaryocytes. As described in Chapter 14 on the immune system, the lymphoid progenitor cells migrate from the bone marrow to the thymus or the lymph nodes, spleen, and other lymphoid structures, where they proliferate and differentiate.

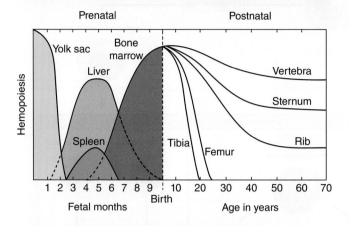

FIGURE **13–1** Shifting locations of hemopoiesis during development and aging.

Hemopoiesis, or blood cell formation, first occurs in a mesodermal cell population of the embryonic yolk sac, and shifts during the second trimester mainly to the developing liver, before becoming concentrated in newly formed bones during the last 2 months of gestation. Hemopoietic bone marrow occurs in many locations through puberty, but then becomes increasingly restricted to components of the axial skeleton.

Progenitor & Precursor Cells

The progenitor cells for blood cells are commonly called **colony-forming units** (**CFUs**), because they give rise to colonies of only one cell type when cultured or injected into a spleen. As shown in Figure 13–2, there are four major types of progenitor cells/CFUs:

- Erythroid lineage of CFU-erythrocytes (CFU-E),
- Thrombocytic lineage of CFU-megakaryocytes (CFU-Meg),
- Granulocyte-monocyte lineage of CFU-granulocytes-monocytes (CFU-GM), and
- Lymphoid lineage of CFU-lymphocytes of all types (CFU-L).

Each progenitor cell/CFU lineage produces **precursor cells** (or blasts) that gradually assume the morphologic characteristics of the mature, functional cell types they will become (Figure 13–2). In contrast, stem and progenitor cells cannot be morphologically distinguished and simply resemble large lymphocytes. While stem cells divide at a rate only sufficient to maintain their relatively small population, progenitor and precursor cells divide more rapidly, producing large numbers of differentiated, mature cells (3×10^9 erythrocytes and 0.85×10^9 granulocytes/kg/d in human bone marrow). The changing potential and activities of cells during hemopoiesis are shown graphically in Figure 13–3.

Hemopoiesis depends on a microenvironment, or niche, with specific endocrine, paracrine, and juxtacrine factors. These requirements are provided largely by the local cells and extracellular matrix (ECM) of the hemopoietic organs, which together create the niches in which stem cells are maintained and progenitor cells develop.

Hemopoietic growth factors, often called **colony-stimulating factors** (**CSF**) or cytokines, are glycoproteins that stimulate proliferation of progenitor and precursor cells and promote cell differentiation and maturation within specific lineages. Cloning of the genes for several important hematopoietic growth factors has significantly advanced study of blood formation and permitted the production of clinically useful factors for patients with hemopoietic disorders. The major activities, target cells, and sources of several well-characterized cytokines promoting hemopoiesis are presented in Table 13–1.

▶▶ MEDICAL APPLICATION

Hemopoietic growth factors are important products of biotechnology companies. They are used clinically to increase marrow cellularity and blood cell counts in patients with conditions such as severe anemia or during chemo- or radiotherapy, which lower white blood cell counts (leukopenia). Such cytokines may also increase the efficiency of marrow transplants by enhancing cell proliferation, enhance host defenses in patients with infectious and immunodeficient diseases, and improve treatment of some parasitic diseases.

▶ BONE MARROW

Under normal conditions, the production of blood cells by the bone marrow is adjusted to the body's needs, increasing its activity several-fold in a very short time. Bone marrow is found in the medullary canals of long bones and in the small cavities of cancellous bone, with two types based on their appearance at gross examination: blood-forming **red bone marrow**, whose color is produced by an abundance of blood and hemopoietic cells, and **yellow bone marrow**, which is filled with adipocytes that exclude most hemopoietic cells. In the newborn all bone marrow is red and active in blood cell production, but as the child grows, most of the marrow changes gradually to the yellow variety. Under certain conditions, such as severe bleeding or hypoxia, yellow marrow reverts to red.

Red bone marrow (Figure 13–4) contains a reticular connective tissue **stroma** (Gr. *stroma*, bed), **hemopoietic cords** or **islands** of cells, and **sinusoidal capillaries**. The stroma is a meshwork of specialized fibroblastic cells called **stromal cells** (also called **reticular** or **adventitial cells**) and a delicate web of reticular fibers supporting the hemopoietic cells and macrophages. The matrix of bone marrow also contains collagen type I, proteoglycans, fibronectin, and laminin, the latter glycoproteins interacting with integrins to bind cells to the matrix. Red marrow is also a site where older, defective erythrocytes undergo phagocytosis by macrophages, which then reprocess heme-bound iron for delivery to the differentiating erythrocytes.

FIGURE **13–2** Origin and differentiative stages of blood cells.

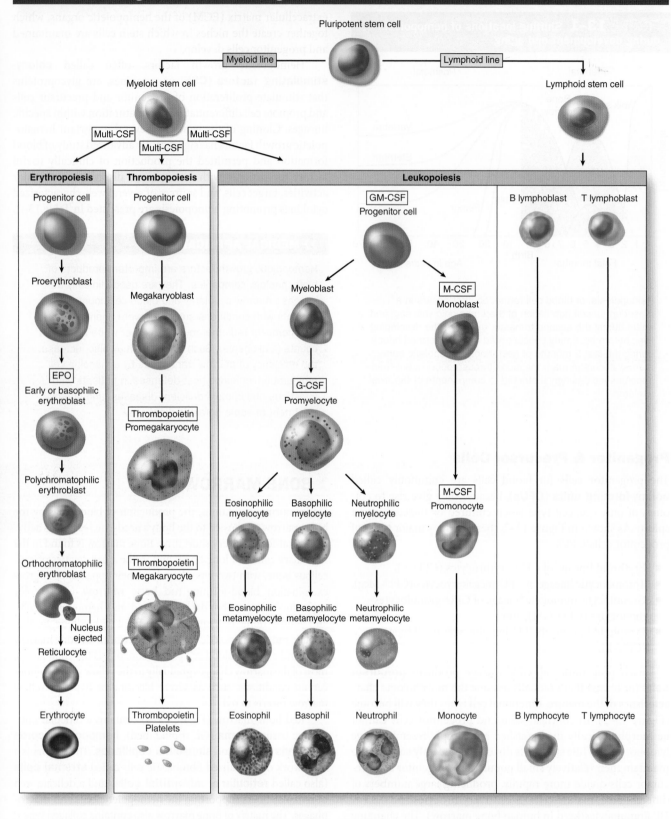

Rare pluripotent stem cells divide slowly, maintain their own population, and give rise to two major cell lineages of progenitor cells: the myeloid and lymphoid stem cells. The myeloid lineage includes precursor cells (blasts) for erythropoiesis, thrombopoiesis, granulopoiesis, and monocytopoiesis, all in the bone marrow. The lymphoid lineage forms lymphopoietic cells, partly in the bone marrow and partly in lymphoid organs.

FIGURE **13–3** Major changes in developing hemopoietic cells.

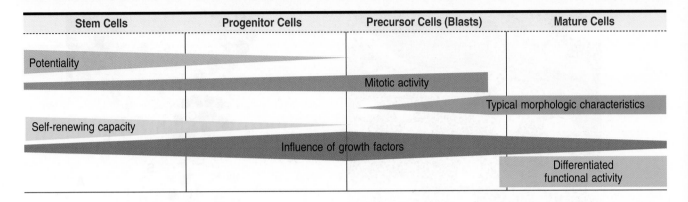

TABLE **13–1** Major hemopoietic cytokines (growth factors or colony-stimulating factors).

Cytokine	Major Activities and Target Cells[a]	Important Sources
Stem cell factor (SCF)	Mitogen for all hemopoietic progenitor cells	Stromal cells of bone marrow
Erythropoietin (EPO)	Mitogen for all erythroid progenitor and precursor cells, also promoting their differentiation	Peritubular endothelial cells of the kidney; hepatocytes
Thrombopoietin (TPO)	Mitogen for megakaryoblasts and their progenitor cells	Kidney and liver
Granulocyte-macrophage colony-stimulating factor (GM-CSF)	Mitogen for all myeloid progenitor cells	Endothelial cells of bone marrow and T lymphocytes
Granulocyte colony-stimulating factor (G-CSF or filgrastim)	Mitogen for neutrophil precursor cells	Endothelial cells of bone marrow and macrophages
Monocyte colony-stimulating factor (M-CSF)	Mitogen for monocyte precursor cells	Endothelial cells of marrow and macrophages
Interleukin-1 (IL-1)	Regulates activities and cytokine secretion of many leukocytes and other cells	Macrophages and T helper cells
Interleukin-2 (IL-2)	Mitogen for activated T and B cells; promotes differentiation of NK cells	T helper cells
Interleukin-3 (IL-3)	Mitogen for all granulocyte and megakaryocyte progenitor cells	T helper cells
Interleukin-4 (IL-4)	Promotes development of basophils and mast cells and B-lymphocyte activation	T helper cells
Interleukin-5 (IL-5) or eosinophil differentiation factor (EDF)	Promotes development and activation of eosinophils	T helper cells
Interleukin-6 (IL-6)	Mitogen for many leukocytes; promotes activation of B cells and regulatory T cells	Macrophages, neutrophils, local endothelial cells
Interleukin-7 (IL-7)	Major mitogen for all lymphoid stem cells	Stromal cells of bone marrow

[a]Most of the cytokines listed here target all the cells of specific lineages, including the progenitor cells and the precursor cells that are committed and maturing but still dividing. Many promote both mitosis and differentiation in target cells.

FIGURE **13–4** Red bone marrow (active in hemopoiesis).

Red bone marrow contains adipocytes but is primarily active in hemopoiesis, with several cell lineages usually present. It can be examined histologically in sections of bones or in biopsies, but its cells can also be studied in smears. Marrow consists of capillary sinusoids running through a stroma of specialized, fibroblastic stromal cells and an ECM meshwork with reticular fibers. Stromal cells produce the ECM; both stromal and bone cells secrete various CSFs, creating the microenvironment for hemopoietic stem cell maintenance, proliferation, and differentiation.

(a) Sections of red bone marrow include trabeculae (**T**) of cancellous bone, adipocytes (**A**), and blood-filled sinusoids (**S**) between hemopoietic cords (**C**) or islands of developing blood cells. X140. H&E. **(b)** At higher magnification the flattened nuclei of sinusoidal endothelial cells (**E**) can be distinguished, as well as the variety of densely packed hemopoietic cells in the cords (**C**) between the sinusoids (**S**) and adipocytes (**A**). Most stromal cells and specific cells of the hemopoietic lineages are difficult to identify with certainty in routinely stained sections of marrow. X400. H&E.

The hematopoietic niche in marrow includes the stroma, osteoblasts, and megakeryocytes. Between the hematopoietic cords run the sinusoids, which have discontinuous endothelium, through which newly differentiated blood cells and platelets enter the circulation (Figure 13–5).

>> **MEDICAL APPLICATION**

Red bone marrow also contains stem cells that can produce other tissues in addition to blood cells. These pluripotent cells may make it possible to generate specialized cells that are not rejected by the body because they are produced from stem cells from the marrow of the same patient. The procedure is to collect bone marrow stem cells, cultivate them in appropriate medium for their differentiation to the cell type needed for transplant, and then use the resulting cells to replace defective cells. These studies in **regenerative medicine** are at early stages, but results with animal models are promising.

› MATURATION OF ERYTHROCYTES

A mature cell is one that has differentiated to the stage at which it can carry out its specific functions. Erythrocyte maturation is an example of terminal cell differentiation involving hemoglobin synthesis and formation of a small, enucleated, biconcave corpuscle. Several major changes take place during **erythropoiesis** (Figures 13–6 and 13–7). Cell and nuclear volumes decrease, while the nucleoli diminish in size and disappear. Chromatin density increases until the nucleus presents a pyknotic appearance and is finally extruded from the cell. There is a gradual decrease in the number of polyribosomes (basophilia), with a simultaneous increase in the amount of hemoglobin (a highly eosinophilic protein). Mitochondria and other organelles gradually disappear.

There are three to five intervening cell divisions between the proerythroblast and the mature erythrocyte. The development of an erythrocyte from its first recognizable progenitor cell to the release of reticulocytes into the blood takes

FIGURE **13–5** Sinusoidal endothelium in active marrow.

The diagram shows that mature, newly formed erythrocytes, leukocytes, and platelets in marrow enter the circulation by passing through the discontinuous sinusoidal endothelium. All leukocytes cross the wall of the sinusoid by their own activity, but the non-motile erythrocytes cannot migrate through the wall actively and enter the circulation pushed by a pressure gradient across the wall. Megakaryocytes form thin processes (proplatelets) that also pass through such apertures and liberate platelets at their tips.

approximately 1 week. The glycoprotein **erythropoietin**, a growth factor produced by cells in the kidneys, stimulates production of mRNA for **globins**, the protein components of hemoglobin, and is essential for the production of erythrocytes.

The distinct progenitor cell of the erythroid series (Figure 13–6) is the **proerythroblast**, a large cell with loose, lacy chromatin, nucleoli, and basophilic cytoplasm. The next stage is represented by the **basophilic erythroblast**, with more strongly basophilic cytoplasm and a condensed nucleus with no visible nucleolus. The basophilia of these two cell types is caused by the large number of polysomes synthesizing hemoglobin. During the next stage cell volume is reduced, polysomes decrease, and some cytoplasmic areas begin to be filled with hemoglobin, producing regions of both basophilia and acidophilia in the cell, now called a **polychromatophilic erythroblast**. In the next stage, the cell and nuclear volumes continue to condense and no basophilia is evident, resulting in a uniformly acidophilic cytoplasm—the **orthochromatophilic erythroblast** (also called a **normoblast**). Late in this stage, this cell ejects its nucleus which is then phagocytosed by macrophages. The cell still has a small number of polyribosomes that, when treated with the dye brilliant cresyl blue, form a faintly stained network and the cell is called the **reticulocyte**. Reticulocytes pass to the circulation (where they may

FIGURE **13–6** Summary of erythrocyte maturation.

The color change in the cytoplasm shows the continuous decrease in basophilia and the increase in hemoglobin concentration from proerythroblast to erythrocyte. There is also a gradual decrease in nuclear volume and an increase in chromatin condensation, followed by extrusion of a pyknotic nucleus. The times indicate the average duration of each cell type. In the graph, 100% represents the highest recorded concentrations of hemoglobin and RNA.

FIGURE **13–7** Erythropoiesis: Major erythrocyte precursors.

(a) Micrographs showing a very large and scarce proerythroblast (**P**), a slightly smaller basophilic erythroblast (**B**) with very basophilic cytoplasm, typical and late polychromatophilic erythroblasts (**Pe** and **LPe**) with both basophilic and acidophilic cytoplasmic regions, and a small orthochromatophilic erythroblast (**Oe**) with cytoplasm nearly like that of the mature erythrocytes in the field. All X1400. Wright.

(b) Micrograph containing reticulocytes (arrows) that have not yet completely lost the polyribosomes used to synthesize globin, as demonstrated by a stain for RNA. X1400. Brilliant cresyl blue.

constitute 1% of the red blood cells), quickly lose the polyribosomes, and mature as erythrocytes.

› MATURATION OF GRANULOCYTES

Granulopoiesis involves cytoplasmic changes dominated by synthesis of proteins for the **azurophilic granules** and **specific granules**. These proteins are produced in the rough ER and the prominent Golgi apparatus in two successive stages (Figure 13–8). Made initially are the azurophilic granules, which contain lysosomal hydrolases, stain with basic dyes, and are basically similar in all three types of granulocytes. Golgi activity then changes to produce proteins for the specific granules, whose contents differ in each of the three types of granulocytes and endow each type with certain different properties (as explained in Chapter 12). In sections of bone marrow, cords of granulopoietic cells can be distinguished from erythropoietic cords by their granule-filled cytoplasm (Figure 13–9).

The **myeloblast** is the most immature recognizable cell in the myeloid series (see Figures 13–2 and 13–10). Typically these have finely dispersed chromatin, and faint nucleoli. In the next stage, the **promyelocyte** is characterized by basophilic cytoplasm and azurophilic granules containing lysosomal enzymes and myeloperoxidase. Different promyelocytes activate different sets of genes, resulting in lineages for the three types of granulocytes (see Figure 13–2). The first visible sign of this differentiation appears in the **myelocyte** stage (Figure 13–11), in which specific granules gradually increase in number and eventually occupy most of the cytoplasm at the **metamyelocyte** stage. These neutrophilic, basophilic, and eosinophilic metamyelocytes mature with further condensations of the nuclei. Before its complete maturation, the

neutrophilic granulocyte passes through an intermediate stage, the **band cell** (or stab cell), in which the nucleus is elongated but not yet polymorphic.

>> MEDICAL APPLICATION

The appearance of large numbers of immature neutrophils (band cells) in the blood, sometimes called a "shift to the left," is clinically significant, usually indicating a bacterial infection.

The vast majority of granulocytes are neutrophils and the total time required for a myeloblast to produce mature, circulating neutrophils ranges from 10 to 14 days. Five mitotic divisions normally occur during the myeloblast, promyelocyte, and neutrophilic myelocyte stages. As diagrammed in Figure 13–12, developing and mature neutrophils exist in four functionally and anatomically defined compartments: (1) the granulopoietic compartment in active marrow; (2) storage as mature cells in marrow until release; (3) the circulating population; and (4) a population undergoing margination, a process in which neutrophils adhere loosely and accumulate transiently along the endothelial surface in venules and small veins. Margination of neutrophils in some organs can persist for several hours and is not always followed by the cells' emigration from the microvasculature.

At sites of injury or infection, neutrophils and other granulocytes enter the connective tissues by migrating through intercellular junctions between endothelial cells of postcapillary venules in diapedesis. Inflamed connective tissues thus form a fifth terminal compartment for neutrophils, where the cells reside for a few days and then die by apoptosis, regardless of whether they have performed their major function of phagocytosis.

FIGURE **13–8** Granulopoiesis: Formation of granules.

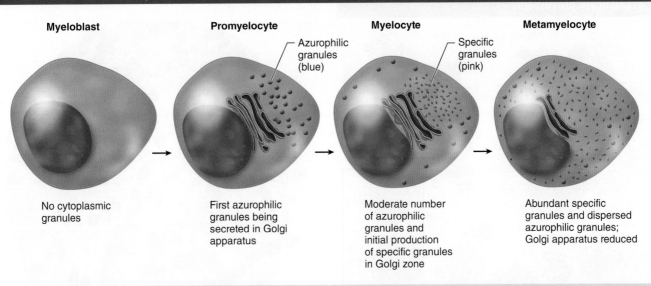

Myeloblast

No cytoplasmic granules

Promyelocyte

Azurophilic granules (blue)

First azurophilic granules being secreted in Golgi apparatus

Myelocyte

Specific granules (pink)

Moderate number of azurophilic granules and initial production of specific granules in Golgi zone

Metamyelocyte

Abundant specific granules and dispersed azurophilic granules; Golgi apparatus reduced

Illustrated is the sequence of cytoplasmic events in the maturation of granulocytes from **myeloblasts**. Modified lysosomes or azurophilic granules form first at the **promyelocyte** stage and are shown in blue; the specific granules of the particular cell type form at the **myelocyte** stage and are shown in pink. All granules are fully dispersed at the **metamyelocyte** stage, when indentation of the nucleus begins.

FIGURE **13–9** Developing erythrocytes and granulocytes in marrow.

Granulopoiesis

Erythropoiesis

Precursor cells of different hemopoietic lineages develop side by side with some intermingling as various cell islands or cords in the bone marrow. This plastic section of red bone marrow shows mitotic figures (arrows) and fairly distinct regions of **erythropoiesis** and **granulopoiesis**. Most immature granulocytes are in the myelocyte stage: their cytoplasm contains large, dark-stained azurophilic granules and small, less darkly stained specific granules. The large white areas shown peripherally are sites of fat cells. X400. Giemsa.

›› MEDICAL APPLICATION

Changes in the number of neutrophils in the blood must be evaluated by taking all their compartments into consideration. Thus, **neutrophilia**, an increase in the number of circulating neutrophils, does not necessarily imply an increase in granulopoiesis. Intense muscular activity or the administration of epinephrine can cause neutrophils in the marginating compartment to move into the circulating compartment, producing neutrophilia even though granulopoiesis has not increased. However, glucocorticoids (adrenal hormones) such as cortisone increase the mitotic activity of neutrophil precursors and this also increases the blood count of neutrophils.

Transitory neutrophilia may also result from liberation of greater numbers of neutrophils from the medullary storage compartment and is typically followed by a recovery period during which no neutrophils are released.

The neutrophilia that occurs during bacterial infections is due to an increase in production of neutrophils and a shorter duration of these cells in the medullary storage compartment. In such cases, immature forms such as band or stab cells, neutrophilic metamyelocytes, and even myelocytes may appear in the bloodstream. The neutrophilia occurring during infection is typically of much longer duration than that occurring as a result of intense muscular activity.

FIGURE **13–10** Granulopoiesis: Major granulocyte precursors.

Two micrographs from smears of bone marrow show the major cells of the neutrophilic granulocyte lineage. Typical precursor cells shown are labeled as follows: myeloblast (**MB**); promyelocyte (**1**); myelocytes (**2**); late myelocyte (**3**); metamyelocytes (**4**); band cells (**5**); nearly mature segmented neutrophils (**6**). Some of the early stages show faint nucleoli (**N**). Inset: Eosinophilic myelocytes (**EM**) and metamyelocytes (**EMm**) with their specific granules having distinctly different staining. These and cells of the basophilic lineage are similar to developing neutrophils, except for their specific staining granules and lack of the stab cell form. Also seen among the erythrocytes of these marrow smears are some orthochromatophilic erythroblasts (**Oe**), a small lymphocyte (**L**), and a cell in mitosis (arrow). All X1400. Wright.

❯ MATURATION OF AGRANULOCYTES

The precursor cells of monocytes and lymphocytes do not show specific cytoplasmic granules or nuclear lobulation, both of which facilitate the distinction of cells in the granulopoietic series. Monocytes and lymphocytes in smear preparations are discriminated mainly on the basis of size and nuclear shape.

Monocytes

The **monoblast** is a committed progenitor cell that is virtually identical to the myeloblast morphologically. Further

FIGURE **13–11** Neutrophilic myelocyte.

At the myelocyte stage lysosomes (azurophilic granules) have formed and production of specific secretory granules is under way. This micrograph shows ultrastructurally a peroxidase-stained section of a neutrophilic myelocyte with cytoplasm containing both large, peroxidase-positive azurophilic granules (**AG**) and smaller specific granules (**SG**), which do not stain for peroxidase. The peroxidase reaction product is present only in mature azurophilic granules and is not seen in the rough ER (**RER**) or Golgi cisternae (**GC**), which are located around the centriole (**C**) near the nucleus (**N**). X15,000.

(*With permission, from Dr Dorothy F. Bainton, Department of Pathology, University of California at San Francisco.*)

differentiation leads to the **promonocyte**, a large cell (up to 18 μm in diameter) with basophilic cytoplasm and a large, slightly indented nucleus (see Figures 13–2 and 12–12). The chromatin is lacy and nucleoli are evident. Promonocytes divide twice as they develop into **monocytes**. Differentiating monocytes contain extensive RER and large Golgi complexes forming lysosomes, which are observed as fine azurophilic granules at maturity. Monocytes circulate in blood for several hours and enter tissues where they mature as **macrophages** (or other phagocytic cells) and function for up to several months.

Lymphocytes

As discussed with the immune system (see Chapter 14), circulating lymphocytes originate mainly in the thymus and the

FIGURE 13–12 Compartments of neutrophils in the body.

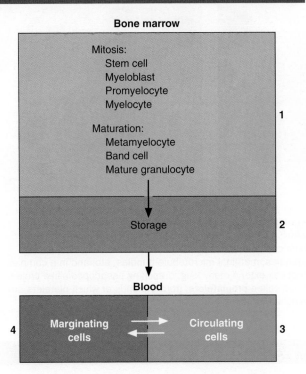

Bone marrow

Mitosis:
   Stem cell
   Myeloblast
   Promyelocyte
   Myelocyte

Maturation:
   Metamyelocyte
   Band cell
   Mature granulocyte

1

Storage   2

Blood

4   Marginating cells   Circulating cells   3

Neutrophils exist in at least four anatomically and functionally distinct compartments, whose sizes reflect the number of cells:

(1) A **granulopoietic** compartment in bone marrow with developing progenitor cells.

(2) A **storage** (reserve) compartment, also in red marrow, acts as a buffer system, capable of releasing large numbers of mature neutrophils as needed. Trillions of neutrophils typically move from marrow to the bloodstream every day.

(3) A **circulating** compartment throughout the blood.

(4) A **marginating** compartment, in which cells temporarily do not circulate but rather accumulate temporarily at the surface of the endothelium in venules and small veins.

The marginating and circulating compartments are actually of about equal size, and there is a constant interchange of cells between them, with the half-life of cells in these two compartments less than 10 hours. The granulopoietic and storage compartments together include cells in approximately the first 14 days of their existence and are about 10 times larger than the circulating and marginating compartments.

peripheral lymphoid organs (eg, spleen, lymph nodes, tonsils, etc). However, all lymphocyte progenitor cells originate in the bone marrow. Some of these lymphocytes migrate to the thymus, where they acquire the properties of T lymphocytes. Subsequently, T lymphocytes populate specific regions of peripheral lymphoid organs. Other bone marrow lymphocytes differentiate into B lymphocytes in the bone marrow and then

migrate to peripheral lymphoid organs, where they inhabit and multiply within their own niches.

The first identifiable progenitor of lymphoid cells is the **lymphoblast**, a large cell capable of dividing two or three times to form **lymphocytes** (see Figures 13–2 and 12–11). As lymphocytes develop, their nuclei become smaller, nucleoli become less visible, and the cells decrease in size overall. In the bone marrow and in the thymus, these cells synthesize the specific cell surface proteins that characterize B or T lymphocytes, respectively. Mature and functionally active B and T cells are generally larger than newly formed lymphocytes. Subsets of lymphocytes acquire distinctive cell surface and other proteins during differentiation that can be detected by immunocytochemical techniques and used to sort the specific lymphocytic types.

>> **MEDICAL APPLICATION**

Abnormal proliferation of stem cells in bone marrow can produce a range of myeloproliferative disorders. **Leukemias** are malignant clones of leukocyte precursors. They can occur in both lymphoid tissue (**lymphoblastic leukemias**) and bone marrow (**myelogenous leukemias**). In these diseases, there is usually a release of large numbers of immature cells into the blood and an overall shift in hemopoiesis, with a lack of some cell types and excessive production of others. The patient is usually anemic and prone to infection.

Diagnosis of leukemias and other bone marrow disturbances involves **bone marrow aspiration**. A needle is introduced through the compact bone, typically at the iliac crest, and a sample of marrow is withdrawn. Immunocytochemistry with labeled monoclonal antibodies specific to membrane proteins of precursor blood cells contributes to a more precise diagnosis of the leukemia.

> **ORIGIN OF PLATELETS**

The membrane-enclosed cell fragments called **platelets** or thrombocytes originate in the red bone marrow by dissociating from mature **megakaryocytes** (Gr. *megas*, big + *karyon*, nucleus, + *kytos*), which in turn differentiate from **megakaryoblasts** in a process driven by **thrombopoietin**. The megakaryoblast is 25 to 50 μm in diameter and has a large ovoid or kidney-shaped nucleus (Figure 13–13), often with several small nucleoli. Before differentiating, these cells undergo endomitosis, with repeated rounds of DNA replication not separated by cell divisions, resulting in a nucleus that is highly polyploid (ie, 64N or >30 times more DNA than in a normal diploid cell). The cytoplasm of this cell is homogeneous and highly basophilic.

Megakaryocytes are giant cells, up to 150 μm in diameter, with large, irregularly lobulated polyploid nuclei, coarse chromatin, and no visible nucleoli. Their cytoplasm contains

FIGURE **13–13** Megakaryoblast and megakaryocytes.

(a) Megakaryoblasts (**Mb**) are very large, fairly rare cells in bone marrow, with very basophilic cytoplasm. X1400. Wright. **(b)** Megakaryoblasts undergo endomitosis (DNA replication without intervening cell divisions), becoming polyploid as they differentiate into megakaryocytes (**M**). These cells are even larger but with cytoplasm that is less intensely basophilic. X1400. Wright. **(c)** Micrograph of sectioned bone marrow in which a megakaryocyte (**M**) is shown near sinusoids (**S**). X400. Giemsa. Megakaryocytes produce all the characteristic components of platelets (membrane vesicles, specific granules, marginal microtubule bundles, etc) and in a complex process extend many long, branching pseudopodia-like projections called **proplatelets**, from the ends of which platelets are pinched off almost fully formed.

numerous mitochondria, a well-developed RER, and an extensive Golgi apparatus from which arise the conspicuous specific granules of platelets (see Chapter 12). They are widely scattered in marrow, typically near sinusoidal capillaries.

To form platelets, megakaryocytes extend several long (>100 μm), wide (2-4 μm) branching processes called **proplatelets**. These cellular extensions penetrate the sinusoidal endothelium and are exposed in the circulating blood of the sinusoids (see Figure 13–5). Internally proplatelets have a framework of actin filaments and loosely bundled, mixed polarity microtubules along which membrane vesicles and specific granules are transported. A loop of microtubules forms a teardrop-shaped enlargement at the distal end of the proplatelet, and cytoplasm within these loops is pinched off to form platelets with their characteristic marginal bundles of microtubules, vesicles, and granules (see Figure 12–13b).

During proplatelet growth microtubules polymerize in both directions. Proplatelet elongation depends less on this polymerization and more on a dynein-based mechanism in which microtubules slide past one another. Mature megakaryocytes have numerous invaginations of plasma membrane ramifying throughout the cytoplasm, called **demarcation membranes** (Figure 13–14), which were formerly considered "fracture lines" or "perforations" for the release of platelets but are now thought to represent a membrane reservoir that facilitates the continuous rapid proplatelet elongation. Each megakaryocyte produces a few thousand platelets, after which the remainder of the cell shows apoptotic changes and is removed by macrophages.

FIGURE **13–14** Megakaryocyte ultrastructure.

This TEM of a megakaryocyte shows the lobulated nucleus (**N**), numerous cytoplasmic granules (**G**), and an extensive system of demarcation membranes (**D**) through the cytoplasm. The system of demarcation membranes is considered to serve as a reservoir to facilitate rapid elongation of the numerous proplatelets extending from the megakaryocyte surface. X10,000.

⟩⟩ MEDICAL APPLICATION

Some bleeding disorders result from **thrombocytopenia**, a reduction in the number of circulating platelets. One cause of thrombocytopenia is **ineffective megakaryopoiesis** resulting from deficiencies of folic acid or vitamin B$_{12}$. In different types of **thrombocytopenic purpura** (L. **purple**, the color of small spots or petechiae in the skin from poorly inhibited bleeding), platelet function is compromised, usually by autoimmune reactions.

Hemopoiesis SUMMARY OF KEY POINTS

- **Pluripotent stem cells** for blood cell formation, or **hemopoiesis**, occur in the bone marrow of children and adults.
- **Progenitor cells**, committed to forming each type of mature blood cell, proliferate and differentiate within microenvironmental niches of **stromal cells**, other cells, and ECM with specific growth factors.
- These progenitor cells are also known as **colony-forming units (CFUs)** and the growth factors are also called **colony-stimulating factors (CSFs)** or cytokines.
- **Red bone marrow** is active in hemopoiesis; **yellow bone marrow** consists mostly of adipose tissue.
- **Erythropoietic islands** or cords within marrow contain the red blood cell lineage: **proerythroblasts**, **erythroblasts** with succeeding developmental stages called **basophilic, polychromatophilic,** and **orthochromatophilic** that reflect the cytoplasmic transition from RNA-rich to hemoglobin-filled.
- At the last stage of erythropoiesis cell nuclei are extruded, producing **reticulocytes** that still contain some polyribosomes but are released into the circulation.

- **Granulopoiesis** includes **myeloblasts**, which have large nuclei and relatively little cytoplasm; **promyelocytes**, in which lysosomal **azurophilic granules** are produced; **myelocytes**, in which **specific granules** for one of the three types of granulocytes are formed; and **metamyelocytes**, in which the characteristic changes in nuclear morphology occur.
- Immature neutrophilic metamyelocytes called **band (stab) cells** are released prematurely when the compartment of circulating neutrophils is deleted during bacterial infections.
- **Monoblasts** produce **monocytes** in red marrow, but **lymphoblasts** give rise to **lymphocytes** primarily in the lymphoid tissues in processes involving acquired immunity.
- **Megakaryocytes**, large polyploid cells of red bone marrow, produce **platelets**, or **thrombocytes**, by releasing them from the ends of cytoplasmic processes called **proplatelets**.
- All these **formed elements** of blood enter the circulation by crossing the **discontinuous endothelium** of sinusoids in the red marrow.

14

The Immune System & Lymphoid Organs

The **immune system** provides defense or **immunity** against infectious agents ranging from viruses to multicellular parasites. Histologically this system consists of a large, diverse population of leukocytes located within every tissue of the body and **lymphoid organs** interconnected only by the blood and lymphatic circulation. Immunity obviously has tremendous medical importance, one part of which focuses on autoimmune diseases in which immune cells begin to function abnormally and attack molecular components of the body's own organs.

Immunologists recognize two partially overlapping lines of defense against invaders and/or other abnormal, potentially harmful cells: **innate immunity** and **adaptive immunity**. The first of these is nonspecific, involves a wide variety of effector mechanisms, and is evolutionarily older than the second type. Among the cells mediating innate immunity are most of the granulocytes and other leukocytes described in Chapters 12 and 13. Conversely, adaptive immunity aims at specific microbial invaders, is mediated by lymphocytes and **antigen-presenting cells (APCs)** discussed in this chapter, and produces memory cells that permit a similar, very rapid response if that specific microbe appears again.

The lymphocytes and APCs for adaptive immunity are distributed throughout the body in the blood, lymph, and epithelial and connective tissues. Lymphocytes are formed initially in **primary lymphoid organs** (the thymus and bone marrow), but most lymphocyte activation and proliferation occur in **secondary lymphoid organs** (the lymph nodes, the spleen, and diffuse lymphoid tissue found in the mucosa of the digestive system, including the tonsils, Peyer patches,

and appendix). The immune cells located diffusely in the digestive, respiratory, or urogenital mucosae comprise what is collectively known as **mucosa-associated lymphoid tissue (MALT)**. Proliferating B lymphocytes in the secondary structures of MALT are arranged in small spherical **lymphoid nodules**. The wide distribution of immune system cells and the constant traffic of lymphocytes through the blood, lymph, connective tissues, and secondary lymphoid structures provide the body with an elaborate and efficient system of surveillance and defense (Figure 14–1).

› INNATE & ADAPTIVE IMMUNITY

The system of defenses termed **innate immunity** involves immediate, nonspecific actions, including **physical barriers** such as the skin and mucous membranes of the gastrointestinal, respiratory, and urogenital tracts that prevent infections or penetration of the host body. Bacteria, fungi, and parasites that manage to penetrate these barriers are quickly removed by **neutrophils** and other leukocytes in the adjacent connective tissue. **Toll-like receptors (TLRs)** on leukocytes allow the recognition and binding of surface components of such invaders. Other leukocytes orchestrate the defenses at sites of penetration. **Natural killer (NK) cells** destroy various unhealthy host cells, including those infected with virus or bacteria, as well as certain potentially tumorigenic cells.

Leukocytes and specific cells of the tissue barriers also produce a wide variety of antimicrobial chemicals that

FIGURE **14–1** The lymphoid organs and main paths of lymphatic vessels.

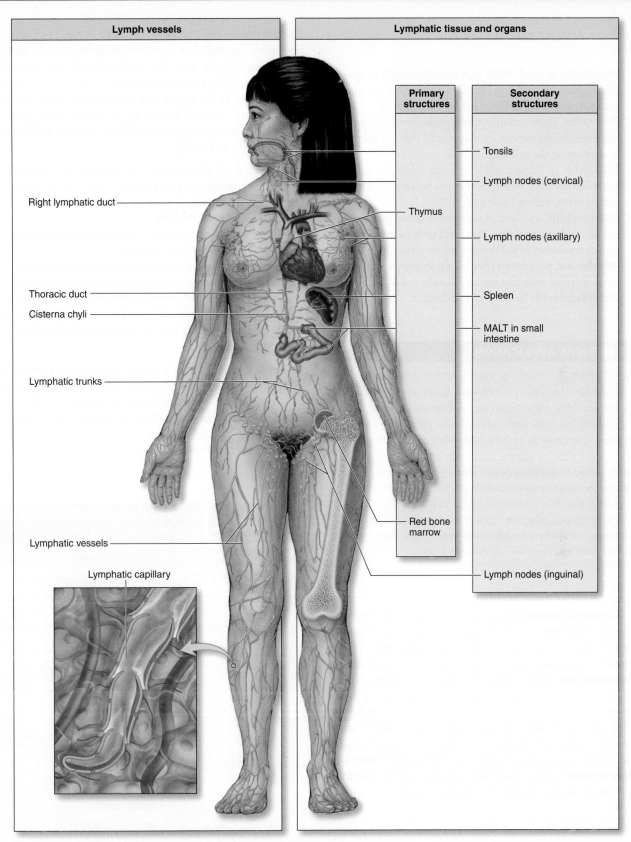

Lymph vessels	Lymphatic tissue and organs	
	Primary structures	Secondary structures

Lymph vessels

Right lymphatic duct

Thoracic duct

Cisterna chyli

Lymphatic trunks

Lymphatic vessels

Lymphatic capillary

Primary structures

Thymus

Red bone marrow

Secondary structures

Tonsils

Lymph nodes (cervical)

Lymph nodes (axillary)

Spleen

MALT in small intestine

Lymph nodes (inguinal)

The lymphatic system is composed of lymphatic vessels that transport interstitial fluid (as lymph) back to the blood circulation, and the lymphoid organs that house lymphocytes and other cells of the body's immune defense system. Primary lymphoid organs are the bone marrow and thymus, where B and T lymphocytes are formed, respectively. The secondary lymphoid organs include the lymph nodes, mucosa-associated lymphoid tissue (MALT), and spleen.

also form a major part of innate immunity, including the following:

- **Hydrochloric acid (HCl) and organic acids** in specific regions lower the pH locally to either kill entering microorganisms directly or inhibit their growth.
- **Defensins**, short cationic polypeptides produced by neutrophils and various epithelial cells that kill bacteria by disrupting the cell walls.
- **Lysozyme**, an enzyme made by neutrophils and cells of epithelial barriers, which hydrolyzes bacterial cell wall components, killing those cells.
- **Complement**, a system of proteins in blood plasma, mucus, and macrophages that react with bacterial surface components to aid removal of bacteria.
- **Interferons**, paracrine factors from leukocytes and virus-infected cells that signal NK cells to kill such cells and adjacent cells to resist viral infection.

›› MEDICAL APPLICATION

Some pathogenic bacteria, such as *Haemophilus influenzae* and *Streptococcus pneumoniae*, **avoid phagocytosis** by granulocytes and macrophages of **innate immunity** by covering their cell walls with a "capsule" of polysaccharide. The capsule inhibits recognition and binding to the phagocytes' receptors. Eventually such bacteria can be removed by antibody-based mechanisms, including phagocytosis after **opsonization**, but in the interim of several days the cells proliferate undisturbed and establish a more dangerous infection. Elderly or immunocompromised patients, with reduced **adaptive immunity**, are particularly susceptible to infections with such bacteria.

Adaptive immunity, acquired gradually by exposure to microorganisms, is more specific, slower to respond, and an evolutionarily more recent development than innate immunity. The adaptive immune response involves **B and T lymphocytes**, whose origins are described in this chapter, which become activated against specific invaders by being presented with specific molecules from those cells by **APCs**, which are usually derived from monocytes. Unlike innate immunity, adaptive immune responses are aimed at specific microbial invaders and involve production of **memory lymphocytes** so that a similar response can be mounted very rapidly if that invader ever appears again.

› CYTOKINES

Within lymphoid organs and during inflammation at sites of infection or tissue injury cells in the immune system communicate with each other primarily via **cytokines** to coordinate

defensive measures. Involved in both innate and adaptive immunity, cytokines are a diverse group of peptides and glycoproteins, usually with low molecular masses (between 8 and 80 kDa) and a paracrine mode of action. They coordinate cell activities in the innate and adaptive immune responses. Examples of several important cytokines are given in Table 14–1. Major responses induced in target cells by such factors are the following:

- Directed cell movements, or **chemotaxis**, toward and cell accumulation at sites of inflammation, for example, during diapedesis. Cytokines producing this effect are also called **chemokines**.
- Increased mitotic activity in certain leukocytes, both locally and in the bone marrow.
- Stimulation or suppression of lymphocyte activities in adaptive immunity. A group of cytokines with such effects were named **interleukins** because they were thought to be produced by and to target only leukocytes.
- Stimulated phagocytosis or directed cell killing by innate immune cells.

Most cytokines have multiple target cells in which they exert several effects. Some are produced by and target cells besides immune cells, including endothelial cells, certain autonomic neurons, and cells of the endocrine system. The broad range of cytokine actions greatly extends the physiologic effects of infections and other stressors.

TABLE **14–1**	Examples of cytokines, grouped by their main function.
Cytokine[a]	**Main Functions**
GM-CSF, M-CSF	Growth and differentiation factors for leukocyte progenitor cells in bone marrow
TNF-α, TGF-β, IL-1	Stimulation of inflammation and fever
IL-12	Stimulation of growth in T lymphocytes and NK cells
IL-2, IL-4	Growth factors for T helper cells and B lymphocytes
IL-5	Eosinophil proliferation, differentiation, and activation
Interferon-γ, IL-4	Activation of macrophages
IL-10	Inhibition of macrophages and specific adaptive immune responses
Interferon-α, interferon-β	Antiviral activity
IL-8	Chemokine for neutrophils and T lymphocytes

[a]GM-CSF, granulocyte-macrophage colony-stimulating factor; IL, interleukin; M-CSF, macrophage colony-stimulating factor; TGF, transforming growth factor; TNF, tumor necrosis factor.

› ANTIGENS & ANTIBODIES

A molecule that is recognized by cells of the adaptive immune system is called an **antigen** and typically elicits a response from these cells. Antigens may consist of soluble molecules (such as proteins or polysaccharides) or molecules that are still components of intact cells (bacteria, protozoa, or tumor cells). Immune cells recognize and react to small molecular domains of the antigen known as antigenic determinants or **epitopes**. The immune response to antigens may be cellular (in which lymphocytes are primarily in charge of eliminating the antigen), humoral (in which antibodies are primarily responsible for the response), or both.

An **antibody** is a glycoprotein of the **immunoglobulin** family that interacts specifically with an antigenic determinant. Antibodies are secreted by plasma cells that arise by terminal differentiation of clonally proliferating B lymphocytes whose receptors recognize and bind specific epitopes. Antibodies either accumulate in the blood plasma and interstitial fluid of tissues or are transported across epithelia into the secretion of glands such as mucous, salivary, and mammary glands. Other antibodies are membrane proteins on the surface of B lymphocytes or other leukocytes. In all these situations each antibody combines with the epitope that it specifically recognizes.

Immunoglobulins of all antibody molecules have a common design, consisting of two identical light chains and two identical heavy chains bound by disulfide bonds (Figure 14–2). The isolated carboxyl-terminal portion of the heavy-chain molecules is called the constant **Fc region**. The Fc regions of some immunoglobulins are recognized by cell surface receptors on basophils and mast cells, localizing these antibodies to the surface of these cells. The first 110 amino acids near the amino-terminal ends of the light and heavy chains vary widely among different antibody molecules, and this region is called the **variable region**. The variable portions of one heavy and one light chain make up an antibody's **antigen-binding site**. DNA sequences coding for these regions undergo recombination and rearrangement after B lymphocytes are activated against a specific antigen and the progeny of those cells all produce antibodies that specifically bind that antigen. Each antibody has two antigen-binding sites, both for the same antigen.

Classes of Antibodies

Immunoglobulins of humans fall into five major classes, listed in Table 14–2 with their structural features, abundance in plasma, major locations, and functions. The classes are called **immunoglobulin G (IgG)**, **IgA**, **IgM**, **IgE**, and **IgD**, and key aspects for each include the following:

- **IgG** is the most abundant class representing 75% to 85% of the immunoglobulin in blood. Production increases during immune responses following infections, etc. Unlike the other classes of antibodies, IgG is highly soluble, stable (half-life >3 weeks), and crosses the placental barrier into the fetal circulation. This confers **passive immunity** against certain infections until the newborn's own adaptive immune system is acquired.

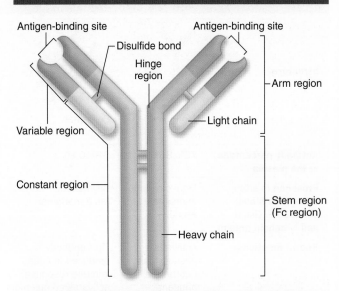

FIGURE 14–2 Basic structure of an immunoglobulin (antibody).

Antigen-binding site
Antigen-binding site
Disulfide bond
Hinge region
Arm region
Light chain
Variable region
Constant region
Stem region (Fc region)
Heavy chain

Two light chains and two heavy chains form an **antibody** molecule ("monomer"). The chains are linked by disulfide bonds. The **variable portions** near the amino end of the light and heavy chains bind the antigen. The **constant region** (or Fc) of the molecule may bind to surface receptors of several cell types.

- **IgA** is present in almost all exocrine secretions as a dimeric form in which the heavy chains of two monomers are united by a polypeptide called the **J chain**. IgA is produced by plasma cells in mucosae of the digestive, respiratory, and reproductive tracts. Another protein bound to this immunoglobulin, the **secretory component**, is released by the epithelial cells as IgA undergoes transcytosis. The resulting structure is relatively resistant to proteolysis and reacts with microorganisms in milk, saliva, tears, and mucus coating the mucosae in which it is made.

- **IgM** constitutes 5% to 10% of blood immunoglobulin and usually exits in a pentameric form united by a J chain. IgM is mainly produced in an initial response to an antigen. IgM bound to antigen is the most effective antibody class in activating the complement system.

- **IgE**, usually a monomer, is much less abundant in the circulation and exists bound at its Fc region to receptors on the surface of mast cells and basophils. When this IgE encounters the antigen that elicited its production, the antigen-antibody complex triggers the liberation of several biologically active substances, such as histamine, heparin, and leukotrienes. This characterizes an **allergic reaction**, which is thus mediated by the binding of cell-bound IgE with the antigens (**allergens**) that stimulated the IgE to be synthesized initially (see Mast Cells in Chapter 5).

TABLE **14–2**	Important features of the antibody classes in humans.				
	IgG	**IgM**	**IgA**	**IgD**	**IgE**
Structure	Monomer	Pentamer	secretory component Dimer with J chain and secretory component	Monomer	Monomer
Antibody percentage in the plasma	75%-85%	5%-10%	10%-15%	0.001%	0.002%
Presence in sites other than blood, connective tissue, and lymphoid organs	Fetal circulation in pregnant women	B lymphocyte surface (as a monomer)	Secretions (saliva, milk, tears, etc)	Surface of B lymphocytes	Bound to the surface of mast cells and basophils
Known functions	Activates phagocytosis, neutralizes antigens	First antibody produced in initial immune response; activates complement	Protects mucosae	Antigen receptor triggering initial B cell activation	Destroys parasitic worms and participates in allergies

■ **IgD**, the least abundant immunoglobulin in plasma, is also the least understood class of antibody. Monomers of IgD are bound to the surface of B lymphocytes where they (along with IgM monomers) act as antigen receptors in triggering B-cell activation.

Actions of Antibodies

As shown in Figure 14–3a, antigen-binding sites of IgG and IgA antibodies are able to bind specifically and **neutralize** certain viral particles and bacterial toxins, **agglutinate** many bacterial cells, and **precipitate** most soluble antigens. In addition, the Fc portions of these and other antibodies also bind receptors for this sequence and thereby optimize three important actions of innate immunity (Figure 14–3b):

■ **Complement activation:** Antigen-antibody complexes containing IgG or IgM bind polypeptides of the **complement system**, a group of around 20 plasma proteins produced mainly in the liver, and activate them through a cascade of enzymatic reactions. After activation, specific complement components bind and rupture membranes of invading cells, clump antigen-bearing bacteria or cells, and elicit arrival of relevant leukocytes.

■ **Opsonization:** This refers to the ability of receptors on macrophages, neutrophils, and eosinophils to recognize and bind the Fc portions of antibodies attached to surface antigens of microorganisms. Opsonization greatly increases the efficiency of **phagocytosis** by these leukocytes at sites of infection.

■ **NK cells activation:** Antibodies bound to antigens on virus-infected cells of the body are recognized by the primitive lymphocytes called **NK cells**, which are then activated to kill the infected cell by releasing **perforin** and various **granzymes**. These two proteins together enter the infected cell via other receptors and cause apoptosis.

❯ ANTIGEN PRESENTATION

Antigens recognized by lymphocytes are often bound to specialized integral membrane protein complexes on cell surfaces. These abundant antigen-presenting proteins are parts of the **major histocompatibility complex (MHC)** that includes the two key types called MHC class I and class II. As the name implies, these proteins were first recognized by their roles in the immune rejection of grafted tissue or organs. Proteins of both classes, which on human cells are often called human leukocyte antigens (HLAs), are encoded by genes in large chromosomal loci having very high degrees of allelic variation between different individuals. T lymphocytes are specialized to recognize both classes of MHC proteins and the antigens they present. If the MHCs on cells of a tissue graft are not similar to those that T lymphocytes encountered during their development, the grafted cells will induce a strong immune reaction by T cells of the recipient. To these lymphocytes, the unfamiliar MHC epitopes on the graft's cells are recognized as markers of potentially tumorigenic, infected, or otherwise abnormal ("non-self") cells that they must eliminate.

Like all integral membrane protein complexes, MHC molecules are made in the rough ER and Golgi apparatus. Before leaving the ER, **MHC class I** proteins bind a wide variety of proteasome-derived peptide fragments representing the range of all proteins synthesized in that cell. All nucleated cells

FIGURE 14–3 Various specific and nonspecific functions of antibodies.

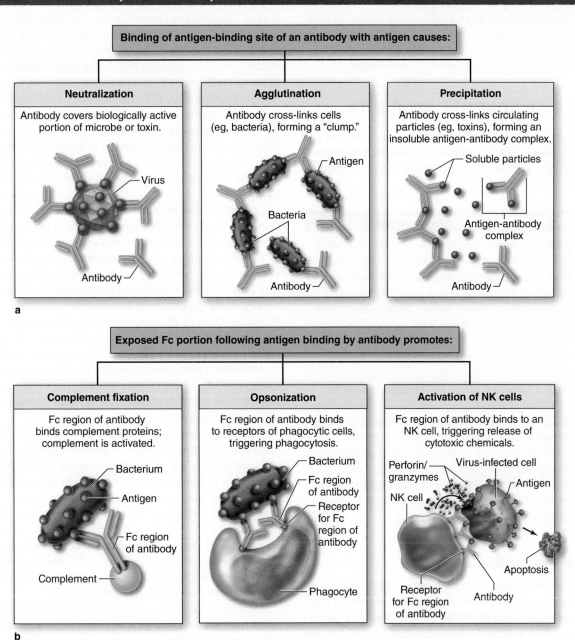

Binding of antigen-binding site of an antibody with antigen causes:

Neutralization

Antibody covers biologically active portion of microbe or toxin.

Virus

Antibody

a

Agglutination

Antibody cross-links cells (eg, bacteria), forming a "clump."

Antigen

Bacteria

Antibody

Precipitation

Antibody cross-links circulating particles (eg, toxins), forming an insoluble antigen-antibody complex.

Soluble particles

Antigen-antibody complex

Antibody

Exposed Fc portion following antigen binding by antibody promotes:

Complement fixation

Fc region of antibody binds complement proteins; complement is activated.

Bacterium

Antigen

Fc region of antibody

Complement

b

Opsonization

Fc region of antibody binds to receptors of phagocytic cells, triggering phagocytosis.

Bacterium

Fc region of antibody

Receptor for Fc region of antibody

Phagocyte

Activation of NK cells

Fc region of antibody binds to an NK cell, triggering release of cytotoxic chemicals.

Perforin/ granzymes

Virus-infected cell

NK cell

Antigen

Apoptosis

Receptor for Fc region of antibody

Antibody

Shown here are important mechanisms by which the most common antibodies act in immunity. **(a)** Specific binding of antigens can **neutralize** or **precipitate** antigens, or cause microorganisms bearing the antigens to clump (**agglutinate**) for easier removal.

(b) Complement proteins and surface receptors on many leukocytes bind the Fc portions of antibodies attached to cell-surface antigens, producing **active complement**, more efficient phagocytosis (**opsonization**), and **NK-cell activation**.

produce and expose on their surfaces MHC class I molecules presenting such "self-antigens," which T cells recognize as a signal to ignore those cells. By this same mechanism, some virally infected cells or cells with proteins altered by gene mutation also have MHC class I proteins displaying peptides that T cells do *not* recognize as "self," helping lead to the elimination of such cells.

MHC class II proteins are synthesized and transported to the cell surface similarly but only in cells of the mononuclear phagocyte system and certain other cells under some conditions. Before joining the plasmalemma, the Golgi-derived vesicles with the MHC class II complexes first fuse with endolysosomal vesicles containing antigens ingested by receptor-mediated endocytosis, pinocytosis, or phagocytosis. This allows the class II proteins to bind fragments of whatever proteins the cells had ingested, including those from dead, infected, or abnormal cells and atypical proteins of all kinds. At the surface of these cells, the class II complexes display the peptides from these potentially pathogenic cells, signaling T lymphocytes and activating their responses against sources of these antigens.

› CELLS OF ADAPTIVE IMMUNITY

Described in Chapter 12 with blood, lymphocytes and the monocyte-derived cells specialized for antigen presentation to lymphocytes are the major players in adaptive immune responses.

> ### ›› MEDICAL APPLICATION
>
> Tissue grafts and organ transplants are classified as **autografts** when the donor and the host are the same individual, such as a burn patient for whom skin is moved from an undamaged to the damaged body region; **isografts** are those involving identical twins. Neither of these graft types is immunologically rejected. **Homografts** (or **allografts**), which involve two related or unrelated individuals, consist of cells with MHC class I molecules and contain dendritic cells with MHC class II molecules, all presenting peptides that the host's T cells recognize as "foreign," leading to immune rejection of the graft.
>
> Development of **immunosuppressive drugs** such as the **cyclosporins** that inhibit the activation of cytotoxic T cells has allowed the more widespread use of allografts or even **xenografts** taken from an animal donor if allografts are in short supply. Such immunosuppression can however lead to other immune-related problems, such as certain opportunistic infections or cancers.

Antigen-Presenting Cells

Most specialized antigen-presenting cells (APCs) are part of the mononuclear phagocyte system, including all types of macrophages and specialized **dendritic cells** in lymphoid organs. Features common to all APCs are an active endocytotic system and expression of MHC class II molecules for presenting peptides of exogenous antigens. Besides dendritic cells (not to be confused with cells of nervous tissue) and all monocyte-derived cells, "professional" APCs include the epithelial reticular cells of the thymus (discussed below) and B lymphocytes.

During inflammation transient expression of MHC class II is induced by interferon-γ in certain local cells that can be considered "nonprofessional" APCs, including fibroblasts and vascular endothelial cells.

Lymphocytes

Lymphocytes both regulate and carry out adaptive immunity. In adults stem cells for all lymphocytes are located in the red bone marrow, but cells of the major lymphoid lineages mature and become functional in two different central or **primary lymphoid organs**. Cells destined to become B lymphocytes remain and differentiate further in the **bone marrow**. Progenitors of T lymphocytes move via the circulation into the developing **thymus**. After maturation in these primary structures, B and T cells circulate to the peripheral **secondary lymphoid organs**, which include the **MALT**, the **lymph nodes**, and the **spleen** (see Figure 14–1). Lymphocytes do not stay long in the lymphoid organs; they continuously recirculate through the body in connective tissues, blood, and lymph. Because of the constant mobility of lymphocytes and APCs, the cellular locations and microscopic details of lymphoid organs differ from one day to the next. However, the relative percentages of T and B lymphocytes in these compartments are relatively steady (Table 14–3).

Lymphoid tissue is usually reticular connective tissue filled with large numbers of lymphocytes. It can be either diffuse within areas of loose connective tissue or surrounded by capsules, forming discrete (secondary) lymphoid organs. Because lymphocytes have prominent basophilic nuclei and very little cytoplasm, lymphoid tissue packed with such cells usually stains dark blue in hematoxylin and eosin (H&E)–stained sections. In all secondary lymphoid tissue the lymphocytes are supported by a rich reticulin fiber network of type III collagen (Figure 14–4a). The fibers are produced by fibroblastic **reticular cells**, which extend numerous processes along and around the fibers (Figure 14–4b). Besides lymphocytes and reticular cells, lymphoid tissue typically contains various APCs and plasma cells.

Although most lymphocytes are morphologically indistinguishable in either the light or electron microscope, various surface proteins ("cluster of differentiation" or **CD markers**) allow them to be distinguished as B cells and subcategories of T cells by immunocytochemical methods. Key features of B and T lymphocytes also include the surface receptors involved in activating their different responses to antigens (Figure 14–5). Receptors of B cells are immunoglobulins that bind antigens directly; those on T cells react only with antigen on MHC molecules and this requires the additional cell surface proteins CD4 or CD8.

Lymphocytes in the marrow and thymus of a newborn infant not yet exposed to antigens are immunocompetent but naive and unable to recognize antigens. After circulating to the various secondary lymphoid structures, lymphocytes are exposed to antigens on APCs and become activated,

TABLE **14–3**	Approximate percentages of B and T cells in lymphoid organs.	
Lymphoid Organ	**T Lymphocytes (%)**	**B Lymphocytes (%)**
Thymus	100	0
Bone marrow	10	90
Spleen	45	55
Lymph nodes	60	40
Blood	70	30

FIGURE **14–4** Reticular fibers and cells of lymphoid tissue.

(a) A three-dimensional framework of reticular fibers (collagen type III) supports the cells of most lymphoid tissues and organs (except the thymus). Areas with larger spaces between the fibers offer more mobility to cells than areas in which the fiber meshwork is denser, such as in trabeculae (**T**) where fewer lymphocytes are aggregated and cells are generally more stationary. X140. Silver impregnation.

(b) Cells of typical lymphoid tissue include the fibroblast-like reticular cells (**R**) that produce and maintain the trabeculae (**T**) and reticulin framework. Many cells are loosely attached to the reticulin fibers, including macrophages (**M**) and many lymphocytes. X240. H&E.

(With permission, from Dr Paulo A. Abrahamsohn, Institute of Biomedical Sciences, University of São Paulo, Brazil.)

FIGURE **14–5** Specific receptors on T and B lymphocytes.

(a) All T lymphocytes have cell surface protein receptors (TCRs) with variable regions that recognize specific antigens. Cell activation requires **costimulation** by the **TCR** and either

CD4 or CD8, which characterize helper and cytotoxic T cells, respectively. **(b)** B-cell receptors (BCRs) are **immunoglobulin** molecules projecting from the plasmalemma.

FIGURE 14–6 Activation of lymphocytes.

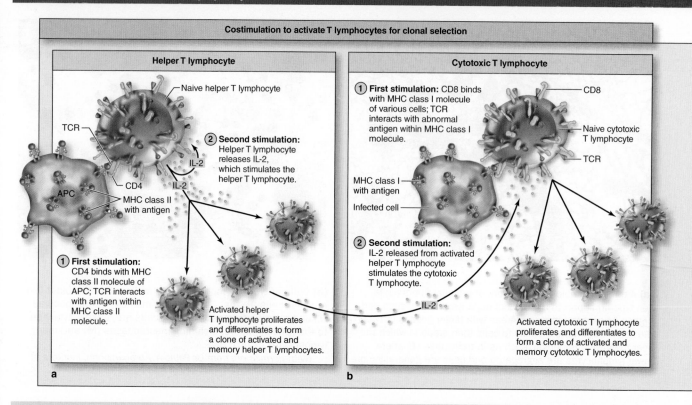

Costimulation to activate T lymphocytes for clonal selection

Helper T lymphocyte

Naive helper T lymphocyte

TCR

② **Second stimulation:** Helper T lymphocyte releases IL-2, which stimulates the helper T lymphocyte.

IL-2

CD4

IL-2

APC

MHC class II with antigen

① **First stimulation:** CD4 binds with MHC class II molecule of APC; TCR interacts with antigen within MHC class II molecule.

Activated helper T lymphocyte proliferates and differentiates to form a clone of activated and memory helper T lymphocytes.

a

Cytotoxic T lymphocyte

① **First stimulation:** CD8 binds with MHC class I molecule of various cells; TCR interacts with abnormal antigen within MHC class I molecule.

CD8

Naive cytotoxic T lymphocyte

TCR

MHC class I with antigen

Infected cell

② **Second stimulation:** IL-2 released from activated helper T lymphocyte stimulates the cytotoxic T lymphocyte.

IL-2

Activated cytotoxic T lymphocyte proliferates and differentiates to form a clone of activated and memory cytotoxic T lymphocytes.

b

Lymphocyte activation requires costimulation of at least two receptors and causes cell proliferation that produces many effector cells and a smaller population of memory cells.
(a) The TCR and CD4 proteins of a **helper T cell** bind antigens presented on MHC class II molecules and with interleukin-2 (IL-2) stimulation, the lymphocyte is activated and proliferates.
(b) Cytotoxic T lymphocytes, or CTLs, recognize and bind abnormal peptides on MHC class I molecules, and triggered by IL-2 from helper T cells the CTLs proliferate.

proliferating to produce a clone of lymphocytes all able to recognize that antigen.

T Lymphocytes

T cells are long-lived lymphocytes and constitute nearly 75% of the circulating lymphocytes. They recognize antigenic epitopes via surface protein complexes termed **T-cell receptors (TCRs)**. Most TCRs include two glycoproteins called the α and β **chains,** each with variable regions produced similarly to those of immunoglobulins. Because TCRs only recognize antigenic peptides when presented as part of MHC molecules (interacting with both the MHC and the peptide it presents), T lymphocytes are said to be **MHC restricted**.

Several types of T lymphocytes exist, with various functions. Important subpopulations of T cells include the following:

▪ **Helper T cells** (Th cells) are characterized by **CD4,** the coreceptor with the TCR for binding MHC class II molecules and the peptides they are presenting (Figure 14–6a). Activated by such binding, helper T cells greatly assist immune responses by producing cytokines

that promote differentiation of B cells into plasma cells, activate macrophages to become phagocytic, activate cytotoxic T lymphocytes (CTLs), and induce many parts of an inflammatory reaction. Some specifically activated helper T cells persist as long-lived memory helper T cells, which allow a more rapid response if the antigen appears again later.

▪ **CTLs** are **CD8**[+]. Their TCRs together with CD8 coreceptors bind specific antigens on foreign cells or virus-infected cells displayed by MHC class I molecules (Figure 14–6b). In the presence of interleukin-2 (IL-2) from helper T cells, cytotoxic T cells that have recognized such antigens are activated and proliferate. Also called killer T cells, they attach to the cell sources of the antigens and remove them by releasing perforins and granzymes, which trigger apoptosis. This represents **cell-mediated immunity** and its mechanism is largely similar to that of NK cells. Activation of cytotoxic T cells also results in a population of memory cytotoxic T cells.

▪ **Regulatory T cells** (T$_{regs}$ or suppressor T cells) are CD4$^+$CD25$^+$ and serve to inhibit specific immune

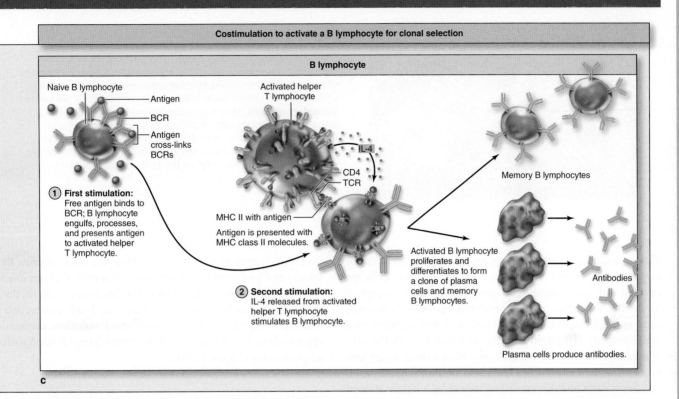

Costimulation to activate a B lymphocyte for clonal selection

B lymphocyte

Naive B lymphocyte

— Antigen
— BCR
— Antigen cross-links BCRs

Activated helper T lymphocyte

IL-4

CD4
TCR

MHC II with antigen —

Antigen is presented with MHC class II molecules.

Memory B lymphocytes

Antibodies

Plasma cells produce antibodies.

① First stimulation: Free antigen binds to BCR; B lymphocyte engulfs, processes, and presents antigen to activated helper T lymphocyte.

② Second stimulation: IL-4 released from activated helper T lymphocyte stimulates B lymphocyte.

Activated B lymphocyte proliferates and differentiates to form a clone of plasma cells and memory B lymphocytes.

c

(c) Antigen bound to the immunoglobulin receptors on B cells (BCRs) is endocytosed, processed, and presented on MCH class II proteins to helper T cells. These then secrete IL-4 and other cytokines that stimulate gene recombination and clonal proliferation of these specific B cells. They differentiate as **plasma cells** producing antibodies against the antigen that was originally bound and processed.

responses. These cells, also identified by the presence of the Foxp3 transcription factor, play crucial roles in allowing immune tolerance, maintaining unresponsiveness to self-antigens and suppressing excessive immune responses. These cells produce **peripheral tolerance**, which acts to supplement the central tolerance that develops in the thymus.

- γδ **T lymphocytes** represent a smaller subpopulation whose TCRs contain γ (gamma) and δ (delta) chains instead of α and β chains. The γδ T cells migrate to the epidermis and mucosal epithelia, becoming largely intraepithelial, and do not recirculate to secondary lymphoid organs. They function in many ways like cells of innate immunity, in the front lines against invading microorganisms.

B Lymphocytes

In B lymphocytes the surface receptors for antigens are monomers of IgM or IgD, with each B cell covered by about 150,000 such **B-cell receptors (BCRs)** (Figure 4–5b). BCRs bind an antigen, which may be free in solution, on an exposed part of an infectious agent, or already bound to antibodies, and the surface complexes then undergo endocytosis. Degraded in endosomes, peptides from the antigens are presented on MHC class II molecules of the B cell. A helper T cell then binds this B cell and activates it further with a cytokine, inducing recombination in the immunoglobulin genes and stimulating several cycles of cell proliferation (see Figure 14–6c).

In all secondary lymphoid tissues B lymphocytes interact with scattered **follicular dendritic cells (FDCs)**, which have long filamentous processes. Unlike other dendritic cells,

FIGURE 14–7 Lymphoid nodules (or follicles).

Large aggregates of B cells called lymphoid nodules or follicles transiently characterize all secondary lymphoid organs. Aggregates of uniform cell density and staining represent **primary nodules**, while those with larger, more euchromatic cells centrally are termed **secondary nodules**. Here two secondary nodules can be seen, with germinal centers (**GC**) at different stages of development. Rapid proliferation of activated B lymphoblasts in the germinal center causes smaller, naive lymphocytes to be pushed aside and crowded together peripherally as the follicular mantle (**M**).

FDCs are mesenchymal in origin and their function does not involve MHC class II molecules. Surfaces of these cells are covered with antibody-antigen complexes bound to receptors for complement proteins and for immunoglobulin Fc regions, causing B cells to attach, become activated, and aggregate as a small **primary lymphoid nodule** (or follicle). With the help of adjacent Th cells, these B cells now form a much larger and more prominent **secondary lymphoid nodule** (Figure 14–7).

Secondary nodules are characterized by a lightly stained **germinal center** filled with large lymphoblasts (or centroblasts) undergoing immunoglobulin gene recombination, rapid proliferation, and quality control. Growth of activated B cells in germinal centers is exuberate and very rapid, causing naive, nonproliferating B cells to be pushed aside and produce the more darkly stained peripheral **mantle** (Figure 14–7). After 2 to 3 weeks of proliferation, most cells of the germinal center and mantle are dispersed and the structure of the secondary lymphoid nodule is gradually lost.

Most of these new, specific B lymphocytes differentiate into **plasma cells** secreting antibodies that will bind the same epitope recognized by the activated B cell. Because the antibodies specified by B cells circulate in lymph and blood throughout the body, B cells are said to provide **humoral immunity**. As with activated T cells, some of the newly formed B cells remain as long-lived **memory B cells**. Formation of long-lived memory lymphocytes is a key feature of adaptive immunity, which allows a very rapid response upon subsequent exposure to the same antigen.

› THYMUS

While immature B lymphocytes emerge from the bone marrow, the primary or central lymphoid organ in which T cells are produced is the **thymus**, a bilobed structure in the mediastinum (Figure 14-8). A main function of the thymus is induction of **central tolerance**, which along with regulatory T cells prevents autoimmunity. The organ originates from the embryo's third pair of pharyngeal pouches (endoderm), with precursor lymphoblasts circulating from the bone marrow to invade and proliferate in this unique thymic epithelium during its development. Fully formed and functional at birth, the thymus remains large and very active in T-cell production until puberty, during which it undergoes **involution**, decreasing greatly in size and activity and becoming largely filled with adipose tissue (Figure 14–8).

>> **MEDICAL APPLICATION**

Failure of the third (and fourth) pharyngeal pouches to develop normally in the embryo leads to **DiGeorge syndrome**, characterized by **thymic hypoplasia** (or aplasia). Lacking many or all thymic epithelial cells, such individuals cannot produce T lymphocytes properly and have severely depressed cell-mediated immunity.

The thymus has a vascularized connective tissue capsule that extends septa into the parenchyma, dividing the organ into many incompletely separated lobules. Each lobule has an outer darkly basophilic **cortex** surrounding a more lightly stained **medulla**. The staining differences reflect the much greater density of lymphoblasts and small lymphocytes in the cortex than the medulla (Figure 14–8b).

The thymic cortex contains an extensive population of T lymphoblasts (or **thymocytes**), some newly arrived via venules, located among numerous macrophages and associated with the unique **thymic epithelial cells** (**TECs**) that have certain features of both epithelial and reticular cells. These cells usually have large euchromatic nuclei but are morphologically and functionally diverse. There are three major types of TECs in the cortex of the thymus:

- Squamous TECs form a layer, joined by desmosomes and occluding junctions, line the connective tissue of the capsule and septa and surround the microvasculature. This creates an isolated cortical compartment and, together with the vascular endothelial cells and pericytes,

FIGURE **14–8** Thymus.

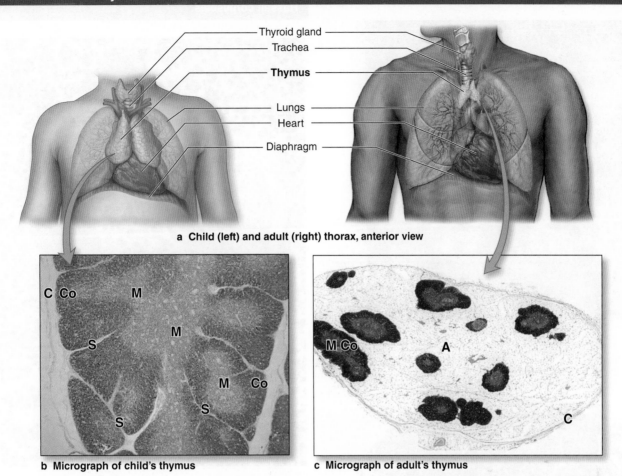

a Child (left) and adult (right) thorax, anterior view

- Thyroid gland
- Trachea
- **Thymus**
- Lungs
- Heart
- Diaphragm

b Micrograph of child's thymus

c Micrograph of adult's thymus

(a) The thymus is a bilobed organ in the mediastinum that is most active and prominent before puberty and undergoes involution with less activity in the adult. **(b)** A child's thymus, showing connective of the capsule (**C**) and septa (**S**) between thymic lobules, each having an outer cortex (**Co**) and incompletely separated medulla (**M**) of lymphoid tissue. H&E, X40. **(c)** After involution the thymus shows only small regions of lymphoid tissue, here still with cortex (**Co**) and medulla (**M**), and these are embedded in adipose tissue (**A**). H&E, X24.

forms a **blood-thymus barrier** preventing unregulated exposure of thymocytes to antigens.

- Throughout this compartment another population of stellate TECs, with processes containing keratin tonofilaments joined by desmosomes, form a **cytoreticulum** to which macrophages and developing lymphocytes attach instead of to reticulin fibers (Figure 14–9). Importantly, these cells are APCs, expressing MHC class II molecules in addition to MHC class I. They also secrete numerous cytokines for T-cell development and other immune functions, justifying this organ's inclusion among endocrine glands.
- Other squamous cortical TECs also express MHC class II molecules but form a sheetlike structure contributing to a functional **corticomedullary barrier** between these two regions of each lobule.

The more lightly stained thymic medulla contains fewer and larger, more mature lymphocytes. Three related types of medullary TECs form the following:

- A second layer of the boundary between cortex and medulla.
- A cytoreticulum that (1) supports less densely packed T lymphocytes, dendritic cells, and macrophages, and (2) expresses many specialized proteins specific to cells of other organs.
- Large aggregates of TECs, sometimes concentrically arranged, called **Hassall corpuscles** (Figure 14–10). Up to 100 μm in diameter, thymic corpuscles are unique to the medulla. Their cells secrete several cytokines that control activity of local dendritic cells, including factors that promote development of regulatory T cells for peripheral tolerance.

FIGURE **14–9** Cortex of the thymus.

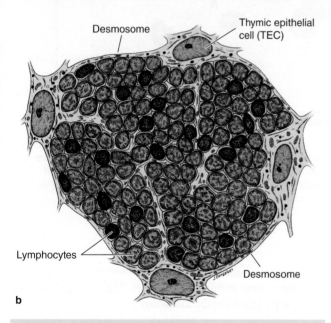

Desmosome

Thymic epithelial cell (TEC)

Lymphocytes

Desmosome

b

(a) The cortical zone of an active thymus is packed with small, highly basophilic lymphoblasts that proliferate as well as undergo positive and negative selection in that region. The lymphoblasts are supported on a meshwork (or cytoreticulum) of unusual thymic epithelial cells (**E**). X400. PT.

(b) The epithelial reticular cells throughout the cortex are APCs and extend long processes bound together by desmosomes to make the framework, the cytoreticulum, for the lymphocytes, having a cytoreticulum consisting of APC cellular processes. rather than the more common network of simple reticulin fibers, allows regulated specificity of lymphocyte binding via the changing antigens on MHC proteins. Some cortical epithelial cells also secrete cytokines that promote T-cell maturation.

FIGURE **14–10** Medulla of the thymus with Hassall corpuscles.

The thymic medulla contains fewer lymphocytes than the cortex, and the epithelial cells (**E**) located here have different morphology and function. The most characteristic feature of the medulla in humans is the presence of thymic (Hassall) corpuscles (**H**). These are of variable size and contain aggregates of thymic epithelial cells releasing many cytokines important within the medullary microenvironment, especially for dendritic cell activity and for the differentiation of regulatory T cells. Dendritic cells on the medulla are difficult to discern without special staining. X200. H&E.

The microvasculature of the medulla is not surrounded by a tight layer of TECs, and mature T lymphocytes exit the thymus by passing through the walls of venules and efferent lymphatics in this region.

Role of the Thymus in T-Cell Maturation & Selection

The thymus is the site of T-lymphocyte differentiation and the selective removal of T cells reactive against self-antigens, a key part of inducing central self-tolerance.

T lymphoblasts arriving in the thymus do not yet express CD4, CD8, or a TCR. These cells populate the cortex and begin

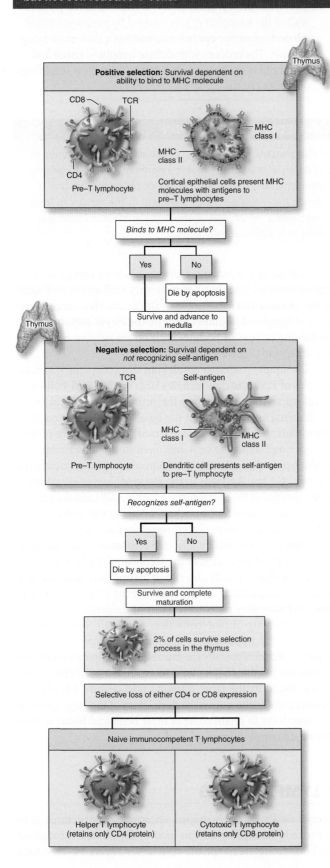

FIGURE **14–11** Thymic selection of functional but not self-reactive T cells.

Positive selection: Survival dependent on ability to bind to MHC molecule

CD8 TCR

MHC class I

MHC class II

CD4

Pre–T lymphocyte

Cortical epithelial cells present MHC molecules with antigens to pre–T lymphocytes

Thymus

Binds to MHC molecule?

Yes No

Die by apoptosis

Survive and advance to medulla

Thymus

Negative selection: Survival dependent on *not* recognizing self-antigen

TCR Self-antigen

MHC class I

MHC class II

Pre–T lymphocyte

Dendritic cell presents self-antigen to pre–T lymphocyte

Recognizes self-antigen?

Yes No

Die by apoptosis

Survive and complete maturation

2% of cells survive selection process in the thymus

Selective loss of either CD4 or CD8 expression

Naive immunocompetent T lymphocytes

Helper T lymphocyte (retains only CD4 protein)

Cytotoxic T lymphocyte (retains only CD8 protein)

to proliferate, recombine variable regions of the TCR α and β chain genes, and then express these TCR proteins as well as both CD4 and CD8. With these key functional components in place, thymocytes begin a stringent, **two-stage selection process** of quality control, which ensures that mature T cells have TCRs that are fully functional but do not recognize and strongly bind MHC with self-antigens. The selection process for each pre–T lymphocyte begins in the cortex, ends in the medulla, and lasts about 2 weeks. Key events are summarized in Figure 14–11, and a simplified account of how the process is currently understood is presented here.

TECs in the cytoreticulum of the cortex present the developing thymocytes with peptides on both MHC class I and class II proteins, which are important for development of CD8+ and CD4+ T cells, respectively. This interaction determines whether the newly made TCR proteins of these cells are functional. The cells are examined by **positive selection**, with a cell's survival depending on whether its TCRs can recognize and bind antigens on the MHC molecules properly. If the cell cannot pass this test, due, for example, to faulty gene recombination and expression of α and β chains, they are nonfunctional and completely useless. Such cells (as many as 80% of the total) undergo apoptosis and are removed by the macrophages. T cells with normal binding to antigens on either MHC class I or class II are positively selected and move to the medullary compartment (Figure 14–11).

In the medulla T cells with functional TCRs encounter antigens presented on both cytoreticular TECs and dendritic cells. Here the focus is on removing T cells whose TCRs strongly bind self-antigens, a process called **negative selection** because survival depends on a cell *not* binding to MHC molecules with such peptides (Figure 14–11). Among the peptides presented in this compartment are those from proteins specific for many tissues other than the thymus. This occurs because medullary thymic epithelial cells express high levels of the gene *Aire* (*autoimmune regulator*), whose product promotes expression of a multitude of such **tissue-specific antigens** in these cells. Most of these proteins are transferred to neighboring dendritic cells, which play the major role in presenting them to developing thymocytes.

T cells that strongly bind MHCs containing these self-peptides undergo apoptosis, which is important because release of any such cells from the thymus would lead to a damaging autoimmune response. Only about 2% of all developing T lymphocytes pass both the positive and negative selection

Positive selection occurs in the cortex and allows survival only of T cells with functional TCRs that recognize MHC class I and class II molecules. **Negative selection** occurs in the medulla and allows survival only of T cells that do *not* tightly bind self-antigens presented on dendritic cells there.

tests and survive to exit the thymus as immunocompetent T cells. Depending on which class of MHC they interacted with, most of these lymphocytes will have stopped expressing *either* CD8 or CD4, and become either helper T cells or cytotoxic T cells (Figure 14–11).

Deletion of self-reactive helper and cytotoxic T lymphocytes in the thymus is the basis for the central immunotolerance produced there. Supplementing this throughout the body is the peripheral tolerance mediated by regulatory T cells, which also develop initially in the thymic medulla under the influence of cytokines from Hassall corpuscles.

MUCOSA-ASSOCIATED LYMPHOID TISSUE

Secondary lymphoid structures, where most lymphocytes are activated by antigen presentation, include the mucosa-associated lymphoid tissue (MALT), the lymph nodes, and the spleen.

The mucosa or inner lining of the digestive, respiratory, and genitourinary tracts is a common site of invasion by pathogens because their lumens open to the external environment. To protect against such invaders mucosal connective tissue of these tracts contains large and diffuse collections of lymphocytes, IgA-secreting plasma cells, APCs, and lymphoid nodules, all of which comprise the MALT. Lymphocytes are also present within the epithelial lining of such mucosae. Most of the immune cells in MALT are dispersed diffusely in the connective tissue; others are found in aggregates that form large, conspicuous structures such as the **tonsils**, the **Peyer patches** in the ileum, and the **appendix**. Collectively the MALT is one of the largest lymphoid organs, containing up to 70% of all the body's immune cells. Most of the lymphocytes here are B cells; among T cells, CD4⁺ helper T cells predominate.

Tonsils are large, irregular masses of lymphoid tissue in the mucosa of the posterior oral cavity and nasopharynx where their cells encounter antigens entering the mouth and nose. Named by their location these masses are the **palatine**, **lingual**, and **pharyngeal tonsils** (Figure 14–12a). In all tonsils the lymphoid tissue is closely associated with the surface epithelium. Other features include the following:

- **Palatine tonsils**, located posteriorly on the soft palate, are covered by stratified squamous epithelium. The surface area of each is enlarged with 10-20 deep invaginations or **tonsillar crypts** in which the epithelial lining is densely infiltrated with lymphocytes and other leukocytes (Figure 14–12). The lymphoid tissue is filled diffusely with lymphocytes, with many secondary lymphoid nodules around the crypts. This tissue is underlain by dense connective tissue that acts as a partial capsule.
- **Lingual tonsils** are situated along the base of the tongue, are also covered by stratified squamous

epithelium with crypts, and have many of the same features as palatine tonsils but lack distinct capsules.
- The single **pharyngeal tonsil** is situated in the posterior wall of the nasopharynx, is covered by pseudostratified ciliated columnar epithelium, and has a thin underlying capsule. The mucosa with diffuse lymphoid tissue and lymphoid nodules is invaginated with shallow infoldings but lacks crypts.

> ## ❯❯ MEDICAL APPLICATION
>
> Inflammation of the tonsils, **tonsillitis**, is more common in children than adults. Chronic inflammation of the pharyngeal lymphoid tissue and tonsils of children often produces hyperplasia and enlargement of the tonsils to form "adenoids," which can obstruct the eustachian tube and lead to middle ear infections.

Diffuse MALT extends from the pharynx along the entire gastrointestinal tract but becomes very well-developed again in the mucosa and submucosa of the ileum. Here large aggregates of lymphoid nodules comprise the **Peyer patches**, each containing dozens of nodules with no underlying connective tissue capsule (Figure 14–13a).

The simple columnar epithelium that covers the lymphoid nodules of Peyer patches includes large epithelial **M cells** with apical microfolds rather than the brush border typical of the neighboring enterocytes. On the basal side M cells have large intracellular pockets that contain transient populations of lymphocytes and dendritic cells and open to the underlying lymphoid tissue through a highly porous basement membrane (Figure 14–13b). Antigens in the intestinal lumen are continuously sampled at the apical surface of these cells and transferred to the immune cells in the pockets. Lymphocytes and dendritic cells leaving the M cell pockets through the basement membrane pores interact and initiate adaptive responses to the antigens, which results in formation of the secondary lymphoid nodules. Locally produced B cells give rise to plasma cells secreting IgA, which is transported by enterocytes into the intestinal lumen to bind and neutralize potentially harmful antigens.

Another significant collection of MALT occurs in the mucosa of the **appendix**, a short, small-diameter projection from the cecum. Typically the mucosa of the appendix is almost completely filled with lymphoid tissue, effacing the glands otherwise found in the large intestine wall (Figure 14–14). The lumen contains the normal bacterial flora of the large intestine and may serve to retain some of these beneficial bacteria there during diarrheal illnesses.

LYMPH NODES

Lymph nodes are bean-shaped, encapsulated structures, generally only 10 mm by 2.5 cm in size, distributed throughout the body along the lymphatic vessels (see Figure 14–1). A total

FIGURE **14–12** Tonsils.

a

Pharyngeal
tonsil
Opening of
auditory tube
Palate
Palatine tonsil
Lingual tonsil

c

b

Masses of lymphoid nodules comprising tonsils are collected in three general locations in the wall of the pharynx.

(a) Palatine tonsils are located in the posterior lateral walls of the oral cavity, and **lingual** tonsils are situated along the surface of the posterior third of the tongue. Both are covered with stratified squamous epithelium. The **pharyngeal tonsil** is a single medial mass situated in the posterior wall of the nasopharynx. It is usually covered by ciliated pseudostratified columnar epithelium, but areas with stratified epithelium can also be observed. Hypertrophied regions of pharyngeal tonsils resulting from chronic inflammation are called **adenoids**.

(b) A section showing several lymphoid nodules (**LN**), collectively covered by stratified squamous epithelium (**E**) on one side and a connective tissue capsule (**CT**) on the other. Some nodules show lighter staining germinal centers (**GC**). Infoldings of the mucosa in some tonsils form crypts (**C**), along which nodules are especially numerous. Lumens of crypts contain desquamated epithelial cells, live and dead lymphocytes, and bacteria. X140. H&E.

(c) Epithelium (**E**) surrounding tonsillar crypts (**C**) often becomes infiltrated with lymphocytes and other leukocytes and can become difficult to recognize histologically. Adjacent connective tissue at the top of the photo also contains numerous lymphocytes. X200. H&E.

(Figure 14-12b and c reproduced with permission, from Dr Paulo A. Abrahamsohn, Institute of Biomedical Sciences, University of São Paulo, Brazil.)

of 400 to 450 lymph nodes are present, most abundantly in the axillae (armpits) and groin, along the major vessels of the neck, and in the thorax and abdomen, especially in mesenteries. The nodes constitute a series of in-line filters of lymph that defend against the spread of microorganisms and tumor cells and provide enclosed environments that facilitate production of plasma cells secreting non-IgA antibodies. Before merging with the bloodstream, all lymph is filtered and has antibodies added by at least one lymph node.

Embedded in loose connective tissue, a lymph node has a convex surface where **afferent lymphatics** enter and a concave depression, the **hilum**, where an **efferent lymphatic**

leaves and where an artery, vein, and nerve penetrate the organ (Figure 14–15). A dense connective tissue capsule surrounds the lymph node, extending trabeculae internally through which the blood vessels branch. Valves in the lymphatics ensure that lymph flow is unidirectional.

The most abundant cells of lymph nodes are lymphocytes of all types, plasma cells, dendritic cells, macrophages, and other APCs. FDCs are present within lymphoid nodules. All of these cells are arranged in a stroma of reticulin fibers and reticular cells to form three major regions: an outer **cortex**, a central **medulla**, and a smaller area between these two called the **paracortex** (Figures 14–15 and 14–16).

FIGURE **14–13** Peyer's patch and M cells.

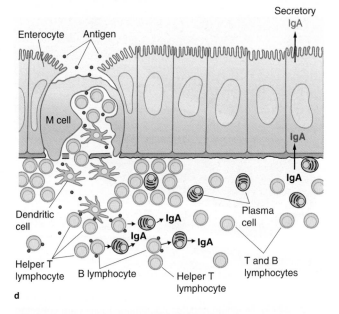

Peyer's patches are very large clusters of lymphoid follicles located in the wall of the ileum which allow close monitoring of microorganisms in the gut.

(a) A section through a Peyer patch shows a few lymphoid nodules (**N**), some with germinal centers (arrow). The mucosa of the small intestine is folded into many projecting villi (**V**). X100. H&E.

(b) With the surface epithelial cells removed, scanning electron microscopy (SEM) shows typical basement membrane over the villi (**V**) but reveals a highly porous covering over lymphoid nodules of the Peyer patch. This sieve-like basement membrane facilitates interactions between immune cells and M cells in the epithelium over the nodules.

(*With permission, from Dr Samuel G. McClugage, Department of Cell Biology and Anatomy, Louisiana State University Health Sciences Center, New Orleans, LA.*)

(c) The TEM shows that the epithelium directly over a Peyer patch lymphoid nodule has unique cells called **M (microfold)**

cells with short apical folds but no brush border. The basal surface of M cells forms a large intracellular pocket that harbors a transient population of T and B lymphocytes (**L**) and dendritic cells (**D**) which move through the openings in the basement membrane (**BM**). Darker cytoplasm of adjacent enterocytes (**E**) with brush borders (**B**) is also seen. X1000.

(*With permission, from Dr Marian R. Neutra, Children's Hospital, Harvard Medical School, Boston, MA.*)

(d) A summary diagram showing that antigens in the gut lumen are bound by **M cells** and undergo transcytosis into their intraepithelial pockets where **dendritic cells** take up the antigen, process it, and present it to **T helper cells**. B lymphocytes stimulated by the Th cells differentiate into **plasma cells** secreting IgA antibodies. The IgA is transported into the gut lumen where it binds its antigen on the surface of microorganisms, neutralizing potentially harmful invaders before they penetrate the mucosa.

FIGURE **14-14** Appendix.

A blind evagination off the cecum, the appendix is a significant part of the MALT with its lamina propria and submucosa filled with lymphocytes and lymphoid follicles (**L**). The small lumen contains a sample of the microbial flora of the intestine, along with undigested material. X20. H&E.

These regions are not physically compartmentalized like those of the thymus.

The **cortex** includes the following components:

- A **subcapsular sinus**, immediately inside the capsule, receives lymph from the afferent lymphatics (Figure 14–17). From this space **cortical sinuses** (or trabecular sinuses) branch internally among the lymphoid nodules along trabeculae. These sinuses are lined by a very thin, discontinuous endothelium penetrated by reticulin fibers and processes of dendritic cells. Lymph containing antigens, lymphocytes, and APCs passes through these sinuses and percolates easily into the surrounding lymphoid tissue.
- **Lymphoid nodules**, with or without germinal centers, fill most cortical areas, formed largely by helper T lymphocytes and proliferating B lymphoblasts (Figures 14–16 and 14–17). Each nodule is organized around the long,

interdigitating processes of follicular dendritic cells (FDCs), but these are not readily seen by routine light microscopy. Numerous macrophages are also present for removal of newly formed defective B cells.

The region between the cortex and medulla, the **paracortex** does not have precise boundaries but can be distinguished from the outer cortex by its lack of B-cell lymphoid nodules (Figure 14–16). Unlike the superficial cortex, the paracortex contains lymphoid tissue rich T cells that can be seen by immunohistochemistry (Figure 14–18).

Specialized postcapillary venules in the paracortex called **high endothelial venules (HEVs)** represent an important entry point for most (90%) lymphocytes into lymph nodes. These vessels have an unusual endothelial lining of cuboidal cells, whose apical surface glycoproteins and integrins facilitate rapid diapedesis of lymphocytes out of the blood into the paracortex of the lymph node (Figure 14–19). HEVs also occur in the large accumulations of MALT discussed previously, but are less well-characterized in those tissues.

The **medulla** of a lymph node has two major components (Figures 14–16 and 14–20):

- **Medullary cords** are branched cordlike masses of lymphoid tissue extending from the paracortex. They contain T and B lymphocytes and many plasma cells.
- **Medullary sinuses** are dilated spaces lined by discontinuous endothelium that separate the medullary cords. As shown in Figure 14–20, the lumens of medullary sinuses include a meshwork of processes from reticular cells, which represent a final lymph filter. These sinuses contain many macrophages and sometimes neutrophils if the lymph node is draining an infected region. They are continuous with the cortical sinuses and converge at the hilum as the efferent lymphatic vessel (Figure 14–15).

›› MEDICAL APPLICATION

Metastatic cancer cells detached from a primary tumor can enter lymphatics and are carried to nearby lymph nodes, especially the **sentinel lymph node** that is the first one downstream of the region with the tumor. Cells from well-established tumors are often immunosuppressive themselves and may continue growth as a **secondary tumor** within lymph nodes. During cancer surgery lymph nodes in the lymphatics draining the tumor area are examined by pathologists for the presence of cancer cells. The presence of such metastatic cells in lymph nodes is a key determinant in most **staging systems** for various types of cancer and an important prognostic indicator.

Role of Lymph Nodes in the Immune Response

The lymph arriving at a lymph node contains antigens free in solution or bound to antibodies or complement, still on

FIGURE **14–15** Lymph node.

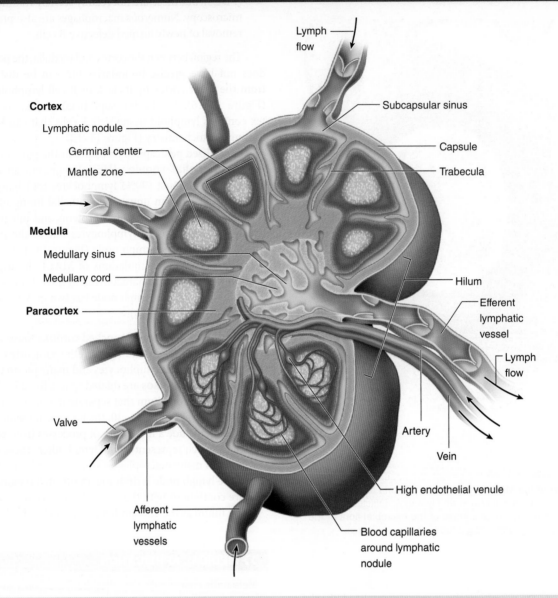

Lymph flow

Cortex
Lymphatic nodule
Germinal center
Mantle zone

Medulla
Medullary sinus
Medullary cord

Paracortex

Valve

Afferent lymphatic vessels

Subcapsular sinus
Capsule
Trabecula

Hilum
Efferent lymphatic vessel
Lymph flow

Artery
Vein

High endothelial venule

Blood capillaries around lymphatic nodule

Lymph nodes are small encapsulated structures positioned along lymphatic vessels to filter lymph and facilitate antibody production. Valves in the lymphatic vessels ensure the one-way flow of lymph, indicated by arrows. The three major regions of a lymph node include the outer **cortex** receiving lymph from the afferent lymphatics, an inner **paracortex** where most lymphocytes enter via high endothelial venules (HEVs), and a central **medulla** with sinuses converging at the efferent lymphatic.

microorganisms, or already internalized and transported by APCs. If draining from an infected or inflamed region, lymph may also contain microorganisms and cytokines. Antigens not yet phagocytosed will be internalized by APCs in the lymph nodes and presented on MHC class II molecules.

Circulating B and T lymphocytes traffic from node to node, entering via the lymph or HEVs, where B cells contact antigens on FDCs and T cells sample antigens presented on dendritic cells and other APCs. Lymphocytes whose receptors recognize such antigens will be activated. B cells will proliferate rapidly in germinal centers of follicles with the help of Th cells, often enlarging the entire lymph node. Activated cytotoxic T cells in the paracortex proliferate to a much lesser extent without forming follicles.

Many newly made B cells, now activated against a specific antigen, differentiate as plasma cells and move to the medulla or to downstream sites beyond the lymph node where they produce antibodies. Specific Th cells, CTLs, and T_{regs} also recirculate in the efferent lymph and with the antibodies spread the immune defenses against those microorganisms

FIGURE **14–16** Regions of a lymph node.

A low-magnification section of a lymph node shows the three functional regions: the cortex (**C**), the paracortex (**P**), and the medulla (**M**). Connective tissue of the capsule (**CT**) completely surrounds each lymph node and extends as several trabeculae (**T**) throughout the lymphoid tissue. Major spaces for lymph flow are present in this tissue under the capsule and along the trabeculae. A changing population of immune cells is suspended on reticular fibers throughout the cortex, paracortex, and medulla. Lymphoid nodules (**LN**) are normally restricted to the cortex, and the medulla is characterized by sinuses (**MS**) and cords (**MC**) of lymphoid tissue. X40. H&E.

(*With permission, from Dr Paulo A. Abrahamsohn, Institute of Biomedical Sciences, University of São Paulo, Brazil.*)

throughout the body. Both B and T memory cells also move elsewhere in the body, providing long-lived protection and proliferating more rapidly upon subsequent exposure to their specific antigen.

›› MEDICAL APPLICATION

Neoplastic proliferation of lymphocytes, producing a malignant **lymphoma**, may occur diffusely but is often located in one or more lymph nodes. Such growth can completely obliterate the normal architecture of the node and convert it to an enlarged, encapsulated structure filled with lymphocytes, a condition called **lymphadenopathy**.

FIGURE **14–17** Lymph node cortex.

The outer regions on the convex sides of a lymph node include the capsule (**C**), subcapsular sinuses (**S**), and diffuse lymphoid tissue with lymphoid nodules (**N**). Afferent lymphatic vessels (which are only rarely shown well in sections) penetrate this capsule, dumping lymph into the sinus where its contents are processed by lymphocytes and APCs. X140. H&E.

(*With permission, from Dr Paulo A. Abrahamsohn, Institute of Biomedical Sciences, University of São Paulo, Brazil.*)

› SPLEEN

The spleen contains the largest single accumulation of lymphoid tissue in the body and is the only lymphoid organ involved in filtration of blood, making it an important organ in defense against blood-borne antigens. It is also the main site of old erythrocyte destruction. As is true of other secondary lymphoid organs, the spleen is a production site of antibodies and activated lymphocytes, which here are delivered directly into the blood.

Located high in the left upper quadrant of the abdomen and typically about 12 × 7 × 3 cm in size, the spleen's volume varies with its content of blood and tends to decrease very slowly after puberty. The organ is surrounded by a capsule of dense connective tissue from which emerge trabeculae to penetrate the parenchyma or **splenic pulp** (Figure 14–21). Large trabeculae originate at the hilum, on the medial surface of the spleen, and carry branches of the splenic artery, vein, lymphatics, and nerves into the splenic pulp.

Functions of Splenic White & Red Pulp

The spleen is filled with reticular tissue containing reticular cells and fibers, many lymphocytes and other blood cells, macrophages, and APCs. This splenic pulp has two components: the **white pulp** (20% of the spleen) and the **red pulp** (Figure 14–21). The small masses of white pulp consist of **lymphoid nodules** and the **periarteriolar lymphoid sheaths**

FIGURE **14–18** Lymph node cortex and paracortex.

The region just inside the cortex is called the **paracortex**. Although most lymphocytes in the cortex are B cells, many located in nodules, the lymphocytes of the paracortex are largely T cells. This separation is indicated in the fluorescence micrographs here using immunohistochemistry on adjacent sections of lymph node. **(a)** Antibody against a B-cell surface marker labels nearly all the lymphocytes in the cortex (**C**), as well as many cells around an HEV (**V**) in the paracortex, but few cells in the paracortex proper (**P**). **(b)** Stained with an antibody against a T-cell marker, the paracortex is heavily labeled, but only a few cells in the cortex (**C**) are stained, possibly T helper cells. X200.

(*With permission, from I. L. Weissman, Stanford University School of Medicine, Palo Alto, CA.*)

(PALS), while the red pulp consists of blood-filled **sinusoids** and **splenic cords**.

As expected of an organ where the blood is monitored immunologically, the splenic microvasculature contains unique regions shown schematically in Figure 14–22. Branching from the hilum, small **trabecular arteries** leave the trabecular connective tissue and enter the parenchyma as arterioles enveloped by the PALS, which consists primarily of T cells with some macrophages, DCs, and plasma cells as part of the white pulp. Surrounded by the PALS, these vessels are known

FIGURE **14–19** High endothelial venules.

HEVs are found in the paracortex of lymph nodes, as shown, as well as in tonsils and Peyer patches. Their endothelial cells are unusually shaped but generally cuboidal and facilitate rapid translocation of lymphocytes from lymph into the lymphoid tissue. L-selectin on the lymphocytes recognizes sugar-rich ligands on the surfaces of these endothelial cells and, as a consequence, the lymphocytes stop there. Integrins promote adhesion between lymphocytes and the endothelial cells, and the lymphocytes cross the vessel wall into the lymph node parenchyma.

(a) HEVs can be difficult to identify in H&E-stained paraffin sections. X400. H&E. **(b)** Plastic sections more clearly reveal the HEVs (arrowheads) and the lymphocytes passing between them (arrows). X400. PT. **(c)** SEM of a sectioned HEV shows five typical lymphocytes adhering to endothelial cells (arrowheads) before migrating between them and joining other lymphocytes in the surrounding paracortex. X500.

(*Figure 14–19 c reproduced, with permission, from Fujita T. Prog Clin Biol Res 1989;295:493.*)

FIGURE **14–20** Lymph node medulla.

(a) The medulla of a lymph node consists mainly of the medullary sinuses (**MS**) separated by intervening medullary cords (**MC**). Lymphocytes and plasma are abundant and predominate in number over other cell types. A blood vessel within a medullary cord is also seen. X200. H&E. **(b)** Higher magnification of a medullary cord (**MC**) shows plasma cells (arrows) with spherical, eccentric nuclei and much more cytoplasm

than lymphocytes. Efferent lymph is rich in newly synthesized antibodies. A medullary sinus (**MS**) with a meshwork of eosinophilic processes from surrounding reticular cells is also seen. X400. H&E.

(*With permission, from Dr Paulo A. Abrahamsohn, Institute of Biomedical Sciences, University of São Paulo, Brazil.*)

FIGURE **14–21** Spleen.

The capsule (**C**) of the spleen connects to trabeculae (**T**) extending into the pulp-like interior of the organ. The red pulp (**R**) occupies most of the parenchyma, with white pulp (**W**) restricted to smaller areas, mainly around the central arterioles. Names of these splenic areas refer to their color in the fresh state: red pulp is filled with blood cells of all types, located both in cords and sinuses; white pulp is lymphoid tissue. Large blood vessels and lymphatics enter and leave the spleen at a hilum. X20. Picro-Sirius-hematoxylin.

FIGURE **14–22** Blood flow in the spleen.

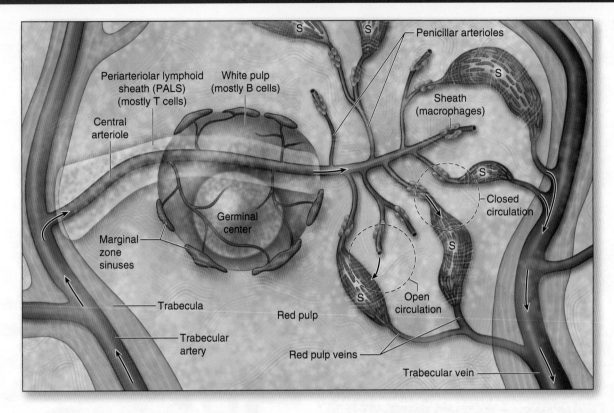

Schematic view of the blood circulation and the structure of the spleen, from the trabecular artery to the trabecular vein. Small branches of these arteries are called **central arterioles** and become enclosed within a sheath of lymphoid cells, the **periarteriolar lymphoid sheath (PALS)** in white pulp. B cells in these sheaths can form nodules as the largest masses of white pulp, and around these nodules are located the marginal zone

sinuses. Emerging from the white pulp, the central arteriole branches as the penicillar arterioles, which lead to sheathed capillaries. From these, blood flows into either a **closed circulation** passing directly into splenic sinuses (**S**) or an **open circulation**, being dumped from the vasculature into the lymphoid tissue of the red pulp's splenic cords. From there viable blood cells reenter the vasculature through the walls of the sinuses.

as **central arterioles** (Figure 14–23). B cells located within the PALS may be activated by a trapped antigen from the blood and form a temporary lymphoid nodule like those of other secondary lymphoid organs (Figure 14–23b). In growing nodules the arteriole is pushed to an eccentric position but is still called the central arteriole. These arterioles send capillaries throughout the white pulp and to small sinuses in a peripheral marginal zone of developing B cells around each lymphoid nodule (Figure 14–22).

Each central arteriole eventually leaves the white pulp and enters the red pulp, losing its sheath of lymphocytes and branching as several short straight **penicillar arterioles** that continue as capillaries (Figure 14–22). Some of these capillaries are sheathed with APCs for additional immune surveillance of blood.

The red pulp is composed almost entirely of **splenic cords** (of Billroth) and **splenic sinusoids** and is the site where effete RBCs in blood are removed (Figure 14–24). The splenic cords contain a network of reticular cells and fibers filled with T and B lymphocytes, macrophages, other leukocytes, and red

blood cells. The splenic cords are separated by the sinusoids (Figure 14–25). Unusual elongated endothelial cells called **stave cells** line these sinusoids, oriented parallel to the blood flow and sparsely wrapped in reticular fibers and highly discontinuous basal lamina (Figure 14–26).

Blood flow through the splenic red pulp can take either of two routes (Figure 14–22):

■ In the **closed circulation**, capillaries branching from the penicillar arterioles connect directly to the sinusoids and the blood is always enclosed by endothelium.

■ In the **open circulation**, capillaries from about half of the penicillar arterioles are uniquely *open-ended*, dumping blood into the stroma of the splenic cords. In this route plasma and all the formed elements of blood must reenter the vasculature by passing through narrow slits between the stave cells into the sinusoids. These small openings present no obstacle to platelets, to the motile leukocytes, or to thin flexible erythrocytes. However stiff or effete, swollen RBCs at their normal life span of 120 days are

FIGURE **14–23** White pulp of the spleen.

The splenic white pulp consists of lymphoid tissue surrounding the central arterioles as the PALS and the nodules of proliferating B cells in this sheath. **(a)** Longitudinal section of white pulp (**W**) in a PALS surrounding a central arteriole (arrowhead). Surrounding the PALS is much red pulp (**R**).

(b) A large nodule with a germinal center forms in the PALS and the central arteriole (arrowhead) is displaced to the

nodule's periphery. Small vascular sinuses can be seen at the margin between white (**W**) and red (**R**) pulp. Both X20. H&E.

(With permission, from Dr Paulo A. Abrahamsohn, Institute of Biomedical Sciences, University of São Paulo, Brazil.)

blocked from passing between the stave cells and undergo selective removal by macrophages (Figure 14–24).

Removal of defective RBCs and recycling of their iron are major functions of the red pulp. Iron released from hemoglobin during the degradation of RBCs is stored by macrophages within complexes of ferritin proteins or bound to transferrin,

returned to the circulation, and reused primarily for erythropoiesis. Iron-free heme is either bound to its transport protein, hemopexin, or is metabolized to bilirubin and excreted in the bile by liver cells. After surgical removal of the spleen (splenectomy), the number of abnormal erythrocytes in the circulation increases although most such cells are then removed by macrophages in sinusoids of the bone marrow and liver.

From the sinusoids blood proceeds to small red pulp veins that converge as the **trabecular veins** (Figure 14–22), which in turn form the splenic vein. The trabecular veins lack significant smooth muscle and resemble endothelium-lined channels hollowed out in the trabecular connective tissue.

Important aspects of the major lymphoid organs (thymus, MALT, lymph nodes, and spleen) are summarized and compared in Table 14–4.

FIGURE **14–24** Erythrocyte removal by splenic macrophages.

A micrograph showing five macrophages in a splenic cord engaged in phagocytosis of effete erythrocytes. X400. PT.

›› MEDICAL APPLICATION

Enlargement of the spleen, **splenomegaly**, can occur from a variety of causes, including lymphoma or other malignant growth, infections such as mononucleosis, or sickle cell disease and other types of anemia. The splenic capsule is relatively thin, and an enlarged spleen is susceptible to traumatic rupture, a potentially life-threatening occurrence due to loss of blood into the abdominal cavity. Such rupture may require prompt surgical removal of the spleen, **splenectomy**, after which most functions of the organ are carried out by other lymphoid organs, with erythrocyte removal occurring in the liver and bone marrow.

FIGURE **14–25** Red pulp of the spleen.

(a) The splenic red pulp is composed entirely of sinusoids (**S**) and splenic cords (**C**), both of which contain blood cells of all types. The cords, often called **cords of Billroth**, are reticular tissue rich in macrophages and lymphocytes. X140. H&E.

(b) Higher magnification shows that the sinusoids (**S**) are lined by endothelial cells (arrows) with large nuclei bulging into the sinusoidal lumens. The unusual endothelial cells are called **stave cells** and have special properties that allow separation of healthy from effete red blood cells in the splenic cords (**C**). X200. H&E.

(*Both with permission, from Dr Paulo A. Abrahamsohn, Institute of Biomedical Sciences, University of São Paulo, Brazil.*)

TABLE **14–4** | Important histologic comparisons of the major lymphoid organs.

	Thymus	MALT	Lymph Nodes	Spleen
Cortex/medulla	Distinctly present	Absent	Present	Absent
Lymphoid nodules	Absent	Present	Present (in cortex only)	Present (in white pulp only)
Lymphatic vessels	No afferents; few efferents in septa	No afferents; efferents present	Afferents at capsule, emptying into subcapsular sinus; efferent at hilum	No afferents; efferents in trabeculae
Unique features	Hassall (thymic) corpuscles in medulla; epithelial-reticular cells in cortex and medulla	Crypts lined by surface mucosa in tonsils; epithelial M cells in mucosa over Peyer patches	Thin paracortical region between cortex and medulla, with high endothelial venules (HEV); medullary cords and sinuses	Minor white pulp component, with central arterioles; major red pulp component, with many sinusoids

FIGURE **14–26** Structure and function of splenic sinusoids.

The endothelial stave cells that line the sinusoids in red pulp are long cells oriented lengthwise along the sinusoids.

(a) SEM clearly shows the parallel alignment of the stave cells **(S)**, as well as many macrophages **(M)** in the surrounding red pulp **(R)**. X500.

(With permission, from Fujita T. Prog Clin Biol Res 1989; 295:493)

(b) A silver-stained section of spleen shows dark reticular fibers in the splenic cords **(C)** and wrapped around the sinusoids **(S)**. The sinusoidal basement membrane is highly discontinuous and open to the passage of blood cells, X400.

(c) Diagram showing these components of splenic sinusoids, with the structures resembling a loosely organized wooden barrel. In the open circulation mode of blood flow, blood cells dumped into the splenic cords move under pressure or by their own motility through the spaces between **stave cells**, reentering the vasculature and soon leaving the spleen via the splenic vein. Cells that cannot move between the stave cells, mainly effete erythrocytes, are removed by macrophages.

The Immune System & Lymphoid Organs SUMMARY OF KEY POINTS

Basic Immunology

- **Innate immunity** is present from birth and involves leukocytes (mainly granulocytes), and proteins such as defensins, complement, lysozyme, and interferons; **adaptive immunity** develops more slowly and is based on antigen presentation to **lymphocytes**.
- Immune cells communicate with one another and regulate one another's activities via polypeptide hormones called **cytokines**.
- **Antigens** are the regions of macromolecules, usually proteins, that are recognized by lymphocytes to elicit a specific immune response against them.
- **Antibodies** are immunoglobulins produced by plasma cells after a progenitor B cell is activated by a specific antigen and rearranges its immunoglobulin genes so the antibody matches the antigen.
- Surfaces of all nucleated cells bear fragments of their constituent proteins on **major histocompatibility complex (MHC) class I** molecules.
- Only **antigen-presenting cells (APCs)**, mostly derived from monocytes, also present fragments of endocytosed foreign (usually from microorganisms) proteins on surface **MHC class II** molecules.

Lymphocyte Origins and Differentiation

- Lymphocytes originate in the **primary lymphoid organs**: bone marrow for **B lymphocytes** and the thymus for **T lymphocytes**.
- B cells produce antibodies for **humoral immunity**; T cells function in **cell-mediated immunity**.
- T cells develop receptors (**TCRs**), usually containing α and β **chains**, that bind antigen along with another surface protein designated by a **CD ("cluster of differentiation") numbering system**.
- Important classes of T cells include **CD4⁺ T helper cells**; **CD8⁺ cytotoxic T cells**; **CD4⁺CD25⁺ regulatory T cells**; and **γδ T cells**, which have those TCR chains and are mainly in epithelia.
- **B-cell receptors (BCRs)** are IgM or IgD antibodies on the cell surface that bind specific antigens whenever they contact them.
- B and T cells are often activated, proliferate, and begin to function in the **secondary lymphoid organs** : the **lymph nodes**, all **mucosa-associated lymphoid tissue (MALT)**, and the **spleen**.
- In these organs lymphocytes are distributed within a meshwork of reticulin produced by fibroblastic **reticular cells**, and most APCs are **dendritic cells** with many processes.
- In secondary lymphoid tissues, BCRs bind antigen not presented in MHC class II molecules of another cell, the **follicular dendritic cell (FDC)**.
- With cytokines from helper T cells, a FDC-activated B cell proliferates clonally to produce temporarily a large **lymphoid nodule** (or follicle), which develops a pale **germinal center**.
- From lymphoid nodules cells produced there disperse as **plasma cells**, various T cells, and **B and T memory cells** that respond and proliferate quickly if their specific antigen reappears.

Thymus

- T lymphoblasts, or **thymocytes**, attach in the **thymus** to a **cytoreticulum** composed of interconnected **epithelioreticular cells**.
- Thymic epithelioreticular cells also secrete many **cytokines**, **compartmentalize** the thymus into a **cortex** and a **medulla**, and in the cortex surround blood vessels in the **blood-thymus barrier**.
- Developing T cells with nonfunctional TCRs are detected and removed in the thymic cortex by a process of **positive selection**; cells with functional TCRs move into the thymic medulla.

- In the thymic medulla T cells whose TCRs bind strongly to "**self-proteins**, " including proteins of many nonthymus cell types made by epithelioreticular cells expressing the **Aire** gene, are induced to undergo apoptosis there in a process of **negative selection**.
- This two-stage thymic selection leads to **central immune tolerance**, producing functional T cells that do not bind to proteins of the host.
- **Peripheral immune tolerance** occurs throughout the body when specific immune reactions are suppressed by **regulatory T cells** that also originate largely in the thymic medulla.
- Regulatory T cells form in the thymus upon interacting with dendritic cells presenting self-antigens in a process promoted by cytokines from epithelioreticular cell aggregates called **Hassall corpuscles**, found only in the thymic medulla.

Mucosa-associated Lymphoid Tissue (MALT)

- **MALT** is found in the mucosa of most tracts but is concentrated in the **palatine**, **lingual** and **pharyngeal tonsils**, **Peyer patches**, and the **appendix**.
- Unlike MALT, **lymph nodes** are completely **encapsulated** and occur along the lymphatic vessels; each has several **afferent lymphatics** and one **efferent lymphatic**.

Lymph Nodes

- Each lymph node **filters lymph** and **provides a site for B-cell activation** and differentiation to antibody-secreting **plasma cells**.
- A lymph node has three functional but not physically separate compartments: an outer **cortex**, a underlying **paracortex**, and an inner **medulla** adjacent to the hilum and efferent lymphatic.
- Lymphatics enter at the **cortex** of a node, where **B cells** encounter antigens, proliferate in **lymphoid nodules**, and then move into the deeper regions of the lymph node.
- Most lymphocytes enter at the **paracortex** of the lymph node via **high endothelial venules (HEVs)** located there only; most lymphocytes in this region are **T helper cells**.
- The medulla has **medullary cords** containing reticular fibers with many plasma cells, macrophages, and other leukocytes; between the cords are lymph-filled **medullary sinuses** that converge at the efferent lymphatic.

Spleen

- The **spleen** is a large lymphoid organ without a cortex/medulla structure; instead, it has two intermingled but functionally different regions: **white pulp** and **red pulp**.
- **White pulp**, only 20% of the spleen, is **secondary lymphoid tissue** associated with small central arterioles that are also enclosed by **periarteriolar lymphoid sheaths (PALS)** of T cells.
- **Red pulp**, which filters blood, removes defective erythrocytes, and recycles hemoglobin iron, consists of **splenic cords** with macrophages and blood cells of all kinds and **splenic sinusoids**.
- The **splenic sinusoids** are lined by unusual endothelial cells called **stave cells** that are elongated and aligned parallel to the blood flow, with open slits between the cells.
- Blood flow in red pulp is either a **closed circulation**, moving from capillaries into the venous sinusoids, or an **open circulation**, with capillaries opening directly into the splenic cords.
- **Blood filtration** in the open circulation involves interaction with splenic cord **macrophages** that remove old, swollen RBCs unable to slip between stave cells to reenter the venous blood flow.

15 Digestive Tract

The digestive system consists of the **digestive tract**—oral cavity, esophagus, stomach, small and large intestines, and anus—and its associated glands—salivary glands, liver, and pancreas (Figure 15–1). Also called the **gastrointestinal (GI) tract** or **alimentary canal**, its function is to obtain from ingested food the molecules necessary for the maintenance, growth, and energy needs of the body. During digestion proteins, complex carbohydrates, nucleic acids, and fats are broken down into their small molecule subunits that are easily absorbed through the small intestine lining. Most water and electrolytes are absorbed in the large intestine. In addition, the inner layer of the entire digestive tract forms an important protective barrier between the content of the tract's lumen and the internal milieu of the body's connective tissue and vasculature.

Structures within the digestive tract allow the following:

- **Ingestion,** or introduction of food and liquid into the oral cavity.
- **Mastication,** or chewing, which divides solid food into digestible pieces.
- **Motility,** muscular movements of materials through the tract.
- **Secretion** of lubricating and protective mucus, digestive enzymes, acidic and alkaline fluids, and bile.
- **Hormone release** for local control of motility and secretion.
- **Chemical digestion** or enzymatic degradation of large macromolecules in food to smaller molecules and their subunits.
- **Absorption** of the small molecules and water into the blood and lymph.
- **Elimination** of indigestible, unabsorbed components of food.

› GENERAL STRUCTURE OF THE DIGESTIVE TRACT

All regions of the GI tract have certain structural features in common. The GI tract is a hollow tube with a lumen of variable diameter and a wall made up of four main layers: the **mucosa, submucosa, muscularis,** and **serosa.** Figure 15–2 shows a general overview of these four layers; key features of each layer are summarized here.

- The **mucosa** consists of an **epithelial lining**; an underlying **lamina propria** of loose connective tissue rich in blood vessels, lymphatics, lymphocytes, smooth muscle cells, and often containing small glands; and a thin layer of smooth muscle called the **muscularis mucosae** separating mucosa from submucosa and allowing local movements of the mucosa. The mucosa is also frequently called a **mucous membrane.**
- The **submucosa** contains denser connective tissue with larger blood and lymph vessels and the **submucosal (Meissner) plexus** of autonomic nerves. It may also contain glands and significant lymphoid tissue.
- The thick **muscularis** (or muscularis externa) is composed of smooth muscle cells organized as two or more sublayers. In the internal sublayer (closer to the lumen), the fiber orientation is generally circular; in the external sublayer it is longitudinal. The connective tissue between the muscle sublayers contains blood and lymph vessels, as well as the **myenteric (Auerbach) nerve plexus** of many autonomic neurons aggregated into small ganglia and interconnected by pre- and postganglionic nerve fibers. This and the submucosal plexus together comprise the **enteric nervous system** of the digestive tract. Contractions of the muscularis, which mix and

FIGURE **15–1** The digestive system.

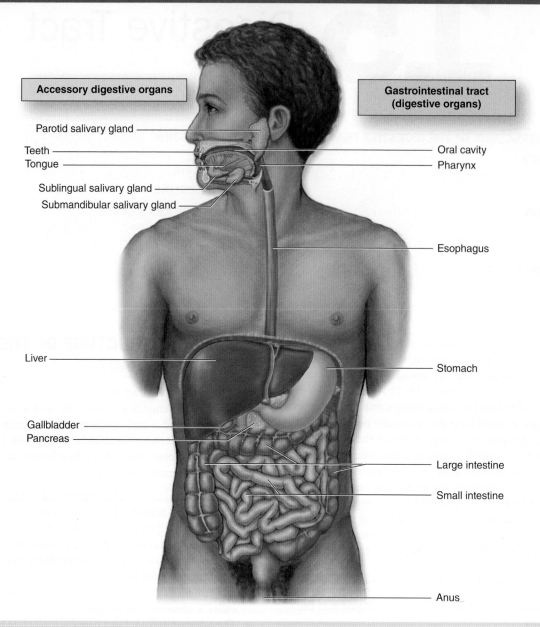

The digestive system consists of the tract from the mouth (oral cavity) to the anus, as well as the digestive glands emptying into this tract, primarily the salivary glands, liver, and pancreas. These accessory digestive glands are described in Chapter 16.

propel the luminal contents forward, are generated and coordinated by the myenteric plexus.

- The **serosa** is a thin layer of loose connective tissue, rich in blood vessels, lymphatics, and adipose tissue, with a simple squamous covering epithelium or **mesothelium**. In the abdominal cavity, the serosa is continuous with **mesenteries**, thin membranes covered by mesothelium on both sides that support the intestines. Mesenteries are continuous with the **peritoneum**, a serous membrane

that lines that cavity. In places where the digestive tract is not suspended in a cavity but bound directly to adjacent structures, such as in the esophagus (Figure 15–1), the serosa is replaced by a thick **adventitia**, a connective tissue layer that merges with the surrounding tissues and lacks mesothelium.

The numerous free immune cells and lymphoid nodules in the mucosa and submucosa constitute the MALT described

FIGURE **15–2** Major layers and organization of the digestive tract.

Mucosa
Epithelium
Lamina propria
Muscularis
mucosae

Submucosa
Submucosal gland
Blood vessel
Submucosal nerve plexus

Muscularis
Inner circular layer
Myenteric nerve plexus
Outer longitudinal layer

Serosa

Mesentery

Vein
Artery
Lymph vessel

Lumen

Diagram showing the structure of the small intestine portion of the digestive tract, with the four main layers and their major components listed on the left. The stomach, small intestine, and large intestine are suspended by mesenteries that are the sites of nerves, blood vessels and lymphatics from the stomach and intestines.

in Chapter 14. The digestive tract normally contains thousands of microbial species, including both useful inhabitants of the gut as well as potential pathogens ingested with food and drink. The mucosa-associated immune defense system provides an essential backup to the thin physical barrier of the epithelial lining. Located just below the epithelium, the lamina propria is rich with macrophages and lymphocytes, many for production of IgA antibodies. Such antibodies undergo transcytosis into the intestinal lumen bound to the secretory protein produced by the epithelial cells. This IgA complex resists proteolysis by digestive enzymes and provides important protection against specific viral and bacterial pathogens.

>> **MEDICAL APPLICATION**

In diseases such as **Hirschsprung disease** (congenital aganglionic megacolon) or **Chagas disease** (trypanosomiasis, infection with the protozoan *Trypanosoma cruzi*), plexuses in the digestive tract's enteric nervous system are absent or severely injured, respectively. This disturbs digestive tract motility and produces dilations in some areas. The rich autonomic innervation of the enteric nervous system also provides an anatomic explanation of the well-known actions of emotional stress on the stomach and other regions of the GI tract.

› ORAL CAVITY

The oral cavity (Figure 15–1) is lined with stratified squamous epithelium, which may be keratinized, partially keratinized, or nonkeratinized depending on the location. Epithelial differentiation, keratinization, and the interface between the epithelium and lamina propria are similar to those features in the epidermis and dermis and are discussed more extensively with skin (see Chapter 18). Like the keratinized surface cells of epidermis, the flattened superficial cells of the oral epithelium undergo continuous desquamation, or loss at the surface. Unlike those of the epidermis, the shed cells of the nonkeratinized or parakeratinized oral epithelium retain their nuclei.

›› MEDICAL APPLICATION

Viral infections with herpes simplex 1 cause death of infected epithelial cells that can lead to vesicular or ulcerating lesions of the oral mucosa or skin near the mouth. In the oral cavity such areas are called **canker sores**, and on the skin they are usually called **cold sores** or **fever blisters**. Such lesions, often painful and clustered, occur when the immune defenses are weakened by emotional stress, fever, illness, or local skin damage, allowing the virus, present in the local nerves, to move into the epithelial cells.

The keratinized cell layers resist damage from abrasion and are best developed in the **masticatory mucosa** on the gingiva (gum) and hard palate. The lamina propria in these regions rests directly on the periosteum of underlying bone. Nonkeratinized squamous epithelium predominates in the **lining mucosa** over the soft palate, cheeks, the floor of the mouth, and the **pharynx**, the posterior region of the oral cavity leading to the esophagus. Lining mucosa overlies a thick submucosa containing many minor salivary glands, which secrete continuously to keep the mucosal surface wet, and diffuse lymphoid tissue. Throughout the oral cavity, the epithelium contains transient antigen-presenting cells and rich sensory innervation.

The well-developed core of striated muscle in the **lips**, or labia, (Figure 15–3) makes these structures highly mobile for ingestion, speech, and other forms of communication. Both lips have three differently covered surfaces:

- The internal mucous surface has lining mucosa with a thick, nonkeratinized epithelium and many minor labial salivary glands.
- The red **vermilion zone** of each lip is covered by very thin keratinized stratified squamous epithelium and is transitional between the oral mucosa and skin. This region lacks salivary or sweat glands and is kept moist with saliva from the tongue. The underlying connective tissue is very rich in both sensory innervation and capillaries, which impart the pink color to this region.

FIGURE **15–3** Lip.

Low-magnification micrograph of a lip section showing one side covered by typical oral mucosa (**OM**), the opposite side covered by skin (**S**) containing hair follicles (**F**) and associated glands. Between the oral portion of the lips and normal skin is the vermilion zone (**V**), where epidermis is very thin, lightly keratinized, and transparent to blood in the rich microvasculature of the underlying connective tissue. Because this region lacks the glands for oil and sweat, it is prone to excessive dryness and chapping in cold, dry weather. Internally, the lips contain much striated muscle (**M**) and many minor salivary glands (**G**). X10. H&E.

- The outer surface has thin skin, consisting of epidermal and dermal layers, sweat glands, and many hair follicles with sebaceous glands.

Tongue

The tongue is a mass of striated muscle covered by mucosa, which manipulates ingested material during mastication and swallowing. The muscle fibers are oriented in all directions, allowing a high level of mobility. Connective tissue between the small fascicles of muscle is penetrated by the lamina propria, which makes the mucous membrane strongly adherent to the muscular core. The lower surface of the tongue is smooth, with typical lining mucosa. The dorsal surface is irregular, having hundreds of small protruding **papillae** of various types on its anterior two-thirds and the massed lingual tonsils on the posterior third, or root of the tongue (Figure 15–4). The papillary and tonsillar areas of the lingual surface are separated by a V-shaped groove called the **sulcus terminalis**.

FIGURE **15–4** Tongue, lingual papillae, and taste buds.

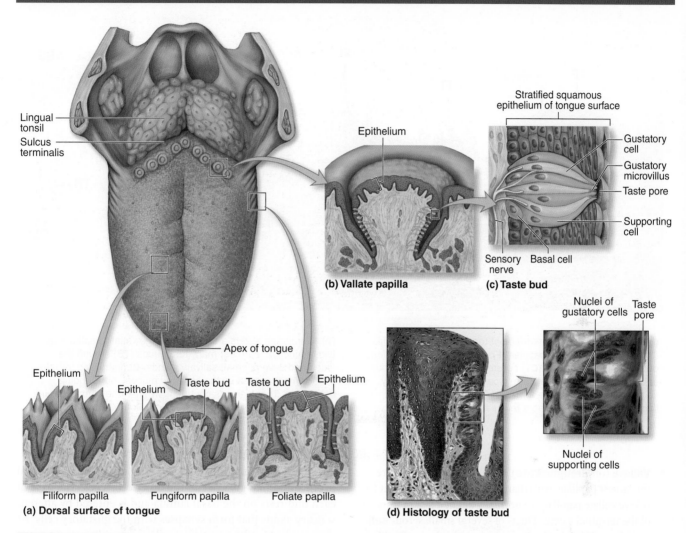

(a) Dorsal surface of tongue

Lingual tonsil

Sulcus terminalis

Apex of tongue

Epithelium

Filiform papilla

Epithelium

Fungiform papilla

Taste bud

Taste bud

Epithelium

Foliate papilla

Epithelium

(b) Vallate papilla

Stratified squamous epithelium of tongue surface

Gustatory cell

Gustatory microvillus

Taste pore

Supporting cell

Sensory nerve   Basal cell

(c) Taste bud

Nuclei of gustatory cells   Taste pore

Nuclei of supporting cells

(d) Histology of taste bud

On its dorsal surface **(a)**, the posterior third of the tongue has the **lingual tonsils** and the anterior portion has numerous **lingual papillae** of four types. Pointed **filiform papillae** provide friction to help move food during chewing. Ridge-like **foliate papillae** on the sides of the tongue are best developed in young children. **Fungiform papillae** are scattered across the dorsal surface, and 8-12 large **vallate papillae (b)** are present in a V-shaped line near the terminal sulcus. **Taste buds** are present on fungiform and foliate papillae but are much more abundant on vallate papillae.

(c) Diagram of a single taste bud shows the **gustatory (taste) cells**, the **supporting cells** whose function is not well understood, and the basal **stem cells**. Microvilli at the ends of the gustatory cells project through an opening in the epithelium, the **taste pore**. Afferent sensory axons enter the basal end of taste buds and synapse with the gustatory cells. In the stratified squamous epithelium of the tongue surface, taste buds form as distinct clusters of cells that are recognizable histologically even at low magnification **(d)**. At higher power the taste pore may be visible, as well as the elongated nuclei of gustatory and supporting cells. 140X and 500X. H&E.

The lingual papillae are elevations of the mucous membrane that assume various forms and functions. There are four types (Figure 15–4):

- **Filiform papillae** (Figure 15–5) are very numerous, have an elongated conical shape, and are heavily keratinized, which gives their surface a gray or whitish appearance. They provide a rough surface that facilitates movement of food during chewing.

- **Fungiform papillae** (Figure 15–5) are much less numerous, lightly keratinized, and interspersed among the filiform papillae. They are mushroom-shaped with well-vascularized and innervated cores of lamina propria.
- **Foliate papillae** consist of several parallel ridges on each side of the tongue, anterior to the sulcus terminalis, but are rudimentary in humans, especially older individuals.

FIGURE **15–5** Lingual papillae.

(a) Section of the dorsal surface of tongue showing both filiform (**FI**) and fungiform papillae (**F**). Both types are elevations of the connective tissue (**CT**) covered by stratified squamous epithelium (**SS**), but the filiform type is pointed and heavily keratinized while the fungiform type is mushroom-shaped, lightly keratinized, and has a few taste buds.

(b) Micrograph shows a single very large vallate papilla with two distinctive features: many taste buds (**TB**) around the sides and several small salivary glands (**GL**) emptying into the cleft or moat formed by the elevated mucosa surrounding the papilla. These glands continuously flush the cleft, renewing the fluid in contact with the taste buds. Both X20. H&E.

- **Vallate** (or **circumvallate**) **papillae** (Figure 15–5) are the largest papillae, with diameters of 1 to 3 mm. Eight to twelve vallate papillae are normally aligned just in front of the terminal sulcus. Ducts of several small, serous **salivary (von Ebner) glands** empty into the deep, moatlike groove surrounding each vallate papilla. This provides a continuous flow of fluid over the taste buds that are abundant on the sides of these papillae, washing away food particles so that the taste buds can receive and process new gustatory stimuli. Secretions from these and other minor salivary glands associated with taste buds contain a lipase that prevents the formation of a hydrophobic film on these structures that would hinder gustation.

Taste buds are ovoid structures within the stratified epithelium on the tongue's surface, which sample the general chemical composition of ingested material (Figures 15–4 and 15–5). Approximately 250 taste buds are present on the lateral surface of each vallate papilla, with many others present on fungiform and foliate (but not the keratinized filiform) papillae. They are not restricted to papillae and are also widely scattered elsewhere on the dorsal and lateral surfaces of the tongue, where they are also continuously flushed by numerous minor salivary glands.

A taste bud has 50 to 100 cells, about half of which are elongated **gustatory (taste) cells**, which turn over with a 7- to 10-day life span. Other cells present are slender **supportive cells**, immature cells, and slowly dividing basal **stem cells** that give rise to the other cell types. The base of each bud rests on the basal lamina and is entered by afferent sensory axons that form synapses with the gustatory cells. At the apical ends of the gustatory cells, microvilli project toward a 2-μm-wide opening in the structure called the **taste pore**. Molecules (tastants) dissolved in saliva contact the microvilli through the pore and interact with cell surface taste receptors (Figure 15–4).

Taste buds detect at least five broad categories of tastants: sodium ions (salty); hydrogen ions from acids (sour); sugars and related compounds (sweet); alkaloids and certain toxins (bitter); and amino acids such as glutamate and aspartate (umami; Jap. *umami*, savory). Salt and sour tastes are produced by ion channels and the other three taste categories are mediated by G-protein–coupled receptors. Receptor binding produces depolarization of the gustatory cells, stimulating the sensory nerve fibers that send information to the brain for processing. Conscious perception of tastes in food requires olfactory and other sensations in addition to taste bud activity.

Teeth

In the adult human there are normally 32 **permanent teeth**, arranged in two bilaterally symmetric arches in the maxillary and mandibular bones (Figure 15–6a). Each quadrant has eight teeth: two incisors, one canine, two premolars, and three permanent molars. Twenty of the permanent teeth are preceded by **primary teeth** (deciduous or milk teeth) that are shed; the others are permanent molars with no deciduous precursors. Each tooth has a **crown** exposed above the gingiva, a constricted **neck** at the gum, and one or more **roots** that fit firmly into bony sockets in the jaws called **dental alveoli** (Figure 15–6b).

The crown is covered by very hard, acellular **enamel** and the roots by a bone-like tissue called **cementum.** These two coverings meet at the neck of the tooth. The bulk of a tooth is composed of another calcified material, **dentin,** which surrounds an internal **pulp cavity** (Figure 15–6b). **Dental pulp** is highly vascular and well-innervated and

consists largely of loose, mesenchymal connective tissue with much ground substance, thin collagen fibers, fibroblasts, and mesenchymal stem cells. The pulp cavity narrows in each root as the **root canal**, which extends to an opening (**apical foramen**) at the tip of each root for the blood vessels, lymphatics, and nerves of the pulp cavity. The **periodontal ligaments** are fibrous connective tissue bundles of collagen fibers inserted into both the cementum and the alveolar bone.

Dentin

Dentin is a calcified tissue harder than bone, consisting of 70% hydroxyapatite. The organic matrix contains type I collagen and proteoglycans secreted from the apical ends of **odontoblasts,** tall polarized cells derived from the cranial neural crest that line the tooth's pulp cavity (Figure 15–7a).

FIGURE **15–6** Teeth.

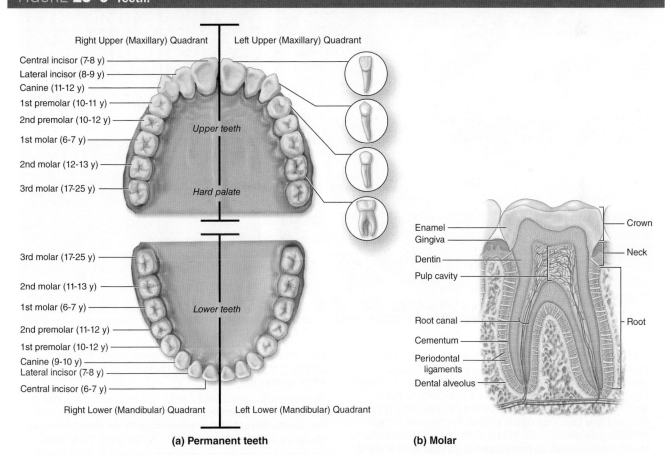

(a) Permanent teeth

(b) Molar

All teeth are similar embryologically and histologically.

(a) The dentition of the permanent teeth is shown, as well as the approximate age at eruption for each tooth.

(b) Diagram of a molar's internal structure is similar to that of all teeth, with an enamel-covered **crown**, cementum-covered **roots** anchoring the tooth to alveolar bone of the jaw, and a slightly constricted **neck** where the **enamel** and **cementum**

coverings meet at the gingiva. Most of the roots and neck consists of **dentin**. A **pulp cavity** extends into the neck and is filled with well-vascularized, well-innervated mesenchymal connective tissue. Blood vessels and nerves enter the tooth through apical foramina at the root tips. **Periodontal ligaments** hold the tooth to bone of the jaw.

FIGURE **15–7** Dentin and odontoblasts.

(a) Odontoblasts (O) are long polarized cells derived from mesenchyme of the developing pulp cavity (PC). Odontoblasts are specialized for collagen and GAG synthesis and are bound together by junctional complexes as a layer, with no basal lamina, so that a collagen-rich matrix called predentin (P) is secreted only from their apical ends at the dentinal surface. Within approximately 1 day of secretion, predentin mineralizes to become dentin (D) as hydroxyapatite crystals form in a process similar to that occurring in osteoid of developing bones (see Chapter 8). In this process the collagen is masked, and calcified matrix becomes much more acidophilic and stains quite differently than that of predentin. When predentin secretion begins, an apical extension from each cell, the odontoblast process (OP), forms and is surrounded by new matrix. As the dentin-predentin layer thickens, these processes lengthen. When tooth formation is complete, odontoblasts persist and

their processes are maintained in canals called **dentinal tubules** that run through the full thickness of the dentin. X400. Mallory trichrome.

(b) Odontoblast processes can be silver-stained and shown to branch near the junction of dentin with enamel (E) and along their length closer to their source (c), with the lateral branches occupying smaller canaliculi within dentin. Both X400. Silver.

(d) These odontoblast process (OP) connections to the odontoblasts (O), shown with stained nuclei here, are important for the maintenance of dentin in adult teeth. X400. Mallory trichrome.

(*Figure 15-7b, c, and d used, with permission, from M. F. Santos, Department of Histology and Embryology, Institute of Biomedical Sciences, University of São Paulo, Brazil.*)

Mineralization of the **predentin** matrix secreted by odontoblasts involves matrix vesicles in a process similar to that occurring in osteoid during bone formation (see Chapter 8).

Long apical **odontoblast processes** extend from the odontoblasts within **dentinal tubules** (Figure 15–7b) that penetrate the full thickness of the dentin, gradually becoming longer as the dentin becomes thicker. Along their length, the processes extend fine branches into smaller lateral branches of the tubules (Figure 15–7c). The odontoblast processes are important for the maintenance of dentin matrix. Odontoblasts continue predentin production into adult life, gradually reducing the size of the pulp cavity, and are stimulated to repair dentin if the tooth is damaged.

Teeth are sensitive to stimuli such as cold, heat, and acidic pH, all of which can be perceived as pain. Pulp is highly innervated, and unmyelinated nerve fibers extend into the dental tubules along with odontoblast processes near the pulp cavity (Figure 15–8). Such stimuli can affect fluid inside the dentinal tubules, stimulating these nerve fibers and producing tooth sensitivity.

›› MEDICAL APPLICATION

Immune defenses in the oral cavity cannot protect against all infections. **Pharyngitis** and **tonsillitis** are often due to the bacterium *Streptococcus pyrogenes*. White excrescences or **leukoplakia** on the sides of the tongue can be caused by Epstein-Barr virus. **Oral thrush**, a white exudate on the tongue's dorsal surface, is due to a yeast (*Candida albicans*) infection and usually affects neonates or immunocompromised patients.

Enamel

Enamel is the hardest component of the human body, consisting of 96% calcium hydroxyapatite and only 2% to 3% organic material including very few proteins and no collagen. Other ions, such as fluoride, can be incorporated or adsorbed by the hydroxyapatite crystals; enamel containing fluorapatite is more resistant to acidic dissolution caused by microorganisms, hence the addition of fluoride to toothpaste and water supplies.

Enamel consists of uniform, interlocking columns called **enamel rods** (or prisms), each about 5 μm in diameter and surrounded by a thinner layer of other enamel. Each rod extends through the entire thickness of the enamel layer, which averages 2 mm. The precise, interlocked arrangement of the enamel rods is crucial for enamel's hardness and resistance to great pressures during mastication.

In a developing tooth bud, the matrix for the enamel rods is secreted by tall, polarized cells, the **ameloblasts** (Figure 15–9a), which are part of a specialized epithelium in the tooth bud called the **enamel organ**. The apical ends of the ameloblasts face those of the odontoblasts producing predentine (Figure 15–10). An apical extension from each ameloblast, the **ameloblast** (or **Tomes**) **process**, contains numerous secretory granules with the proteins of the enamel matrix. The secreted matrix undergoes very rapid mineralization. Growth of the hydroxyapatite crystals to produce each elongating enamel rod is guided by a small (20 kDa) protein **amelogenin**, the main structural protein of developing enamel.

Ameloblasts are derived from the ectodermal lining of the embryonic oral cavity, while odontoblasts and most tissues of the pulp cavity develop from neural crest cells and

---

FIGURE **15–8** Ultrastructure of dentinal tubule.

(a) TEM shows the calcification of dentin (**D**) at its border with not-yet calcified predentin (**P**). An odontoblast process (**OP**) with microtubules and a few secretory vesicles is seen in the fluid-filled space (**S**) in the dentinal tubule. A process extends from each odontoblast, and the tubules continue completely across the dentin layer. X32,000.

(b) TEM cross section of an odontoblast process (**OP**) near predentin (**P**) shows its close association with an unmyelinated nerve fiber (**N**) extending there from fibers in the pulp cavity. These nerves respond to various stimuli, such as cold temperatures, reaching the nerve fibers through the dentinal tubules. X61,000.

FIGURE 15–9 Ameloblasts and enamel.

(a) In a section of tooth bud ameloblasts (**A**) are tall polarized cells whose apical ends initially contact dentin (**D**). Ameloblasts are joined to form a cell layer surrounded basally by connective tissue (**CT**). As odontoblasts secrete predentin, ameloblasts secrete a matrix lacking collagens, but rich in proteins such as amelogenin that quickly initiate calcium hydroxyapatite formation to make enamel (**E**), the hardest material in the body. Enamel forms a layer but consists of enamel rods or prisms, solidly fused together by more enamel. Each enamel rod represents the product of one ameloblast. No cellular processes occur in enamel, and the layer of ameloblasts

surrounding the developing crown is completely lost during tooth eruption. Teeth that have been decalcified for histologic sectioning typically lose their enamel layer completely. X400. H&E.

(b) Micrograph of a thin preparation of a tooth prepared by grinding. Fine, long tubules can be observed in the dentin (**D**), and rods aligned the same way can be very faintly observed (arrows) in the enamel (**E**). The more prominent lines that cross enamel diagonally represent incremental growth lines produced as the enamel matrix is secreted cyclically by the ameloblast layer. X400. Unstained.

mesoderm, respectively. Together, these tissues produce a series of 52 tooth buds in the developing oral cavity, 20 for the primary teeth and 32 for the secondary or permanent teeth. Primary teeth complete development and begin to erupt about 6 months after birth. Development of the secondary tooth buds arrests at the "bell stage," shown in Figure 15–10a, until about 6 years of age, when these teeth begin to erupt as the primary teeth are shed.

>> **MEDICAL APPLICATION**

Periodontal diseases include **gingivitis**, inflammation of the gums, and **periodontitis**, which involves inflammation at deeper sites, both of which are caused most commonly by bacterial infections with poor oral hygiene. Chronic periodontitis weakens the periodontal ligament and can lead to loosening of the teeth. The depth of the gingival sulcus, measured during clinical dental examinations, is an important indicator of potential periodontal disease.

Periodontium

The **periodontium** comprises the structures responsible for maintaining the teeth in the maxillary and mandibular bones, and includes the **cementum**, the **periodontal ligament**, and the **alveolar bone** with the associated **gingiva** (Figure 15–6b; Figure 15–11).

Cementum covers the dentin of the root and resembles bone, but it is avascular. It is thickest around the root tip where **cementocytes** reside in lacunae with processes in canaliculi, especially near the cementum surface. Although less labile than bone, cementocytes maintain their surrounding matrix and react to stresses by gradually remodeling.

The **periodontal ligament** is fibrous connective tissue with bundled collagen fibers (Sharpey fibers) binding the cementum and the alveolar bone (Figure 15–11). Unlike typical ligaments, it is highly cellular and has a rich supply of blood vessels and nerves, giving the periodontal ligament sensory and nutritive functions in addition to its role in supporting the tooth. It permits limited movement of the tooth within the alveolus and helps protect the alveolus from the

FIGURE **15–10** Tooth formation.

Tooth formation begins in the embryo when ectodermal epithelium lining the oral cavity grows into the underlying mesenchyme of the developing jaws. At a series of sites corresponding to each future tooth, these epithelial cells proliferate extensively and become organized as **enamel organs**, each shaped like a wine glass with its stem initially still attached to the oral lining. **Ameloblasts** form from the innermost layer of cells in the enamel organ. Mesenchymal cells inside the concave portion of the enamel organ include neural crest cells that differentiate as the layer of **odontoblasts** with their apical ends in contact with the apical ends of the ameloblasts.

(a) A section of enamel organ in which production of dentin and enamel has begun. The ameloblast layer (**A**) is separated from the outer enamel epithelium (**OEE**) by a thick intervening region rich in GAGs but with few, widely separated cells. Surrounding the enamel organ is mesenchyme, some parts of which begin to undergo intramembranous bone formation (**B**). Inside the cavity of each enamel organ, mesenchymal cells comprise the dental papilla (**DP**), in which the outermost cells are the layer of odontoblasts (**O**) facing the ameloblasts.

These two cell layers begin to move apart as the odontoblasts begin to produce the layer of predentin (**PD**). Contact with dentin induces each ameloblast to begin secretion of an enamel rod. More slowly, calcifying interprismatic enamel fuses all the enamel rods into a very strong, solid mass. X20. H&E.

(b) Detail of an enamel organ showing the layers of predentin (**PD**) and dentin (**D**) and a layer of enamel (**E**), along with the organized cell layers that produced this material. Odontoblasts (**O**) are in contact with the very cellular mesenchyme of the dental papilla (**DP**) that will become the pulp cavity. Ameloblasts (**A**) are prominent in the now much thinner enamel organ, which is very close to developing bone (**B**). Enamel formation continues until shortly before tooth eruption; formation of dentin continues after eruption until the tooth is fully formed. Odontoblasts persist around the pulp cavity, with processes penetrating the dental layer, producing factors to help maintain dentin. Mesenchymal cells immediately around the enamel organ differentiate into the cells of cementum and other periodontal tissues. X120. H&E.

recurrent pressure exerted during mastication. Its thickness (150-350 μm) is fairly uniform along the root but decreases with aging.

The **alveolar bone** lacks the typical lamellar pattern of adult bone but has osteoblasts and osteocytes engaging in continuous remodeling of the bony matrix. It is surrounded by the periodontal ligament, which serves as its periosteum. Collagen fiber bundles of the periodontal ligament penetrate this bone, binding it to the cementum (Figure 15–11c).

Around the peridontium the keratinized oral mucosa of the **gingiva** is firmly bound to the periosteum of the maxillary and mandibular bones (Figure 15–11). Between the enamel and the gingival epithelium is the **gingival sulcus**, a groove up to 3 mm deep surrounding the neck (Figure 15–11a). A

specialized part of this epithelium, the **junctional epithelium**, is bound to the tooth enamel by means of a cuticle, which resembles a thick basal lamina to which the epithelial cells are attached by numerous hemidesmosomes.

› ESOPHAGUS

The **esophagus** is a muscular tube, about 25 cm long in adults, which transports swallowed material from the pharynx to the stomach. The four layers of the GI tract (Figure 15–12) first become well-established and clearly seen in the esophagus. The esophageal mucosa has nonkeratinized stratified squamous epithelium, and the submucosa contains small mucus-secreting

FIGURE **15–11** Periodontium.

The periodontium of each tooth consists of the **cementum**, **periodontal ligament**, **alveolar bone**, and **gingiva**.

(a) Micrograph of decalcified tooth shows the gingiva. The free gingiva (**FG**) is against the dentin (**D**), with little of the gingival sulcus apparent. Gingiva stratified squamous epithelium over connective tissue of the lamina propria (**LP**). The connective tissue is continuous with that of the periosteum (**P**) covering the alveolar bone (**B**) and with the periodontal ligament (**PL**). X10. H&E.

(b) Micrograph shows the periodontal ligament (**L**) with its many blood vessels (**V**) and insertions into the alveolar bone (**B**). This ligament serves as the periosteum of the alveolar in tooth sockets and is also continuous with developing layers of cementum (**C**) that covers the dentin. Cementum forms a thin layer of bone-like material secreted by large, elongated cells called **cementoblasts**. X100. H&E.

(c) Polarizing light micrograph shows the continuity of collagen fibers in alveolar bone (**B**), with the bundles in the periodontal ligament (**L**). X200. Picrosirius in polarized light.

FIGURE **15–12** Esophagus.

Mucosa

Submucosa

Muscularis

Adventitia

E

LP

MM

(a) In cross section the four major layers of the GI tract are clearly seen. The esophageal mucosa is folded longitudinally, with the lumen largely closed. X10. H&E. **(b)** Higher magnification of the mucosa shows the stratified squamous epithelium (**E**), the lamina propria (**LP**) with scattered lymphocytes, and strands of smooth muscle in the muscularis mucosae (**MM**). X65. H&E.

FIGURE **15–13** Esophagus.

(a) Longitudinal section of esophagus shows mucosa consisting of nonkeratinized stratified squamous epithelium (**SS**), lamina propria (**LP**), and smooth muscles of the muscularis mucosae (**MM**). Beneath the mucosa is the submucosa containing esophageal mucous glands (**GL**) that empty via ducts (**D**) onto the luminal surface. X40. H&E.

(b) Transverse section showing the muscularis halfway along the esophagus reveals a combination of large skeletal or striated muscle fibers (**St**) and smooth muscle fibers (**Sm**) in the outer layer, which is cut transversely here. This transition from muscles under voluntary control to the type controlled autonomically is important in the swallowing mechanism. X200. H&E.

glands, the **esophageal glands**, which lubricate and protect the mucosa (Figure 15–13a). Near the stomach the mucosa also contains groups of glands, the **esophageal cardiac glands**, which secrete additional mucus.

❯❯ MEDICAL APPLICATION

The lubricating mucus produced in the esophagus offers little protection against acid that may move there from the stomach. Such movement can produce **heartburn** or **reflux esophagitis**. An incompetent inferior esophageal sphincter may result in chronic heartburn, which can lead to erosion of the esophageal mucosa or **gastro-esophageal reflux disease (GERD)**. Untreated GERD can produce metaplastic changes in the stratified squamous epithelium of the esophageal mucosa, a condition called **Barrett esophagus**.

Swallowing begins with voluntary muscle action but finishes with involuntary peristalsis. In approximately the upper one-third of the esophagus, the muscularis is exclusively skeletal muscle like that of the tongue. The middle portion of the esophagus has a combination of skeletal and smooth muscle fibers (Figure 15–13b), and in the lower third the muscularis is exclusively smooth muscle. Only the distal 1 to 2 cm of the esophagus, in the peritoneal cavity, is covered by serosa; the rest is enclosed by the loose connective tissue of the adventitia, which blends into the surrounding tissue.

❯ STOMACH

The stomach is a greatly dilated segment of the digestive tract whose main functions are:

- To continue the digestion of carbohydrates initiated by the amylase of saliva,
- To add an acidic fluid to the ingested food and mixing its contents into a viscous mass called **chyme** by the churning activity of the muscularis,
- To begin digestion of triglycerides by a secreted lipase, and
- To promote the initial digestion of proteins with the enzyme **pepsin**.

❯❯ MEDICAL APPLICATION

For various reasons, including autoimmunity, parietal cells may be damaged to the extent that insufficient quantities of intrinsic factor are secreted and **vitamin B$_{12}$** is not absorbed adequately. This vitamin is a cofactor required for DNA synthesis; low levels of vitamin B$_{12}$ can reduce proliferation of erythroblasts, producing **pernicious anemia**.

Four major regions make up the stomach: the cardia, fundus, body, and pylorus (Figure 15–14a). The **cardia** is a narrow transitional zone, 1.5-3 cm wide, between the esophagus and the stomach; the **pylorus** is the funnel-shaped region that

FIGURE **15–14** Stomach.

(a) **Stomach regions, anterior view**

(c) **Stomach wall, sectional view**

The stomach is a muscular dilation of the digestive tract where mechanical and chemical digestion occurs. **(a)** The major stomach regions are the **cardia, fundus, body**, and **pylorus**, all with longitudinal gastric folds, or rugae. The muscularis has three layers.

(b) At the esophagogastric junction, stratified squamous epithelium (**SSE**) lining the esophagus is abruptly replaced by simple columnar epithelium (**SCE**) of the stomach. Also seen here are the mucous esophageal cardiac glands (**ECG**) beneath the lamina propria (**LP**) and muscularis mucosae (**MM**). X60. H&E.

(c) The mucosa of the stomach wall contains invaginations called **gastric pits** that lead into **gastric glands**. These structures are lined by simple columnar epithelium containing five functional cell types.

(d) A histologic section of the gastric mucosa shows the gastric pits (**P**) and glands (**GG**) surrounded by cells of the lamina propria. The underlying muscularis mucosae (**MM**) is also seen. X60. H&E.

opens into the small intestine. Both these regions are primarily involved with mucus production and are similar histologically. The much larger **fundus** and **body** regions are identical in microscopic structure and are the sites of gastric glands releasing acidic gastric juice. The mucosa and submucosa of the empty stomach have large, longitudinally directed folds called **rugae**, which flatten when the stomach fills with food. The wall in all regions of the stomach is made up of all four major layers (Figures 15–14c and 15–15).

Mucosa

Changing abruptly at the esophagogastric junction (Figures 15–14b), the mucosal surface of the stomach is a simple columnar epithelium that invaginates deeply into the lamina propria. The invaginations form millions of **gastric pits**, each with an opening to the stomach lumen (see Figure 15–14; Figure 15–16). The **surface mucous cells** that line the lumen and gastric pits secrete a thick, adherent, and highly viscous mucous layer that is rich in bicarbonate ions and protects the mucosa from both abrasive effects of intraluminal food and the corrosive effects of stomach acid.

The gastric pits lead to long, branched, tubular glands that extend through the full thickness of the lamina propria. **Stem cells** for the epithelium that lines the glands, pits, and stomach lumen are found in a narrow segment (isthmus) between each gastric pit and the gastric glands. The pluripotent stem cells divide asymmetrically, producing progenitor cells for all the other epithelial cells. Some of these move upward to replace surface mucous cells, which have a turnover time of 4 to 7 days. Other progenitor cells migrate more deeply and differentiate into the secretory cells of the glands that turn over much more slowly than the surface mucous cells.

The vascularized **lamina propria** that surrounds and supports the gastric pits and glands contains smooth muscle fibers, lymphoid cells, capillaries, and lymphatics. Separating the mucosa from the underlying submucosa is a layer of smooth muscle, the **muscularis mucosae** (Figure 15–15).

In the fundus and body the **gastric glands** themselves fill most of the mucosa, with several such glands formed by branching at the isthmus or neck of each gastric pit. Secretory epithelial cells of the gastric glands are distributed unevenly and release products that are key to the stomach's functions. These cells are of four major types and important properties of each are as follows:

■ **Mucous neck cells** are present in clusters or as single cells among the other cells in the necks of gastric glands and include many progenitor and immature surface mucous cells (Figure 15–17). Less columnar than the surface mucous cells lining the gastric pits, mucous neck cells are often distorted by neighboring cells, but they have round nuclei and apical secretory granules. Their mucus secretion is less alkaline than that of the surface epithelial mucous cells.

FIGURE **15–15** Wall of the stomach with rugae.

A low-magnification micrograph of the stomach wall at the fundus shows the relative thickness of the four major layers: the mucosa (**M**), the submucosa (**SM**), the muscularis externa (**ME**), and the serosa (**S**). Two rugae (folds) cut transversely and consisting of mucosa and submucosa are included. The mucosa is packed with branched tubular glands penetrating the full thickness of the lamina propria so that this sublayer cannot be distinguished at this magnification. The **muscularis mucosae** (arrows), immediately beneath the basal ends of the gastric glands, is shown. The submucosa is largely loose connective tissue, with blood vessels (**V**) and lymphatics. X12. H&E.

FIGURE **15–16** Gastric pits and glands.

(a) SEM of the stomach lining cleared of its mucous layer reveals closely placed gastric pits (**P**) surrounded by polygonal apical ends of surface mucous cells. X600.

(b) A section of the same lining shows that these surface mucous cells are part of a simple columnar epithelium continuous with the lining of the pits (**P**). Each pit extends into the lamina propria and then branches into several tubular glands. These glands coil and fill most of the mucosa. Around the various cells of the closely-packed gastric glands are cells, capillaries, and small lymphatics of the connective tissue lamina propria. X200. H&E.

- **Parietal** (oxyntic) **cells** produce hydrochloric acid (HCl) and are present among the mucous neck cells and throughout deeper parts of the gland. They are large cells, usually appearing rounded or pyramidal, each with one (sometimes two) central round nucleus. The cytoplasm is intensely eosinophilic due to the high density of mitochondria (Figure 15–17). A striking ultrastructural feature of an active parietal cell is a deep, circular invagination of the apical plasma membrane to form an **intracellular canaliculus** with a large surface area produced by thousands of microvilli (Figure 15–18). As shown in Figure 15–19, **carbonic anhydrase** catalyzes the conversion of cytoplasmic water and CO_2 into HCO_3^+ and H^+. The HCO_3^+ is transported from the basal side of the cell and H^+ is pumped from the cell apically, along with Cl^-. In the lumen the H^+ and Cl^- ions combine to form HCl. While the gastric secretion becomes highly acidic, the mucosa itself remains at a more neutral pH partly because of the bicarbonate released into the lamina propria. The abundant mitochondria provide energy primarily for operating the cells' ion pumps.

  Parietal cells also secrete **intrinsic factor**, a glycoprotein required for uptake of vitamin B_{12} in the small intestine.

  Parietal cell secretory activity is stimulated both by parasympathetic innervation and by paracrine release of histamine and the polypeptide **gastrin** from enteroendocrine cells.

- **Chief (zymogenic) cells** predominate in the lower regions of the gastric glands (Figure 15–17) and have all the characteristics of active protein-secreting cells. Ultrastructurally chief cells show abundant RER and numerous apical secretory granules (Figure 15–20). The granules contain inactive enzyme **pepsinogens**, precursors which are converted in the acid environment of the stomach into active **pepsins** (Gr. *peptein*, to digest). Pepsins are endoproteinases with broad specificity and maximal activity at a pH between 1.8 and 3.5. Pepsins initiate the hydrolysis of ingested protein in the stomach. Chief cells also produce **gastric lipase**, which digests many lipids.

- **Enteroendocrine cells** are scattered epithelial cells in the gastric mucosa with endocrine or paracrine functions. In the fundus small enteroendocrine cells secreting **serotonin** (5-hydroxytryptamine) are found at the basal lamina of the gastric glands (Figure 15-20). In the pylorus other enteroendocrine cells are located in contact with the glandular lumens, including **G cells** producing the peptide **gastrin**.

Various enteroendocrine cells secreting different hormones, usually peptides, are also found in the intestinal mucosa and are of major importance for function of the digestive tract. Important examples are summarized in Table 15–1. Seldom seen by routine light microscopy, these cells can be visualized by TEM tissue treatment with chromium or silver salts. This provided the alternative

FIGURE **15–17** Gastric glands.

(a)   **(b)**   **(c)**   **(d)**

Throughout the **fundus** and **body** regions of the stomach, the gastric pits lead to gastric glands with various cell types.
(a) The long, coiled gastric glands penetrate the complete thickness of the mucosa, from the gastric pits (**GP**) to the muscularis mucosae (**MM**).

(b) In the neck of a gastric gland, below the surface mucous cells (**SM**) lining the gastric pit, are small mucous neck cells (**MN**), scattered individually or clustered among parietal cells (**P**) and stem cells that give rise to all epithelial cells of the glands. The numerous parietal cells (**P**) are large distinctive cells often bulging from the tubules, with central nuclei surrounded by intensely eosinophilic cytoplasm with unusual ultrastructure. These cells produce HCl, and the numerous

mitochondria required for this process cause the eosinophilia. Chief cells (**C**) begin to appear in the neck region. Around these tubular glands are various cells and microvasculature in connective tissue.

(c) Near the muscularis mucosae (**MM**), the bases of these glands contain fewer parietal cells (**P**) but many more zymogenic chief cells (**C**). Chief cells are found in clusters, with basal nuclei and basophilic cytoplasm. From their apical ends chief cells secrete pepsinogen, the zymogen precursor for the major protease pepsin. Zymogen granules are often removed or stain poorly in routine preparations. Both X200. H&E.

(d) Diagram showing general morphology and functions of major gastric gland cells.

names **enterochromaffin (EC) cells** and **argentaffin cells,** respectively. Now usually visualized immunohistochemically using antibodies against their product, they are named with the initial letter of the main hormone they produce (see Table 15–1). Most of these cells process amines and are also collectively called **APUD cells** for their "amine precursor uptake and decarboxylation" activity. All such cells are more generally considered part of the **diffuse neuroendocrine system (DNES),** which is discussed further in Chapter 20.

FIGURE **15–18** Ultrastructure of parietal cells.

(a) A TEM of an active parietal cell shows abundant microvilli (**MV**) protruding into the intracellular canaliculi, near the lumen and deep in the cell. The cytoplasm contains numerous mitochondria (**M**). X10,200.

(b) Composite diagram of a parietal cell shows the ultrastructural differences between a resting cell (left) and an active cell (right). In the resting cell, a number of tubulovesicular structures (**TV**) can be below the apical plasmalemma (left), but the cell has few microvilli and only a short intracellular canaliculus (**IC**) among the mitochondria (**M**) and Golgi vesicles (**G**). When stimulated to produce HCl (right), the tubular vesicles fuse with the cell membrane to form the large intracellular canaliculus (**IC**) and microvilli (**MV**), thus providing a generous increase in the surface of the cell membrane for diffusion and ion pumps. Prolonged activity may produce more mitochondria (**M**).

(*Figure 15–18a, with permission, from Dr Susumu Ito, Department of Cell Biology, Harvard Medical School, Boston, MA.*)

FIGURE **15–19** Synthesis of HCl by parietal cells.

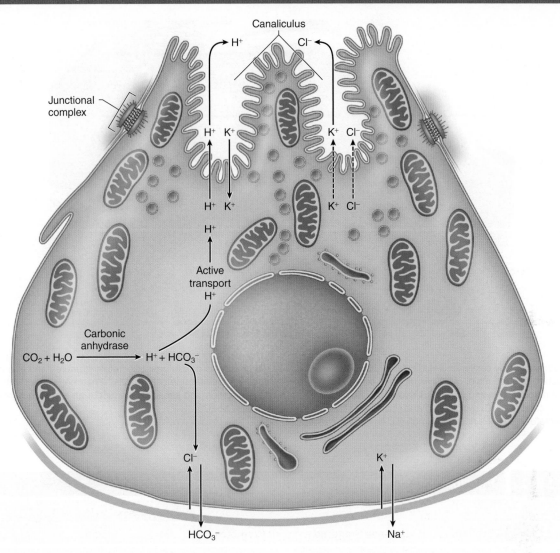

Diagram shows the main steps in the synthesis of HCl. Active transport by ATPase is indicated by arrows and diffusion is indicated by dotted arrows. Under the action of **carbonic anhydrase**, carbonic acid is produced from CO_2. Carbonic acid dissociates into a **bicarbonate ion** and a **proton (H^+)**, which is pumped into the stomach lumen in exchange for K^+. A high concentration of intracellular K^+ is maintained by the Na^+, K^+ ATPase, while HCO_3^- is exchanged for Cl^- by an antiport.

Chloride ions diffuse from the cell into the canaliculi and combine with protons in the lumen of the gastric gland to form HCl.

The tubulovesicles of the cell apex are seen to be related to HCl secretion, because their number decreases after parietal cell stimulation as microvilli increase. Most of the bicarbonate ion returns to the blood locally and is important for maintaining the neutral pH of the mucosa. Other HCO_3^- is taken up by surface mucous cells and used to raise the pH of mucus.

Upon stimulation, these cells release their hormone products that then exert paracrine (local) or endocrine (systemic) effects via the vasculature. Cells of the digestive tract DNES fall into two classes: a "closed" type, in which the cellular apex is covered by neighboring epithelial cells (Figure 15–20), and an "open" type, in which the constricted apical end of the cell contacts the lumen and bears chemoreceptors that sample the lumen's contents. Effects of the hormones include regulation of peristalsis and tract motility; secretion of digestive enzymes, water, and electrolytes; and the sense of being satiated after eating.

In the cardia and pylorus regions of the stomach, the mucosa also contains tubular glands, with long pits, branching into coiled secretory portions, called **cardial glands** and **pyloric glands** (Figure 15–21). These glands lack both parietal and chief cells, primarily secreting abundant mucus.

Other Layers

The other major layers of the stomach wall are summarized in Figures 15–14 and 15–15. In all stomach regions the **submucosa**

TEM of a transversely sectioned gastric gland shows the ultrastructure of three major cell types. Parietal cells (**P**) contain abundant mitochondria and intracellular canaliculi (**IC**). Also shown are chief cells (**C**), which have extensive rough ER and apical secretory granules near the lumen (**L**). An enteroendocrine cell (**E**) shows dense basal secretory granules and is a closed-type enteroendocrine cell; that is, it has no contact with the gland's lumen and secretes product in an endocrine/paracrine manner. X1200.

TABLE 15–1   Principal enteroendocrine cells in the gastrointestinal tract.

Cell Type	Major Location	Hormone Produced	Major Action	
			Promotes	Inhibits
D cells	Pylorus, duodenum, and pancreatic islets	Somatostatin		Secretion from other DNES cells nearby
EC cells	Stomach, small and large intestines	Serotonin and substance P	Increased gut motility	
G cells	Pylorus	Gastrin	Gastric acid secretion	
I cells	Small intestine	Cholecystokinin (CCK)	Pancreatic enzyme secretion, gallbladder contraction	Gastric acid secretion
K cells	Duodenum and jejunum	Gastric inhibitory polypeptide (GIP)		Gastric acid secretion
L cells	Ileum and colon	Glucagon-like peptide (GLP-1)	Insulin secretion	Gastric acid secretion Sense of hunger
L cells	Ileum and colon	Peptide YY	H_2O and electrolyte absorption in large intestine	Gastric acid secretion
Mo cells	Small intestine	Motilin	Increased gut motility	
N cells	Ileum	Neurotensin		Gastric acid secretion
S cells	Small intestine	Secretin	Pancreatic and biliary bicarbonate and water secretion	Gastric acid secretion Stomach emptying

FIGURE **15–21** Pyloric glands.

The pyloric region of the stomach has deep gastric pits (**P**) leading to short, coiled pyloric glands (**G**) in the lamina propria (**LP**). Cardial glands are rather similar histologically and functionally. Cells of these glands secrete mucus and lysozyme primarily, with a few enteroendocrine G cells also present. The glands and pits are surrounded by cells of the lamina propria connective tissue containing capillaries, lymphatics and MALT. Immediately beneath the glands is the smooth muscle layer of the muscularis mucosae. X140. H&E.

mucus, HCl, and digestive enzymes from the gastric mucosa. At the pylorus the middle layer is greatly thickened to form the **pyloric sphincter**. The stomach is covered by a thin **serosa**.

› SMALL INTESTINE

The small intestine is the site where the digestive processes are completed and where the nutrients (products of digestion) are absorbed by cells of the epithelial lining. The small intestine is relatively long—approximately 5 m—and consists of three segments: the **duodenum**, **jejunum**, and **ileum**. These segments have most histologic features in common and are discussed together.

>> **MEDICAL APPLICATION**

Leiomyomas, benign tumors of smooth muscle cells, are the most common type of tumor in the stomach and small intestine and may become large. Autopsy records suggest that the muscularis of the stomach may include leiomyomas in up to 50% of the population older than 50 years.

Mucosa

Viewed macroscopically, the lining of the small intestine shows a series of permanent circular or semilunar folds (**plicae circulares**), consisting of mucosa and submucosa (Figures 15–22a and 15–23), which are best developed in the jejunum. Densely covering the entire mucosa of the small intestine are short (0.5- to 1.5-mm) mucosal outgrowths called **villi** that project into the lumen (Figure 15–22). These finger- or leaflike projections are covered by a simple columnar epithelium of absorptive cells called **enterocytes**, with many interspersed **goblet cells**. Each villus has a core of loose connective tissue that extends from the lamina propria and contains fibroblasts, smooth muscle fibers, lymphocytes and plasma cells, fenestrated capillaries, and a central lymphatic called a **lacteal**.

>> **MEDICAL APPLICATION**

Celiac disease (celiac sprue) is a disorder of the small intestine mucosa that causes **malabsorption** and can lead to damage or destruction of the villi. The cause of celiac disease is an immune reaction against gluten or other proteins in wheat and certain other types of grain. The resulting inflammation affects the enterocytes, leading to reduced nutrient absorption.

Between the villi are the openings of short tubular glands called **intestinal glands** or **crypts** (or **crypts of Lieberkühn**) and the epithelium of each villus is continuous with that of the intervening glands (Figure 15–22c). The epithelium of the intestinal glands includes differentiating cells

is composed of connective tissue with large blood and lymph vessels and many lymphoid cells, macrophages, and mast cells. The **muscularis** has three poorly defined layers of smooth muscle: an outer longitudinal layer, a middle circular layer, and an innermost oblique layer. Rhythmic contractions of the muscularis thoroughly mix ingested food and chyme with

FIGURE **15–22** Absorptive surface of the small intestine.

(a) Layers

Mucosa
Submucosa
Muscularis
Inner circular layer
Outer longitudinal layer
Serosa

Circular folds
Circular fold

(b) Section of small intestine

Intestinal villi
Submucosa
Serosa
Inner circular layer
Outer longitudinal layer
Muscularis

(c) Intestinal villus

Capillary network
Goblet cells
Lacteal
Intestinal gland
Lymphatic nodule
Enterocyte (absorbs nutrients)
Paneth cells (innate immunity)
Muscularis mucosae
Venule
Lymph vessel
Arteriole

(d) Intestinal villi

Intestinal lumen
Villi
Simple columnar epithelium
Lamina propria
Goblet cells

(e) Microvilli

Simple columnar cell
Microvilli
Intestinal lumen

(a) The **mucosa** and **submucosa** are the inner two of the gut's four concentric layers. **(b)** They form circular folds or **plicae circulares**, which increase the absorptive area. **(c)** They are lined by a dense covering of fingerlike projections called **villi**. Internally each villus contains lamina propria connective tissue with microvasculature and lymphatics called **lacteals**.

(d) Villi are covered with a simple columnar epithelium composed of absorptive enterocytes and goblet cells. X70. H&E.
(e) At the apical cell membrane of each enterocyte are located dense **microvilli**, which serve to increase greatly the absorptive surface of the cell. X18,000. TEM.

FIGURE **15–23** Circular folds (plicae circulares) of the jejunum.

The mucosa and submucosa (**SM**) of the small intestine form distinct projecting folds called plicae (**P**), which encircle or spiral around the inner circumference and are best developed in the jejunum. On each fold the mucosa forms a dense covering of projecting structures called **villi** (**V**). In this longitudinal section the two layers of the muscularis (**M**) are clearly

distinguished. The inner layer has smooth muscle encircling the submucosa; the outer layer runs lengthwise just inside the serosa (**S**), the gut's outer layer. This arrangement of smooth muscle provides for strong peristaltic movement of the gut's contents. X12. H&E.

and pluripotent stem cells for all the cell types of the small intestine. These include the following:

- **Enterocytes**, the absorptive cells, are tall columnar cells, each with an oval nucleus located basally (Figure 15–24). The apical end of each enterocyte displays a prominent ordered region called the **striated** (or **brush**) **border**. Ultrastructurally the striated border is seen to be a layer of densely packed **microvilli** covered by **glycocalyx** through which nutrients are taken into the cells (Figures 15–22e and 15–24c). As discussed in Chapter 4, each microvillus is a cylindrical protrusion of the apical cytoplasm approximately 1 μm tall and 0.1 μm in diameter containing actin filaments and enclosed by the cell membrane. Each enterocyte has an average of 3000 microvilli and each 1 mm² of mucosal surface contains about 200 million of these structures. Microvilli, villi, and the plicae circulares all greatly increase

the mucosal surface area in contact with nutrients in the lumen, which is an important feature in an organ specialized for nutrient absorption. It is estimated that plicae increase the intestinal surface area 3-fold, the villi increase it 10-fold, and the microvilli increase it another 20-fold, resulting in a total absorptive area of over 200 m² in the small intestine!

The mechanism of nutrient absorption varies with the different molecules produced by digestion. Disaccharidases and peptidases secreted by the enterocytes and located within the glycocalyx hydrolyze disaccharides and dipeptides into monosaccharides and amino acids. These are easily absorbed by active transport and immediately released again from the enterocytes for uptake by the capillaries. Digestion of fats by gastric and pancreatic lipases produces lipid subunits, including glycerol, monoglycerides, and fatty acids, which are emulsified by bile salts into small (2 nm) micelles

FIGURE **15–24** Cells covering the villi.

(a) The columnar epithelium that covers intestinal villi consists mainly of the tall absorptive enterocytes (**E**). The apical ends of these cells are joined and covered by a **brush border** of microvilli. Covered by a coating of glycoproteins, the brush border, along with the mucus-secreting goblet cells (**G**), stains with carbohydrate staining methods. Other cells of the epithelium are scattered enteroendocrine cells, which are difficult to identify in routine preparations, and various immune cells such as intraepithelial lymphocytes. The small spherical nuclei of lymphocytes can be seen between the enterocytes. X250. PAS-hematoxylin.

(b) At higher magnification individual **microvilli** of enterocytes are better seen and the striated appearance of the border is apparent. X500. **(c)** TEM shows microvilli and densely packed mitochondria of enterocytes (**E**), and enteroendocrine cells (**EC**) with basal secretory granules can be distinguished along the basal lamina. X2500.

from which lipids enter enterocytes by passive diffusion and membrane transporters. These lipids are reesterified into triglycerides in the enterocyte smooth ER and then complexed with apoproteins in the Golgi apparatus, producing **chylomicrons** that are discharged from the cell's basolateral surface for uptake by the lacteal. Figure 15–25 summarizes basic aspects of lipid absorption.

- **Goblet cells** are interspersed among the absorptive enterocytes (see Figures 15–22d and 15–24a, b). They secrete glycoprotein mucins that are then hydrated to form mucus, whose main function is to protect and lubricate the lining of the intestine.
- **Paneth cells**, located in the basal portion of the intestinal crypts below the stem cells, are exocrine cells with large,

eosinophilic secretory granules in their apical cytoplasm (Figure 15–26). Paneth cell granules release lysozyme, phospholipase A_2, and hydrophobic peptides called **defensins**, all of which bind and break down membranes of microorganisms and bacterial cell walls. Paneth cells have an important role in innate immunity and in regulating the microenvironment of the intestinal crypts.

- **Enteroendocrine cells** are present in varying numbers throughout the length of the small intestine, secreting various peptide hormones (see Table 15–1). Many of these are of the "open" type, in which the constricted apical end of the cell contacts the intestinal lumen and has chemoreceptors similar to those of taste buds, sampling levels of certain nutrients such as sugars to regulate hormone release basally (Figure 15–27).

FIGURE **15–25** Lipid absorption and processing by enterocytes.

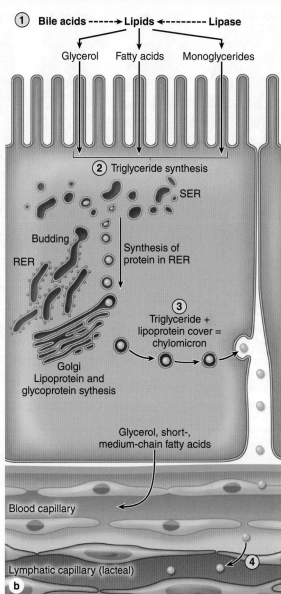

(a) TEM shows that enterocytes involved in lipid absorption accumulate many small lipid droplets in vesicles of the smooth ER (**SER**). These vesicles fuse near the nucleus, forming larger globules that are moved laterally and cross the cell membrane to the extracellular space (**arrows**) for eventual uptake by lymphatic capillaries (lacteals) in the lamina propria. X3000.

(b) Diagram showing lipid processing by enterocytes. Ingested fats are emulsified by **bile acids** to form a suspension of lipid droplets from which lipids are digested by **lipases** to produce glycerol, fatty acids, and monoglycerides ①. The products of hydrolysis diffuse passively across the microvilli membranes and are collected in the cisternae of the smooth ER, where they are resynthesized as **triglycerides** ②. Processed through the RER and Golgi, these triglycerides are surrounded by a thin layer of proteins and packaged in vesicles containing **chylomicrons** (0.2-1 μm in diameter) of lipid complexed with protein ③. Chylomicrons are transferred to the lateral cell membrane, secreted by exocytosis, and flow into the extracellular space in the direction of the lamina propria, where most enter the lymph in **lacteals** ④.

(*Figure 15–25a, with permission, from Dr Robert R. Cardell, Jr, Department of Cancer and Cell Biology, University of Cincinnati College of Medicine, Cincinnati, OH.*)

FIGURE 15–26 Intestinal crypts or glands, with Paneth cells.

(a) Between villi (**V**) throughout the small intestine, the covering epithelium invaginates into the lamina propria (**LP**) to form short tubular glands called intestinal glands or intestinal crypts (**IC**). The lining near the openings of the crypts contains a population of stem cells for the entire epithelial lining of the small intestine. Daughter cells slowly move with the growing epithelium out of the crypts, differentiating as **goblet cells, enterocytes,** and **enteroendocrine cells**. These cells continue to move up each villus and within a week are shed at the tip, with billions

shed throughout the small intestine each day. At the base of the crypts are many Paneth cells (**P**) with an innate immune function. The submucosa (**S**) has many lymphatics draining lacteals. X200. H&E.

(b) Higher magnification at the base of an intestinal gland shows the typical eosinophilic granules of Paneth cells (**P**), along with an open-type enteroendocrine cell (**EC**) and a differentiating goblet cell (**G**). X400. H&E.

▪ **M (microfold) cells** are specialized epithelial cells in the mucosa of the ileum overlying the lymphoid follicles of Peyer patches. As discussed in Chapter 14, these cells are characterized by the presence of basal membrane invaginations or pockets containing many intraepithelial lymphocytes and antigen-presenting cells (see Figure 14–13). M cells selectively endocytose antigens and transport them to the underlying lymphocytes and dendritic cells, which then migrate to lymph nodes for an appropriate immune response.

Other Layers

Along the entire small intestine loose connective tissue of the mucosal lamina propria contains extensive blood and lymph

microvasculature, nerve fibers, smooth muscle cells, and diffuse lymphoid tissue. The lamina propria penetrates the core of each intestinal villus, bringing with it microvasculature, lymphatics, and nerves (see Figure 15–22c; Figure 15–28). Smooth muscle fibers extending from the muscularis mucosae produce rhythmic movements of the villi that increase the absorption efficiency. Fibers of the muscularis mucosae also produce local movements of plicae circulares that help propel lymph from the lacteals into submucosal and mesenteric lymphatics.

The submucosa has larger blood and lymph vessels and the diffuse, interconnected neurons of the **submucosal (Meissner) nerve plexus**. The proximal part of the duodenum has in the submucosa and mucosa large clusters of branched tubular mucous glands, the **duodenal (or Brunner) glands**, with

FIGURE **15–27** Enteroendocrine cell.

TEM of an open-type enteroendocrine cell in the epithelium of the duodenum shows microvilli at its apical end in contact with the lumen. The microvilli have components of nutrient-sensing and signal transduction systems similar in some components to those of taste bud gustatory cells. Activation of these cells by nutrients triggers the release at the baso-lateral membranes of peptide factors, including satiation peptides, which diffuse through extracellular fluid to enter capillaries (endocrine) or to bind receptors on nearby nerve terminals, smooth muscle fibers, or other cells (paracrine). Hormones from the various enteroendocrine cells act in a coordinated manner to control gut motility, regulate secretion of enzymes, HCl, bile and other components for digestion, and produce the sense of satiety in the brain. X4500.

(With permission, from A.G.E. Pearse, Department of Histochemistry, Royal Postgraduate Medical School, London, UK.)

FIGURE **15–28** Microvasculature, lymphatics, and muscle in villi.

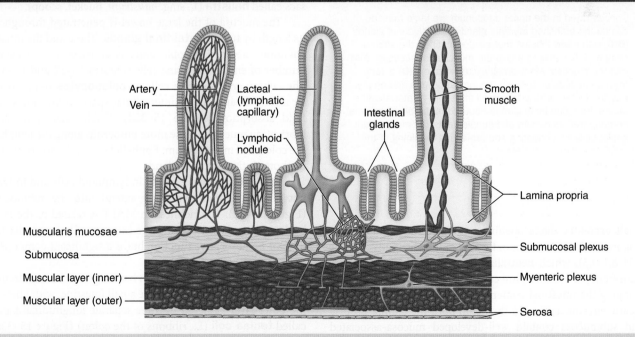

The villi of the small intestine contain blood microvasculature (left), lymphatic capillaries called lacteals (center), and both innervation and smooth muscle fibers (right).

FIGURE **15–29** Duodenal (Brunner) glands.

Concentrated in the upper duodenum are large masses of compound branched **mucous glands**, the duodenal glands (**DG**), with many lobules that occupy much of the submucosa and may extend above the muscularis mucosae (**MM**) into the mucosa. Many small excretory ducts (**D**) extend from these lobules through the lamina propria and empty into the lumen among the small intestinal crypts. Alkaline mucus from duodenal glands neutralizes the pH of material entering the duodenum and supplements the mucus from goblet cells in lubricating and protecting the lining of the small intestine. X100. H&E.

small excretory ducts opening among the intestinal crypts (Figure 15–29). Mucus from these glands is distinctly alkaline (pH 8.1-9.3), which neutralizes chyme entering the duodenum from the pylorus, protecting the mucous membrane, and bringing the intestinal contents to the optimum pH for pancreatic enzyme action. In the ileum both the lamina propria and submucosa contain well-developed mucosa-associated lymphoid tissue (MALT), consisting of the large lymphoid nodule aggregates known as **Peyer patches** underlying the epithelial M cells.

The muscularis is well developed in the small intestine, composed of an internal circular layer, an external longitudinal layer, and between them the neurons of the **myenteric (Auerbach) nerve plexus** which produce peristalsis (Figure 15–30). Neurons of both the submucosal and myenteric plexuses are largely autonomic and collectively make up the large enteric nervous system. The small intestine is covered by a thin serosa with mesothelium continuous with that of mesenteries (see Figure 15–22a).

>> **MEDICAL APPLICATION**

Crohn disease is a chronic inflammatory bowel disease that occurs most commonly in the ileum or colon, resulting from a poorly understood combination of immune, environmental, and genetic factors. Excessive lymphocytic activity and inflammation occur in any or all layers of the tract wall, producing pain, localized bleeding, malabsorption, and diarrhea.

> **LARGE INTESTINE**

The large intestine or bowel, which absorbs water and electrolytes and forms indigestible material into feces, has the following regions: the short **cecum**, with the **ileocecal valve** and the **appendix**; the ascending, transverse, descending, and sigmoid **colon**; and the **rectum**, where feces is stored prior to evacuation (Figure 15–31). The mucosa lacks villi and except in the rectum has no major folds. Less than one-third as long as the small intestine, the large intestine has a greater diameter (6-7 cm). The wall of the colon is puckered into a series of large sacs called **haustra** (L. sing. *haustrum*, bucket, scoop).

The mucosa of the large bowel is penetrated throughout its length by tubular **intestinal glands**. These and the intestinal lumen are lined by goblet and absorptive cells, with a small number of enteroendocrine cells (Figures 15–32 and 15–33). The columnar absorptive cells or **colonocytes** have irregular microvilli and dilated intercellular spaces indicating active fluid absorption (Figure 15–33d). Goblet cells producing lubricating mucus become more numerous along the length of the colon and in the rectum. Epithelial stem cells are located in the bottom third of each gland.

The lamina propria is rich in lymphoid cells and in lymphoid nodules that frequently extend into the submucosa (Figure 15–32). The richness in MALT is related to the large bacterial population of the large intestine. The appendix has little or no absorptive function but is a significant component of MALT (see Chapter 14).

The muscularis of the colon has longitudinal and circular layers but differs from that of the small intestine, with fibers of the outer layer gathered in three separate longitudinal bands called **teniae coli** (L., ribbons of the colon) (Figure 15–32a). Intraperitoneal portions of the colon are covered by serosa, which is characterized by small, pendulous protuberances of adipose tissue.

FIGURE **15–30** Small intestine muscularis and myenteric plexus.

(a) Transverse sections of the small intestinal wall show the orientation of the internal (**IM**) and external (**EM**) smooth muscle layers. The inner layer is predominantly circular while the outer layer is longitudinal. The serosa (**S**) is a thin connective tissue covered here by a mesothelium of cuboidal cells. X200. PT.

(b) Between the internal and external layers of muscularis (**IM** and **EM**) are ganglia of pale-staining neurons and other cells of the myenteric plexus (**MP**). X100. H&E.

>> MEDICAL APPLICATION

Colorectal cancer is an **adenocarcinoma** that develops initially from benign **adenomatous polyps** in the mucosal epithelium. Such polyps usually occur in epithelium of rectum, sigmoid colon, or distal descending colon and are more common in individuals with low-fiber diets, which reduce the bulk of fecal material, and this in turn prolongs contact of the mucosa with toxins in feces. Screens for colorectal cancer include **sigmoidoscopy** or **colonoscopy** to see polyps and tests for **fecal occult blood** resulting from mucosal bleeding as an adenocarcinoma invades more deeply into the mucosa.

>> MEDICAL APPLICATION

Swollen blood vessels in the mucosa or submucosa of the anal canal can cause a painful disorder called **hemorrhoids**. This common condition typically results from a low-fiber diet, **constipation**, prolonged sitting, or straining at defecation, conditions that produce increased pressure on these blood vessels.

The distal end of the GI tract is the **anal canal**, 3-4 cm long. At the **rectoanal junction** the simple columnar mucosal lining of the rectum is replaced by stratified squamous epithelium (Figure 15–34). The mucosa and submucosa of the anal canal form several longitudinal folds, the **anal columns** (Figure 15–31b), in which the lamina propria and submucosa include sinuses of the rectal venous plexus. Near the anus the circular layer of the rectum's muscularis forms the **internal anal sphincter**. Defecation involves the action of voluntary muscle comprising the **external anal sphincter** (Figure 15–31b).

Table 15–2 summarizes the histologic features distinguishing each region of the digestive tract.

>> MEDICAL APPLICATION

Herniation or outpocketing of the mucosa and submucosa of the colon can occur between the teniae coli, forming bulges (diverticula) and a condition called **diverticulosis**. This disorder can result from structural defects in the colon wall or from high intraluminal pressure or **constipation**. Fecal material can become immobilized in the diverticula and cause localized inflammation or **diverticulitis**.

FIGURE **15–31** Large intestine.

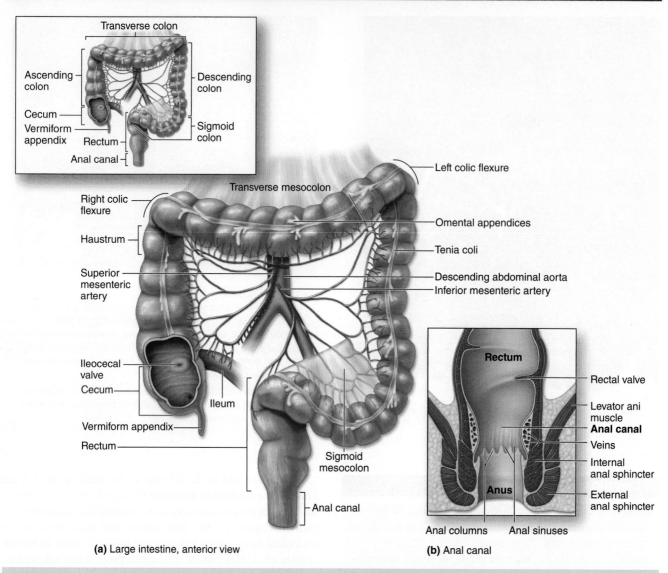

(a) Large intestine, anterior view **(b)** Anal canal

As shown at the top, the large intestine consists of the cecum; the ascending, transverse, descending, and sigmoid regions of the colon; and the rectum. **(a)** Anterior view of the large intestine with the proximal end exposed shows the **ileocecal valve** at its attachment to the ileum, along with the sac called the **cecum** and its extension, the **appendix**. The mucosa has only shallow plicae and no villi. The muscularis has two layers, but the outer longitudinal layer consists only of three distinct bundles of muscle fibers called **teniae coli** that produce the haustra in the colon wall. The serosa of the colon is continuous with that of the supporting mesenteries and displays a series of suspended masses of adipose tissue called **omental appendages**.

(b) At the distal end of the rectum, the anal canal, the mucosa, and submucosa are highly vascularized, with venous sinuses, and are folded as a series of longitudinal folds called **anal columns** (of Morgagni) with intervening **anal sinuses**. Fecal material accumulates in the rectum is eliminated by muscular contraction, including action of an **internal anal sphincter** continuous with the circular layer of the muscularis and an **external sphincter** of striated (voluntary) muscle.

FIGURE **15–32** Wall of the large intestine.

(a) Large intestine tunics

Opening to intestinal gland
Simple columnar epithelium
Intestinal gland
Lamina propria
Lymphatic nodule
Muscularis mucosae
Goblet cells
Lumen
Mucosa
Submucosa
Muscularis
Circular layer
Longitudinal layer (tenia coli)
Nerves
Arteriole
Venule
Serosa

(b) Large intestine mucosa and submucosa

Lumen
Opening to intestinal gland
Goblet cells
Simple columnar epithelium
Intestinal gland
Muscularis mucosae

(a) Diagram shows the wall of the large intestine composed of the four typical layers. The **submucosa** is well vascularized. The **muscularis** has a typical inner circular layer, but the outer longitudinal muscle is only present in three equally spaced bands, the **teniae coli.**

(b) The **mucosa** is occupied mostly by tubular **intestinal glands** extending as deep as the muscularis mucosae and by lamina propria rich in MALT. X80. H&E.

Digestive Tract SUMMARY OF KEY POINTS

Oral Cavity

- The **oral cavity** is lined primarily by **mucosa** with **nonkeratinized stratified squamous epithelium**, with **keratinized stratified squamous epithelium** on the **hard palate** and **gingiva**.
- The dorsal surface mucosa of the tongue has projecting **lingual papillae** of four types: **filiform** papillae with keratinized epithelium and nonkeratinized **foliate, fungiform,** and large **vallate** papillae.
- All lingual papillae, except the filiform type, have epithelial **taste buds** on their sides, with chemosensory **gustatory cells** with synapses to basal sensory innervation, **support cells,** and an apical **taste pore.**
- Each tooth has **enamel** covering its **crown** and **neck** and a vascularized, innervated central **pulp cavity** within the **dentin** that makes up the **roots** and extends into the neck.
- Enamel calcifies as parallel **enamel rods** in a process guided by the protein **amelogenin** after secretion from columnar epithelial cells called **ameloblasts** in the **enamel organ** of the embryonic **tooth bud**.
- **Predentin** is secreted as elongated **dentinal tubules** from tall **odontoblasts** that line the pulp cavity and persist in the fully formed tooth, with apical **odontoblast processes** extending between the tubules.

- The **periodontium** of each tooth consists of a thin layer of bone-like **cementum** surrounding dentin of the roots and the **periodontal ligament** binding the cementum to **alveolar bone** on the jaw socket.

Layers of the Digestive Tract

- From the esophagus to the rectum, the digestive tract has **four major layers**: a lining **mucosa**, a **submucosa**, a **muscularis**, and an outermost **adventitia** or mesothelium-covered **serosa**.
- The **mucosa** varies regionally along the tract but always consists of a lining **epithelium** on a **lamina propria** of loose connective tissue and smooth muscle fibers extending from **muscularis mucosae** layer.

Esophagus

- The mucosa of the **esophagus** has **nonkeratinized stratified squamous epithelium**; its muscularis is striated at its superior end with smooth muscle at its inferior end, with mixed fiber types in the middle.
- Most of the outer layer of the esophagus is **adventitia**, merging with other tissues of the mediastinum.

FIGURE **15–33** Colon mucosa.

(a) Transverse section of the colon shows the muscularis externa (**ME**), including a **tenia coli** cut transversely in the lower part of the figure, the submucosa (**S**), the mucosa (**M**) filled with **tubular intestinal glands**. Some of these glands are cut longitudinally, but most seen here are cut transversely. X14. H&E.

(b) Transversely cut glands are seen to consist of simple columnar epithelium surrounded by a tubular lumen (**L**) and embedded in lamina propria (**LP**) with many free lymphocytes. Lymphocytes can also be seen penetrating the epithelium (**arrow**). X200. H&E.

(c) Longitudinal section of one intestinal gland stained for glycoproteins shows **mucus** in the lumen and two major cell types in the epithelium: goblet cells (**G**) and the neighboring columnar cells specialized for water absorption. X400. PAS.

(d) TEM of the absorptive cells, or **colonocytes**, reveals short **microvilli** at their apical ends and dilated **intercellular spaces** with interdigitating leaflets of cell membrane (**L**), a sign of active water transport. The absorption of water is passive, following the active transport of sodium from the basolateral surfaces of the epithelial cells. X2500.

FIGURE **15–34** Mucosa of the rectoanal junction.

The simple columnar epithelium with tubular **intestinal glands** in the rectum (left side of photo) changes abruptly to stratified squamous epithelium in the **anal canal** (right side of photo), as seen in this longitudinal section. The connective tissue of the lamina propria is seen to contain many free lymphocytes. X40. H&E.

TABLE **15–2**	Summary of distinguishing digestive tract features, by region and layers.			
Region and Subdivisions	Mucosa (Epithelium, Lamina Propria, Muscularis Mucosae)	Submucosa (with Submucosal Plexuses)	Muscularis (Inner Circular and Outer Longitudinal Layers, with Myenteric Plexuses Between Them)	Adventitia/Serosa
Esophagus (upper, middle, lower)	Nonkeratinized **stratified squamous epithelium**; **cardiac glands** at lower end	Small **esophageal glands** (mainly mucous)	Both layers **striated muscle** in upper region; both layers **smooth muscle** in lower region; **smooth and striated muscle** fascicles mingled in middle region	Adventitia, except at lower end with serosa
Stomach (cardia, fundus, body, pylorus)	**Surface mucous cells** and **gastric pits** leading to **gastric glands** with **parietal and chief cells**, (in the fundus and body) or to mucous **cardiac glands** and **pyloric glands**	No distinguishing features	**Three indistinct layers** of smooth muscle (inner oblique, middle circular, and outer longitudinal)	Serosa
Small intestine (duodenum, jejunum, ileum)	**Plicae circulares**; **villi**, with **enterocytes** and **goblet cells**, and **crypts/glands** with **Paneth cells** and **stem cells**; **Peyer patches** in ileum	**Duodenal (Brunner) glands** (entirely mucous); possible extensions of Peyer patches in ileum	No distinguishing features	Mainly serosa
Large intestine (cecum, colon, rectum)	**Intestinal glands** with **goblet cells** and **absorptive cells**	No distinguishing features	Outer longitudinal layer separated into three bands, the **teniae coli**	Mainly serosa, with adventitia at rectum
Anal canal	**Stratified squamous epithelium**; longitudinal anal columns	Venous sinuses	Inner circular layer thickened as **internal sphincter**	Adventitia

- At the **esophagogastric junction**, stratified squamous epithelium changes abruptly to **simple columnar epithelium** invaginating into the lamina propria as many branched tubular glands.

Stomach

- The **stomach** has four major regions: the superior **cardia** and inferior **pylorus**, which are rather similar histologically, and the intervening **fundus** and **body**, which are also similar.
- The mucosa of the stomach fundus and body is penetrated by numerous **gastric pits**, which are lined like the stomach lumen with **surface mucous cells** and which lead into branching **gastric glands**.
- The surface mucous cells secrete a thick layer of **viscous mucus with bicarbonate ions**, which protects these cells and the underlying lamina propria.
- The **gastric glands** are lined by epithelium with four **major cell types**, as well as their pluripotent **stem cells** that are located in the narrow neck regions of these glands:
  - **Mucous neck cells** include immature precursors of the surface mucous cells but produce less alkaline mucus while migrating up into the gastric pits.
  - **Parietal cells** are large cells with many mitochondria and **large intracellular canaliculi** for production of HCl in the gastric secretion; they also secrete **intrinsic factor** for vitamin B$_{12}$ uptake.
  - **Chief (zymogenic) cells**, clustered mainly in the lower half of the gastric glands, secrete the protein **pepsinogen** that is activated by the low pH in the lumen to form the major protease **pepsin**.

- **Enteroendocrine cells** are scattered epithelial cells of the **diffuse neuroendocrine system**, which release **peptide hormones** to regulate activities of neighboring tissues during food digestion.
- The mucosa of the stomach cardiac and pyloric regions has branching **cardial and pyloric glands** that consist almost entirely of columnar **mucous cells**, lacking parietal and chief cells.

Small Intestine

- The **small intestine** has three regions: the **duodenum** with large mucous glands in the submucosa called **duodenal glands**; the **jejunum**; and the **ileum** with the large mucosal and submucosal **Peyer patches**.
- In all regions of small intestine the mucosa has millions of projecting **villi**, with simple columnar epithelium over cores of lamina propria, and intervening simple tubular **intestinal glands** (or crypts).
- Stem cells in these glands produce the columnar epithelial cells of villi, mainly **goblet cells** and **enterocytes** for nutrient absorption, as well as defensin-producing **Paneth cells** deep in the glands.
- **Sugars** and **amino acids** produced by final steps of digesting carbohydrates and polypeptides in the **glycocalyx** undergo transcytosis through **enterocytes** for uptake by **capillaries**.
- Products of **lipid** digestion associate with bile salts, are taken up by enterocytes, and are converted to **triglycerides** and **lipoproteins** for release as **chylomicrons** and uptake by a lymphatic called a **lacteal** in the core of each villus.
- **Smooth muscle** of the **lamina propria** and **muscularis mucosae**, under the control of the autonomic **submucosal (Meissner) plexus**, moves the villi and helps propel lymph through the lacteals.

- **Smooth muscle** in the **inner circular layer** and the **outer longitudinal layer** of the muscularis, under the control of the autonomic **myenteric (Auerbach) plexus**, produces strong **peristalsis**.

Large Intestine

- The **large intestine** has three major regions: the short **cecum**, with the appendix; the long **colon**, with its ascending, transverse, descending, and sigmoid portions; and the **rectum**.
- Along its entire length, the mucosa of the large intestine has millions of short simple tubular **intestinal glands**, lined by lubricant **goblet cells** and **absorptive cells** for the uptake of water and electrolytes.

- The **muscularis** of the colon has its outer longitudinal layer subdivided into three bands of smooth muscle called **teniae coli**, which act in the peristaltic movement of feces to the rectum.

Anal Canal

- At the **anal canal** the simple columnar epithelium lining the rectum shifts abruptly to **stratified squamous epithelium** of the skin at the **anus**.
- Near the anus the circular layer of the rectum's muscularis forms the **internal anal sphincter**, with further control exerted by **striated muscle** of the **external anal sphincter**.

16 Organs Associated with the Digestive Tract

The organs associated with the digestive tract include the major salivary glands, the pancreas, the liver, and the gallbladder. Products of these organs facilitate transport and digestion of food within the gastrointestinal tract. The main functions of the salivary glands are to moisten and lubricate ingested food and the oral mucosa, to initiate the digestion of carbohydrates and lipids with amylase and lipase, and to secrete innate immune components such as lysozyme and lactoferrin.

The pancreas secretes digestive enzymes that act in the small intestine and hormones important for the metabolism of the absorbed nutrients. Bile, whose components are necessary for digestion and absorption of fats, is made in the liver but stored and concentrated in the gallbladder. The liver also plays a major role in carbohydrate and protein metabolism, inactivates many toxic substances and drugs, and synthesizes most plasma proteins and factors necessary for blood coagulation.

› SALIVARY GLANDS

Exocrine glands in the mouth produce saliva, which has digestive, lubricating, and protective functions. With a normal pH of 6.5 to 6.9, saliva also has an important buffering function and in some species is also important for evaporative cooling. There are three pairs of large salivary glands: the **parotid, submandibular,** and **sublingual glands** (Figure 16–1), in addition to the numerous minor mucosal salivary glands throughout the oral cavity, which secrete about 10% of the total saliva volume.

›› MEDICAL APPLICATION

Inadequate saliva production, leading to **dry mouth** or **xerostomia,** can be caused by various factors affecting the major salivary glands, such as **mumps** viral infection, radiation of the glands, or the normal side effect of drugs such as **antihistamines.**

A connective tissue capsule surrounds each major salivary gland. The parenchyma of each consists of secretory units on a branching duct system arranged in lobules, separated by septa of connective tissue. The secretion of each gland is either serous, seromucous, or mucous, depending on its content of the glycoprotein mucin. Saliva from the parotids is serous and watery. The submandibular and sublingual glands produce a seromucous secretion, while that of the minor glands is mostly mucous. Saliva is modified by the cells of the duct system draining the secretory units, with much Na^+ and Cl^- reabsorbed while certain growth factors and digestive enzymes are added.

Three epithelial cell types comprise the salivary secretory units:

- **Serous cells** are polarized protein-secreting cells, usually pyramidal in shape, with round nuclei, well-stained RER, and apical secretory granules (Figures 16–2 through 16–4). Joined apically by tight and adherent junctions, serous cells form a somewhat spherical unit called an **acinus** (L. grape), with a very small central lumen (Figure 16–2). Serous acinar cells secrete enzymes and other proteins.
- **Mucous cells** are somewhat more columnar in shape, with more compressed basal nuclei (Figures 16–2 and 16–4). Mucous cells contain apical granules with hydrophilic mucins that provide lubricating properties in saliva but cause poor cell staining in routine preparations (Figure 16–5). Mucous cells are most often organized as cylindrical **tubules** rather than acini. Mixed salivary glands have tubuloacinar secretory units with both serous and mucous secretion.
- **Myoepithelial cells,** described in Chapter 4, are found inside the basal lamina surrounding acini, tubules, and the proximal ends of the duct system (Figures 16–2 and 16–4). These small, flattened cells extend several contractile processes around the associated secretory

FIGURE **16-1** Major salivary glands.

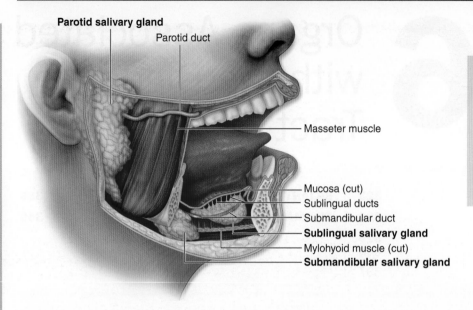

Parotid salivary gland

Parotid duct

Masseter muscle

Mucosa (cut)
Sublingual ducts
Submandibular duct
Sublingual salivary gland
Mylohyoid muscle (cut)
Submandibular salivary gland

About 90% of saliva is produced by three bilateral pairs of salivary glands: the **parotid, submandibular**, and **sublingual glands**. Locations and relative sizes of these glands are shown here diagrammatically. These glands plus microscopic minor salivary glands throughout the oral mucosa produce 0.75-1.50 L of saliva daily.

FIGURE **16-2** Epithelial components of a submandibular gland lobule.

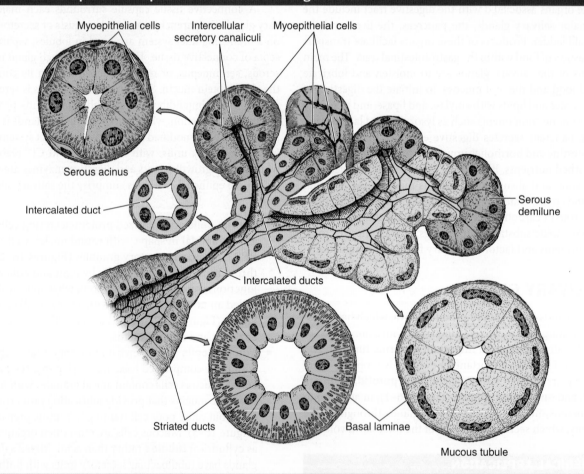

Myoepithelial cells

Intercellular secretory canaliculi

Myoepithelial cells

Serous acinus

Intercalated duct

Serous demilune

Intercalated ducts

Striated ducts

Basal laminae

Mucous tubule

The secretory portions are composed of pyramidal serous (violet) and mucous (tan) cells. **Serous cells** are typical protein-secreting cells, with rounded nuclei, accumulation of rough ER in the basal third, and an apex filled with protein-rich secretory granules. The nuclei of **mucous cells**, flattened with condensed chromatin, are located near the bases of the cells.

The short intercalated ducts are lined with cuboidal epithelium. The **striated ducts** are composed of columnar cells with characteristics of ion-transporting cells: basal membrane invaginations with mitochondrial accumulations. **Myoepithelial cells** are shown around the serous acini.

FIGURE **16–3** Parotid gland.

The large parotid gland consists entirely of serous acini with cells producing amylase and other proteins for storage in secretory granules. **(a)** Micrograph of a parotid gland shows densely packed serous acini (**A**) with ducts. Secretory granules of serous cells are clearly shown in this plastic section, as well as an intercalated duct (**ID**) and striated duct (**SD**), both cut transversely. X400. PT.

(b) Striations of a duct (**SD**) are better seen here, along with a septum (**CT**) and numerous serous acini (**A**). The connective tissue often includes adipocytes. X200. H&E.

unit or duct and their activity is important for moving secretory products into and through the ducts.

›› MEDICAL APPLICATION

Excessive saliva production, or **sialorrhea**, is associated with the autonomic activity of **nausea**, inflammation within the oral cavity, and **rabies** viral infection.

In the **intralobular duct system**, secretory acini and tubules empty into short **intercalated ducts**, lined by cuboidal epithelial cells, and several of these ducts join to form a **striated duct** (Figure 16–2). The more columnar striated duct cells have many infoldings of their basolateral membrane, all aligned with numerous mitochondria that, by light microscopy, appear as faint basal striations radiating toward the nuclei (Figure 16–6). Striated ducts reabsorb Na^+ ions from the initial secretion and their folded cell membranes present a large surface area with ion transporters, facilitating rapid ion transcytosis and making the secretion slightly hypotonic.

Plasma cells in the connective tissue surrounding the small intralobular ducts release **IgA**, which forms a complex with the secretory component synthesized by the epithelial cells of the serous acini and intralobular ducts. Transferred into the saliva, the IgA complex released into the saliva provides defense against specific pathogens in the oral cavity.

Ducts from each lobule converge and drain into interlobular **excretory ducts** with increasing size and thicker

FIGURE **16–4** Ultrastructure of serous and mucous cells.

A micrograph of a mixed acinus from a submandibular gland shows both serous and mucous cells surrounding the small lumen (**L**). Mucous cells (**M**) have large, hydrophilic granules like those of goblet cells, while serous cells (**S**) have small, dense granules. Small myoepithelial cells (**My**) extend contractile processes around each acinus. X2500.

(*With permission, from Dr John D. Harrison, King's College London Dental Institute, London, UK.*)

connective tissue layers. The lining of these ducts is unusual, combining various epithelial types, including simple cuboidal or columnar, stratified cuboidal or columnar, and pseudostratified epithelia, distributed in no apparent pattern. These atypical epithelia may reflect their composition of cells with many diverse functions, including cells for ion reabsorption, cells for secretion of mucin and other proteins, enteroendocrine cells, and basal stem cells, all in highly branched ducts of small diameter. Before emptying into the oral cavity, the main duct of each gland is lined with nonkeratinized stratified squamous epithelium.

Vessels and nerves enter the large salivary glands at a hilum and gradually branch into the lobules. A rich vascular and nerve plexus surrounds the secretory and duct components of each lobule. The capillaries surrounding the secretory units provide fluid important for saliva production, which is stimulated by the autonomic nervous system. Parasympathetic stimulation, usually elicited through the smell or taste of food, provokes a copious watery secretion with relatively little organic content. Sympathetic stimulation inhibits such secretion and produces the potential for dry mouth often associated with anxiety.

Features specific to each group of major salivary glands include the following:

- **Parotid glands**, located in each cheek near the ear, are branched acinar glands with exclusively serous acini (Figure 16–3). Serous cells of parotid glands secrete abundant α-**amylase** that initiates hydrolysis of carbohydrates and proline-rich proteins with antimicrobial and other protective properties.
- **Submandibular glands**, which produce two-thirds of all saliva, are branched tubuloacinar glands, having primarily serous acini, but with many mixed tubuloacinar secretory units (Figures 16–4 and 16–5a). Serous cells of these mixed units are mostly in peripheral crescent-shaped groups called **serous demilunes** (Figure 16–5a), aggregates formed at least in part artifactually when the adjacent mucous cells swell during routine tissue preparation. Basolateral membrane infoldings of the serous cells facilitate electrolyte and water transport. In addition to α-amylase and proline-rich proteins, serous cells of the submandibular gland secrete other enzymes, including **lysozyme** for bacterial wall hydrolysis.
- **Sublingual glands**, the smallest of the major glands, are also considered branched tubuloacinar glands, but here secretory tubules of mucous cells predominate and the main product of the gland is mucus (Figure 16–6b). The few serous cells present in demilunes add amylase and lysozyme to the secretion.

As described in Chapter 15, small, nonencapsulated salivary glands are distributed throughout the oral mucosa and submucosa with short ducts to the oral cavity. These minor salivary glands are usually mucous, except for the small serous glands at the bases of circumvallate papillae. Plasma cells releasing IgA are also common within the minor salivary glands.

› PANCREAS

The **pancreas** is a mixed exocrine-endocrine gland that produces both digestive enzymes and hormones. It is an elongated retroperitoneal organ, with a large head near the duodenum and more narrow body and tail regions that extend to the left (Figure 16–7). The pancreas has a thin capsule of connective tissue, from which septa extend to cover the larger vessels and ducts and to separate the parenchyma into lobules (Figure 16–8). The secretory acini are surrounded by a basal lamina that is supported only by a delicate sheath of reticular fibers with a rich capillary network. Endocrine function of the pancreas involves primarily smaller cells similar to enteroendocrine cells located in variously sized clusters called the **pancreatic islets** (islets of Langerhans). These are described with the endocrine organs in Chapter 20.

FIGURE **16–5** Submandibular gland and sublingual gland.

(a) The submandibular gland is a mixed serous and mucous gland (serous cells predominate), and shows well-stained serous acini (**A**) and serous demilunes (**S**) and pale-staining mucous cells (**M**) grouped as tubules in this tubuloacinar gland. Small intralobular ducts (**ID**) drain each lobule. X340. H&E.

(b) The sublingual gland is a mixed but largely mucous gland with a tubuloacinar arrangement of poorly stained mucous cells (**M**). Small intralobular ducts (**ID**) are seen in connective tissue, as well as small fascicles of lingual striated muscle (**SM**). X140. H&E.

›› MEDICAL APPLICATION

Pancreatic cancer, which is usually a carcinoma of duct cells, can arise anywhere in the gland but occurs most often in the head of the organ near the duodenum. The tumor is usually asymptomatic until growth and metastasis are well advanced, leading to the low rate of early detection and subsequent high rate of mortality. Metastasis may be facilitated by the relatively sparse connective tissue around the ducts and vasculature of the pancreas.

The digestive enzymes are produced by cells of serous acini in the larger exocrine portion of the pancreas (Figure 16–9a). This somewhat resembles the parotid gland histologically, although the pancreas lacks striated ducts and the parotid glands lack islets of endocrine tissue. Each pancreatic acinus consists of several serous cells surrounding a very small lumen, without myoepithelial cells (Figure 16–9). The acinar cells are polarized, with round basal nuclei, and numerous zymogen granules apically, typical of protein-secreting cells (Figure 16–10).

Each acinus is drained by a short **intercalated duct** of simple squamous epithelium. The initial cells of these small ducts extend into the lumen of the acinus as small pale-staining **centroacinar cells** that are unique to the pancreas. Cells of the intercalated ducts secrete a large volume of fluid, rich in HCO_3^- (bicarbonate ions), which alkalinizes and transports hydrolytic enzymes produced in the acini. The intercalated

FIGURE **16–6** Striated ducts.

(a) A striated duct (**SD**) shows very faint striations in the basal half of the columnar cells, which represent mitochondria located in the folds of the lateral cell membrane. X200. H&E.

(b) SEM indicates that the apical ends of the cells are joined together near the small lumen (**L**), with interdigitating folds of cell membrane best developed at the basal end (**B**). X4000.

(c) SEM shows the bases (**B**) of several such cells with the basal lamina removed, revealing the interlocking of folded membrane between neighboring cells. Mitochondria within the folds supply energy for rapid ion uptake from saliva. X4000.

ducts merge with **intralobular ducts** and larger **interlobular ducts**, which have increasingly columnar epithelia before joining the main pancreatic duct that runs the length of the gland.

The exocrine pancreas secretes approximately 1.5 L of alkaline pancreatic juice per day and delivers it directly into the duodenum where the HCO_3^- ions neutralize the acidic chyme entering there from the stomach and establish the pH for optimal activity of the pancreatic enzymes. These digestive enzymes include several **proteases**, α-**amylase**, **lipases**, and **nucleases** (DNAase and RNAase). The proteases are secreted as inactive zymogens (**trypsinogen, chymotrypsinogen**, proelastase, kallikreinogen, and procarboxipeptidases). Trypsinogen is cleaved and activated by enteropeptidases in the duodenum, generating trypsin that activates the other proteases in a cascade. Pancreatic tissue is protected against autodigestion by the following:

- Restricting protease activation to the duodenum,
- Trypsin inhibitor, which is copackaged in the secretory granules with trypsinogen, and

- The low pH in the acini and duct system due to HCO_3^- secreted by the centroacinar and intercalated duct cells, which helps keep all the enzymes inactive.

›› MEDICAL APPLICATION

In **acute pancreatitis**, the proenzymes may be activated and digest pancreatic tissues, leading to very serious complications. Possible causes include infection, gallstones, alcoholism, drugs, and trauma. **Chronic pancreatitis** can produce progressive fibrosis and loss of pancreatic function.

Exocrine secretion in the pancreas is regulated mainly through two polypeptide hormones produced by enteroendocrine cells of the small intestine:

- **Cholecystokinin (CCK)** stimulates enzyme secretion by the acinar cells.

FIGURE **16–7** Pancreas and duodenum.

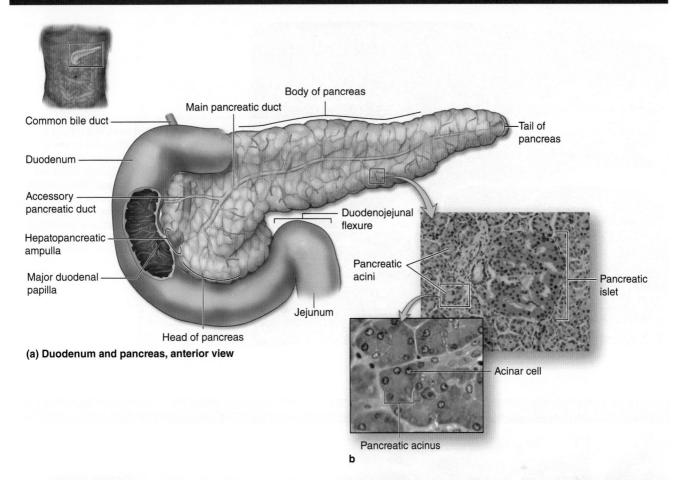

(a) Duodenum and pancreas, anterior view

Common bile duct

Duodenum

Accessory pancreatic duct

Hepatopancreatic ampulla

Major duodenal papilla

Head of pancreas

Main pancreatic duct

Body of pancreas

Tail of pancreas

Duodenojejunal flexure

Jejunum

Pancreatic acini

Pancreatic islet

Acinar cell

Pancreatic acinus

b

(a) The main regions of the pancreas are shown in relation to the two pancreatic ducts and the duodenum.

(b) Micrographs show a pancreatic islet and several pancreatic acini. X75 and X200. H&E.

- **Secretin** promotes water and HCO_3^- secretion by the duct cells.

Autonomic (parasympathetic) nerve fibers also stimulate secretion from both acinar and duct cells.

›› MEDICAL APPLICATION

In the normal liver most dense connective tissue is found only in the portal areas, surrounding the blood vessels and bile ductule. In liver **cirrhosis**, which occurs late in **chronic liver disease**, fibrosis and proliferation of fibroblasts and hepatic stellate cells occur beyond the portal areas. The excessive connective tissue may disrupt the normal hepatic architecture and interfere with liver function.

› LIVER

The **liver** is the largest internal organ, in adults averaging about 1.5 kg or 2% of the body weight. Located in the right upper quadrant of the abdomen just below the diaphragm (see Figure 15–1), the liver has major left and right lobes with two smaller inferior lobes, most of which are covered by a thin capsule and mesothelium of the visceral peritoneum. The capsule thickens at the hilum (or porta hepatis) on the inferior side, where the **dual blood supply** from the **hepatic portal vein** and **hepatic artery** enters the organ and where the hepatic vein, lymphatics, and common hepatic (bile) duct exit.

The main digestive function of the liver is production of **bile**, a complex substance required for the emulsification, hydrolysis, and uptake of fats in the duodenum. The liver is also the major interface between the digestive system and the blood, as the organ in which nutrients absorbed in the small

FIGURE **16–8** Pancreas.

Low-power view of pancreas includes several islets (**I**) surrounded by many serous acini (**A**). The larger intralobular ducts (**D**) are lined by simple columnar epithelium. The ducts and blood vessels (**V**) are located in connective tissue, which also provides a thin capsule to the entire gland and thin septa separating the lobules of secretory acini. X20. H&E.

FIGURE **16–9** Pancreatic acini.

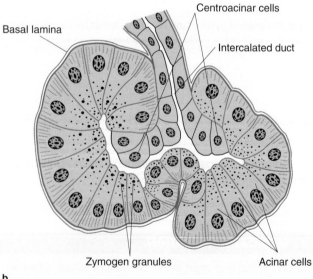

(a) Micrograph of exocrine pancreas shows the serous, enzyme-producing cells arranged in small acini (**A**) with very small lumens. Acini are surrounded by only small amounts of connective tissue with fibroblasts (**F**). Each acinus is drained by an intercalated duct with its initial cells, the centroacinar cells (**arrow**), inserted into the acinar lumen. X200. H&E.

(b) The diagram shows the arrangement of cells more clearly. Under the influence of secretin, the **centroacinar** and **intercalated duct cells** secrete a copious HCO_3^--rich fluid that hydrates, flushes, and alkalinizes the enzymatic secretion of the acini.

FIGURE **16–10** Pancreatic acinar cell ultrastructure.

TEM of a pancreatic acinar cell shows its pyramidal shape and the round, basal nucleus (**N**) surrounded by cytoplasm packed with cisternae of rough ER (**RER**). The Golgi apparatus (**G**) is situated at the apical side of the nucleus and is associated with condensing vacuoles (**C**) and numerous secretory granules (**S**) with zymogen. The small lumen (**L**) of the acinus contains proteins recently released from the cell by exocytosis. Exocytosis of digestive enzymes from secretory granules is promoted by CCK, released by enteroendocrine cells of the duodenum when food enters that region from the stomach. X8000.

intestine are processed before distribution throughout the body. About 75% of the blood entering the liver is nutrient-rich (but O$_2$-poor) blood from the portal vein arising from the stomach, intestines, and spleen; the other 25% comes from the hepatic artery and supplies the organ's O$_2$.

Hepatocytes (Gr. *hepar*, liver), the key cells of this organ, are among the most functionally diverse cells of the body. In addition to an exocrine function in the secretion of bile components, hepatocytes and other liver cells process the contents of blood, with many specific functions:

- Synthesis and endocrine secretion into the blood of the major **plasma proteins**, including albumins, fibrinogen, apolipoproteins, transferrin, and many others
- Conversion of amino acids into glucose (**gluconeogenesis**)
- Breakdown (**detoxification**) and conjugation of ingested toxins, including many drugs
- Amino acid **deamination**, producing **urea** removed from blood in kidneys
- **Storage of glucose** in glycogen granules and **triglycerides** in small lipid droplets

- Storage of vitamin A (in **hepatic stellate cells**) and other fat-soluble vitamins
- Removal of effete erythrocytes (by specialized macrophages, or **Kupffer cells**)
- Storage of iron in complexes with the protein **ferritin**

Hepatocytes & Hepatic Lobules

The liver's unique histologic organization and microvasculature allow hepatocytes to perform their diverse metabolic, exocrine, and endocrine functions. Hepatocytes are large cuboidal or polyhedral epithelial cells, with large, round central nuclei and eosinophilic cytoplasm rich in mitochondria. The cells are frequently binucleated and about 50% of them are polyploid, with two to eight times the normal chromosome number.

The liver parenchyma is organized as thousands of small (~0.7 × 2 mm) **hepatic lobules** in which hepatocytes form hundreds of irregular plates arranged radially around a small **central vein** (Figures 16–11 through 16–13). The hepatocyte

FIGURE **16–11** Liver.

(a) Hepatic lobules

(b) Hepatocytes and sinusoids

(c) Portal triad and hepatic lobule

The liver, a large organ in the upper right quadrant of the abdomen, immediately below the diaphragm, is composed of thousands of polygonal structures called **hepatic lobules**, which are the basic functional units of the organ. **(a)** Diagram showing a small **central vein** in the center of a hepatic lobule and several sets of blood vessels at its periphery. The peripheral vessels are grouped in connective tissue of the **portal tracts** and include a branch of the portal vein, a branch of the hepatic artery, and a branch of the bile duct (the **portal triad**).

(b) Both blood vessels in this triad branch as **sinusoids**, which run between plates of **hepatocytes** and drain into the central vein.

(c) Micrograph of a lobule shows the central vein (**C**), plates of hepatocytes (**H**), and in an adjacent portal area a small lymphatic (**L**) and components of the portal triad: a portal venule (**PV**), hepatic arteriole (**HA**), and bile ductule (**B**). X220. H&E.

FIGURE **16–12** Hepatic lobule.

Cut transversely, hepatic lobules are polygonal units showing plates of epithelial cells called **hepatocytes** radiating from a central venule (**C**). (a) Hepatic lobules of some mammals, such as the pig, are delimited on all sides by connective tissue. (b) In humans these lobules have much less connective tissue and their boundaries are more difficult to distinguish. In both cases peripheral connective tissue of portal areas contains the portal triad: small bile ductules (**D**), venule (**V**) branches of the portal vein, and arteriole (**A**) branches of the hepatic artery. Both X150. H&E.

plates are supported by a delicate stroma of reticulin fibers (Figure 16–13b). Peripherally each lobule has three to six portal areas with more fibrous connective tissue, each of which contains three interlobular structures that comprise the **portal triad** (Figures 16–11 and 16–13d):

- A **venule** branch of the portal vein, with blood rich in nutrients but low in O_2,
- An **arteriole** branch of the hepatic artery that supplies O_2,
- One or two small **bile ductules** of cuboidal epithelium, branches of the bile conducting system.

Most of the peripheral portal areas also contain lymphatics and nerve fibers and in some species (eg, pigs) extend thin sheets of fibrous connective tissue completely around the lobules, making individual lobules easier to distinguish than in humans (Figure 16–12).

Between all of the anastomosing plates of hepatocytes of a hepatic lobule are important vascular **sinusoids** that emerge from the peripheral branches of the portal vein and hepatic artery and converge on the lobule's **central vein** (Figures 16–11 through 16–13c). The venous and arterial blood mixes in these irregular hepatic sinusoids. The anastomosing sinusoids have thin, discontinuous linings of fenestrated endothelial cells surrounded by sparse basal lamina and reticular fibers. The discontinuities and fenestrations allow plasma to fill a narrow **perisinusoidal space** (or **space of Disse**) and directly bathe the many irregular microvilli projecting from the hepatocytes into this space (Figure 16–14). This direct contact between hepatocytes and plasma facilitates most key hepatocyte functions that involve uptake and release of nutrients, proteins, and potential toxins.

Two other functionally important cells are found with the sinusoids of hepatic lobules:

- Numerous specialized **stellate macrophages**, usually called **Kupffer cells**, are found within the sinusoid lining (Figure 16–15). These cells recognize and phagocytose aged erythrocytes, freeing heme and iron for reuse or storage in ferritin complexes. Kupffer cells are also antigen-presenting cells and remove any bacteria or debris present in the portal blood.
- In the perisinusoidal space are **hepatic stellate cells** (or **Ito cells**) with small lipid droplets that store vitamin A

FIGURE **16–13** Hepatic lobule microvasculature.

(a) Hepatocytes (**H**) are polygonal epithelial cells that form branching, irregular plates separated by venous sinusoids (**S**). H&E X400.

(b) Reticulin (collagen type III) fibers (**R**) running along the plates of hepatocytes (**H**), supporting these and the intervening sinusoids. Most connective tissue in the liver is found in the septa and portal tracts. X400. Silver.

(c) With plates of hepatocytes (**H**) appearing to radiate from it, the central vein (**C**) of the lobule has more collagen than

the smaller sinusoids (**S**) that drain into it from all directions (arrows). X200. Mallory trichrome.

(d) Peripheral portal areas contain more connective tissue and are the sites of the portal triad: a portal venule (**PV**), an arteriole branching off the hepatic artery (**HA**), and one or two bile ductules (**BD**). X200. H&E.

and other fat-soluble vitamins (Figure 16–15b). These mesenchymal cells, which are difficult to see in routine preparations, also produce extracellular matrix (ECM) components (becoming myofibroblasts after liver injury) and cytokines that help regulate Kupffer cell activity.

The endothelium of the central vein in the middle of each hepatic lobule is supported by a very thin layer of fibrous connective tissue (Figure 16–13c). Central venules from each lobule converge into larger veins, which eventually form two or more large **hepatic veins** that empty into the inferior vena cava.

FIGURE **16–14** Ultrastructure of hepatocytes, perisinusoidal space, and bile canaliculi.

(a) TEM of hepatocytes shows small bile canaliculi (**BC**) between tight junctions (**TJ**) joining two cells. A hepatocyte nucleus (**H**) is in the lower right corner, surrounded by small tubular vesicles of smooth ER (**SER**), much rough ER (**RER**), many mitochondria (**M**), small electron-dense glycogen granules, and Golgi complexes (**G**). Between the hepatocytes and the fenestrated endothelial cell (**E**) of the sinusoid (**S**) is the very small perisinusoidal space (**PS**) almost filled with **microvilli**. X9500.

(*Figure 16–14a, with permission, from Douglas L. Schmucker, Department of Anatomy, University of California, San Francisco, CA.*)

(b) SEM of the luminal surface of the endothelium lining a hepatic sinusoid shows grouped fenestrations (**F**). At the border are seen cut edges of endothelial cells (**E**) in this discontinuous sinusoid and hepatocytes (**H**). Between these two cells is the thin perisinusoidal space (**PS**), into which project **microvilli** from the hepatocytes surface. X6500.

(*Figure 16–14b, with permission from Eddie Wisse, Electron Microscopy Unit, Department of Pathology, University of Maastricht, Maastricht, the Netherlands.*)

(c) SEM of hepatocytes (**H**) broken apart from one another reveals the length of a bile canaliculus (**BC**) along the cell's surface. Such canaliculi run between the cells of the hepatocyte plates in the hepatic lobules and carry bile toward the portal areas where the canaliculi join cuboidal bile ductules. X8000.

Blood always flows from the periphery to the center of each hepatic lobule. Consequently, oxygen and metabolites, as well as all other toxic or nontoxic substances absorbed in the intestines, reach the lobule's peripheral cells first and then the more central cells. This direction of blood flow partly explains why the properties and function of the periportal hepatocytes differ from those of the centrolobular cells. Hepatocytes near the portal areas can rely on aerobic metabolism and are often more active in protein synthesis, while the more central cells are exposed to lower concentrations of nutrients and

FIGURE 16–15 Hepatic sinusoids.

In the endothelial lining of the hepatic sinusoids are numerous specialized stellate macrophages or **Kupffer cells** that detect and phagocytose effete erythrocytes. **(a)** Kupffer cells (**K**) are seen as black cells in a liver lobule from a rat injected with particulate India ink. X200. H&E.

(b) In a plastic section, Kupffer cells (**K**) are seen in the sinusoid (**S**) between two groups of hepatocytes (**H**). They are larger than the flattened endothelial cells (**E**). Between the endothelium and the hepatocytes is a very thin space called the perisinusoidal space (**PS**) of Disse, in which are located small hepatic stellate cells (**HS**), or Ito cells, that maintain the very sparse ECM of this compartment and also store vitamin A in small lipid droplets. These cells are numerous but are difficult to demonstrate in routine histologic preparations. X750. PT.

oxygen and are more involved with detoxification and glycogen metabolism.

While the sinusoidal (basolateral) domains of hepatocytes process nutrients and other blood components and secrete the plasma proteins, the smaller apical surfaces of the hepatocytes form **bile canaliculi** and are involved in exocrine secretion bile (Figures 16–14 and 16–16). Within the hepatic plates hepatocytes adhere firmly with desmosomes and junctional complexes. The apical surfaces of two adherent hepatocytes are grooved and juxtaposed to form the canaliculus, sealed by tight junctions, into which bile components are secreted (Figure 16–14). These canaliculi are elongated spaces (total length >1 km) with lumens only 0.5-1μm in diameter with large surface areas due to the many short microvilli from the constituent hepatocytes (Figures 16–14 and 16–16).

The bile canaliculi form a complex anastomosing network of channels through the hepatocyte plates that end near the portal tracts (Figures 16–11b and 16–17). The bile flow therefore progresses in a direction opposite to that of the blood, that is, from the center of the lobule to its periphery. Bile canaliculi are the smallest branches of the biliary tree or bile conducting system. They empty into bile **canals of Hering** (Figure 16–17) composed of cuboidal epithelial cells called **cholangiocytes**.

The short bile canals quickly merge in the portal areas with the **bile ductules** lined by cuboidal or columnar cholangiocytes and with a distinct connective tissue sheath. Bile ductules gradually merge, enlarge, and form right and left **hepatic ducts** leaving the liver.

Into the canaliculi hepatocytes continuously secrete bile, a mixture of **bile acids** (organic acids such as cholic acid), **bile salts** (the deprotonated forms of bile acids), electrolytes, fatty acids, phospholipids, cholesterol, and **bilirubin**. Some bile components are synthesized in hepatocyte SER, but most are taken up from the perisinusoidal space; all are quickly secreted into the bile canaliculi (Figure 16–16). Bile acids/salts have an important function in emulsifying the lipids in the duodenum, promoting their digestion and absorption.

Bilirubin is a pigmented breakdown product of heme that is released from splenic macrophages primarily, but also from Kupffer cells, and carried to hepatocytes bound to albumen. Released into the duodenum with bile, bilirubin is converted by intestinal bacteria into other pigmented products, some of which are absorbed in the intestinal mucosa to be processed and excreted again in the liver or excreted into urine by the kidneys. These bilirubin-related compounds give feces and urine their characteristic colors.

FIGURE **16–16** Hepatocyte ultrastructure and major functions.

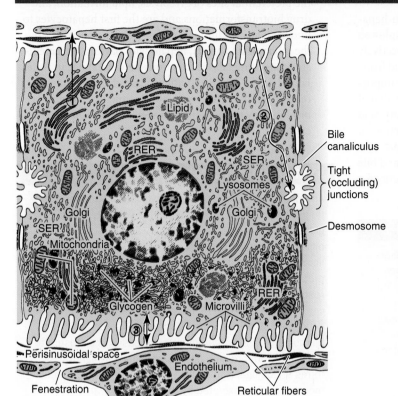

A diagram of hepatocyte cytoplasmic organization, with major functions localized. (**1**) RER is primarily engaged in synthesis of **plasma proteins** for release into the perisinusoidal space. (**2**) Potentially toxic compounds, bilirubin (bound to albumin) and bile acids are taken up from the perisinusoidal space, processed by enzymes in the tubulovesicular system of the SER, and secreted into the **bile canaliculi**. (**3**) Glucose is taken up from the perisinusoidal space and stored in **glycogen granules**, with the process reversed when glucose is needed.

FIGURE **16–17** Bile ductules.

Near the periphery of each hepatic lobule, many bile canaliculi join with the much larger bile canals of Hering, which are lined by cuboidal epithelial cells called **cholangiocytes**. These canals soon join the bile ductules in the portal areas and drain into the biliary tree.

Structure & Function in the Liver

As mentioned previously, hepatocytes are highly versatile cells with diverse functions that are reflected in their structure (Figure 16–16). Abundant **rough ER** is focused on synthesis of plasma proteins and causes cytoplasmic basophilia, which is often more pronounced in hepatocytes near the portal areas (Figure 16–12). Abundant **smooth ER**, distributed more evenly throughout the cytoplasm, contains the enzyme systems for the biotransformation or detoxification of substances in blood, which are then usually excreted with bile. These include enzymes responsible for oxidation, methylation, and conjugation of steroids, barbiturates, antihistamines, anticonvulsants, and other drugs. Under some conditions prolonged presence of drugs can lead to increased amounts of SER in hepatocytes, thus improving the liver's detoxification capacity. Other SER enzymes (glucuronosyl transferases) conjugate bilirubin to glucuronate, rendering it more soluble and facilitating its excretion in bile.

Glycogen granules and small **lipid droplets** in hepatocytes, and very small electron-dense **ferritin complexes** (hemosiderin) primarily in the Kupffer cells, respectively mediate temporary storage of glucose, triglycerides, and iron.

Hepatocyte **peroxisomes** are also abundant and important for oxidation of excess fatty acids, catalase-mediated breakdown of the hydrogen peroxide generated by fatty acid oxidation (by means of catalase activity), and conversion of excess purines to uric acid. Many Golgi complexes are also present, involved in synthesis of both plasma proteins and bile components. The numerous mitochondria provide energy for all these activities (Figure 16–16).

> **>> MEDICAL APPLICATION**
>
> **Fatty liver disease** is a reversible condition in which large lipid droplets containing triglycerides accumulate abnormally in hepatocytes via the process called **steatosis**. This disorder has multiple causes, but it occurs most commonly in individuals with **alcoholism** or **obesity**. Accumulation of fat in hepatocytes may produce a progressive inflammation of the liver, or **hepatitis**, in this case called **steatohepatitis**.

The different categories of hepatocyte functions—including secretion of proteins into blood, the exocrine secretion of bile, and the removal of diverse small compounds from blood—have led to three ways of considering liver lobule structure, which are summarized in Figure 16–18.

- The classic **hepatic lobule** (Figure 16–18a), with blood flowing past hepatocytes from the portal areas to a central venule, emphasizes the endocrine function of the structure producing factors for uptake by plasma.
- The concept of **portal lobules** of hepatocytes is more useful when considering the exocrine function of these cells, that is, bile secretion. The portal area has the bile ductule at the center, and bile, moving in the opposite direction as the blood, flows toward it from all the surrounding hepatocytes. The tissue draining bile into each portal area duct is roughly triangular in shape, with the central veins of three classic lobules at its angles (Figure 16–18b).
- The **hepatic acinus**, a third way of viewing liver cells, emphasizes the nature of the blood supply to the hepatocytes and the oxygen gradient from the hepatic artery branch to the central vein. In a liver acinus hepatocytes make up an irregular oval or diamond-shaped area extending from two portal triads to the two closest central veins (Figure 16–18c). Periportal hepatocytes nearest the hepatic arteriole, comprising zone I in the acinus, get the most oxygen and nutrients and can most readily carry out functions requiring oxidative metabolism such as protein synthesis. Hepatocytes in zone III, near the central vein, get the least oxygen and nutrients. They are the preferential sites of glycolysis, lipid formation, and drug biotransformations and are the first hepatocytes to undergo fatty accumulation and ischemic necrosis. In the intervening zone II, hepatocytes have an intermediate range of metabolic functions between those in zones I and III. The major activities in any given hepatocyte result from the cell adapting to the microenvironment produced by the contents of the blood to which it is exposed.

> **>> MEDICAL APPLICATION**
>
> An important function of hepatocyte SER is the conjugation of hydrophobic (water-insoluble), yellow bilirubin by glucuronosyl transferases to form water-soluble, nontoxic bilirubin glucuronide, which is excreted into the bile canaliculi. When bilirubin glucuronide is not formed or excreted properly, various diseases characterized by jaundice can result.
>
> A frequent cause of jaundice in newborns is an underdeveloped state of the hepatocyte SER (neonatal hyperbilirubinemia). A treatment in these cases is exposure to blue light from ordinary fluorescent tubes, which transforms unconjugated bilirubin into a water-soluble photoisomer that can be excreted by the kidneys.

Unlike the salivary glands and pancreas, the liver has a strong capacity for **regeneration** despite its normal slow rate of cell renewal. Hepatocyte loss from the action of toxic substances triggers mitosis in the remaining healthy hepatocytes in a process of **compensatory hyperplasia** that maintains the original tissue mass. Surgical removal of a liver portion produces a similar response in the hepatocytes of the remaining lobe(s). The regenerated liver tissue is usually well organized, with the typical lobular arrangement, and replaces the functions of the destroyed tissue. This regenerative capacity is important clinically because one major liver lobe can sometimes be donated by a living relative for surgical transplant and full liver function restored in both donor and recipient.

Besides proliferation of existing hepatocytes, a role for **liver stem cells** in regeneration has been shown in some experimental models. Such cells, often called **oval cells**, are present among cholangiocytes of the bile canals near portal areas and produce progenitor cells for both hepatocytes and cholangiocytes.

> **>> MEDICAL APPLICATION**
>
> Most malignant tumors of the liver derive from hepatocytes or cholangiocytes of the hepatic ducts. The pathogenesis of **liver carcinoma** is associated with a variety of acquired disorders, such as **chronic viral hepatitis** (B or C) and cirrhosis.

FIGURE **16–18** Concepts of structure-function relationships in liver.

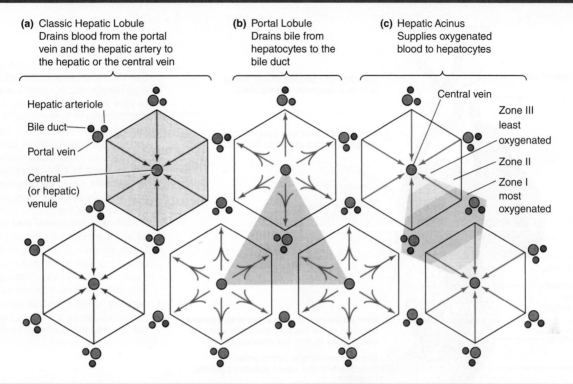

(a) Classic Hepatic Lobule
Drains blood from the portal vein and the hepatic artery to the hepatic or the central vein

Hepatic arteriole
Bile duct
Portal vein
Central (or hepatic) venule

(b) Portal Lobule
Drains bile from hepatocytes to the bile duct

(c) Hepatic Acinus
Supplies oxygenated blood to hepatocytes

Central vein
Zone III least oxygenated
Zone II
Zone I most oxygenated

Studies of liver microanatomy, physiology, and pathology have given rise to three related ways to view the liver's organization, which emphasize different aspects of hepatocyte activity.

(a) The **classic lobule** concept offers a basic understanding of the structure-function relationship in liver organization and emphasizes the endocrine function of hepatocytes as blood flows past them toward the central vein.

(b) The **portal lobule** emphasizes the hepatocytes' exocrine function and the flow of bile from regions of three classic lobules toward the bile duct in the portal triad at the center here. The area drained by each bile duct is roughly triangular.

(c) The **hepatic acinus** concept emphasizes the different oxygen and nutrient contents of blood at different distances along the sinusoids, with blood from each portal area supplying cells in two or more classic lobules. Major activity of each hepatocyte is determined by its location along the oxygen/nutrient gradient: periportal cells of zone I get the most oxygen and nutrients and show metabolic activity generally different from the pericentral hepatocytes of zone III, exposed to the lowest oxygen and nutrient concentrations. Many pathologic changes in the liver are best understood from the point of view of liver acini.

(*Reproduced, with permission, from Boron WF, Boulpaep EL. Medical Physiology: A Cellular and Molecular Approach. Philadelphia, PA: Saunders Elsevier, 2005.*)

› BILIARY TRACT & GALLBLADDER

The bile produced by the hepatocytes flows through the **bile canaliculi**, **bile ductules**, and **bile ducts**. These structures gradually merge, forming a converging network that ultimately forms the **common hepatic duct** that joins the **cystic duct** from the gallbladder and continues to the duodenum as the **common bile duct** (Figure 16–19).

The hepatic, cystic, and common bile ducts are lined with a mucous membrane having a simple columnar epithelium of cholangiocytes. The lamina propria and submucosa are relatively thin, with mucous glands in some areas of the cystic duct, and surrounded by a thin muscularis. This muscle layer becomes thicker near the duodenum and finally, in the duodenal papilla, forms a sphincter that regulates bile flow into the small bowel.

The gallbladder is a hollow, pear-shaped organ (Figure 16–19) attached to the lower surface of the liver, capable of storing 30-50 mL of bile that is concentrated during storage. The wall of the gallbladder consists of a mucosa composed of simple columnar epithelium and lamina propria, a thin muscularis with bundles of muscle fibers oriented in several directions, and an external adventitia or serosa (Figure 16–20a). The mucosa has numerous folds that are particularly evident when the gallbladder is empty.

The lining epithelial cells of the gallbladder have prominent mitochondria, microvilli, and large intercellular spaces, all indicative of cells actively transporting water, in this case for concentrating bile (Figure 16–20b). The mechanism for this includes activity of Na^+ pumps in the basolateral membranes, followed by passive movement of water from the bile. To move stored bile into the duodenum, contraction of the gallbladder

FIGURE 16–19 Biliary tract and gallbladder.

Left and right hepatic ducts

Common hepatic duct

Cystic duct

① **Left and right hepatic ducts merge to form a common hepatic duct.**

② **Common hepatic and cystic ducts merge to form a common bile duct.**

Common bile duct

Accessory pancreatic duct

Stored bile

Gallbladder

Minor duodenal papilla

Hepatopancreatic ampulla with hepatopancreatic sphincter

Main pancreatic duct

Major duodenal papilla

Duodenum

③ **Main pancreatic duct merges with common bile duct at the hepatopancreatic ampulla, which extends into the duodenum.**

④ **Bile and pancreatic juices enter duodenum at the major duodenal papilla.**

Bile leaves the liver in the left and right hepatic ducts, which merge to form the common hepatic duct, which connects to the cystic duct serving the gallbladder. The latter two ducts merge to form a common bile duct. All these ducts carrying bile are lined by cuboidal or low columnar cells called **cholangiocytes**, similar to those of the small bile ductules in the liver.

The main pancreatic duct merges with the common bile duct at the hepatopancreatic ampulla, which enters the wall of the duodenum at a major papilla (of Vater); the accessory pancreatic duct enters the duodenum at a minor papilla. Bile and pancreatic juices are mixed before release into the duodenal lumen.

muscularis is induced by cholecystokinin (CCK) released from enteroendocrine cells of the small intestine. Release of CCK is, in turn, stimulated by the presence of ingested fats in the small intestine. Gallbladder removal due to obstruction or chronic inflammation leads to the direct flow of bile from liver to gut, with few major consequences on digestion.

›› MEDICAL APPLICATION

Reabsorption of water from bile in the gallbladder is involved in the formation of **gallstones** in the lumen of the gallbladder or biliary ducts, a condition called **cholelithiasis**.

This disorder usually originates with bile that already contains excessive amounts of normal bile components. Supersaturation of cholesterol in bile can lead to the formation of **cholesterol stones**, the most common form. Brown or black **pigment stones** can form when bile contains excessive amounts of unconjugated bilirubin, which can result from chronic hemolysis associated with disorders such as sickle cell anemia. Gallstones can lead to biliary obstruction or more commonly to inflammation in **acute or chronic cholecystitis**.

Organs Associated with the Digestive Tract SUMMARY OF KEY POINTS

Salivary Glands

- **Salivary glands** have secretory units of either **protein-secreting serous cells**, usually organized in round or oval **acini**, or of **mucin-secreting mucous cells** in elongated **tubules**.
- **Parotid glands** have only serous acini; **sublingual glands** are mixed but have primarily mucous tubules, some with **serous demilunes**; **submandibular glands** are also mixed but have mainly serous acini.
- Salivary secretory units are drained by simple cuboidal **intercalated ducts** that merge as simple columnar **striated ducts**, which merge as larger interlobular or **excretory ducts**.

- Cells of **striated ducts** have mitochondria-lined, basolateral membrane folds specialized for electrolyte re-absorption from the secretion; **excretory ducts** are unusual in having **stratified cuboidal or columnar** cells.

Pancreas

- **Pancreatic islets** of endocrine cells are embedded in exocrine **serous acinar tissue**, which comprises most of the pancreas and in which the cells secrete hydrolytic **digestive enzymes** for delivery to the duodenum.

FIGURE **16–20** Gallbladder.

The gallbladder is a saclike structure that stores and concentrates bile, and releases it into the duodenum after a meal. **(a)** Its wall consists largely of a highly folded mucosa, with a simple columnar epithelium (arrows) overlying a typical lamina propria (**LP**); a muscularis (**M**) with bundles of muscle fibers oriented in all directions to facilitate emptying of the organ; and an external adventitia (**A**) where it is against the liver and a serosa where it is exposed. X60. H&E.

(b) TEM of the epithelium shows cells specialized for water uptake across apical microvilli (**MV**) and release into the intercellular spaces (**arrows**) along the folded basolateral cell membranes. From these spaces water is quickly removed by capillaries in the lamina propria. Abundant mitochondria provide the energy for this pumping process. Scattered apical secretory granules (**G**) contain mucus. X5600.

- Each pancreatic **acinar cell** is pyramidal, with **secretory (zymogen) granules** in the narrow apical end and Golgi complexes, much rough ER, and a large nucleus at the basal end.
- **Intercalated ducts** draining pancreatic acini, including their initial **centroacinar cells** that insert into the acinar lumen, **secrete bicarbonate** ions (HCO_3^-) to neutralize chyme entering the duodenum from the stomach.

Liver

- Liver **hepatocytes** are large epithelial cells with large central nuclei (polyploid and often binucleated), much smooth and rough ER, and many small Golgi complexes.
- **Hepatocytes** have many functions, including endocrine (**plasma protein** secretion), exocrine (**bile** secretion), glucose storage (**glycogen granules**), and **detoxification** (using SER and peroxisomes).

- In the liver **hepatocytes** are organized into irregular plates to form polygonal **hepatic lobules** in which the hepatocyte plates radiate toward a small **central vein**.
- Each hepatic lobule is surrounded by sparse connective tissue that is more abundant in the **portal areas** at the corners.
- **Portal areas** or tracts contain a small lymphatic and the **portal triad**: a **portal venule** branch from the portal vein, a **hepatic arteriole** branch of the hepatic artery, and a **bile ductule** branch of the biliary tree.
- In the lobules the portal venule and hepatic arteriole both branch into irregular **sinusoids** between the hepatic plates where the nutrient-rich and O_2-rich blood mixes, flows past hepatocytes, and drains to the central vein.
- The endothelium of the hepatic **sinusoids** is **discontinuous and fenestrated**; between it and the hepatocytes is the **perisinusoidal**

space (of Disse) where exchange occurs between the hepatocytes and blood plasma.

- The sinusoidal endothelium includes many specialized **stellate macrophages** or **Kupffer cells**, which recognize and remove effete erythrocytes, **releasing iron and bilirubin** for uptake by hepatocytes.
- Also present in the perisinusoidal spaces are **hepatic stellate cells** (or Ito cells) containing many small lipid droplets for **storage of vitamin A** and other fat-soluble vitamins.
- Between adherent hepatocytes in the hepatic plates are grooves called **bile canaliculi**, sealed by tight junctions, into which hepatocytes secrete water and **bile components**, including **bilirubin** and **bile acids**.
- In each hepatic lobule, all bile canaliculi converge on the **bile canals (of Hering)**, which join the **bile ductules** in the portal areas and eventually all merge to form the left and right **hepatic ducts**.

Biliary Tract and Gallbladder

- All bile-conducting ducts after the bile canaliculi are lined by simple cuboidal or columnar cells called **cholangiocytes**.
- The common hepatic duct leads to the cystic duct that carries bile to the **gallbladder** for temporary **bile storage** and concentration.
- The mucosa of the **gallbladder** has many **folds** with a large surface area, a well-vascularized lamina propria, and a lining of **columnar cholangiocytes** specialized for water uptake from bile.
- Contraction of the gallbladder **muscularis** sends bile to the duodenum via the **common bile duct** and is induced by **cholecystokinin (CCK)** from enteroendocrine cells in the duodenum when food is present.

17 The Respiratory System

The respiratory system provides for exchange of O_2 and CO_2 to and from the blood. Respiratory organs include the **lungs** and a branching system of bronchial tubes that link the sites of gas exchange with the external environment. Air is moved through the lungs by a ventilating mechanism, consisting of the thoracic cage, intercostal muscles, diaphragm, and elastic components of the lung tissue. The system is divided anatomically into structures of the upper and lower respiratory tracts (Figure 17–1). Functionally, the system has two components:

- The **conducting portion**, which consists of the nasal cavities, nasopharynx, larynx, trachea, bronchi (Gr. *bronchos*, windpipe), bronchioles, and terminal bronchioles
- The **respiratory portion,** where the system's main function of gas exchange occurs, consisting of respiratory bronchioles, alveolar ducts, and alveoli

Alveoli, the cellular sites of the exchange of O_2 and CO_2 between inspired air and blood, are saclike structures that make up most of the lungs.

The conducting portion cleans and humidifies the inspired air and provides a conduit through which air moves to and from the lungs. To ensure an uninterrupted supply of air, a combination of cartilage, elastic and collagen fibers, and smooth muscle provides the conducting portion with rigid structural support and the necessary flexibility and extensibility.

› NASAL CAVITIES

The left and right nasal cavity each has two components: the external, dilated **vestibule** and the internal **nasal cavity**.

Skin of the nose enters the **nares** (nostrils) partway into the vestibule and has sweat glands, sebaceous glands, and coarse, moist **vibrissae** (hairs) that filter out particulate material from the inspired air. Within the vestibule, the epithelium loses its keratinized nature and undergoes a transition to typical pseudostratified columnar epithelium before entering the nasal cavities.

The nasal cavities lie within the skull as two cavernous chambers separated by the osseous **nasal septum**. Extending from each lateral wall are three bony shelflike projections (Figure 17–1) called **conchae**, or turbinates. The mucosa covering these and other parts of the nasal cavity walls has a lamina propria with important roles in conditioning inhaled air. A complex vasculature with loops of capillaries near the epithelial surface carries blood in a general direction counter to the flow of inspired air and releases heat to warm that air while it is humidified by water released from small seromucous glands. The thin layer of mucus produced by these glands and the goblet cells also serves to trap particulate and gaseous air impurities that are then removed. Immunoglobulin A (IgA) from plasma cells in the lamina propria is also present in nasal secretions.

The middle and inferior conchae are covered with **respiratory epithelium**; the roof of the nasal cavities and the superior conchae are covered with specialized **olfactory epithelium**.

Respiratory Epithelium

Most of the nasal cavities and the respiratory system's conducting portion is lined with mucosa having ciliated pseudostratified columnar epithelium, described with epithelia in

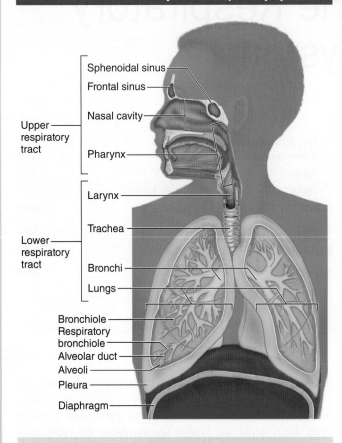

FIGURE **17–1** Anatomy of the respiratory system.

Sphenoidal sinus
Frontal sinus
Nasal cavity
Upper respiratory tract
Pharynx
Larynx
Trachea
Lower respiratory tract
Bronchi
Lungs
Bronchiole
Respiratory bronchiole
Alveolar duct
Alveoli
Pleura
Diaphragm

Anatomically, the respiratory tract has upper and lower parts. Histologically and functionally, the respiratory system has a **conducting portion**, which consists of all the components that condition air and bring it into the lungs, and a **respiratory portion**, where gas exchange actually occurs, consisting of respiratory bronchioles, alveolar ducts, and alveoli in the lungs. Portions of two sets of paranasal sinuses are also shown here.

Chapter 4 and commonly known as **respiratory epithelium** (Figure 17–2). This epithelium has five major cell types, all of which contact an unusually thick basement membrane:

- **Ciliated columnar cells** are the most abundant, each with 250-300 cilia on its apical surface (Figure 17–2).
- **Goblet cells** are also numerous and predominate in some areas (Figure 17–2), with basal nuclei and apical domains filled with granules of mucin glycoproteins.
- **Brush cells** are a much less numerous, columnar cell type, in which a small apical surface bears sparse, blunt microvilli (Figure 17–2c). Brush cells are **chemosensory receptors** resembling gustatory cells, with similar signal transduction components and synaptic contact with afferent nerve endings on their basal surfaces.
- **Small granule cells** (or Kulchitsky cells) are difficult to distinguish in routine preparations, but possess numerous dense core granules 100 to 300 nm in diameter. Like

enteroendocrine cells of the gut, they are part of the **diffuse neuroendocrine system** (DNES; see Chapter 20). Like brush cells, they represent only about 3% of the cells in respiratory epithelium.
- **Basal cells** are mitotically active stem and progenitor cells that give rise to the other epithelial cell types.

>> MEDICAL APPLICATION

The chronic presence or accumulation of toxins that occur with heavy cigarette smoking or industrial air pollution affects the respiratory epithelium beginning in the nasal cavities. Immobilization of the cilia causes failure to clear mucus containing filtered material and exacerbates the problem, leading eventually to the likelihood of **squamous metaplasia** of the epithelium. A change from pseudostratified ciliated columnar to stratified squamous epithelium can occur, particularly in the mucosa of bronchi. This can produce precancerous **cell dysplasia** in this tissue.

Olfactory Epithelium

The olfactory chemoreceptors for the sense of smell are located in the **olfactory epithelium**, a specialized region of the mucous membrane covering the superior conchae at the roof of the nasal cavity. In adult humans, it is about 10 cm² in area and up to 100 μm in thickness. This thick, pseudostratified columnar epithelium has three major cell types (Figure 17–3):

- **Olfactory neurons** are bipolar neurons present throughout this epithelium. Their nuclei form an irregular row near the middle of this thick epithelium. The apical (luminal) pole of each olfactory cell is its dendrite end and has a knoblike swelling with about a dozen basal bodies. From the basal bodies emerge long cilia with nonmotile axonemes but considerable surface areas for membrane chemoreceptors. These receptors respond to odoriferous substances by generating an action potential along the axons extending from the basal ends of these neurons. The axons leave the epithelium and unite in the lamina propria as very small nerves that then pass to the brain through foramina in the cribriform plate of the ethmoid bone (Figure 17–3). There they form the olfactory nerve, cranial nerve I, and eventually synapse with other neurons in the olfactory bulb.
- **Supporting cells** are columnar, with broad, cylindrical apexes containing the nuclei and narrower bases. On their free surface are microvilli submerged in a fluid layer. Well-developed junctional complexes bind the supporting cells to the olfactory cells. The supportive role of these cells is not well understood, but they express abundant ion channels that help maintain a microenvironment conducive to olfactory function and survival.
- **Basal cells** are small, spherical or cone-shaped cells near the basal lamina. These are the stem cells for the other two types, replacing the olfactory neurons every 2 to 3 months and support cells less frequently.

FIGURE 17–2 Respiratory epithelium.

Respiratory epithelium is the classic example of **pseudostratified ciliated columnar epithelium. (a)** Details of its structure vary in different regions of the respiratory tract, but it usually rests on a very thick basement membrane (**BM**) and has several cell types, some columnar, some basal, and all contacting the basement membrane. Ciliated columnar cells are most abundant, with hundreds of long robust cilia (**C**) on each of their bulging apical ends that provide a lush cover of cilia on the luminal surface. Most of the small rounded cells at the basement membrane are stem cells and their differentiating progeny, which together make up about 30% of the epithelium. Mucus-secreting goblet cells (**G**) and intraepithelial lymphocytes and dendritic cells are also present in respiratory epithelium. The lamina propria is well-vascularized (**V**). X400. Mallory trichrome.

(b) Scanning electron microscopy (SEM) shows the luminal surface of goblet cells (**G**) among the numerous ciliated cells.

(c) SEM of another region shows that goblet cells (**G**) predominate in some areas, with subsurface accumulations of mucus evident in some (**arrows**). The film of mucus traps most airborne dust particles and microorganisms, and the ciliary movements continuously propel the sheet of mucus toward the pharynx for elimination. Other columnar cells, representing only about 3% of the cells in respiratory epithelium, are brush cells (**B**) with small apical surfaces bearing a tuft of short, blunt microvilli. Both X3000.

(*Figure 17-2b and 17-2c reprinted, with permission, from John Wiley & Sons, Inc., Andrews P. Am J Anat 1974;139:421.*)

The lamina propria of the olfactory epithelium possesses large serous glands, the **olfactory glands** (of Bowman), which produce a constant flow of fluid surrounding the olfactory cilia and facilitating the access of new odoriferous substances.

>> **MEDICAL APPLICATION**

The loss or reduction of the ability to smell, **anosmia** or **hyposmia**, respectively, can be caused by traumatic damage to the ethmoid bone that severs olfactory nerve axons or by damage to the olfactory epithelium caused by intranasal drug use.

The olfactory neurons are the best-known neurons to be replaced regularly because of **regenerative activity** of the epithelial stem cells from which they arise. For this reason, loss of the sense of smell due to toxic fumes or physical injury to the olfactory mucosa itself is usually temporary.

Paranasal Sinuses

The **paranasal sinuses** are bilateral cavities in the frontal, maxillary, ethmoid, and sphenoid bones of the skull (Figure 17–1). They are lined with a thinner respiratory epithelium with fewer goblet cells. The lamina propria contains only a few small glands and is continuous with the underlying periosteum. The paranasal sinuses communicate with the nasal cavities through small openings; mucus produced there is moved into the nasal passages by the activity of the ciliated epithelial cells.

>> **MEDICAL APPLICATION**

Sinusitis is an inflammatory process of the sinuses that may persist for long periods of time, mainly because of obstruction of drainage orifices. Chronic sinusitis and **bronchitis** are components of **primary ciliary dyskinesia**, or Kartagener syndrome, an inherited genetic disorder characterized by defective ciliary action.

FIGURE **17–3** Olfactory mucosa.

(a) The olfactory mucosa covers the superior conchae bilaterally and sends axons from throughout its entire 10 cm² area to the brain via small openings in the cribriform plate of the ethmoid bone. It is a pseudostratified epithelium, containing basal stem cells and columnar support cells in addition to the bipolar olfactory neurons. The dendrites of these neurons are at the luminal ends and have cilia specialized with many membrane receptors for odor molecules. Binding such ligands causes depolarization which passes along basal axons to the olfactory bulb of the brain.

(b) Only a thin basement membrane separates the olfactory basal cells (**B**) from the underlying lamina propria (**LP**). Nuclei of the bipolar olfactory neurons (**ON**) lie in the middle of the pseudostratified olfactory epithelium, with a zone of supporting cell (**S**) nuclei above it. At the apical end of the cells are the nonmotile cilia (**C**), or olfactory hairs, and a layer of mucus (**M**). X200. H&E.

❯ NASOPHARYNX

The nasal cavities open posteriorly into the **nasopharynx**, which is the first part of the pharynx and continuous caudally with the oropharynx, the posterior part of the oral cavity leading to the larynx (Figure 17–1). The nasopharynx is lined with respiratory epithelium, and its mucosa contains the medial pharyngeal tonsil and the bilateral openings of the auditory tubes connected to each middle ear cavity.

❯ LARYNX

The **larynx** is a short (4 cm × 4 cm) passage for air between the pharynx and the trachea (Figure 7–1). Its rigid wall is reinforced by hyaline cartilage (in the thyroid, cricoid, and the inferior arytenoid cartilages) and smaller elastic cartilages (in the epiglottis, cuneiform, corniculate, and the superior arytenoid cartilages), all of which are connected by ligaments. In addition to maintaining an open airway, movements of these cartilages by skeletal muscles participate in sound production during phonation.

The **epiglottis**, a flattened structure projecting from the upper rim of the larynx, serves to prevent swallowed food or fluid from entering that passage. Its upper, or lingual, surface has stratified squamous epithelium; at variable points on its laryngeal surface this epithelium undergoes a transition to ciliated pseudostratified columnar (respiratory) epithelium. Mixed mucous and serous glands are found in the lamina propria beneath the epithelium.

Below the epiglottis and laryngeal vestibule, the mucosa projects into the lumen bilaterally with two pairs of folds separated by a narrow space or ventricle (Figure 17–4). The upper pair, the immovable **vestibular folds**, is partly covered with typical respiratory epithelium overlying numerous seromucous glands and occasional lymphoid nodules. The lower pair of folds, the **vocal folds** (or cords), have features important for phonation or sound production:

FIGURE **17–4** Larynx.

The larynx is a short air passage between the pharynx and trachea. Its wall contains skeletal muscles and pieces of cartilage, all of which make the larynx specialized for sound production, or phonation. This low-power micrograph shows the laryngeal vestibule (**LV**), which is surrounded by seromucous glands (**G**). The lateral walls of this region bulge as a pair of vestibular folds (**VF**). These also contain seromucous glands and areolar tissue with MALT, often with lymphoid nodules (**L**) and are largely covered by respiratory epithelium, with regions near the epiglottis having stratified squamous epithelium.

Below each large vestibular fold is a narrow space or ventricle (**V**), below which is another pair of lateral folds, the vocal folds or cords (**VC**). These are covered by stratified squamous epithelium and project more sharply into the lumen, defining the rim of the opening into the larynx itself. Each contains a large striated vocalis muscle (**VM**) and nearer the surface a small ligament, which is cut transversely and therefore difficult to see here. Variable tension of these ligaments caused by the muscles produces different sounds as air is expelled across the vocal cords. All the structures and spaces above these folds add resonance to the sounds, assisting phonation. X15. H&E.

- They are covered with stratified squamous epithelium that protects the mucosa from abrasion and desiccation from rapid air movement.
- A dense regular bundle of elastic connective tissue, the vocal ligament, supports the free edge of each vocal fold.
- Deep to the mucosa of each vocal fold are large bundles of striated fibers that comprise the **vocalis muscle**.

During phonation the vocalis muscles draw the paired vocal folds together (adduction), narrowing the intervening luminal space, the **rima glottidis**, and air expelled from the lungs causes the adducted vocal folds to vibrate and produce sound.

The pitch and other qualities of the sound are altered by changing the tension on the vocal folds, the width of the rima glottidis, the volume of air expelled, etc. The vestibular folds and ventricles, along with other structures and spaces higher in the respiratory tract, contribute to the resonance of sound produced in the larynx. Speech is produced when sounds made in the larynx are modified by movements of the pharynx, tongue, and lips. The larynx is larger in males than in females after puberty, causing men's voices to be typically deeper than women's voices.

▶ TRACHEA

The **trachea**, 10 to 12 cm long in adults, is lined with typical respiratory mucosa in which the lamina propria contains numerous seromucous glands producing watery mucus (Figure 17–5). A series with about a dozen C-shaped rings of hyaline cartilage in the submucosa reinforces the wall and keeps the tracheal lumen open (Figure 17–6). The open ends of the cartilage rings are on the posterior surface, against the esophagus, and are bridged by a bundle of smooth muscle called the **trachealis muscle** and a sheet of fibroelastic tissue attached to the perichondrium. The entire organ is surrounded by adventitia.

The trachealis muscle relaxes during swallowing to facilitate the passage of food by allowing the esophagus to bulge into the lumen of the trachea, with the elastic layer preventing excessive distention of the lumen. The muscle strongly contracts in the cough reflex to narrow the tracheal lumen and provide for increased velocity of the expelled air and better loosening of material in the air passage.

FIGURE **17–5** Trachea.

The trachea is lined by typical respiratory epithelium (**RE**) underlain by connective tissue of the lamina propria (**LP**) and seromucous glands (**G**) in the lamina propria and submucosa. The submucosa also contains C-shaped rings of hyaline cartilage (**C**) covered by perichondrium (**P**). X50. H&E.

Major features of all upper respiratory tract structures are summarized in Table 17–1.

▶ BRONCHIAL TREE & LUNG

The trachea divides into two **primary bronchi** that enter each lung at the hilum, along with arteries, veins, and lymphatic

FIGURE **17–6** Bronchial tree.

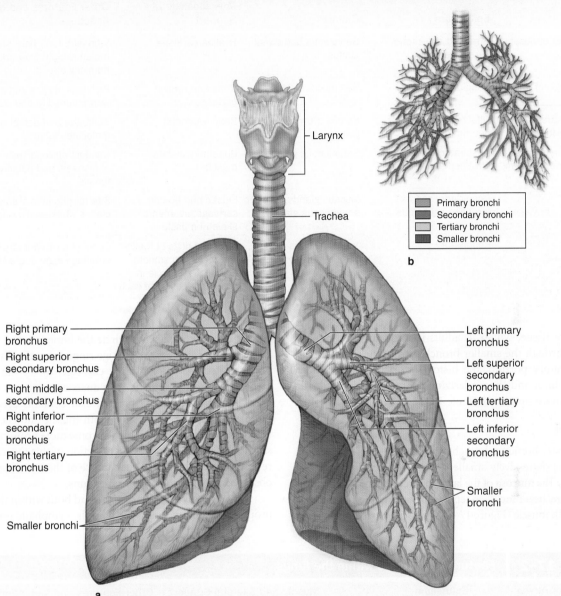

Larynx

Trachea

Primary bronchi
Secondary bronchi
Tertiary bronchi
Smaller bronchi

b

Right primary bronchus

Right superior secondary bronchus

Right middle secondary bronchus

Right inferior secondary bronchus

Right tertiary bronchus

Smaller bronchi

Left primary bronchus

Left superior secondary bronchus

Left tertiary bronchus

Left inferior secondary bronchus

Smaller bronchi

a

The **trachea** bifurcates as right and left **primary bronchi** that enter the hilum on the posterior side of each **lung** along with the pulmonary vessels, lymphatics, and nerves. **(a)** Within each lung, bronchi subdivide further to form the **bronchial tree**, the last component of the air conducting system. **(b)** The small diagram shows the color-coded major branches of the bronchial tree.

vessels. After entering the lungs, the primary bronchi course downward and outward, giving rise to three **secondary (lobar) bronchi** in the right lung and two in the left lung (Figure 17–6), each of which supplies a pulmonary lobe. These lobar bronchi again divide, forming **tertiary (segmental) bronchi**. Each of the tertiary bronchi, together with the smaller branches it supplies, constitutes a **bronchopulmonary segment**—approximately 10% to 12% of each lung with its own connective tissue capsule and blood supply.

The existence of such lung segments facilitates the specific surgical resection of diseased lung tissue without affecting nearby healthy tissue.

The tertiary bronchi give rise to smaller and smaller bronchi, whose terminal branches are called **bronchioles**. Each bronchiole enters a pulmonary lobule, where it branches to form five to seven **terminal bronchioles**. The pulmonary lobules are each pyramid-shaped, with the apex aimed at the pulmonary hilum, and each is delineated by a thin layer of

TABLE 17–1	Histologic features of the upper respiratory tract, larynx, and trachea.			
Region	Epithelium	Glands	Musculoskeletal Support	Other Features and Major Functions
Vestibules of nasal cavities	Stratified squamous, keratinized to nonkeratinized	Sebaceous and sweat glands	Hyaline cartilage	Vibrissae (stiff hairs) and moisture both filter and humidify air
Most areas of nasal cavities	Respiratory	Seromucous glands	Bone and hyaline cartilage	Rich vasculature and glands warm, humidify, and clean air
Superior areas of nasal cavities	Olfactory, with bipolar neurons	Serous (Bowman) glands	Bone (ethmoid)	Solubilize and detect odorant molecules in air
Nasopharynx and posterior oropharynx	Respiratory and stratified squamous	Seromucous glands	Bone and skeletal muscle	Conduct air to larynx; pharyngeal and palatine tonsils
Larynx	Respiratory and stratified squamous	Mucous glands, smaller seromucous glands	Elastic and hyaline cartilage, ligaments, skeletal muscle	Site for phonation; epiglottis closes while swallowing
Trachea	Respiratory	Mainly mucous glands, some serous or mixed glands	C-shaped rings of hyaline cartilage, with smooth (trachealis) muscle in posterior opening of each	Conduct air to primary bronchi entering lungs; some MALT

connective tissue, which in adults is frequently incomplete. Moving through the smaller bronchi and bronchioles toward the respiratory portion, the histologic organization of both the epithelium and the underlying lamina propria gradually becomes more simplified (Table 17–2).

Bronchi

Each primary bronchus branches repeatedly, with each branch becoming progressively smaller until it reaches a diameter of 1 to 2 mm. The mucosa of the larger bronchi is structurally similar to the tracheal mucosa except for the organization of cartilage and smooth muscle (Figure 17–7). In the primary bronchi most

cartilage rings completely encircle the lumen, but as the bronchial diameter decreases, cartilage rings are gradually replaced with isolated plates of hyaline cartilage. Small mucous and serous glands are abundant, with ducts opening into the bronchial lumen. The lamina propria also contains crisscrossing bundles of spirally arranged smooth muscle and elastic fibers (Figures 17–7 and 17–8), which become more prominent in the smaller bronchial branches. Contraction of this muscle layer is responsible for the folded appearance of the bronchial mucosa observed histologically in cross sections.

Numerous lymphocytes are found both within the lamina propria and among the epithelial cells. Lymphatic nodules are

TABLE 17–2	Features of airways within the lungs.		
Region of Airway	Epithelium	Muscle and Skeletal Support	Other Features and Major Functions
Bronchi	Respiratory	Prominent spiral bands of smooth muscle; irregular hyaline cartilage plates	Repeated branching; conduct air deeper into lungs
Bronchioles	Simple ciliated cuboidal to columnar, with Clara cells	Prominent circular layer of smooth muscle; no cartilage	Conduct air; important in bronchoconstriction and bronchodilation
Terminal bronchioles	Simple cuboidal, ciliated and Clara cells	Thin, incomplete circular layer of smooth muscle; no cartilage	Conduct air to respiratory portions of lungs; Clara cells with several protective functions
Respiratory bronchioles	Simple cuboidal, ciliated and Clara cells, with scattered alveoli	Fewer smooth muscle fibers, mostly around alveolar openings	Conduct air deeper, with some gas exchange and protective Clara cells
Alveolar ducts and sacs	Simple cuboidal between many alveoli	Bands of smooth muscle around alveolar openings	Conduct air, with much gas exchange
Alveoli	Types I and II alveolar cells (pneumocytes)	None (but with network of elastic and reticular fibers)	Sites of all gas exchange; surfactant from type II pneumocytes; dust cells

FIGURE **17–7** Tertiary (segmental) bronchus.

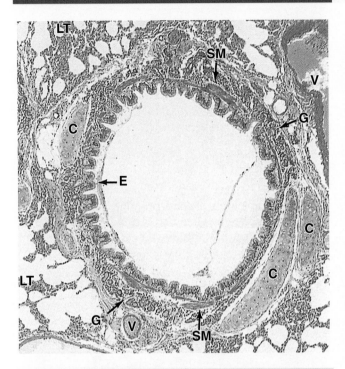

In a cross section of a large bronchus, the lining of respiratory epithelium (**E**) and the mucosa are folded due to contraction of its smooth muscle (**SM**). At this stage in the bronchial tree, the wall is also surrounded by many pieces of hyaline cartilage (**C**) and contains many seromucous glands (**G**) in the submucosa which drain into the lumen. In the connective tissue surrounding the bronchi can be seen arteries and veins (**V**), which are also branching as smaller and smaller vessels in the approach to the respiratory bronchioles. All bronchi are surrounded by distinctive lung tissue (**LT**) showing the many empty spaces of pulmonary alveoli. X56. H&E.

present, especially at the branching points of the bronchial tree. Like the smooth muscle and elastic fibers, mucosa-associated lymphoid tissue (MALT) also becomes relatively more abundant as bronchi become smaller and the cartilage and other connective tissue are reduced.

Bronchioles

Bronchioles are typically designated as the intralobular airways with diameters of 1 mm or less, formed after about the 10th generation of branching; they lack both mucosal glands and cartilage, although dense connective tissue is associated with the smooth muscle (Figure 17–9). In the larger bronchioles, the epithelium is still ciliated pseudostratified columnar, but this decreases in height and complexity to become ciliated simple columnar or simple cuboidal epithelium in the smallest **terminal bronchioles**, which are the last parts of the air conducting system. The ciliated epithelial lining of bronchioles

begins the **mucociliary apparatus** or escalator, important in clearing debris and mucus by moving it upward along the bronchial tree and trachea.

Most numerous in the cuboidal epithelium of terminal bronchioles are **Clara cells**, or **exocrine bronchiolar cells**, which have nonciliated, dome-shaped apical ends with secretory granules (Figure 17–10). Clara cells have various functions, including the following:

- **Secretion of surfactant** lipoproteins and mucins in the fluid layer on the epithelial surface
- **Detoxification** of inhaled xenobiotic compounds by enzymes of the SER
- Secretion of **antimicrobial peptides** and cytokines for local immune defense
- In a **stem cell** subpopulation, injury-induced mitosis for replacement of the other bronchiolar cell types.

Also present in the terminal bronchiole epithelium are small mucous cells and ciliated cells, as well as chemosensory **brush cells** and **DNES small granule cells** like those of the respiratory epithelium higher in the system.

The bronchiolar lamina propria still contains elastic fibers and smooth muscle, producing folds in the mucosa. Muscular contraction in both the bronchi and the bronchioles is controlled primarily by nerves of the autonomic nervous system.

FIGURE **17–8** Bronchial wall.

(a) The epithelial lining (E) of bronchi is mainly pseudostratified ciliated columnar cells with a few goblet cells. The lamina propria (LP) contains the distinct layer of smooth muscle (SM) surrounding the entire bronchus. The submucosa is the site of the supporting cartilage (C) and the adventitia includes blood vessels (V) and nerves (N). Lung tissue (LT) directly surrounds the adventitia of bronchi. X140. H&E.

(b) In the smaller bronchi the epithelium is primarily of columnar cells with cilia (arrows), with fewer goblet cells. The lamina propria has both smooth muscle (SM) and small serous glands (G) near cartilage (C). X400. H&E.

Respiratory Bronchioles

Each terminal bronchiole subdivides into two or more **respiratory bronchioles** that include saclike **alveoli** and represent, therefore, the first-part respiratory region of this organ system (Figure 17–11). The respiratory bronchiolar mucosa is structurally identical to that of the terminal bronchioles, except for a few openings to the alveoli where gas exchange occurs. The mucosa lining consists of Clara cells and ciliated cuboidal cells, with simple squamous cells at the alveolar openings and extending into the alveolus. Proceeding distally along the respiratory bronchioles, alveoli are more numerous and closer together. Smooth muscle and elastic connective tissue make up the lamina propria.

❯❯ MEDICAL APPLICATION

Obstruction of the air supply in bronchi due to excess mucus or to aspirated material can lead to collapse of pulmonary lobules as circulating blood absorbs gases from the affected alveoli. This condition, called **atelectasis**, is normally reversible when the blockage is relieved but, if persistent, can cause fibrosis and loss of respiratory function.

Alveolar Ducts

Distal ends of respiratory bronchioles branch into tubes called **alveolar ducts** that are completely lined by the openings of alveoli (Figures 17–11 and 17–12). Both the alveolar ducts

FIGURE **17–9** Bronchioles.

The smallest branches of the bronchial tree are the bronchioles, which lack supporting cartilage and glands.

(a) A large bronchiole has the characteristically folded respiratory epithelium (**E**) and prominent smooth muscle (arrows), but it is supported only by fibrous connective tissue (**CT**). X140. H&E.

(b) Staining for elastic fibers reveals the high elastic content of the smooth muscle (**arrowhead**) associated with the muscle of a smaller bronchiole in which the epithelium is

simple columnar but still ciliated. Darkly stained elastic fibers are also present in the tunica media of a large arteriole (**A**) nearby and to a lesser extent in the accompanying venule (**V**). The connective tissue includes many lymphocytes (**L**) of diffuse MALT and lymphoid nodules. X180. Elastic stain.

(c) In very small bronchioles the epithelium (**E**) is reduced to simple cuboidal cells with cilia. Several layers of smooth muscle cells (**arrows**) comprise a high proportion of the wall. X300. H&E.

and the alveoli themselves are lined with extremely attenuated squamous cells. In the thin lamina propria, a strand of smooth muscle cells surrounds each alveolar opening and a matrix of elastic and collagen fibers supports both the duct and its alveoli.

Larger clusters of alveoli called **alveolar sacs** form the ends of alveolar ducts distally and occur occasionally along

their length (Figures 17–11 and 17–12). The lamina propria is now extremely thin, consisting essentially of a network of **elastic** and **reticular fibers** that encircles the alveolar openings and closely surrounds each alveolus. Prominent in this sparse connective tissue, another network of **capillaries** also surrounds each alveolus.

FIGURE **17–10** Terminal bronchiole and Clara cells.

The last parts of the air conducting system before the sites of gas exchange appear are called the **terminal bronchioles**. **(a)** A terminal bronchiole has only one or two layers of smooth muscle (**SM**) cells surrounded by connective tissue (**CT**). The epithelium (**E**) contains ciliated cuboidal cells and many low columnar nonciliated cells. Alveoli (**A**) are seen in the surrounding lung tissue. X300. PT.

(b) The nonciliated Clara cells (**C**) with bulging domes of apical cytoplasm contain granules, as seen better here in a plastic section. Named after Dr Max Clara, the histologist who first described them in 1937, these cells have several important functions. They secrete components of surfactant which reduces surface tension and helps prevent collapse of the bronchioles. The P450 enzyme system of their smooth ER detoxifies potentially harmful compounds in air. In other defensive functions, Clara cells also produce the secretory component for the transfer of IgA into the bronchiolar lumen; lysozyme and other enzymes active against bacteria and viruses; and several cytokines that regulate local inflammatory responses. Also included among Clara cells are the occasional stem cells that give rise to all of the cells within the bronchiolar epithelium. X500. PT.

›› MEDICAL APPLICATION

Diffuse alveolar damage or **adult respiratory distress syndrome** can be produced by various types of injuries to the alveolar epithelial and the capillary endothelial cells. Common causes of such injuries include viral and bacterial **respiratory tract infections**; inhalation of **toxic gases**, chemicals, or air with **excessive oxygen**; and **fat embolism syndrome**, in which adipocytes enter the blood during surgery, circulate, and later block the capillary beds. With removal of the initiating factors, normal alveolar wall components can often be restored and at least partial function restored.

FIGURE 17–11 Terminal bronchioles, respiratory bronchioles, and alveoli.

a

b

c

Terminal bronchioles branch into **respiratory bronchioles**, which then branch further into **alveolar ducts** and individual **alveoli**. Respiratory bronchioles are similar in most respects to terminal bronchioles except for the presence of scattered alveoli along their length. **(a)** The diagram shows this branching relationship, as well as the pulmonary blood vessels that travel with the bronchioles and the dense layer of branching capillaries and elastic fibers that surround each alveolus.

(b) The micrograph shows the branching nature of the air passages in two dimensions: respiratory bronchiole (**RB**), alveolar ducts (**AD**), alveolar sacs (**AS**), and individual alveoli (**A**). X60. H&E.

(c) SEM shows in three dimensions the relationship of a terminal bronchiole (**TB**), respiratory bronchiole (**RB**), alveolar duct (**AD**), alveolar sacs (**AS**), and individual alveoli (**A**). X180.

FIGURE 17–12 Respiratory bronchioles, alveolar ducts, and alveoli.

Lung tissue has a spongy structure because of the abundant air passages and pockets called alveoli. **(a)** Typical section of lung tissue includes many bronchioles, some of which are respiratory bronchioles (**RB**) cut lengthwise, and shows the branching continuity with alveolar ducts (**AD**) and sacs (**AS**). Respiratory bronchioles still have a layer of smooth muscle and some regions of cuboidal epithelium, but alveolar ducts consist of a linear series of alveoli, each with smooth muscle fibers around the opening. Individual alveoli (**A**) all open to the sacs or ducts. The respiratory bronchiole runs along a thin-walled

branch of the pulmonary artery (**PA**), while branches of the pulmonary vein (**V**) course elsewhere in the parenchyma. X14. H&E.

(b) Higher magnification shows the relationship of the many rounded, thin-walled alveoli (**A**) to alveolar ducts (**AD**). Alveolar ducts end in two or more clusters of alveoli called alveolar sacs (**AS**). Smooth muscle around the alveolar openings appears as eosinophilic "knobs" between adjacent alveoli. The alveoli here that do not show openings to the ducts or the sacs have their connections in planes of adjacent sections. X140. H&E.

Alveoli

Alveoli are saclike evaginations, each about 200 μm in diameter, from the respiratory bronchioles, alveolar ducts, and alveolar sacs. Along with the airways, alveoli are responsible for the spongy structure of the lungs (Figures 17–11 and 17–12). Each adult lung has approximately 200 million alveoli with a total internal surface area of 75 m². Each alveolus resembles a small rounded pouch open on one side to an alveolar duct or alveolar sac. Air in these structures exchanges O_2 and CO_2 with the blood in surrounding capillaries, through thin specialized alveolar walls that enhance diffusion between the external and internal environments.

Between neighboring alveoli lie thin **interalveolar septa** consisting of scattered fibroblasts and sparse extracellular matrix (ECM), notably elastic and reticular fibers, of connective tissue. The arrangement of elastic fibers enables alveoli to expand with inspiration and contract passively with expiration; reticular fibers prevent both collapse and excessive distention of alveoli. The interalveolar septa are vascularized with the richest capillary networks in the body (Figure 17–11).

The densely anastomosing pulmonary capillaries within the interalveolar septa are supported by the meshwork of reticular and elastic fibers, which also provide the primary structural support of the alveoli. Air in the alveoli is separated from capillary blood by three components referred to collectively as

the respiratory membrane or **blood-air barrier** (Figures 17–13 through 17–15):

- two to three highly attenuated, thin cells lining the alveolus,
- the fused basal laminae of these cells and of the capillary endothelial cells, and
- the thin endothelial cells of the capillary.

The total thickness of these layers varies from 0.1 to 1.5 μm. Macrophages and other leukocytes can also be found within the septa (Figures 17–13 and 17–14). **Alveolar pores** (of Kohn), ranging 10-15 μm in diameter, penetrate the interalveolar septa (Figure 17–13) and connect neighboring alveoli that open to different bronchioles. The pores equalize air pressure in these alveoli and permit collateral circulation of air when a bronchiole is obstructed.

O_2 from the alveolar air diffuses through the blood-air barrier into the capillary blood and binds **hemoglobin** in erythrocytes; CO_2 diffuses into the alveolar air from the pulmonary blood. Most CO_2 arrives in the lungs as part of H_2CO_3 inside erythrocytes and is liberated through the action of carbonic anhydrase.

Capillary endothelial cells are extremely thin but continuous and not fenestrated (Figure 17–15). Clustering of most organelles around the nucleus allows the remaining areas of

FIGURE **17–13** Alveoli and the blood-air barrier.

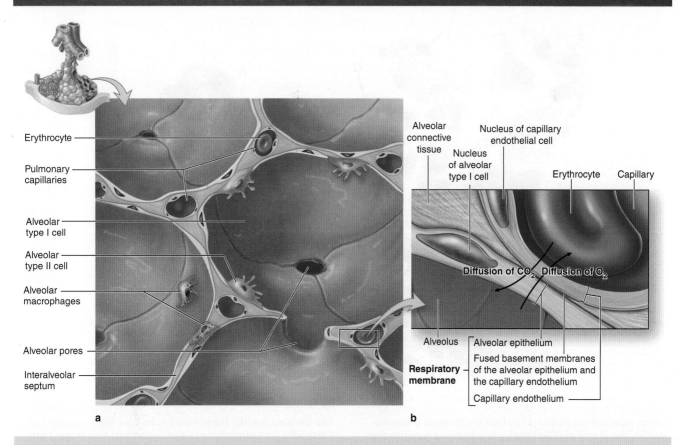

Erythrocyte

Pulmonary capillaries

Alveolar type I cell

Alveolar type II cell

Alveolar macrophages

Alveolar pores

Interalveolar septum

a

Alveolar connective tissue

Nucleus of alveolar type I cell

Nucleus of capillary endothelial cell

Erythrocyte   Capillary

Diffusion of CO_2 Diffusion of O_2

Alveolus

Respiratory membrane

Alveolar epithelium

Fused basement membranes of the alveolar epithelium and the capillary endothelium

Capillary endothelium

b

Gas exchange between air and blood occurs at a membranous barrier between each alveolus and the capillaries surrounding it. **(a)** The diagram shows the relationship between capillaries in the interalveolar septa and the saclike alveoli.

(b) The air-blood barrier consists of an alveolar type I cell, a capillary endothelial cell, and their fused basement membranes.

Oxygen diffuses from alveolar air into capillary blood and carbon dioxide moves in the opposite direction. The inner lining of alveoli is covered by a layer of surfactant, not depicted here, which lowers fluid surface tension and helps prevent collapse of alveoli.

the cell to become very thin and demonstrate highly efficient gas exchange. Ultrastructurally, the most prominent features in the flattened portions of the cell are numerous pinocytotic vesicles.

Type I alveolar cells (or **type I pneumocytes**) are also extremely attenuated cells that line the alveolar surfaces. Type I cells maintain the alveolar side of the blood-air barrier and cover about 95% of the alveolar surface; type II alveolar cells (described below) cover the remainder. These cells are so thin that the TEM was needed to prove that all alveoli have an epithelial lining (Figure 17–15). Organelles are grouped around the nucleus, reducing the thickness of the cytoplasm at the blood-air barrier to as little as 25 nm. Pinocytotic vesicles in the attenuated cytoplasm may play a role in the turnover of surfactant and the removal of small particulate contaminants from the outer surface. In addition to desmosomes, all type I epithelial cells have occluding junctions that prevent the leakage of tissue fluid into the alveolar air space (Figure 17–16).

Type II alveolar cells (**type II pneumocytes** or septal cells) are cuboidal cells that bulge into the air space, interspersed among the type I alveolar cells and bound to them with occluding junctions and desmosomes (Figure 17–16). Type II cells often occur in groups of two or three along at points where two or more alveolar walls unite. These epithelial cells rest on the same basal lamina and have the same origin as the type I cells that line most of the alveolus. Type II cells divide to replace their own population after injury and to provide progenitor cells for the type I cell population. Type II cell nuclei are rounded and may have nucleoli, and their cytoplasm is typically lightly stained with many vesicles.

Many vesicles of type II alveolar cells are **lamellar bodies**, which TEM reveals to be membrane-bound granules about 1 to 2 μm in diameter that contain closely stacked parallel membrane lamellae (Figures 17–16 and 17–17). Lamellar bodies can be considered markers for type II cells.

FIGURE **17-14** Alveolar walls.

The septa between alveoli (**A**) contain several cell types. As seen here, the capillaries (**C**) include erythrocytes and leukocytes. The alveoli are lined mainly by squamous type I alveolar cells (**I**), which line almost the entire alveolus surface and across which gas exchange occurs. Type II alveolar cells line a bit of each alveolus and are large rounded cells, often bulging into the alveolus (**II**). These type II cells have many functions of Clara cells, including production of surfactant. Also present are alveolar macrophages (**M**), sometimes called **dust cells**, which may be in the alveoli or in the interalveolar septa.

They contain various lipids, phospholipids, and proteins that are continuously synthesized and released at the apical cell surface. The secreted material spreads over the entire inner alveolar surface as a film of complexed lipoproteins and water that acts as **pulmonary surfactant**. The surfactant film lowers surface tension at the air-epithelium interface, which helps prevent alveolar collapse at exhalation and allows alveoli to be inflated with less inspiratory force, easing the work of breathing.

Critical components of the surfactant layer produced by type II alveolar cells include the phospholipid **dipalmitoylphosphatidylcholine (DPPC)**, cholesterol, and four surfactant proteins (Figure 17–17). Surfactant protein A (SP-A), a very abundant hydrophilic glycoprotein, and SP-D are important for innate immune protection within the lungs. SP-B and SP-C are required for the maturation of DPPC and its proper orientation in the surfactant film inside the alveolus.

The surfactant layer turns over constantly, with lipoproteins gradually removed by pinocytosis in both types of alveolar cells and by macrophages. In fetal development, surfactant appears in the last weeks of gestation as type II cells differentiate and form lamellar bodies. Lack of adequate surfactant is a major cause of respiratory distress in premature neonates.

>> **MEDICAL APPLICATION**

Infant respiratory distress syndrome, the leading cause of death in premature babies, is due to incomplete differentiation of type II alveolar cells and a resulting deficit of surfactant and difficulty in expanding the alveoli in breathing. Treatment involves insertion of an endotracheal tube to provide both **continuous positive airway pressure (CPAP)** and **exogenous surfactant**, either synthesized chemically or purified from lungs of cattle.

Alveolar macrophages, also called **dust cells**, are found in alveoli and in the interalveolar septum (Figures 17–13 and 17–14). Tens of millions of monocytes migrate daily from the microvasculature into the lung tissue, where they phagocytose erythrocytes lost from damaged capillaries and airborne particulate matter that has penetrated as far as the alveoli. Active macrophages in alveoli can often be distinguished from

FIGURE 17–15 Ultrastructure of the blood-air barrier.

TEM of a capillary (**C**) in an interalveolar septum shows areas for gas exchange between blood and air in three alveoli (**A**). The endothelium is continuous but extremely thin, and its basal lamina (**B**) fuses with that of the type I alveolar cells (**I**) and type II cells. A fibroblast (**F**) can be seen in the septum, and the thickened nuclear regions of two endothelial cells (**E**) are also included. The nucleus at the bottom belongs to an endothelial cell or a circulating leukocyte. X30,000.

type II pneumocytes because they are slightly darker due to their content of dust and carbon from air and complexed iron (hemosiderin) from erythrocytes (Figure 17–14). Filled macrophages have various fates: most migrate into bronchioles where they move up the mucociliary apparatus for removal in the pharynx; others exit the lungs in the lymphatic drainage; and some remain in the interalveolar septa connective tissue for years.

Important histologic features and major functions at each level of airways in lungs are summarized in Table 17–2.

Alveolar lining fluids are also removed via the conducting passages as a result of ciliary activity. As the secretions pass up through the airways, they combine with bronchial mucus to form **bronchoalveolar fluid**, which helps remove particulate components from inspired air. The bronchoalveolar fluid is bacteriostatic, containing lysozyme and other protective agents produced by Clara cells, type II alveolar cells, and alveolar macrophages.

>> MEDICAL APPLICATION

In congestive heart failure, the lungs become congested with blood, and erythrocytes pass into the alveoli, where they are phagocytized by alveolar macrophages. In such cases, these macrophages are called **heart failure cells** when present in the lung and sputum; they are identified by a positive histochemical reaction for iron pigment (hemosiderin).

FIGURE **17–16** Ultrastructure of type II alveolar cells.

TEM of a type II alveolar cell protruding into the alveolar lumen shows unusual lamellar bodies (**L**) that contain newly synthesized pulmonary surfactant after processing of its components in rough ER (**RER**) and the Golgi apparatus (**G**). Smaller multivesicular bodies (**MVB**) with intralumenal vesicles are also often present. Short microvilli (**M**) cover the apical cell surface at the alveolus (**A**) lumen. The type II cell is attached via junctional complexes (**JC**) to the neighboring type I cell (**I**). Reticular fibers (**RF**) are prominent in the ECM. X17,000.

(*Reproduced, with permission, from Dr Mary C. Williams, Pulmonary Center Boston University School of Medicine, MA.*)

Regeneration in the Alveolar Lining

Inhalation of toxic gases or similar materials can kill types I and II cells lining pulmonary alveoli. Death of the first cells results in increased mitotic activity in the remaining type II cells, the progeny of which become both cell types. The normal turnover rate of type II cells is estimated to be 1% per day and results in a continuous renewal of both alveolar cells. With increased toxic stress, some Clara cells can also be stimulated to divide and give rise to alveolar cells.

› LUNG VASCULATURE & NERVES

Blood circulation in the lungs includes both the **pulmonary circulation**, carrying O_2-depleted blood for gas exchange,

FIGURE 17–17 Type II alveolar cell function.

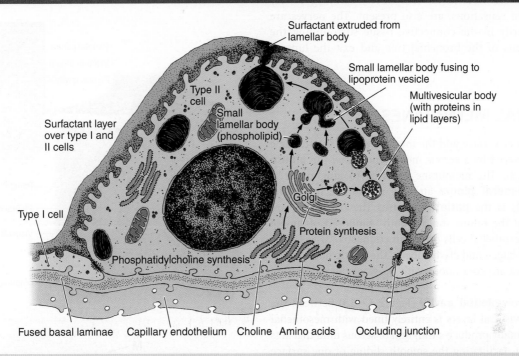

Surfactant extruded from lamellar body

Small lamellar body fusing to lipoprotein vesicle

Multivesicular body (with proteins in lipid layers)

Type II cell

Small lamellar body (phospholipid)

Surfactant layer over type I and II cells

Golgi

Protein synthesis

Type I cell

Phosphatidylcholine synthesis

Fused basal laminae   Capillary endothelium   Choline   Amino acids   Occluding junction

The diagram illustrates **surfactant production** by a type II cell. Surfactant contains protein-lipid complexes synthesized initially in the ER and Golgi apparatus, with further processing and storage in large organelles called **lamellar bodies**. Also present are smaller multivesicular bodies that form when membrane components of an early endosome are sorted, invaginate, and pinch off into smaller vesicles inside the endosome's lumen. In surfactant-producing cells the vesicles in multivesicular bodies are added to the lamellar bodies. Surfactant is secreted continuously by exocytosis and forms an oily film containing phospholipids and surfactant proteins.

and **bronchial circulation**, carrying systemic, nutrient-rich blood. The pulmonary arteries and veins are relatively thin-walled as a result of the low pressures (25 mm Hg systolic, 5 mm Hg diastolic) within the pulmonary circuit. Within the lung, the pulmonary artery branches and accompanies the bronchial tree (Figures 17–11 and 17–12), with its branches sharing the adventitia of the bronchi and bronchioles. At the level of the alveolar duct, the branches of this artery form the dense capillary networks in the interalveolar septa that contact the alveoli.

>> MEDICAL APPLICATION

Emphysema, a chronic lung disease most commonly caused by cigarette smoking, involves dilation and permanent enlargement of the bronchioles leading to pulmonary acini and accompanying loss of cells in the alveoli and other parts of the airway walls, leading to an irreversible loss of respiratory function. Any type of infection in the respiratory regions of the lung produces the local inflammatory condition called **pneumonia**.

Venules arising from the capillary networks are found singly in the lung parenchyma, somewhat removed from the airways (Figures 17–11 and 17–12), supported by a thin covering of connective tissue. After small pulmonary veins leave a lobule, they follow the bronchial tree toward the hilum.

Bronchial arteries branch along with and follow the bronchial tree, distributing blood to most of the lung down to the level of the respiratory bronchioles, at which point they anastomose with small branches of the pulmonary artery and mix their blood with that entering the capillary networks drained by pulmonary venules. Bronchial veins only occur in and around the hilum.

The lymphatic vessels originate in the connective tissue of bronchioles. They follow the bronchioles, bronchi, and pulmonary vessels and all drain into lymph nodes in the region of the hilum. This deep network of lymphatics parallels a superficial network draining areas near the lung surfaces located in the visceral pleura. Lymphatic vessels are not found in the terminal portions of the bronchial tree beyond the alveolar ducts.

Both parasympathetic and sympathetic autonomic fibers innervate the lungs and control reflexes regulating smooth muscle contractions which determine the diameters of the airways. General visceral afferent fibers, carrying poorly localized pain sensations, are also present. The nerves are found primarily in the connective tissue surrounding the larger elements of the bronchial tree and exit the lung at the hilum.

› PLEURAL MEMBRANES

The lung's outer surface and the internal wall of the thoracic cavity are covered by a serous membrane called the **pleura** (Figure 17–18). The membrane attached to lung tissue is called the **visceral pleura** and the membrane lining the thoracic walls is the **parietal pleura**. The two layers are continuous at the hilum and are both composed of simple squamous mesothelial cells on a thin connective tissue layer containing collagen and elastic fibers. The elastic fibers of the visceral pleura are continuous with those of the pulmonary parenchyma.

The narrow **pleural cavity** (Figure 17–18) between the parietal and visceral layers is entirely lined with mesothelial cells that normally produce a thin film of serous fluid that acts as a lubricant, facilitating the smooth sliding of one surface over the other during respiratory movements.

In certain pathologic states, the pleural cavity may contain liquid or air. Like the walls of the peritoneal and pericardial cavities, the serosa of the pleural cavity is water-permeable and fluid exuded from blood plasma commonly accumulates (as a pleural effusion) in this cavity during inflammation and other abnormal conditions.

›› MEDICAL APPLICATION

The condition **pneumothorax** is a partially or completely **collapsed lung** caused by air trapped in the pleural cavity, typically resulting from blunt or penetrating trauma to the chest and producing shortness of breath and hypoxia. Inflammation of the pleura, a condition called either **pleuritis** or **pleurisy**, is most commonly caused by an acute viral infection or pneumonia. **Pleural effusion** or fluid buildup in the pleural cavity produces shortness of breath and can be one result of inflamed pleura.

› RESPIRATORY MOVEMENTS

During inhalation, contraction of the **intercostal muscles** elevates the ribs and contraction of the **diaphragm** lowers the bottom of the thoracic cavity, increasing its diameter and resulting in pulmonary expansion. The bronchi and bronchioles increase in diameter and length during inhalation. The respiratory portion also enlarges, mainly as a result of expansion of the alveolar ducts. Individual alveoli enlarge

FIGURE **17–18** Pleura.

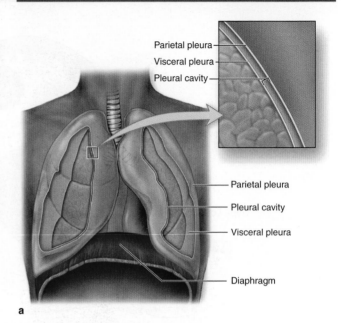

Parietal pleura
Visceral pleura
Pleural cavity

Parietal pleura
Pleural cavity
Visceral pleura

Diaphragm

a

b

The pleura are serous membranes (serosa) associated with each lung and thoracic cavity. **(a)** The diagram shows the **parietal pleura** lining the inner surface of the thoracic cavity and the **visceral pleura** covering the outer surface of the lung. Between these layers is the narrow space of the pleural cavity. **(b)** Both layers are similar histologically and consist of a simple squamous mesothelium (**M**) on a thin layer of connective tissue, as shown here for visceral pleura covering alveoli (**A**). The connective tissue is rich in both collagen and elastic fibers and contains both blood vessels (**V**) and lymphatics (**L**). X140.

only slightly. The elastic fibers of the pulmonary parenchyma are stretched by this expansion. During exhalation, the lungs retract passively because of muscle relaxation and the elastic fibers' return to the unstretched condition.

>> MEDICAL APPLICATION

Lung cancer is one of the most common forms of this disease. **Squamous cell carcinoma**, which is closely correlated with a history of smoking, arises most often from epithelial cells of segmental bronchi. **Adenocarcinoma**, the most common lung cancer in nonsmokers, usually arises from epithelial cells more peripherally, in bronchioles and alveoli. **Small cell carcinoma**, a less common but highly malignant form of lung cancer, develops after neoplastic transformation of small granule Kulchitsky cells in bronchial respiratory epithelium.

The Respiratory System SUMMARY OF KEY POINTS

- The function of the respiratory system is to provide **oxygen to the blood**, with a secondary function of sound production in the larynx.
- The respiratory system consists of an air **conducting region** (the upper respiratory tract in the head, as well as the larynx, trachea, bronchi, and most bronchioles) and a **respiratory region** with alveoli.

Nasal Cavities

- The left and right **nasal cavities** of the upper respiratory tract have **vestibules** where air enters and three projections called **conchae** from their medial walls, which create turbulence in inspired air.
- Moist **vibrissae** in the vestibular openings, the **nares** or nostrils, filter some material from inspired air.
- Deeper areas of the vestibules and the floor, lateral walls, and most of the conchae of the nasal cavities themselves are lined by **respiratory epithelium: pseudostratified ciliated columnar epithelium**.
- **Respiratory epithelium** includes **goblet cells** secreting mucus, **ciliated columnar cells** sweeping the mucus along the surface, chemosensory **brush cells**, scattered **endocrine cells**, and basal **stem cells**.
- The roof and part of the superior concha in each nasal cavity are covered by **olfactory epithelium**, which is pseudostratified epithelium containing bipolar **olfactory neurons**, **support cells**, and **stem cells**.
- The mucosa of the **nasal cavities** and **nasopharynx** also contains a rich **vasculature** and many **seromucous glands**, which help warm, humidify, and clean inspired air.

Larynx, Trachea, and Bronchial Tree

- Within the lumen of the **larynx**, bilateral projecting **vocal folds** (or cords) can be placed under variable tension by the underlying **vocalis muscles** and caused to vibrate by expelled air, producing sounds.
- The **trachea** is completely lined by **respiratory epithelium** and is supported by C-shaped rings of **hyaline cartilage** in the mucosa, with smooth **trachealis muscles** in the posterior opening of the rings.
- Left and right **primary bronchi** enter the two lungs and bifurcate repeatedly as **secondary**, **tertiary**, and **smaller segmental bronchi** with the lung tissue as the **bronchial tree**.

- **Bronchi** and their branches are lined by **respiratory mucosa**, with prominent spiraling bands of **smooth muscle** and increasingly smaller pieces of **hyaline cartilage**.
- Branches of the bronchial tree with diameters of 1 mm or less are generally called **bronchioles**, which are lined by **simple columnar** or **cuboidal ciliated cells**, with circular smooth muscle but **no cartilage**.
- **Terminal bronchioles** are the last branches to lack alveoli and are lined by **simple cuboidal epithelium** consisting mainly of **Clara cells**, which have **innate immune** and **surfactant secretory functions**.

Respiratory Region

- Terminal bronchioles subdivide into two or three **respiratory bronchioles**, lined by simple cuboidal epithelium and **Clara cells** and interrupted by scattered squamous evaginations called **alveoli**, the sites of gas exchange.
- A respiratory bronchiole leads to an **alveolar duct**, which is lined by a continuous series of alveoli and which ends in a cluster of alveoli called the **alveolar sac**.
- All alveoli are surrounded by sparse connective tissue in **interalveolar septa** that consist primarily of **elastic and reticular fibers** and a dense **capillary network**.
- The wall of each alveolus consists of two cell types: extremely **thin type I alveolar cells** (pneumocytes) and **cuboidal type II alveolar cells** with **surfactant** secreting and **innate immune** properties.
- **Type II alveolar cells** are characterized ultrastructurally by unique cytoplasmic **lamellar bodies**, large granules with closely stacked layers of membrane involved in **surfactant synthesis**.
- The **blood-air barrier** allowing gas exchange at each alveolus consists of the **thin type I alveolar cell**, the **thin capillary endothelial cells**, and the **fused basal laminae** of these two cells.
- The **surfactant material** secreted by Clara cells and type II alveolar cells is an oily mixture of **phospholipids** and **surfactant proteins**, which forms a film and **lowers surface tension** in alveoli.
- Each lung is covered by **visceral pleura**, a layer of thin connective tissue and mesothelium, and is continuous with **parietal pleura**, a similar tissue layer that lines the pleural cavity.

The skin is the largest single organ of the body, typically accounting for 15% to 20% of total body weight and, in adults, presenting 1.5 to 2 m² of surface to the external environment. Also known as the **integument** (L. *integumentum*, covering) or **cutaneous layer**, the skin is composed of the **epidermis**, an epithelial layer of ectodermal origin, and the **dermis**, a layer of mesodermal connective tissue (Figure 18–1). At the irregular junction between the dermis and epidermis, projections called **dermal papillae** interdigitate with invaginating **epidermal ridges** to strengthen adhesion of the two layers. Epidermal derivatives include hairs, nails, and sebaceous and sweat glands. Beneath the dermis lies the **subcutaneous tissue** or **hypodermis** (Gr. *hypo*, under + *derma*, skin), a loose connective tissue layer usually containing pads of adipocytes. The subcutaneous tissue binds the skin loosely to the underlying tissues and corresponds to the superficial fascia of gross anatomy.

The specific functions of the skin fall into several broad categories.

- **Protective:** It provides a physical barrier against thermal and mechanical insults such as friction and against most potential pathogens and other material. Microorganisms that do penetrate skin alert resident lymphocytes and antigen-presenting cells (APCs) in skin and an immune response is mounted. The dark pigment melanin in the epidermis protects cell nuclei from ultraviolet (UV) radiation. Skin is also a permeability barrier against excessive loss or uptake of water, which has allowed for terrestrial life. Skin's selective permeability allows some lipophilic drugs such as certain steroid hormones and medications to be administered via skin patches.
- **Sensory:** Many types of sensory receptors allow skin to constantly monitor the environment, and various skin mechanoreceptors help regulate the body's interactions with physical objects.
- **Thermoregulatory:** A constant body temperature is normally easily maintained thanks to the skin's insulating components (eg, the fatty layer and hair on the head) and its mechanisms for accelerating heat loss (sweat production and a dense superficial microvasculature).
- **Metabolic:** Cells of skin synthesize vitamin D₃, needed in calcium metabolism and proper bone formation, through the local action of UV light on the vitamin's precursor. Excess electrolytes can be removed in sweat, and the subcutaneous layer stores a significant amount of energy in the form of fat.
- **Sexual signaling:** Many features of skin, such as pigmentation and hair, are visual indicators of health involved in attraction between the sexes in all vertebrate species, including humans. The effects of sex pheromones produced by the apocrine sweat glands and other skin glands are also important for this attraction.

The dermal-epidermal interdigitations are of the peg-and-socket variety in most skin (Figure 18–1), but they occur as well-formed ridges and grooves in the thick skin of the palms and soles, which is more subject to friction. These ridges and the intervening sulci form distinctive patterns unique for each individual, appearing as combinations of loops, arches, and whorls, called dermatoglyphs, also known as fingerprints and footprints. Skin is elastic and can expand rapidly to cover swollen areas and, like the gut lining, is self-renewing throughout life. In healthy individuals injured skin is repaired rapidly. The molecular basis of skin healing is increasingly well understood and provides a basis for better understanding of repair and regeneration in other organs.

FIGURE **18–1** Layers and appendages of skin.

Epidermal ridges

Dermal papillae

Tactile (sensory) receptor

Artery

Vein

Areolar connective tissue

Adipose connective tissue

Epidermis

Papillary layer

Dermis

Reticular layer

Subcutaneous layer

Diagrammatic overview of skin, showing the major layers and epidermal appendages (hair follicles, sweat, and sebaceous glands), the vasculature, and the major sensory receptors.

› EPIDERMIS

The epidermis consists mainly of a stratified squamous keratinized epithelium composed of cells called **keratinocytes**. There are also three much less abundant epidermal cell types: pigment-producing **melanocytes**, antigen-presenting **Langerhans cells**, and tactile epithelial cells called **Merkel cells** (Figure 18–2).

The epidermis forms the major distinction between **thick skin** (Figure 18–2a), found on the palms and soles, and **thin skin** (Figure 18–3) found elsewhere on the body. The designations "thick" and "thin" refer to the thickness of the epidermal layer, which alone varies from 75 to 150 μm for thin skin and from 400 to 1400 μm (1.4 mm) for thick skin. Total skin thickness (epidermis plus dermis) also varies according to the site. For example, full skin on the back is about 4 mm thick, whereas that of the scalp is about 1.5 mm thick. Like all epithelia, the stratified squamous epidermis lacks microvasculature, its cells receiving nutrients and O_2 by diffusion from the dermis.

From the dermis, the epidermis consists of four layers of keratinocytes (or five layers in thick skin, Figure 18–2):

- The **basal layer** (**stratum basale**) is a single layer of basophilic cuboidal or columnar cells on the basement membrane at the dermal-epidermal junction (Figures 18–2 and 18–3). Hemidesmosomes in the basal cell membranes join these cells to the basal lamina, and desmosomes bind the cells of this layer together in their lateral and upper surfaces. The stratum basale is characterized by intense mitotic activity and contains, along with the deepest part of the next layer, progenitor cells for all the epidermal layers. In addition to the basal stem cells for keratinocytes found here, a niche for such cells

FIGURE **18–2** Layers (strata) of epidermis in thick skin.

(a) Micrograph shows the sequence of the epidermal layers in thick skin and the approximate sizes and shape of keratinocytes in these layers. Also shown are the coarse bundles of collagen in the dermis and on the far left, the duct from a sweat gland entering the epidermis from a dermal papilla and

coiling to a surface pore through all the strata. X100. H&E.
(b) Diagram illustrating the sequence of the epidermal layers also indicates the normal locations of three important nonkeratinocyte cells in the epidermis: melanocytes, a Langerhans cell, and a tactile Merkel cell.

also occurs in the hair follicle sheaths that are continuous with the epidermis. The human epidermis is renewed about every 15 to 30 days, depending on age, the region of the body, and other factors. An important feature of all keratinocytes in the stratum basale is the cytoskeletal **keratins**, intermediate filaments about 10 nm in diameter. During differentiation, the cells move upward and the amount and types of keratin filaments increase until they represent half the total protein in the superficial keratinocytes.

>> MEDICAL APPLICATION

Friction blisters are lymph-filled spaces created between the epidermis and dermis of thick skin by excessive rubbing, as with ill-fitting shoes or hard use of the hands. If continued, such activity produces protective thickening and hardening of the outer cornified epidermal layers, seen as corns and calluses.

■ The **spinous layer** (**stratum spinosum**) is normally the thickest layer, especially in the epidermal ridges (Figures 18–2 and 18–3), and consists of generally polyhedral cells having central nuclei with nucleoli and cytoplasm actively synthesizing keratins. Just above the basal layer,

some cells may still divide and this combined zone is sometimes called the **stratum germinativum**. The keratin filaments assemble here into microscopically visible bundles called **tonofibrils** that converge and terminate at the numerous desmosomes holding the cell layers together. The cells extend slightly around the tonofibrils on both sides of each desmosome (and the extensions elongate if the cells shrink slightly during histologic processing), leading to the appearance of many short "spines" or prickles at the cell surfaces (Figure 18–4). The epidermis of thick skin subject to continuous friction and pressure (such as the foot soles) has a thicker stratum spinosum with more abundant tonofibrils and desmosomes.

>> MEDICAL APPLICATION

In adults, one-third of all cancers originate in the skin. Most of these derive from cells of the basal or spinous layers, producing, respectively, basal cell carcinomas and squamous cell carcinomas. Fortunately, both types of tumors can be diagnosed and excised early and consequently are rarely lethal. Skin cancer shows an increased incidence in fair-skinned individuals residing in regions with high amounts of solar radiation.

FIGURE **18-3** Layers of epidermis in thin skin.

The interface between dermis and epidermis in thin skin is held together firmly by interlocking epidermal ridges or pegs (**EP**) and dermal papillae (**DP**). The dermis (**D**) of thin skin is more cellular and well vascularized than that of thick skin, with elastin and less coarse bundles of collagen. The epidermis usually shows only four layers in thin skin: the one-cell thick stratum basale (**B**) containing most mitotic cells; the stratum spinosum (**S**) where synthesis of much keratin and other proteins takes place; the stratum granulosum (**G**); and the stratum corneum (**C**), consisting of dead squames composed mostly of keratin. X240. H&E.

- The **granular layer (stratum granulosum)** consists of three to five layers of flattened cells, now undergoing the terminal differentiation process of **keratinization**. Their cytoplasm is filled with intensely basophilic masses (Figures 18–2 and 18–3; Figure 18–5) called **keratohyaline granules**. These are dense, non–membrane-bound masses of **filaggrin** and other proteins associated with the keratins of tonofibrils, linking them further into large cytoplasmic structures. Characteristic ultrastructural features in cells of the granular layer are the membranous, Golgi-derived **lamellar granules**, small ovoid (100 by 300 nm) structures with many lamellae containing various lipids. Among the last activities of the keratinocytes, the lamellar granules undergo exocytosis, producing a lipid-rich, impermeable layer around the cells. This material forms a major part of the skin's barrier against water loss. Formation of this barrier, which appeared first in ancestral reptiles, was a key evolutionary process that permitted animals to develop on land. Together, keratinization and production of the lipid-rich layer also have a crucial sealing effect in skin, forming the barrier to penetration by most foreign materials.

- The **stratum lucidum**, found only in thick skin, consists of a thin, translucent layer of flattened eosinophilic keratinocytes held together by desmosomes (Figures 18–1 and 18–5). Nuclei and organelles have been lost, and the cytoplasm consists almost exclusively of packed keratin filaments embedded in an electron-dense matrix.

- The **stratum corneum** (Figures 18–2 and 18–3) consists of 15 to 20 layers of squamous, keratinized cells filled with birefringent filamentous keratins. Keratin filaments contain at least six different polypeptides with molecular

FIGURE **18-4** Keratinocytes of the stratum spinosum.

(**a**) A section of epidermal stratum spinosum of thick skin, showing cells with numerous short cytoplasmic projections (**arrow**). X400. PT.

(**b**) TEM of a single spinous keratinocyte with surface projections (**arrows**). X8400.

(**c**) Detail of the desmosomes joining two cells showing intermediate filaments associated with desmosomes. X40,000.

FIGURE **18–5** Stratum granulosum and stratum lucidum: thick skin.

In keratinocytes moving upward from the stratum spinosum (**S**), differentiation proceeds with the cells becoming filled with numerous large, amorphous masses of protein called **keratohyaline granules**.

Cells with these basophilic granules make up the stratum granulosum (**G**), where keratin filaments are cross-linked with filaggrin and other proteins from these granules to produce tight bundles filling the cytoplasm and flattening the cells. Smaller organelles called **lamellar granules** undergo exocytosis in this layer, secreting a lipid-rich layer around the cells which makes the epidermis impermeable to water. Together, the lipid envelope and the keratin-filled cells determine most of the physical properties of the epidermis.

The cells leaving the stratum granulosum, still bound together by desmosomes, undergo terminal differentiation and in thick skin appear as a dense, thin layer called the **stratum lucidum** (**L**). Here proteins are dispersed through the tonofibril bundles, giving this layer a regular, "clear" appearance. In the most superficial stratum corneum (**C**), the cells have lost nuclei and cytoplasm, consisting only of flattened, keratinized structures called **squames** bound by hydrophobic, lipid-rich intercellular cement. At the surface they are worn away (thick skin) or flake off (thin skin). X560. H&E.

masses ranging from 40 to 70 kDa, synthesized during cell differentiation in the immature layers. As they form, keratin tonofibrils become heavily massed with filaggrin and other proteins in keratohyaline granules. By the end of keratinization, the cells contain only amorphous, fibrillar proteins with plasma membranes surrounded by the lipid-rich layer. These fully keratinized or cornified cells called **squames** are continuously shed at the epidermal surface as the desmosomes and lipid-rich cell envelopes break down.

Important features of the epidermal strata are summarized in Table 18–1.

Melanocytes

The color of the skin is the result of several factors, the most important of which are the keratinocytes' content of **melanin** and **carotene** and the number of blood vessels in the dermis.

Eumelanins are brown or black pigments produced by the **melanocyte** (Figures 18–6 and 18–7), a specialized cell of the epidermis found among the cells of the basal layer and in hair follicles. The similar pigment found in red hair is called **pheomelanin** (Gr. *phaios*, dusky + *melas*, black). Melanocytes are neural crest derivatives that migrate into the embryonic epidermis' stratum basale, where eventually one melanocyte accumulates for every five or six basal keratinocytes (600-1200/mm^2 of skin). They have pale-staining, rounded cell bodies attached by hemidesmosomes to the basal lamina, but lacking attachments to the neighboring keratinocytes. Several long irregular cytoplasmic extensions from each melanocyte cell body penetrate the epidermis, running between the cells of the basal and spinous layers and terminating in invaginations of 5 to 10 keratinocytes. Ultrastructurally a melanocyte has numerous small mitochondria, short cisternae of RER, and a well-developed Golgi apparatus (Figure 18–6).

The first step in melanin synthesis is catalyzed by **tyrosinase**, a transmembrane enzyme in Golgi-derived vesicles (Figure 18–7a). Tyrosinase activity converts tyrosine into **3,4-dihydroxyphenylalanine** (**DOPA**), which is then further transformed and polymerized into the different forms of melanin. Melanin pigment is linked to a matrix of structural proteins and accumulates in the vesicles until they form mature elliptical granules about 1 μm long called **melanosomes** (Figure 18–7b).

Melanosomes are then transported via kinesin to the tips of the cytoplasmic extensions. The neighboring keratinocytes phagocytose the tips of these dendrites, take in the melanosomes, and transport them by dynein toward their nuclei. The melanosomes accumulate within keratinocytes as a supranuclear cap that prior to keratinization absorbs and scatters sunlight, protecting DNA of the living cells from the ionizing, mutagenic effects of UV radiation.

Although melanocytes produce melanosomes, the keratinocytes are the melanin depot and contain more of this pig-

TABLE **18–1**	Skin layers and the subcutaneous layer.	
Layer	**Specific Layer**	**Description**
Epidermis 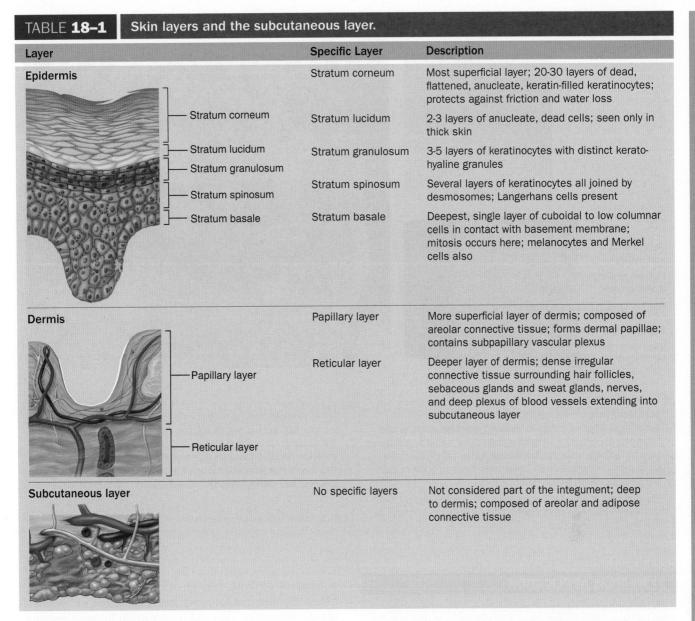	Stratum corneum	Most superficial layer; 20-30 layers of dead, flattened, anucleate, keratin-filled keratinocytes; protects against friction and water loss
	Stratum lucidum	2-3 layers of anucleate, dead cells; seen only in thick skin
	Stratum granulosum	3-5 layers of keratinocytes with distinct kerato-hyaline granules
	Stratum spinosum	Several layers of keratinocytes all joined by desmosomes; Langerhans cells present
	Stratum basale	Deepest, single layer of cuboidal to low columnar cells in contact with basement membrane; mitosis occurs here; melanocytes and Merkel cells also
Dermis	Papillary layer	More superficial layer of dermis; composed of areolar connective tissue; forms dermal papillae; contains subpapillary vascular plexus
	Reticular layer	Deeper layer of dermis; dense irregular connective tissue surrounding hair follicles, sebaceous glands and sweat glands, nerves, and deep plexus of blood vessels extending into subcutaneous layer
Subcutaneous layer	No specific layers	Not considered part of the integument; deep to dermis; composed of areolar and adipose connective tissue

ment than the cells that make it. One melanocyte plus the keratinocytes into which it transfers melanosomes make up an **epidermal-melanin unit**. The density of such units in skin is similar in all individuals. Melanocytes of people with ancestral origins near the equator, where the need for protection against the sun is greatest, produce melanin granules more rapidly and accumulate them more abundantly in keratinocytes.

›› MEDICAL APPLICATION

Albinism is a congenital disorder producing skin **hypopigmentation** due to a defect in tyrosinase or some other component of the melanin-producing pathway. An acquired condition called **vitiligo** involves skin **depigmentation**, often only in affected patches, due to the loss or decreased activity of melanocytes. The causes of melanocyte loss are not clear, but they may include environmental, genetic, or autoimmune conditions.

In regions with much less sunlight such as northern Europe, the small amount of UV radiation penetrating dark skin barely sustains adequate vitamin D_3 synthesis. Individuals with ancestry there have one or more genetic polymorphisms that affect steps in melanin formation and cause more lightly pigmented keratinocytes that have increased UV penetration and vitamin D_3 synthesis.

Darkening of the skin, or tanning, after exposure to solar radiation at wavelengths of 290 to 320 nm is a two-step process. A physicochemical reaction darkens preexisting melanin. At the same time, paracrine factors secreted by keratinocytes experiencing increased UV radiation accelerate melanin synthesis and its accumulation in the epidermis.

FIGURE **18–6** Melanocytes.

(a) Micrograph shows melanocytes (**M**) in the epidermal basal layer which synthesize **melanin granules** and transfer them into neighboring **keratinocytes** of the basal and spinous layers. Typically melanocytes are pale-staining cells on the basement membrane, with lower total melanin content than the keratinocytes. X400. H&E.

(b) Diagram of a melanocyte shows the irregular cytoplasmic processes between neighboring keratinocytes for transfer of melanin to those cells.

(c) Ultrastructurally, a melanocyte is located on the basal lamina (**BL**) and has well-developed Golgi complexes (**G**) producing the vesicles in which melanin is synthesized. As they fill, these vesicles become melanin granules (**MG**), which accumulate at the tips of the dendritic cytoplasmic extensions (**CE**) before transfer to keratinocytes (**K**). X14,000.

>> MEDICAL APPLICATION

Melanocytes can normally proliferate in skin to produce **moles**, or **benign melanocytic nevi** of various types. Changes in the size or appearance of moles are sometimes indicative of dysplasia that can progress further to **malignant melanoma**. Dividing rapidly, malignantly transformed melanocytes often penetrate the basal lamina, enter the dermis, and metastasize by invading blood and lymphatic vessels.

Langerhans Cells

Antigen-presenting cells (APCs) called **Langerhans cells**, which are usually most clearly seen in the spinous layer, represent 2% to 8% of the epidermal cells. Cytoplasmic processes extend from these dendritic cells between keratinocytes of all the layers, forming a fairly dense network in the epidermis (Figure 18–8). Langerhans cells bind, process, and present antigens to T lymphocytes in the same manner as immune dendritic cells in other organs (see Chapter 14). Microorganisms cannot penetrate the epidermis without alerting these dendritic cells and triggering an immune response. Langerhans cells, along with more scattered epidermal lymphocytes and other APCs in the dermis, make up a major component of the skin's adaptive immunity.

Because of its location, the skin is continuously in close contact with many antigenic molecules. Various epidermal features participate in both innate and adaptive immunity (see Chapter 14), providing an important immunologic component to the skin's overall protective function.

Merkel Cells

Merkel cells, or **epithelial tactile cells**, are sensitive mechanoreceptors essential for light touch sensation. Joined by desmosomes to keratinocytes of the basal epidermal layer, Merkel cells resemble the surrounding cells but with few, if any, melanosomes. They are abundant in highly sensitive skin like that of fingertips and at the bases of some hair follicles. Merkel cells originate from the same stem cells as keratinocytes and are characterized by

FIGURE **18–7** Melanosome formation.

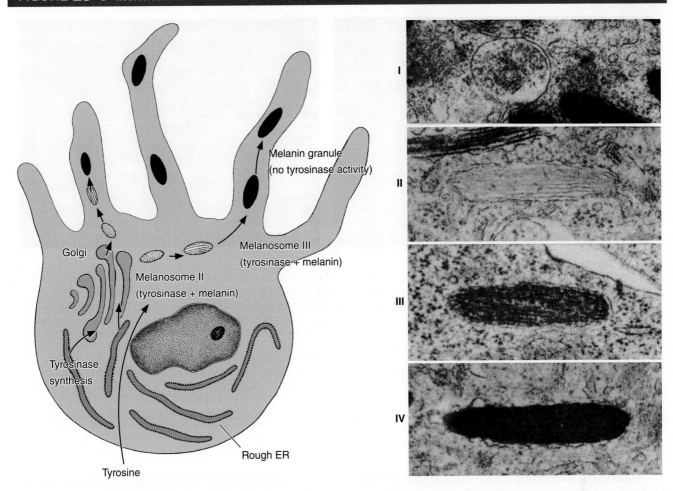

The diagram of a melanocyte shows the main features of melanin formation. The granules containing melanin mature through four stages that are characterized ultrastructurally, as shown on the right. **Tyrosinase** is synthesized in the rough ER, processed through the Golgi apparatus, and accumulates in vesicles that also have a fine granular matrix of other proteins (**stage I** melanosomes). Melanin synthesis begins in the ovoid **stage II** melanosomes, in which the matrix has been organized into parallel filaments on which polymerized melanin is deposited and accumulates in **stage III**. A mature melanin granule (**stage IV**) has lost tyrosinase and other activities and has the internal matrix completely filled with melanin. The mature granules are ellipsoid, approximately 0.5 by 1 μm in size, and visible by light microscopy.

Melanin granules are transported to the tips of the processes of melanocyte and are then transferred to the neighboring keratinocytes of the basal and spinous layers. In keratinocytes the melanin granules are transported to a region near the nucleus, where they accumulate as a supra-nuclear cap shading the DNA against the harmful effects of UV radiation.

small, Golgi-derived dense-core neurosecretory granules containing peptides (Figure 18–9). The basolateral surfaces of the cells contact expanded terminal discs of unmyelinated sensory fibers penetrating the basal lamina (Figure 18–9).

›› MEDICAL APPLICATION

Merkel cells are of clinical importance because Merkel cell carcinomas, though uncommon, are very aggressive and difficult to treat. Merkel cell carcinoma is 40 times less common than malignant melanoma but has twice the mortality of that disease.

› DERMIS

The **dermis** is the layer of connective tissue (Figures 18–1 and 18–2) that supports the epidermis and binds it to the subcutaneous tissue (hypodermis). The thickness of the dermis varies with the region of the body and reaches its maximum of 4 mm on the back. The surface of the dermis is very irregular and has many projections (dermal papillae) that interdigitate with projections (epidermal pegs or ridges) of the epidermis (see Figure 18–1), especially in skin subject to frequent pressure, where they reinforce the dermal-epidermal junction.

FIGURE **18–8** Langerhans cells.

Langerhans cells are dendritic APCs of the epidermis where they comprise an important defense against pathogens and environmental insults. Like other APCs, they develop in the bone marrow, move into the blood circulation, and finally migrate into stratified squamous epithelia where they are difficult to identify in routinely stained sections. **(a)** Section of immunostained skin shows Langerhans cells (yellow) abundant in hair follicles (**F**), where many microorganisms live, and throughout the epidermis (**E**). Keratin of the epidermis and follicles is stained green. X40. Antibodies against langerin/CD207 and keratin.

(b) Face-on view of an epidermal sheet stained using the same antibody showing the network of Langerhans cells among the other epidermal cells, which detects invading microorganisms. After sampling the invaders' antigens, Langerhans cells leave the epidermis and travel to the nearest lymph node to elicit lymphocytes that can mount a collective immune response. X200. Anti-langerin/CD207.

(*Reproduced, with permission, from Romani N et al.* Acta Path Micro Immunol Scandinavica. *2003;111:725.*)

A **basement membrane** always occurs between the stratum basale and the dermis, and follows the contour of the interdigitations between these layers. As described in Chapter 4, this membrane is a composite structure consisting of the **basal lamina** and the **reticular lamina**, and can usually be seen with the light microscope. Nutrients for keratinocytes diffuse into the avascular epidermis from the dermal vasculature through this basement membrane.

›› MEDICAL APPLICATION

Abnormalities of the dermal-epidermal junction can lead to one type of blistering disorder (bullous pemphigoid). Another type of blistering disorder (pemphigus) is caused by autoimmune damage to intercellular junctions between keratinocytes.

The dermis contains two sublayers with indistinct boundaries (see Figure 18–1; Table 18–1):

■ The thin **papillary layer**, which includes the dermal papillae, consists of loose connective tissue, with types I and III collagen fibers, fibroblasts and scattered mast cells, macrophages, and other leukocytes. From this layer,

anchoring fibrils of type VII collagen insert into the basal lamina, helping to bind the dermis to the epidermis.

■ The underlying **reticular layer** is much thicker, consists of dense irregular connective tissue (mainly bundles of type I collagen), with more fibers and fewer cells than the papillary layer. A network of elastic fibers is also present (Figure 18–10), providing elasticity to the skin. Between the collagen and elastic fibers are abundant proteoglycans rich in dermatan sulfate.

›› MEDICAL APPLICATION

With age, collagen fibers thicken and collagen synthesis decreases. In old age, extensive cross-linking of collagen fibers and the loss of elastic fibers, especially after excessive exposure to the sun (solar elastosis), cause the skin to become more fragile, lose its suppleness, and develop wrinkles. The epidermis also normally thins and becomes more transparent during aging. In several disorders, such as cutis laxa and Ehlers-Danlos syndromes, there is a considerable increase in skin and ligament extensibility caused by defective collagen-fibril processing.

FIGURE **18–9** Merkel or tactile cell.

Merkel cells in the basal epidermal layer have high tactile sensitivity and function as mechanoreceptors. This TEM of a Merkel cell shows a mass of dense-core cytoplasmic granules (**G**) near the basolateral cell membrane, which is in direct contact with the expanded, disc-like ending of a sensory nerve (**N**). X14,000. Inset: Granules are similar in morphology and content to the granules of many neuroendocrine cells. X61,500.)

Both dermal regions contain a rich network of blood and lymphatic vessels. Nutritive vessels form two major plexuses (see Figure 18–1):

- Between the papillary and reticular dermal layers lies the microvascular **subpapillary plexus**, from which capillary branches extend into the dermal papillae and form a rich, nutritive capillary network just below the epidermis.
- A deep plexus with larger blood and lymphatic vessels lies near the interface of the dermis and the subcutaneous layer.

In addition to the nutritive function, dermal vasculature has a thermoregulatory function, which involves numerous **arteriovenous anastomoses** or shunts (see Chapter 11) located between the two major plexuses. The shunts decrease blood flow in the papillary layer to minimize heat loss in cold conditions and increase this flow to facilitate heat loss when it is hot, thus helping maintain a constant body temperature. Lymphatic vessels begin in the dermal papillae and converge to form two plexuses located with the blood vessels.

The dermis is also richly innervated. Sensory afferent nerve fibers form a network in the papillary dermis and around hair follicles, ending at epithelial and dermal receptors shown in Figure 18–11. Autonomic effector nerves to dermal sweat glands and smooth muscle fibers in the skin of some areas are postganglionic fibers of sympathetic ganglia; no parasympathetic innervation is present.

❯ SUBCUTANEOUS TISSUE

The **subcutaneous layer** (see Figure 18–1) consists of loose connective tissue that binds the skin loosely to the subjacent organs, making it possible for the skin to slide over them. This layer, also called the **hypodermis** or **superficial fascia**, contains adipocytes that vary in number in different body regions and vary in size according to nutritional state. The extensive vascular supply at the subcutaneous layer promotes rapid uptake of insulin or drugs injected into this tissue.

❯ SENSORY RECEPTORS

With its large surface and external location, the skin functions as an extensive receiver for various stimuli from the environment. Diverse sensory receptors are present in skin, including both simple nerve endings with no Schwann cell or collagenous coverings and more complex structures with sensory fibers enclosed by glia and delicate connective tissue capsules (Figure 18–11). The unencapsulated receptors include the following:

- The **Merkel cells**, each associated with expanded nerve endings (Figure 18–9), which function as tonic receptors for sustained light touch and for sensing an object's texture.
- **Free nerve endings** in the papillary dermis and extending into lower epidermal layers, which respond primarily to high and low temperatures, pain, and itching, but also function as tactile receptors.
- **Root hair plexuses**, a web of sensory fibers surrounding the bases of hair follicles in the reticular dermis that detects movements of the hairs.

The encapsulated receptors are all phasic mechanoreceptors, responding rapidly to stimuli on the skin. Four are recognized in human skin, although only the first two are seen in routine preparations:

- **Meissner corpuscles** are elliptical structures, 30 to 75 μm by 50 to 150 μm, consisting of sensory axons winding among flattened Schwann cells arranged perpendicular to the epidermis in the dermal papillae (Figure 18–12a). They initiate impulses when light-touch or low-frequency stimuli against skin temporarily deform their shape. They are numerous in the fingertips, palms, and soles but decline slowly in number during aging after puberty.

FIGURE **18–10** Elastic fibers of dermis.

A section of thin skin stained for elastic fibers shows the extensive distribution of these darkly stained fibers among the eosinophilic collagen bundles. In the dermal papillary layer, the diameter of fibers decreases as they approach the epidermis and insert into the basement membrane. X100. Weigert elastic stain.

›› MEDICAL APPLICATION

The density of tactile Meissner corpuscles in skin can be determined approximately by **two-point discrimination tests**. Such neurologic measurements indicate that the number of tactile corpuscles in skin normally declines during adult life. Loss of tactile corpuscles or reduction in their activity can also be detected in **scleroderma** and certain other connective tissue disorders that lead to **sclerosis (hardening)** of the dermis and tightening of the skin.

- **Lamellated (pacinian) corpuscles** are large oval structures, approximately 0.5 mm by 1 mm, found deep in the reticular dermis and hypodermis, with an outer capsule and 15-50 thin, concentric lamellae of

flattened Schwann cells and collagen surrounding a highly branched, unmyelinated axon (Figure 18–12b). Lamellated corpuscles are specialized for sensing coarse touch, pressure (sustained touch), and vibrations, with distortion of the capsule amplifying a mechanical stimulus to the axonal core where an impulse is initiated. Pacinian corpuscles are also found in the connective tissue of organs located deep in the body, including the wall of the rectum and urinary bladder, where they also produce the sensation of pressure when the surrounding tissue is distorted.

- **Krause end bulbs** are simpler encapsulated, ovoid structures, with extremely thin, collagenous capsules penetrated by a sensory fiber. They are found primarily in the skin of the penis and clitoris where they sense low-frequency vibrations.
- **Ruffini corpuscles** have collagenous, fusiform capsules anchored firmly to the surrounding connective tissue, with sensory axons stimulated by stretch (tension) or twisting (torque) in the skin.

› HAIR

Hairs are elongated keratinized structures that form within epidermal invaginations, the **hair follicles** (Figure 18–13). The color, size, shape, and texture of hairs vary according to age, genetic background, and region of the body. All skin has at least minimal hair except the glabrous skin of the palms, soles, lips, glans penis, clitoris, and labia minora. The face has about 600 hairs/cm² and the remainder of the body has about 60/cm². Hairs grow discontinuously, with periods of growth followed by periods of rest, and this growth does not occur synchronously in all regions of the body or even in the same area.

The growing hair follicle has a terminal dilation called a **hair bulb** (Figure 18–13a). A **dermal papilla** inserts into the base of the hair bulb and contains a capillary network required to sustain the hair follicle. Keratinocytes continuous with those of the basal epidermis cover the dermal papilla. These cells form the matrix of the elongating **hair root**; the part of a hair extending beyond the skin surface is the **hair shaft**.

The keratinocytes of the hair bulb are generally similar to those in the basal and spinous layers of epidermis. They divide rapidly in the region immediately around the dermal papilla and then undergo keratinization, melanin accumulation, and terminal differentiation. Melanocytes in the hair bulb matrix transfer melanosomes into the epithelial cells that will later differentiate to form the hair. Unlike the epidermis in which all keratinocytes give rise to the stratum corneum, cells in the hair root matrix differentiate with variable amounts and types of keratin. The keratin of hair is harder and more compact than that of the stratum corneum, maintaining its structure as the hair shaft much longer.

In most thick hairs large, vacuolated, and moderately keratinized cells form the central **medulla** of the hair root

FIGURE **18–11** Tactile receptors.

Skin contains several types of **sensory receptors**, with or without capsules of collagen and modified Schwann cells. Most are difficult to see in routine preparations. In the epidermis are **free nerve endings** and tactile discs of nerve fibers associated with **Merkel cells** in the basal layer. Both have unencapsulated nerve fibers, as does the **root hair plexus** around the bases of hair follicles in the dermis. They detect light touch or movement of hair, although epidermal free nerve endings also detect pain and temperature extremes.

More complex, encapsulated tactile receptors are located in the dermis and hypodermis, and include **Meissner corpuscles** for light touch, **lamellated (pacinian) corpuscles** detecting pressure and high-frequency vibration, **Krause end bulbs** for low-frequency vibrations/movements, and **Ruffini corpuscles** detecting tissue distortion. The latter two receptors are less widely distributed in skin and less commonly seen.

(Figures 18–13b and 18–14). Heavily keratinized, densely packed cells make up the **cortex** around the medulla. The most peripheral cells of the hair root comprise the **cuticle**, a thin layer of heavily keratinized, squamous cells covering the cortex (Figures 18–13c and 18–14).

The outermost cells of the hair bulb are continuous with the epithelial root sheath, in which two layers can be recognized. The **internal root sheath** completely surrounds the initial part of the hair root but degenerates above the level of the attached sebaceous glands. The **external root sheath** covers the internal sheath and extends all the way to the epidermis, where it is continuous with the basal and spinous layers. Separating the hair follicle from the dermis is an acellular hyaline layer, the thickened basement membrane called the **glassy membrane** (Figure 18–14b). The surrounding dermis forms a connective tissue sheath.

FIGURE **18–12** Meissner and lamellated (pacinian) corpuscles.

Micrographs show the two most commonly seen sensory receptors of skin. **(a)** Meissner tactile corpuscles (**TC**) are specialized to detect light touch and are frequently located in dermal papillae (**DP**), partially surrounded by epidermis (**E**). They are elliptical, approximately 150 μm long, with an outer capsule (from the perineurium) and thin, stacked inner layers of modified Schwann cells, around which course nerve fibers. X400. H&E.

(b) Lamellated (pacinian) corpuscles (**PC**) detect coarse touch or pressure and are large oval structures, frequently 1 mm in length, found among adipose tissue **(A)** deep in the reticular dermis or in the subcutaneous tissue. Here the outer connective tissue capsule surrounds 15-50 thin, concentric layers of modified Schwann cells, each separated by slightly viscous interstitial fluid. Several axons enter one end of the corpuscle and lie in the cylindrical, inner core of the structure. Movement or pressure of this corpuscle from any direction displaces the inner core, leading to a nerve impulse. X40. H&E.

The **arrector pili muscle**, a small bundle of smooth muscle cells, extends from the midpoint of the fibrous sheath to the dermal papillary layer (Figure 18–13a). Contraction of these muscles pulls the hair shafts to a more erect position, usually when it is cold in an effort to trap a layer of warm air near the skin. In regions where hair is fine, contraction of arrector pili muscles is seen to produce tiny bumps on the skin surface ("goose bumps") where each contracting muscle distorts the attached dermis.

As mentioned earlier hairs grow asynchronously, cyclically, and at different rates in different regions of the body. The hair growth cycle has three major phases:

- A generally long period of mitotic activity and growth (**anagen**),
- A brief period of arrested growth and regression of the hair bulb (**catagen**), and
- A final long period of inactivity (**telogen**) during which the hair may be shed.

At the beginning of the next anagen phase, epidermal stem cells located in small bulge of the external root sheath near the arrector pili muscle produce progenitor cells for the matrix of a new hair bulb. Hair growth on the face and pubis is strongly influenced by sex hormones, especially androgens, and begins at puberty.

FIGURE **18–13** Hair.

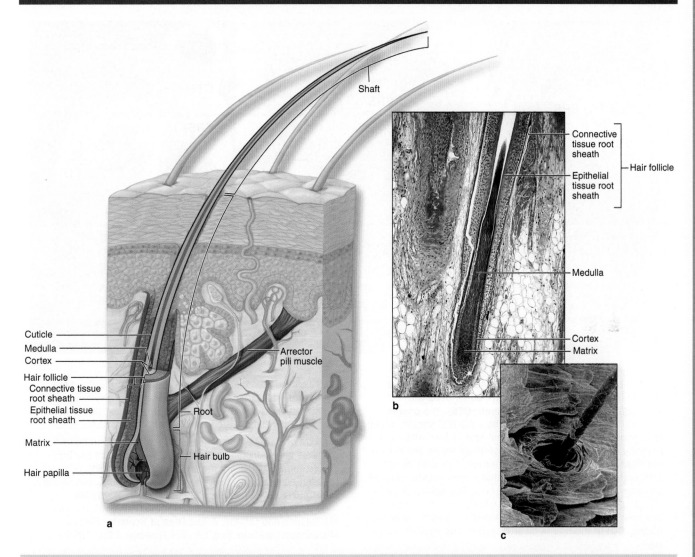

All types of body hair have a similar composition and form in hair follicles derived from the epidermis but extending deep into the dermis. **(a)** The diagram shows major parts of a hair and its follicle, including vascularized, nutritive hair dermal **papilla** and the **arrector pili muscle** that pulls the hair erect.

(b) A longitudinal section of a hair root and bulb shows the **matrix**, **medulla** and **cortex** in the root and the surrounding

epithelial and connective tissue sheaths. Cells of the hair bulb matrix proliferate, take up melanin granules, and undergo keratinization to differentiate as the three concentric layers of the hair. X70. H&E.

(c) The outermost layer of the hair is the thin **cuticle**, composed of shingle-like cells, shown in this SEM of a hair shaft emerging at the stratum corneum. X260.

›› MEDICAL APPLICATION

Loss of hair to produce **baldness** or **alopecia** results from a complex combination of genetic and hormonal factors that is not well understood. Arresting mitotic activity in the hair matrix during cancer **chemotherapy** disrupts both the function and the structural integrity of hair follicles and usually leads to rapid, reversible alopecia.

› NAILS

A similar process of keratinization also produces the **nails**, which are hard plates of keratin on the dorsal surface of each distal phalanx (Figure 18–15). The proximal part of the nail is the **nail root** and is covered by a fold of skin, from which the epidermal stratum corneum extends as the **cuticle**, or **eponychium**. The **nail plate** is bound to a bed of epidermis, the **nail bed**, which contains only the basal and spinous epidermal layers.

FIGURE 18–14 Layers of a hair and its follicle.

(a) The base of a hair follicle sectioned obliquely shows the vascularized dermal papilla (**DP**) continuous with the surrounding connective tissue sheath (**CTS**). The papilla is enclosed by the deepest part of the epithelial sheath, which is continuous with both the internal root sheath (**IRS**) and external root sheath (**ERS**). Both of these layers are in turn continuous with the stratified epidermis. Just outside the ERS is the glassy membrane (**G**) that is continuous with the basement membrane of the epidermis. The epithelial cells (keratinocytes) around the papilla proliferate and differentiate as the root of the hair itself. Above the papilla, only the cortex (**CO**) of the hair is clearly seen in this section. X140. H&E.

(b) A hair root sectioned more transversely shows the same layers of the follicular sheath, but the layers of the hair root are now seen to include the medulla (**M**), cortex (**CO**), and cuticle (**CU**). Other labels are like those of part (a). X140. H&E.

(c) SEM of a similar specimen gives a different perspective on these layers, including the shingle-like nature of the thin cuticle surface (**CU**), and the small blood vessel (**BV**) and collagen bundles (**CB**) near the surrounding connective tissue sheath (**CTS**). Other labels are like those of (a). X2600.

(*Figure 18–14c, with permission, from Kessel RG, Kardon RH.* Tissues and Organs: A Text-Atlas of Scanning Electron Microscopy. *San Francisco, CA: W.H. Freeman & Co.; 1979.*)

The nail root forms from the **nail matrix** in which cells divide, move distally, and become keratinized in a process somewhat similar to hair formation but without keratohyaline granules. The nail root matures and hardens as the nail plate (Figure 18–15). Continuous growth in the matrix pushes the nail plate forward over the nail bed (which makes no contribution to the plate) at a rate of about 3 mm/mo for fingernails and 1 mm/mo for toenails. The distal end of the plate becomes free of the nail bed at the epidermal fold called the **hyponychium**. The nearly transparent nail plate and the thin epithelium of the nail bed provide a useful window on the amount of oxygen in the blood by showing the color of blood in the dermal vessels.

⟩ SKIN GLANDS

Sebaceous Glands

Sebaceous glands are embedded in the dermis over most of the body, except in the thick, glabrous skin of the palms and soles. There is an average of about 100 such glands per square centimeter of skin, but the frequency increases to 400-900/cm² in the face and scalp. Sebaceous glands are branched acinar glands with several acini converging at a short duct that usually empties into the upper portion of a hair follicle (Figure 18–16). A hair follicle and its associated sebaceous glands make up a **pilosebaceous unit**. The stem cell niche of the follicle's bulge region also forms the progenitor cells of

FIGURE **18–15** Nails.

Nails are hard, keratinized derivatives formed in a process similar to that of the stratum corneum and hair. **(a)** Surface view of a finger shows the nail's major parts, including the crescent-shaped white area called the **lunula**, which derives its color from the opaque nail matrix and immature nail plate below it.

(b) A diagrammatic sagittal section includes major internal details of the growing nail and the hyponychium where the free end of the nail plate is bound to epidermis.

(c) A sagittal section from a finger shows the proximal nail fold (**PNF**) and its epidermal extension, the eponychium (**E**) or cuticle. The nail root (**NR**), the most proximal region of the nail plate (**NP**), is formed like the hair root by a matrix of proliferating, differentiating keratinocytes. These cells make up the dorsal nail matrix (**DNM**) and ventral nail matrix (**VNM**), which contribute keratinized cells to the nail root. The mature nail plate remains attached to the nail bed (**NB**), which consists of basal and spinous epidermal layers over dermis (**D**), but is pushed forward on this bed by continuous growth in the nail matrix. X100. Mallory trichrome.

the associated sebaceous glands. In certain hairless regions, such as the penis, clitoris, eyelids, and nipples, sebaceous ducts open directly onto the epidermal surface.

The acini of sebaceous glands are the classic example of holocrine secretion. They have a basal layer of flattened epithelial cells on the basal lamina, which proliferate and are displaced centrally, undergoing terminal differentiation as large, lipid-producing **sebocytes** filled with small fat droplets (Figure 18–17). Their nuclei shrink and undergo autophagy along with other organelles, and near the duct the cells disintegrate, releasing the lipids as the main secretory product. This product, called **sebum**, gradually covers the surfaces of both the epidermis and hair shafts.

Sebum is a complex mixture of lipids that includes wax esters, squalene, cholesterol, and triglycerides that are hydrolyzed by bacterial enzymes after secretion. Secretion from sebaceous glands increases greatly at puberty, stimulated primarily by testosterone in men and by ovarian and adrenal androgens in women. Sebum helps maintain the stratum corneum and hair shafts and exerts weak antibacterial and antifungal properties.

> ## ❯❯ MEDICAL APPLICATION
>
> **Acne vulgaris** is an inflammatory disorder of the pilosebaceous unit, which can be expected to occur during adolescence. It involves excessive keratinization within this unit and excess sebum production, both of which contribute to the blockage of ducts in the follicle. Anaerobic bacteria, typically *Propionibacterium acnes*, grow in the accumulated sebum, leading to localized inflammation and neutrophil infiltration. The resulting enlarged follicle is called a **comedone**.

Sweat Glands

Sweat glands develop as long epidermal invaginations embedded in the dermis (see Figure 18–1). There are two types of sweat glands, eccrine and apocrine, with distinct functions, distributions, and structural details.

Eccrine sweat glands (Figures 18–16 and 18–18a) are widely distributed in the skin and are most numerous on the foot soles (620/cm²). Collectively the 3 million eccrine sweat glands of the average person approximately equal the mass of a kidney and produce as much as 10 L/d, a secretory rate far exceeding that of other exocrine glands. Sweating is a physiologic response to increased body temperature during physical exercise or thermal stress and is the most effective means of temperature regulation of humans.

Both the secretory components and ducts of eccrine sweat glands are coiled and have small lumens. The **secretory part** is generally more pale-staining than the ducts and has stratified cuboidal epithelium with three cell types (Figure 18–19):

- Pale-staining **clear cells** produce the sweat, having abundant mitochondria and microvilli to provide large surface areas. Interstitial fluid from the capillary-rich dermis around the gland is transported through the clear cells, either directly into the gland's lumen or into intercellular canaliculi that open to the lumen.
- **Dark cells** filled with strongly eosinophilic granules (Figure 18–18a) line most of the lumen and do not contact the basal lamina (Figure 18–19). The granules undergo merocrine secretion to release a poorly understood mixture of glycoproteins with bactericidal activity.
- **Myoepithelial cells** on the basal lamina (Figure 18–19) contract to move the watery secretion into the duct.

The **ducts** of eccrine sweat glands have two layers of more acidophilic cells filled with mitochondria and having cell membranes rich in Na⁺, K⁺-ATPase. These duct cells absorb Na⁺ ions from the secreted water to prevent excessive loss of this electrolyte. At the epidermis each duct merges with the stratum basale and sweat flow continues in a spiraling channel through the five epidermal strata to an excretory **sweat pore** in the skin surface (Figures 18–2a and 18–16). Sweat quickly evaporates upon release, cooling the skin and the blood present there. Eccrine sweat glands also function as auxiliary excretory organs, eliminating small amounts of nitrogenous waste and excess salts.

Apocrine sweat glands are largely confined to skin of the axillary and perineal regions. Their development depends on sex hormones and is not complete and functional until after puberty. The secretory components of apocrine glands have much larger lumens than those of the eccrine glands (Figure 18–18) and consist of simple cuboidal, eosinophilic cells with numerous secretory granules that also undergo exocytosis. Thus the glands are misnamed: their cells show merocrine, not apocrine, secretion.

The ducts of apocrine glands are similar to those of the eccrine glands, but they usually open into hair follicles at the epidermis (Figure 18–16) and may contain the protein-rich product. The slightly viscous secretion is initially odorless but may acquire a distinctive odor as a result of bacterial activity. The production of pheromones by apocrine glands is well established in many mammals and is likely in humans, although in a reduced or vestigial capacity. Apocrine sweat glands are innervated by adrenergic nerve endings, whereas eccrine sweat glands receive cholinergic fibers.

> ## ❯❯ MEDICAL APPLICATION
>
> The sweat of infants with cystic fibrosis (CF) is often salty and is commonly taken as indicative of this genetic disease. CF patients have defects in a transmembrane conductance regulator (CFTR) of epithelial cells that lead to disruptive accumulations of thick mucus in the respiratory and digestive tracts. Failure to remove salt from sweat is related to the same genetic defect.

FIGURE **18–16** Glands of skin.

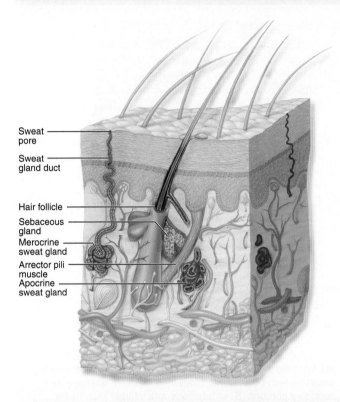

Sweat pore

Sweat gland duct

Hair follicle

Sebaceous gland

Merocrine sweat gland

Arrector pili muscle

Apocrine sweat gland

Skin includes three major types of exocrine glands. **Sebaceous glands** are usually part of a pilosebaceous unit with a hair follicle and secrete oily sebum into the space around the hair root. Thermoregulatory **eccrine sweat glands** empty their secretion onto the skin surface via sweat pores. **Apocrine sweat glands** secrete a more protein-rich sweat into the follicles of hair in skin of the axillae and perineum.

FIGURE **18–17** Sebaceous glands.

Sebaceous glands secrete a complex, oily mixture of lipids called **sebum** into short ducts that in most areas open into hair follicles. Sebum production is the classic example of holocrine secretion, in which the entire cell dies and contributes to the secretory product. **(a)** A section of a pilosebaceous unit shows acini composed of large sebocytes (**S**), which undergo terminal differentiation by filling with small lipid droplets and

then disintegrating near the ducts (**D**) opening at the hair (**H**) shaft. X122. H&E.

(b) A micrograph shows the gland's capsule (**C**) and differentiates sebocytes (**S**) at higher magnification. Proliferation of the small progenitor cells just inside the capsule continuously forces sebum into the ducts; myoepithelial cells are not present. X400. H&E.

FIGURE **18–18** Eccrine and apocrine sweat glands.

(a) Histologically eccrine glands have small lumens in the secretory components (**S**) and ducts (**D**), both of which have an irregular stratified cuboidal appearance. Both clear and acidophilic cells are seen in the stratified cuboidal epithelium of the secretory units.

(b) Apocrine sweat glands, which produce a more protein-rich secretion with pheromonal properties, are characterized by secretory portions (**S**) with lumens much larger than those of eccrine glands. Their ducts (**D**) open into hair follicles (**H**) rather than to the epidermal surface. Both X200. Mallory trichrome.

FIGURE **18–19** Eccrine sweat gland secretory cells.

TEM of these important thermoregulatory structures reveals three cell types in their secretory portions. Myoepithelial cells (**M**) are present at the basal lamina (**BL**) to propel sweat into the duct. Irregular pyramidal cells called **dark cells** (**D**) border the lumen (**L**) and are filled with the electron-dense, eosinophilic secretory granules that release bactericidal peptides and other components of innate immunity. Columnar clear cells (**C**) on the basal lamina rapidly transport water from interstitial fluid in the capillary-rich dermis directly into the lumen or into intercellular canaliculi (**IC**) continuous with the lumen. Na⁺ ions are recovered from this fluid through the action of cells in the ducts. X6500.

› SKIN REPAIR

Skin has a good capacity for repair, which is important in this exposed and easily damaged organ. The process of **cutaneous**

wound healing, whether initiated surgically or accidentally, involves several overlapping stages that vary in duration with the size of the wound (Figure 18–20). In the first phase blood from cut vessels coagulates in the wound, releasing polypep-

FIGURE **18–20** Major stages of cutaneous wound healing.

① Cut blood vessels bleed into the wound.

② Blood clot forms, and leukocytes clean wound.

③ Blood vessels regrow, and granulation tissue forms.

④ Epithelium regenerates, and connective tissue fibrosis occurs.

Skin repair occurs in overlapping stages shown here schematically. The process begins with blood quickly clotting at the wound site, releasing platelet-derived growth factors and other substances (**1**). Macrophages and neutrophils enter the wound as inflammation begins, and epithelial cells from the cut edges of the stratum basale begin to migrate beneath and through the blood clot (**2**).

Under the influence of growth factors and hydrolytic enzymes released in part from macrophages, fibroblasts proliferate and produce much new collagen to form "granulation tissue" containing many new, growing capillaries (**3**). The epidermis gradually reestablishes continuity over the wound site, but excessive collagen usually remains in the dermis as scar tissue (**4**).

tide growth factors and chemokines from the disintegrating platelets. Neutrophils and macrophages undergo diapedesis locally and remove bacteria and debris from the wound. These are major events of **inflammation** that typically lasts 2 to 3 days.

Before this phase is completed, **epithelialization** begins as cells of the epidermal basal layer remove their desmosomes and hemidesmosomes and migrate laterally beneath the blood clot that becomes an increasingly desiccated eschar, or scab. If much epidermis has been lost, new cells may migrate from the bulge region of surviving hair follicles. Growth of epidermal cells and fibroblasts is stimulated by several different growth factors released from macrophages and other cells and from their binding sites in ECM proteoglycans. Matrix metalloproteinases and other proteases from the migrating cells and macrophages facilitate cell migration.

Proliferating fibroblasts and newly sprouted capillaries produce new collagen-rich, well-vascularized tissue in the dermis called **granulation tissue**, which gradually replaces the blood clot (Figure 18–20). In the final stage the epidermis reestablishes continuity but has lost the ability to form new hair or glands. The granulation tissue undergoes **remodeling** and a more normal vasculature is reestablished. Collagen bundles and fibroblasts in this new connective tissue are at least initially much more abundant and disorganized than in uninjured skin, producing **scar tissue** at the wound site.

Skin SUMMARY OF KEY POINTS

- Skin consists mainly of a superficial stratified squamous epithelium, the **epidermis**, and a thicker layer of connective tissue, the **dermis**, which overlies a **subcutaneous hypodermis**.

Epidermis

- The epidermis consists of **keratinocytes** that undergo a terminal differentiation process called **keratinization** in a series of steps that form distinct epidermal strata or layers.
- The **stratum basale** is one layer of mitotically active cuboidal cells attached by **hemidesmosomes** and integrins to the basement membrane and to each other by **desmosomes**.
- The **stratum spinosum** has several layers of polyhedral cells attached to each other by desmosomes at the tips of short projections containing **bundled keratin**, or **tonofibrils**.
- The **stratum granulosum** is a thinner layer of keratinocytes, now flattened and filled densely with **keratohyaline granules** containing **filaggrin** and other proteins binding the tonofibrils.
- The superficial **stratum corneum** protects against water loss, friction, and microbial invasion, and consists of flattened, terminally differentiated cells, or **squames**, which are slowly lost.
- The epidermis-dermis interface is enlarged and strengthened by interdigitating **epidermal ridges** or **pegs** and **dermal papillae** in which microvasculature also supplies nutrients and O_2 for the epidermis.
- **Melanocytes** in the basal epidermis synthesize dark melanin pigment in **melanosomes** and transport these to adjacent keratinocytes, which accumulate them to protect nuclear DNA from UV damage.
- Antigen-presenting cells (APCs) called **Langerhans cells** form a network through the epidermis, intercepting and sampling microbial invaders before moving to lymph nodes in an adaptive immune response.

Dermis

- The **dermis** has two major layers: a superficial **papillary layer** or loose connective tissue with a microvascular plexus, and a thicker dense irregular **reticular layer** containing larger blood vessels.

Cutaneous Sensory Receptors

- Sensory receptors in the epidermis include **free nerve endings**, which detect pain and temperature extremes, and basal **Merkel cells**, light-touch (tactile) receptors associated with sensory fibers.
- Other cutaneous sensory structures include **Meissner corpuscles**, encapsulated elliptical mechanoreceptors that surround sensory axons and also detect light touch.
- Deeper in the dermis and subcutaneous layer are **lamellated or pacinian corpuscles**, which are ovoid and much larger than Meissner corpuscles, for detection of pressure or firm touch.

Epidermal Appendages

- **Hairs** form in **hair follicles**, in which keratinocytes comprising the matrix of the deep **hair bulb** proliferate rapidly and undergo keratinization to form the medulla, cortex, and cuticle of a **hair root**.
- A large dermal **hair papilla** penetrates the base of the hair bulb, and its vasculature supplies nutrients and O_2 for proliferating and differentiating cells.
- The growing **hair root** is surrounded by **internal and external root sheaths** continuous with the epidermis, a **glassy membrane** formed in part by the basal lamina, and a **connective tissue sheath**.
- **Nails** are formed in a manner similar to hairs: keratinocytes proliferate in the matrix of the **nail root** and differentiate with the formation of **hard keratin** as a growing **nail plate** with edges covered by skin folds.
- **Sebaceous glands** produce **sebum** by terminal differentiation of **sebocytes**, the classic example of **holocrine secretion**, secreting this oily substance onto hair in the follicles or **pilosebaceous units**.
- **Eccrine sweat glands** in the dermis produce sweat that is mostly water onto the skin surface, where its evaporation provides an important mechanism for cooling the body.
- **Apocrine sweat glands** are restricted to skin of the axillae and perineum, have much wider lumens than eccrine glands, develop after puberty, and secrete protein-rich sweat onto the hair of hair follicles.

CHAPTER

19 The Urinary System

The urinary system consists of the paired kidneys and ureters, the bladder, and the urethra. This system's primary role is to ensure optimal properties of the blood, which the kidneys continuously monitor. This general role of the kidneys involves a complex combination of renal functions:

- Regulation of the balance between water and electrolytes (inorganic ions) and the acid-base balance
- Excretion of metabolic wastes along with excess water and electrolytes in urine
- Excretion of many bioactive substances, including many drugs
- Regulation of arterial blood pressure by secretion of **renin**

Renin is a protease secreted into the blood that helps regulate blood pressure by cleaving circulating angiotensinogen to angiotensin I. Other renal functions include the following:

- Secretion of **erythropoietin**, a glycoprotein growth factor that stimulates erythrocyte production in red marrow when the blood O_2 level is low;
- Conversion of the steroid prohormone vitamin D, initially produced in the epidermis, to the active form (**1,25-dihydroxyvitamin D$_3$** or calcitriol); and
- **Gluconeogenesis** during starvation or periods of prolonged fasting, making glucose from amino acids to supplement this process in the liver.

Urine, the excretory product of the kidneys, passes through the ureters to the bladder for temporary storage and is then released to the exterior through the urethra.

❯ KIDNEYS

Each kidney has a concave medial border, the **hilum**—where nerves enter, the ureter exits, and blood and lymph vessels enter and exit—and a convex lateral surface, both covered by a thin fibrous capsule (Figure 19–1). Within the hilum the upper end of the ureter expands as the **renal pelvis** and divides into two or three **major calyces**. Smaller branches, the **minor calyces**, arise from each major calyx. The area surrounding the renal pelvis and calyces contains adipose tissue.

The kidney has an outer **cortex**, a darker region with many corpuscles and cross sections of tubules, and an inner **medulla** consisting of straight, aligned structures (Figure 19–1). In humans, the renal medulla consists of 8-12 conical structures called **renal pyramids**, which are separated by extensions from the cortex called **renal columns**. Each pyramid plus the cortical tissue at its base and along its sides constitutes a **renal lobe**. Striations extending from the medulla into the cortex are called **medullary rays**; these plus the attached cortical tissue are considered lobules. The tip of each pyramid, called the **renal papilla**, projects into a minor calyx that collects urine formed by tubules in the pyramid (Figure 19–1).

Each kidney contains around 1 million functional units called **nephrons** (Figure 19–2) that consist of simple, single-layered epithelium along their entire lengths. The major divisions of each nephron are the following:

- **Renal corpuscle**, an initial dilated part enclosing a tuft of capillary loops and the site of blood filtration, always located in the cortex;
- **Proximal tubule**, a long convoluted part, located entirely in the cortex, with a shorter straight part that enters the medulla;
- **Loop of Henle** (or nephron loop), in the medulla, with a **thin descending** and a **thin ascending** limb;
- **Distal tubule,** consisting of a thick straight part ascending from the loop of Henle back into the cortex and a convoluted part completely in the cortex; and
- **Connecting tubule**, a short final part linking the nephron to collecting ducts.

FIGURE **19–1** Kidney.

Renal cortex
Renal medulla
Renal column
Renal pyramid
Corticomedullary junction
Renal papilla
Renal lobe
Fibrous capsule

Minor calyx
Major calyx
Renal pelvis
Renal artery
Renal vein

Ureter

Each kidney is bean-shaped, with a concave **hilum** where the ureter and the renal artery and veins enter. The ureter divides and subdivides into several **major and minor calyces**, around which is located the renal sinus containing adipose tissue. Attached to each minor calyx is a medullary **pyramid**, a conical region of medulla delimited by extensions of **cortex**. The cortex and hilum are covered with a fibrous capsule.

Connecting tubules from several nephrons merge to form **collecting tubules** that then merge as larger **collecting ducts**. These converge in the renal papilla, where they deliver urine to a minor calyx. **Cortical nephrons** are located almost completely in the cortex while **juxtamedullary nephrons** (about one-seventh of the total) lie close to the medulla and have long loops of Henle.

›› MEDICAL APPLICATION

Polycystic kidney disease is an inherited disorder in which normal cortical organization of both kidneys is lost due to the formation of multiple, large, fluid-filled cysts. The cysts may arise from any epithelial cells of the nephron and can lead to gross kidney enlargement and loss of renal function.

› BLOOD CIRCULATION

As expected for an organ specialized to process the blood, the kidney vasculature is large, well-organized, and closely associated with all components of the nephron. Blood vessels of the kidneys are named according to their locations or shapes (Figure 19–3).

Each kidney's **renal artery** divides into two or more segmental arteries at the hilum. Around the renal pelvis, these branch further as the **interlobar arteries**, which extend between the renal pyramids toward the corticomedullary junction (Figure 19–3). Here the interlobar arteries divide again to form the **arcuate arteries** that run in an arc along this junction at the base of each renal pyramid. Smaller **interlobular arteries** (or cortical radial arteries) radiate from the arcuate arteries, extending deeply into the cortex.

From the interlobular arteries arise the microvascular **afferent arterioles**, which divide to form a plexus of capillary loops called the **glomerulus**, each of which is located within a renal corpuscle where the blood is filtered (Figures 19–3 and 19–4). Blood leaves the glomerular capillaries, not via venules, but via **efferent arterioles**, which at once branch again to form another capillary network, usually the **peritubular capillaries** profusely distributed throughout the cortex. From the juxtaglomerular corpuscles near the medulla, efferent arterioles do not form peritubular capillaries, but instead branch repeatedly to form parallel tassel-like bundles of capillary loops called the **vasa recta** (L. *recta*, straight) that penetrate deep into the medulla in association with the loops of Henle and collecting ducts. Collectively, the cortex receives over 10 times more blood than the medulla.

Blood leaves the kidney in veins that follow the same courses as arteries and have the same names (Figure 19–3). The outermost peritubular capillaries and capillaries in the kidney capsule converge into small stellate veins that empty into the interlobular veins.

FIGURE 19–2 Nephrons.

Each kidney contains approximately 1 million functional units called **nephrons**. Each nephron originates in the cortex, at the **renal corpuscle** surrounding a small tuft of glomerular capillaries. Extending from the corpuscle is the long **proximal convoluted tubule** which leads to short **proximal straight tubule** that enters the outer medulla. This tubule continues as the **thin descending limb** and the **thin ascending limb** of the nephron's loop of Henle in the medulla. The loop of

Henle ends with a **thick ascending limb**, a straight tubule that reenters the cortex and ends at its thickened **macula densa** area where it contacts the arterioles entering the glomerulus. Beyond the macula densa this tubule is the **distal convoluted tubule**, the end of which is the short **connecting tubule**. Connecting tubules from many nephrons merge into cortical collecting tubules and a **collecting duct** that transports urine to the calyx.

> ## RENAL FUNCTION: FILTRATION, SECRETION, & REABSORPTION

All the major functions of the kidneys—the removal of metabolic wastes and excess water and electrolytes from blood—are performed by various specialized epithelial cells of the nephrons and collecting systems. Renal function involves specific activities:

- **Filtration**, by which water and solutes in the blood leave the vascular space and enter the lumen of the nephron;

FIGURE **19–3** Blood supply to the kidneys.

A coronal view (left) shows the major blood vessels diagrammatically, with their names. An expanded diagram (right) includes the microvascular components extending into the cortex, and medulla from the interlobular vessels are shown on the right. Pink boxes indicate vessels with arterial blood and light blue indicate the venous return. The intervening lavender boxes and vessels are intermediate sites where most reabsorbed material reenters the blood.

- Tubular **secretion**, by which substances move from epithelial cells of the tubules into the lumens, usually after uptake from the surrounding interstitium and capillaries; and
- Tubular **reabsorption**, by which substances move from the tubular lumen across the epithelium into the interstitium and surrounding capillaries.

Along the length of the nephron tubule and collecting system, the filtrate receives various secreted molecules while others are reabsorbed and then enters the minor calyces as **urine** and undergoes **excretion**.

The number of nephrons decreases slightly in older adults, a process accelerated by high blood pressure. If a kidney is donated for transplant (unilateral nephrectomy), the remaining kidney undergoes compensatory growth, with cellular hypertrophy in the proximal parts of the nephron tubules and an increase in the rate of filtration, which allow normal renal function to continue.

>> **MEDICAL APPLICATION**

Inflammation within the glomeruli, or **glomerulonephritis**, which can range from acute or chronic, usually stems from humoral immune reactions. Varieties of this condition involve the deposition of circulating antibody-antigen complexes within glomeruli or circulating antibodies binding to either glomerular antigens or extraneous antigens deposited in the glomeruli. Regardless of the source the accumulating immune complexes can then elicit a local inflammatory response.

Renal Corpuscles & Blood Filtration

At the beginning of each nephron is a renal corpuscle, about 200 μm in diameter and containing a tuft of glomerular capillaries, surrounded by a double-walled epithelial capsule called

FIGURE **19-4** Microvasculature of the renal cortex.

Cortical vasculature is revealed in a section of the kidney with the renal artery injected with carmine dye before fixation. Small interlobular arteries (**I**) branch from the arcuate arteries and radiate out through the cortex giving off the afferent arterioles (**A**) that bring blood to the glomerular capillaries. Each glomerulus (**G**) contains a mass of capillary loops that drain into an efferent arteriole. These then branch as a large, diffuse network of peritubular capillaries (**PT**) throughout the cortex. X125.

the **glomerular** (**Bowman**) **capsule** (Figures 19–2 and 19–5). The internal or **visceral layer** of this capsule closely envelops the glomerular capillaries, which are finely fenestrated. The outer **parietal layer** forms the surface of the capsule. Between

the two capsular layers is the **capsular** (or **urinary**) **space**, which receives the fluid filtered through the capillary wall and visceral layer. Each renal corpuscle has a **vascular pole**, where the afferent arteriole enters and the efferent arteriole leaves, and a **tubular pole**, where the proximal convoluted tubule (PCT) begins (Figure 19–5).

The outer parietal layer of a glomerular capsule consists of a simple squamous epithelium supported externally by a basal lamina. At the tubular pole, this epithelium changes to the simple cuboidal epithelium that continues and forms the proximal tubule (Figure 19–5).

The visceral layer of a renal corpuscle consists of unusual stellate epithelial cells called **podocytes** (Figures 19–5c, d), which together with the capillary endothelial cells compose the apparatus for renal filtration. From the cell body of each podocyte several **primary processes** extend and curve around a length of glomerular capillary. Each primary process gives rise to many parallel, interdigitating secondary processes or **pedicels** (L. *pedicellus*, little foot; Figures 19–5c, d). The pedicels cover much of the capillary surface, in direct contact with the basal lamina (Figures 19–5c and 19–6).

Between the interdigitating pedicels are elongated spaces, or filtration slit pores, 25 to 30 nm wide (Figures 19–5c and 19–6). Spanning adjacent pedicels and bridging the slit pores are zipper-like **slit diaphragms** (Figure 19–6). Slit diaphragms are modified and specialized occluding or tight junctions composed of **nephrins**, other proteins, glycoproteins, and proteoglycans important for renal function. Projecting from the cell membrane on each side of the filtration slit, these polyanionic glycoproteins and proteoglycans interact to form a series of openings within the slit diaphragm, with a surface that is negatively charged.

Between the highly fenestrated endothelial cells of the capillaries and the covering podocytes is the thick (300-360 nm) glomerular basement membrane (GBM) (Figure 19–6). This membrane is the most substantial part of the filtration barrier that separates the blood from the capsular space and forms by fusion of the capillary- and podocyte-produced basal laminae. Laminin and fibronectin in this fused basement membrane bind integrins of both the podocyte and endothelial cell membranes, and the meshwork of cross-linked type IV collagen and large proteoglycans restricts passage of proteins larger than about 70 kDa. Smaller proteins that are filtered from plasma are degraded, and the amino acids reabsorbed in the proximal tubule. Polyanionic GAGs in the glomerular membrane are abundant and their negative charges, like those of the slit diaphragms, tend to restrict filtration of organic anions.

Filtration, therefore, occurs through a structure with three parts:

- The fenestrations of the capillary endothelium, which blocks blood cells and platelets;
- The thick, combined basal laminae, or GBM, which restricts large proteins and some organic anions; and
- The filtration slit diaphragms between pedicels, which restrict some small proteins and organic anions.

FIGURE **19–5** Renal corpuscles.

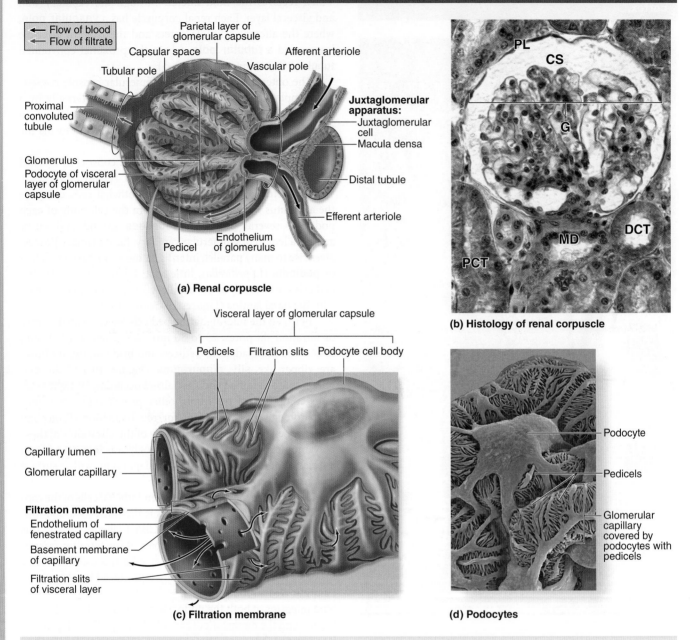

(a) Renal corpuscle

(b) Histology of renal corpuscle

(c) Filtration membrane

(d) Podocytes

(a) The renal corpuscle is a small mass of capillaries called the **glomerulus** housed within a bulbous glomerular capsule. The internal lining of the capsule is composed of complex epithelial cells called **podocytes**, which cover each capillary, forming slit-like spaces between interdigitating processes called **pedicels**. Blood enters and leaves the glomerulus through the afferent and efferent arterioles, respectively.

(b) The micrograph shows the major histologic features of a renal corpuscle. The glomerulus (**G**) of capillaries is surrounded by the capsular space (**CS**) covered by the simple squamous parietal layer (**PL**) of Bowman capsule. Near the corpuscle is that nephron's macula densa (**MD**) and sections

of proximal convoluted tubules (**PCT**) and distal convoluted tubules (**DCT**). H&E. X300.

(c) Filtrate is produced in the corpuscle when blood plasma is forced under pressure through the **capillary fenestrations**, across the filtration **membrane** or GBM surrounding the capillary, and through the **filtration slit** diaphragms located between the podocyte pedicels.

(d) The scanning electron microscopy (SEM) shows the distinctive appearance of podocytes and their pedicel processes that cover glomerular capillaries. X800

FIGURE **19–6** Glomerular filtration barrier.

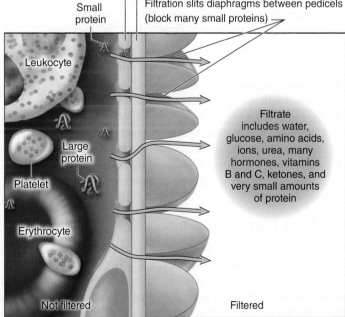

(c) Substances filtered by filtration membrane

The glomerular filtration barrier consists of three layered components: the fenestrated **capillary endothelium**, the **glomerular basement membrane (GBM)**, and **filtration slit** diaphragms between pedicels. The major component of the filter is formed by fusion of the basal laminae of a podocyte and a capillary endothelial cell. **(a)** TEM shows cell bodies of two podocytes (**PC**) and the series of pedicels on the capillary (**C**) basement membrane separated by the filtration slit diaphragms. Around the capillaries and podocytes is the capsular space (**CS**) into which the filtrate enters. The enclosed area is shown in part **b**. X10,000.

(b) At higher magnification, both the fenestrations (**F**) in the endothelium (**E**) of the capillary (**C**) and the filtration slits (**FS**) separating the pedicels (**P**) are clearly seen on the two sides of the thick, fused basement membrane (**BM**). Thin slit diaphragms (**SD**) bridge the slits between pedicels. X45,750.

(c) Diagram shows the three parts of the glomerular filter and their major functions.

Normally about 20% of the blood plasma entering a glomerulus is filtered into the capsular space. The initial glomerular filtrate has a chemical composition similar to that of plasma except that it contains very little protein. The glomerular filter blocks filtration of most plasma proteins, but smaller proteins, including most polypeptide hormones, are removed into the filtrate.

Capillaries of each glomerulus have a total length of approximately 1 cm and are uniquely situated between two arterioles—afferent and efferent—the muscle of which allows increased hydrostatic pressure in these vessels, favoring movement of plasma across the glomerular filter. The glomerular filtration rate (GFR) is constantly regulated by neural and hormonal inputs affecting the degree of constriction in each of these arterioles. The total glomerular filtration area of an adult has been estimated at 500 cm² and the average GFR at 125 mL/min or 180 L/d. Because the total amount of circulating plasma averages 3 L, it follows that the kidneys typically filter the entire blood volume 60 times every day.

In addition to capillary endothelial cells and podocytes, renal corpuscles also contain **mesangial cells** (Gr. *mesos*, in the midst + *angion*, vessel), most of which resemble vascular pericytes in having contractile properties and producing components of an external lamina. Mesangial cells are difficult to distinguish in routine sections from podocytes, but often stain more darkly. They and their surrounding matrix comprise the mesangium (Figure 19–7), which fills interstices between capillaries that lack podocytes. Functions of the mesangium include the following:

- Physical support of capillaries within the glomerulus;
- Adjusted contractions in response to blood pressure changes, which help maintain an optimal filtration rate;
- Phagocytosis of protein aggregates adhering to the glomerular filter, including antibody-antigen complexes abundant in many pathological conditions; and
- Secretion of several cytokines, prostaglandins, and other factors important for immune defense and repair in the glomerulus.

Proximal Convoluted Tubule

Cells in many parts of the nephron tubule and collecting system reabsorb water and electrolytes, but other activities are restricted mainly to specific tubular regions. Table 19–1 summarizes major functions of parts within nephrons and collecting ducts, along with the histologic features involved in these activities.

FIGURE 19–7 Mesangium.

(a) Diagram shows that mesangial cells in renal corpuscles are located between capillaries and cover those capillary surface not covered by podocyte processes. (b) The TEM shows one mesangial cell (**MC**) and the surrounding mesangial matrix (**MM**). This matrix appears similar to and in many places continuous with basement membrane (**BM**) and supports capillaries where podocytes are lacking. Mesangial cells extend contractile processes (arrows) along capillaries that help regulate blood flow in the glomerulus. Some mesangial processes appear to pass between endothelial cells (**EC**) into the capillary lumen (asterisks) where they may help remove or endocytose adherent protein aggregates. The capillary at the left contains an erythrocyte (**E**) and a lymphocyte (**L**). Podocytes (**P**) and their pedicels (**PD**) open to the urinary space (**US**) and associate with the capillary surfaces not covered by mesangial cells. X3500.

At the tubular pole of the renal corpuscle, the simple squamous epithelium of the capsule's parietal layer is continuous with the simple cuboidal epithelium of the **proximal convoluted tubule** (PCT) (Figures 19–8 and 19–9). These long, tortuous tubules fill most of the cortex. PCT cells are specialized for both reabsorption and secretion. Over half of the water and electrolytes, and all of the organic nutrients

TABLE **19–1**	Histologic features and major functions of regions within renal tubules.		
Region of Tubule	**Histological Features**	**Locations**	**Major Functions**
PCT	Simple cuboidal epithelium; cells well-stained, with numerous mitochondria, prominent basal folds and lateral interdigitations; long microvilli, lumens often occluded	Cortex	Reabsorption of all organic nutrients, all proteins, most water and electrolytes; secretion of organic anions and cations, H^+, and NH_4^+
Loop of Henle			
Thin limbs	Simple squamous epithelium; few mitochondria	Medulla	Passive reabsorption of Na^+ and Cl^-
TAL	Simple cuboidal epithelium; no microvilli	Medulla and medullary rays	Active reabsorption of various electrolytes
DCT	Simple cuboidal epithelium; cells smaller than in PCT, short microvilli and basolateral folds, more empty lumens	Cortex	Reabsorption of electrolytes
Collecting system			
Principal cells	Most abundant, cuboidal to columnar; pale-staining, distinct cell membranes	Medullary rays and medulla	Regulated reabsorption of water & electrolytes; regulated secretion of K^+
Intercalated cells	Few and scattered; slightly darker staining	Medullary rays	Reabsorption of K^+ (low-K^+ diet); help maintain acid-base balance

DCT, distal convoluted tubule; PCT, proximal convoluted tubule; TAL, thick ascending limb.

(glucose, amino acids, vitamins, etc), filtered from plasma in the renal corpuscle are normally reabsorbed in the PCT. These molecules are transferred directly across the tubular wall for immediate uptake again into the plasma of the peritubular capillaries.

Transcellular **reabsorption** involves both active and passive mechanisms, with the cells having a large variety of transmembrane ion pumps, ion channels, transporters, enzymes, and carrier proteins. Water and certain solutes can also move passively between the cells (paracellular transport) along osmotic gradients through leaky apical tight junctions.

Small proteins in the filtrate are either reabsorbed by receptor-mediated endocytosis and degraded in the cuboidal cells, or degraded by peptidases on the luminal surface. In both cases the amino acids are released at the basolateral cell surfaces for uptake by capillaries.

Conversely, organic anions and cations not filtered in the renal corpuscle (because of the polyanions in the filter or binding to plasma proteins) may be released in the peritubular capillaries, taken up by the cells of the proximal tubules and undergo **secretion** into the filtrate (Table 19–1). Organic anion and cation transporters allow the kidneys to dispose of such substances at a higher rate than by glomerular filtration alone. Because these molecules include important substances (such as bile salts, creatinine, etc) and many antibiotics and other drugs, this process of tubular secretion is of great pharmacologic importance as a key mechanism of drug clearance.

The cells of the proximal tubules have central nuclei and very acidophilic cytoplasm (Figures 19–8 and 19–9) because of the abundant mitochondria. The cell apex has very many long microvilli that form a prominent **brush border** in the lumen that facilitates reabsorption (Figures 19–8 through 19–10). Because the cells are large, each transverse section of a PCT typically contains only three to five nuclei. In routine histologic preparations, the long brush border may be disorganized and give the lumens a fuzz-filled appearance. Peritubular capillaries are abundant in the sparse surrounding connective tissue interstitium, which fills only about 10% of the cortex (Figure 19–8).

Ultrastructurally the apical cytoplasm of these cells has numerous pits and **vesicles** near the bases of the microvilli, indicating active endocytosis and pinocytosis (Figure 19–10). These vesicles contain the small, reabsorbed proteins that will be degraded in lysosomes, with the amino acids released to the circulation. Proximal tubular cells also have many long basal **membrane invaginations** and lateral interdigitations with neighboring cells (Figure 19–10). Both the brush border and the basolateral folds contain the many types of transmembrane proteins that mediate tubular reabsorption and secretion. Long mitochondria concentrated along the basal invaginations (Figure 19–10) supply ATP locally for the membrane proteins involved in active transport. Because of the extensive interdigitations of the lateral membranes, discrete limits between cells of the proximal tubule are difficult to see with the light microscope.

Besides their major roles in reabsorption and secretion, cells of the proximal tubule also perform hydroxylation of vitamin D and release to the capillaries. Moreover, fibroblastic

FIGURE 19–8 Renal cortex: proximal and distal convoluted tubules.

(a) The micrograph shows the continuity at a renal corpuscle's tubular pole (**TP**) between the simple cuboidal epithelium of a proximal convoluted tubule (**P**) and the simple squamous epithelium of the capsule's parietal layer. The urinary space (**U**) between the parietal layer and the glomerulus (**G**) drains into the lumen of the proximal tubule. The lumens of the proximal tubules appear filled, because of the long microvilli of the brush border and aggregates of small plasma proteins bound to this structure. By contrast, the lumens of distal convoluted tubules (**D**) appear empty, lacking a brush border and protein.

(b) Here the abundant peritubular capillaries and draining venules (arrows) that surround the proximal (**P**) and distal (**D**) convoluted tubules are clearly seen. Both X400. H&E.

interstitial cells in cortical areas near the proximal tubules produce erythropoietin, the growth factor secreted in response to a prolonged decrease in local oxygen concentration.

>> **MEDICAL APPLICATION**

Diabetic glomerulosclerosis, the thickening and loss of function in the GBM produced as part of the systemic microvascular sclerosis in diabetes mellitus, is the leading cause of (irreversible) **end-stage kidney disease** in the United States. Treatment requires either a **kidney transplant** or regular **artificial hemodialysis**.

Loop of Henle

The PCT continues with the much shorter proximal straight tubule that enters the medulla and continues the nephron's **loop of Henle** (see Figure 19–2). This is a U-shaped structure with a **thin descending limb** and a **thin ascending limb**, both composed of simple squamous epithelia. The straight part of the proximal tubule has an outer diameter of about 60 μm, but it narrows abruptly to about 30 μm in the thin limbs of the loop. The wall of the thin segments consists only of squamous cells with few organelles (indicating a primarily passive role in transport) and the lumen is prominent

FIGURE 19–9 Convoluted tubules, nephron loops, and collecting ducts.

(b) Renal cortex

(c) Convoluted tubule epithelia

(a) Nephron components

(d) Cross section of renal medulla

(a) Diagram of a nephron shows levels of the sections in the photos.

(b) A section of cortical tissue shows one renal corpuscle (**RC**), the wide, eosinophilic proximal convoluted tubules (**PCT**) with the smaller, less well-stained distal convoluted tubules (**DCT**). X160. H&E.

(c) Diagram shows the major structural differences between the cuboidal cells of proximal and distal tubules. Cells of both tubules have basal membrane invaginations associated with mitochondria.

(d) A cross section through a medullary pyramid shows the simple squamous epithelium of the thin descending and ascending limbs of loops of Henle (**T**) and its thick ascending limbs (**A**), as well as the pale columnar cells of collecting ducts (**CD**). Note also the homogeneous interstitium with capillaries smaller than the thin limbs. X160. Mallory trichrome.

(Figures 19–9 and 19–11). The thin ascending limb of the loop becomes the **thick ascending limb** (**TAL**), with simple cuboidal epithelium and many mitochondria again, in the outer medulla and extends as far as the macula densa near the nephron's glomerulus.

The loops of Henle and surrounding interstitial connective tissue are involved in further adjusting the salt content of the filtrate. Cuboidal cells of the loops' TALs actively transport sodium and chloride ions out of the tubule against a concentration gradient into the hyaluronate-rich interstitium,

FIGURE 19–10   Ultrastructure of proximal convoluted tubule (PCT) cells.

TEM reveals important features of the cuboidal cells of the proximal convoluted epithelium: the long, dense apical microvilli (**MV**), the abundant endocytotic pits and vesicles (**V**) in the apical regions near lysosomes (**L**). Small proteins brought into the cells nonspecifically by pinocytosis are degraded in lysosomes and the amino acids released basally. Apical ends of adjacent cells are sealed with zonula occludens, but the basolateral sides are characterized by long invaginating folds of membrane along which many long mitochondria (**M**) are situated. Water and the small molecules released from the PCTs are taken up immediately by the adjacent peritubular capillaries (**C**). Between the basement membranes of the tubule and the capillary shown here is an extension of a fibroblast (**F**). X10,500.

making that compartment hyperosmotic. This causes water to be withdrawn passively from the thin descending part of the loop, thus concentrating the filtrate. The thin ascending limbs reabsorb sodium chloride (NaCl) but are impermeable to water. The countercurrent flow of the filtrate (descending, then immediately ascending) in the two parallel thin limbs establishes a gradient of osmolarity in the interstitium of the medullary pyramids, an effect that is "multiplied" at deeper levels in the medulla. Countercurrent blood flow in the descending and ascending loops of the vasa recta helps maintain the hyperosmotic interstitium. The interstitial osmolarity at the pyramid tips is about four times that of the blood. The **countercurrent multiplier system** established by the

nephron loop and vasa recta is an important aspect of renal physiology in humans

Distal Convoluted Tubule & Juxtaglomerular Apparatus

The ascending limb of the nephron is straight as it enters the cortex and forms the macula densa, and then becomes tortuous as the **distal convoluted tubule** (**DCT**) (see Figure 19–2). Much less tubular reabsorption occurs here than in the proximal tubule. The simple cuboidal cells of the distal tubules differ from those of the proximal tubules in being smaller and having no brush border and more empty lumens (Figure 19–9). Because distal tubule cells are flatter and smaller than those of the proximal tubule, more nuclei are typically seen in sections of distal tubules than in those of proximal tubules (Figure 19–8). Cells of the DCT also have fewer mitochondria than cells of proximal tubules, making them less acidophilic (Figure 19–9). The rate of Na$^+$ absorption here is regulated by **aldosterone** from the adrenal glands.

Where the initial, straight part of the distal tubule contacts the arterioles at the vascular pole of the renal corpuscle of its parent nephron, its cells become more columnar and closely packed, forming the **macula densa** (L. thicker spot). This is part of a specialized sensory structure, the **juxtaglomerular apparatus** (**JGA**) that utilizes feedback mechanisms to regulate glomerular blood flow and keep the rate of glomerular filtration relatively constant. The JGA is shown in Figures 19–5 and 19–12. Cells of the macula densa typically have apical nuclei, basal Golgi complexes, and a more elaborate and varied system of ion channels and transporters. Adjacent to the macula densa, the tunica media of the afferent arteriole is also modified. The smooth muscle cells are modified as **juxtaglomerular granular** (**JG**) **cells**, with a secretory phenotype including more rounded nuclei, rough ER, Golgi complexes, and zymogen granules with **renin** (Figures 19–5 and 19–12). Also at the vascular pole are **lacis cells** (Fr. *lacis*, lacework), which are extraglomerular mesangial cells that have many of the same supportive, contractile and defensive functions as these cells inside the glomerulus.

Basic functions of the JGA in the autoregulation of the GFR and in controlling blood pressure include the following activities. Elevated arterial pressure increases glomerular capillary blood pressure, which increases the GFR. Higher GFR leads to higher luminal concentrations of Na$^+$ and Cl$^-$ in the

FIGURE 19–11 Renal medulla: nephron loops and collecting ducts.

(a) A micrograph of a medullary pyramid cut transversely shows closely packed cross sections of the many nephron loops' thin descending and ascending limbs (**T**) and thick ascending limbs (**A**), intermingled with parallel vasa recta capillaries containing blood (**C**) and collecting ducts (**CD**). All these structures are embedded in the interstitium (**I**) that contains sparse myofibroblast-like cells in a matrix very rich in hydrophilic hyaluronate. The specialized nature of the interstitial tissue helps maintain the osmolarity gradient established by differential salt and water transport across the wall of the nephron

loop which is required to concentrate urine and conserve body water. X400. Mallory trichrome.

(b) The TEM reveals the slightly fibrous nature of the interstitium (**I**) and shows that the simple squamous epithelium of the thin limbs (**T**) is slightly thicker than that of the nearby vasa recta capillaries (**C**). X3300.

(Figure 19–11b, with permission, from Dr Johannes Rhodin, Department of Cell Biology and Anatomy, University of South Florida College of Medicine, Tampa.)

TAL of the nephron, which are monitored by cells of the macula densa. Increased ion levels in the lumen cause these cells to release ATP, adenosine, and other vasoactive compounds that trigger contraction of the afferent arteriole, which lowers glomerular pressure and decreases the GFR. This lowers tubular ion concentrations, which turns off the release of vasoconstrictors from the macula densa.

Decreased arterial pressure leads to increased autonomic stimulation to the JGA as a result of baroreceptor function, including local baroreceptors in the afferent arteriole, possibly the JG cells themselves. This causes the JG cells to release renin, an aspartyl protease, into the blood. There renin cleaves the plasma protein **angiotensinogen** into the inactive decapeptide **angiotensin I**. Angiotensin-converting enzyme (ACE) on lung capillaries clips this further to **angiotensin II**, a potent vasoconstrictor that directly raises systemic blood pressure and stimulates the adrenals to secrete **aldosterone**. Aldosterone promotes Na^+ and water reabsorption in the distal convoluted and connecting tubules, which raises blood

volume to help increase blood pressure. The return of normal blood pressure turns off secretion of renin by JG cells.

Collecting Ducts

The last part of each nephron, the **connecting tubule**, carries the filtrate into a collecting system that transports it to a minor calyx and in which more water is reabsorbed if needed by the body. As shown in Figures 19–13, a connecting tubule extends from each nephron and several join together in the cortical medullary rays to form **collecting ducts** of simple cuboidal epithelium and an average diameter of 40 μm. In the outer medulla these merge further as larger, straight collecting ducts (of Bellini), which run to the tips of the medullary pyramids with increasingly columnar cells and overall diameters reaching 200 μm (Figures 19–11 and 19–14). In the apex of the pyramid, several collecting ducts merge further as a **papillary duct** which delivers urine to the minor calyx (Figure 19–13). Running parallel with the descending and ascending limbs of

FIGURE **19–12** Juxtaglomerular apparatus (JGA).

The JGA forms at the point of contact between a nephron's distal tubule (**D**) and the vascular pole of its glomerulus (**G**). At that point cells of the distal tubule become columnar as a thickened region called the macula densa (**MD**). Smooth muscle cells of the afferent arteriole's (**AA**) tunica media are converted from a contractile to a secretory morphology as juxtaglomerular granule cells (**JG**). Also present are lacis cells (**L**), which are extraglomerular mesangial cells adjacent to the macula densa, the afferent arteriole, and the efferent arteriole (**EA**). In this specimen the lumens of proximal tubules (**P**) appear filled and the urinary space (**US**) is somewhat swollen. X400. Mallory trichrome.

the loops of Henle and vasa recta, medullary collecting ducts lie in the area with very high interstitial osmolarity (Figures 19–2 and 19–11).

Collecting ducts are composed mainly of pale-staining **principal cells** with few organelles, sparse microvilli, and unusually distinct cell boundaries (Figure 19–14). Ultrastructurally the principal cells can be seen to have basal membrane infoldings, consistent with their role in ion transport, and a primary cilium among the microvilli. The medullary collecting ducts are the final site of water reabsorption from the filtrate. Principal cells are particularly rich in **aquaporins**, the integral membrane pore proteins that function as specific channels for water molecules, but here most aquaporins are sequestered in membranous cytoplasmic vesicles.

Antidiuretic hormone (ADH), released from the pituitary gland as the body becomes dehydrated, makes collecting ducts more permeable to water and increases the rate at which water molecules are pulled osmotically from the filtrate. Upon binding, ADH receptors on the basolateral cell surface stimulate the movement and insertion of vesicles with aquaporins into the apical (luminal) membranes, increasing the number of membrane channels and water movement through the cells. The high osmolarity of the interstitium draws water passively from the collecting ducts, concentrating the filtrate. The water thus saved immediately enters the blood in the vasa recta.

Scattered among the principal cells are variably darker **intercalated cells**, or IC cells, with more abundant mitochondria and projecting apical folds. Intercalated cells, a few of which also occur in the DCTs, help maintain acid-base balance by secreting either H^+ or HCO_3^-.

Histologic features and major functions of the nephron's parts and collecting ducts are summarized in Table 19–1.

›› MEDICAL APPLICATION

A common problem involving the ureters is their obstruction by **renal calculi** (**kidney stones**) formed in the renal pelvis or calyces, usually from calcium salts (oxalate or phosphate) or uric acid. While urate stones are usually smooth and small, calcium stones can become large and irritate the mucosa. Most kidney stones are asymptomatic, but besides causing an obstruction that can lead to renal problems, movement of stones from the renal pelvis into the ureter can cause extreme pain on the affected side of the body. Problems caused by such stones can be corrected by either surgical removal of the stone or its disintegration using focused ultrasonic shock waves in a procedure called **lithotripsy**, although this treatment can cause significant renal damage.

› URETERS, BLADDER, & URETHRA

Urine is transported by the **ureters** from the renal pelvis to the **urinary bladder** where it is stored until emptying by micturition via the **urethra**. The calyces, renal pelvis, ureter, and bladder have somewhat similar histologic structure, with the walls becoming gradually thicker closer to the bladder. The mucosa of these organs is lined by the unique stratified **transitional epithelium** or urothelium introduced in Chapter 4 (Figures 19–15 and 19–16). Cells of this epithelium are organized as three layers:

- A single layer of small basal cells resting on a very thin basement membrane;
- An intermediate region containing from one to several layers of more columnar cells; and
- A superficial layer of very large, bulbous cells called **umbrella cells** that are occasionally bi- or multinucleated and are highly differentiated to protect underlying cells against the cytotoxic effects of hypertonic urine.

FIGURE **19–13** Fluid transport in the urinary system.

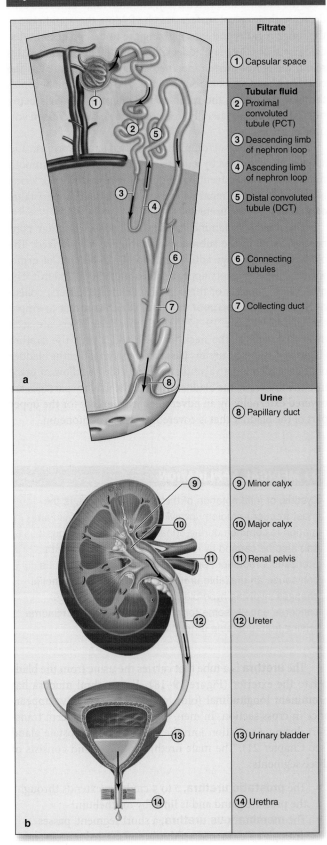

Filtrate

① Capsular space

Tubular fluid

② Proximal convoluted tubule (PCT)

③ Descending limb of nephron loop

④ Ascending limb of nephron loop

⑤ Distal convoluted tubule (DCT)

⑥ Connecting tubules

⑦ Collecting duct

Urine

⑧ Papillary duct

⑨ Minor calyx

⑩ Major calyx

⑪ Renal pelvis

⑫ Ureter

⑬ Urinary bladder

⑭ Urethra

a

b

FIGURE **19–14** Collecting ducts.

Pale-staining columnar **principal cells**, in which ADH-regulated aquaporins of the cell membrane allow more water reabsorption, are clearly seen in these transversely sectioned collecting ducts (**CD**), surrounded by interstitium with vasa recta (**VR**). X600. PT.

≫ MEDICAL APPLICATION

Bacterial infections of the urinary tract can lead to inflammation of the renal pelvis and calyces, or **pyelonephritis**. In acute pyelonephritis bacteria often move from one or more minor calyx into the associated renal papilla, causing accumulation of neutrophils in the collecting ducts.

(Left) (a) Diagram of a nephron and collecting system shows the flow of filtrate. **(b)** Upon delivery at a minor calyx, filtrate is no longer modified by reabsorption or secretion and is called **urine**. It flows passively into the renal pelvis but moves by peristalsis along the ureters for temporary storage in the urinary bladder, which is emptied through the urethra.

FIGURE **19–15** Renal papilla, collecting ducts, and minor calyx.

A sagittal section of a renal papilla shows numerous collecting ducts (also called the **ducts of Bellini** at this level) converging at the end of the renal papilla (**RP**) where they empty into the minor calyx (**MC**). The mucosa of the calyx contains dense connective tissue stained blue here and adipose tissue (**A**). The ducts are embedded in interstitial tissue that also contains thin limbs of the nephron loops. X50. Mallory trichrome. Inset: An enlarged area shows the columnar epithelium of the collecting ducts (**CD**), the interstitium (**I**) and thin limbs (**T**), and the protective urothelium (**U**) that lines the minor calyx. X200.

Umbrella cells are especially well developed in the bladder (Figure 19–17) where contact with urine is greatest. These cells, up to 100 μm in diameter, have extensive intercellular junctional complexes surrounding unique apical membranes. Most of the apical surface consists of **asymmetric unit membranes** in which regions of the outer lipid layer appear ultrastructurally to be twice as thick as the inner leaflet. These regions are composed of lipid rafts containing mostly integral membrane proteins called **uroplakins** that assemble into paracrystalline arrays of stiffened plaques 16 nm in diameter. These membranous plaques are impermeable to water and protect cytoplasm and underlying cells from the hyperosmotic effects of urine.

Plaques are hinged together by more narrow regions of typical membrane. When the bladder is emptied, not only does the mucosa fold extensively, but individual umbrella cells decrease their apical surface area by folding the membrane at the hinge regions and internalizing the folded plaques in discoidal vesicles. As the bladder fills again, the discoidal vesicles rejoin the apical membrane, increasing its surface area as the cell shape changes from round to flat. The urothelium becomes thinner, apparently the result of the intermediate cells being pushed and pulled laterally to accommodate the increased volume of urine.

Urothelium is surrounded by a folded lamina propria and submucosa, followed by a dense sheath of interwoven smooth muscle layers and adventitia (Figures 19–16 and 19–17). Urine is moved from the renal pelvises to the bladder by peristaltic contractions of the ureters.

The bladder's lamina propria and dense irregular connective tissue of the submucosa are highly vascularized. The bladder in an average adult can hold 400 to 600 mL of urine, with the urge to empty appearing at about 150 to 200 mL. The muscularis consists of three poorly delineated layers, collectively called the **detrusor muscle**, which contract to empty the bladder (Figure 19–17). Three muscular layers are seen most distinctly at the neck of the bladder near the urethra (Figure 19–17). The ureters pass through the wall of the bladder obliquely, forming a valve that prevents the backflow of urine into the ureters as the bladder fills. All the urinary passages are covered externally by an adventitial layer, except for the upper part of the bladder that is covered by serous peritoneum.

>> MEDICAL APPLICATION

Cystitis, or inflammation of the bladder mucosa, is the most frequent problem involving this organ. Such inflammation is common during urinary tract infections, but it can also be caused by immunodeficiency, urinary catheterization, radiation, or chemotherapy. Chronic cystitis can cause an **unstable urothelium,** with **benign urothelial changes** involving hyperplasia or metaplasia. Bladder cancer is usually some form of **transitional cell carcinoma** arising from unstable urothelium.

The **urethra** is a tube that carries the urine from the bladder to the exterior (Figure 19–18). The urethral mucosa has prominent longitudinal folds, giving it a distinctive appearance in cross section. In men, the two ducts for sperm transport during ejaculation join the urethra at the prostate gland (see Chapter 21). The male urethra is longer and consists of three segments:

- The **prostatic urethra,** 3 to 4 cm long, extends through the prostate gland and is lined by urothelium.
- The **membranous urethra,** a short segment, passes through an **external sphincter** of striated muscle and is

FIGURE **19–16** Ureters.

(a) Ureter cross section

(b)

(a) Diagram of a ureter in cross section shows a characteristic pattern of longitudinally folded mucosa, surrounded by a thick muscularis that moves urine by regular waves of peristalsis. The lamina propria is lined by a unique stratified epithelium called **transitional epithelium** or **urothelium** that is resistant

to the potentially deleterious effects of contact with hypertonic urine.

(b) Histologically the muscularis (**Mu**) is much thicker than the mucosa (**M**) and adventitia (**A**). X18. H&E.

FIGURE **19–17** Bladder wall and urothelium.

(a) In the neck of the bladder, near the urethra, the wall shows four layers: the mucosa with urothelium (**U**) and lamina propria (**LP**); the thin submucosa (**S**); inner, middle, and outer layers of smooth muscle (**IL**, **ML**, and **OL**); and the adventitia (**A**). X15. H&E.

(b) When the bladder is empty, the mucosa is highly folded and the urothelium (**U**) has bulbous umbrella cells. X250. PSH.
(c) When the bladder is full, the mucosa is pulled smooth, the urothelium (**U**) is thinner, and the umbrella cells are flatter. X250. H&E.

FIGURE 19–18 Urethra.

The urethra is a fibromuscular tube that carries urine from the bladder to the exterior of the body.

(a) A transverse section shows that the mucosa has large longitudinal folds around the lumen (**L**). X50. H&E.

(b) A higher magnification of the enclosed area shows the unusual stratified columnar nature of the urethral epithelium (**E**).

This thick epithelial lining varies between stratified columnar in some areas and pseudostratified columnar elsewhere, but it becomes stratified squamous at the distal end of the urethra. X250. H&E.

lined by stratified columnar and pseudostratified epithelium.

■ The **spongy urethra**, about 15 cm in length, is enclosed within erectile tissue of the penis (see Chapter 21) and is lined by stratified columnar and pseudostratified columnar epithelium (Figure 19–18), with stratified squamous epithelium distally.

In women, the urethra is exclusively a urinary organ. The female urethra is a 4- to 5-cm-long tube, lined initially with transitional epithelium, then by stratified squamous epithelium and some areas of pseudostratified columnar epithelium.

The middle part of the female urethra is surrounded by the external striated muscle sphincter.

›› MEDICAL APPLICATION

Urinary tract infections, usually involving coliform bacteria or *Chlamydia*, often produce **urethritis** and in women often lead to cystitis because of the short urethra. Such infections are usually accompanied by a persistent or more frequent urge to urinate, and urethritis may produce pain or difficulty during urination (**dysuria**).

The Urinary System SUMMARY OF KEY POINTS

Kidney

- Each kidney has a thick outer **cortex**, surrounding a **medulla** that is divided into 8 to 12 renal pyramids; each pyramid and its associated cortical tissue comprises a **renal lobe**.
- The apical papilla of each renal pyramid inserts into a **minor calyx**, a subdivision of two or three **major calyces** extending from the **renal pelvis**.
- The **ureter** carries urine from the renal pelvis and exits the **renal hilum**, where the **renal artery and vein** are also located.

Renal Vasculature

- Renal arteries branch to form smaller arteries between the renal lobes, with **interlobular arteries** entering the cortex to form the microvasculature; venous branches parallel the arterial supply.
- In the cortex **afferent arterioles** enter capillary clusters called **glomeruli**, which are drained by **efferent arterioles**, instead of venules, an arrangement that allows higher hydrostatic pressure in the capillaries.
- The **efferent arterioles** from cortical glomeruli branch diffusely as **peritubular capillaries**, while those from juxtamedullary glomeruli branch as long microvascular loops called **vasa recta** in the medulla.

Nephrons

- Functional units of the kidney are the **nephrons**, numbering about 1 million, each with a **renal corpuscle** and a long **renal tubule**, and a system of **collecting ducts**.
- The renal corpuscle has a simple squamous parietal layer of the **glomerular (Bowman's) capsule**, continuous with the proximal tubule, and a specialized visceral layer of **podocytes** surrounding the glomerular capillaries.
- **Podocytes** extend large primary processes that curve around a capillary and extend short, interdigitating secondary processes or **pedicels**, between which are narrow spaces called **slit pores**.
- The elevated pressure in the capillaries forces water and small solutes of blood plasma through the **glomerular filter** into the **capsular (or urinary) space** inside the glomerular capsule.
- In each glomerulus the filter has three parts: the finely **fenestrated capillary endothelium**; the thick (330 nm) **fused basal laminae** of type IV collagen and other proteins produced by the endothelial cells and podocytes; and the **slit pores** between the pedicels, covered by thin filtration **slit diaphragms**.
- From the renal corpuscle, filtrate enters the long **nephron tubule** that extends through both the cortex and medulla, with epithelial cells for both **reabsorption** and **secretion** of substances into the filtrate.
- The first tubular part, the **proximal convoluted tubule (PCT)**, is mainly cortical, has **simple cuboidal** cells with **long microvilli**

in the lumen, **abundant mitochondria**, and large, interdigitating **basolateral folds**.
- In the **PCT**, all glucose and other organic nutrients, all small proteins and peptides (which are degraded to amino acids), and much water and electrolytes are reabsorbed from the filtrate and transferred to the peritubular capillaries.
- From the PCT filtrate flows into the **loop of Henle**, located in the medulla, which has squamous **thin descending** and **ascending limbs**; the latter extends as a **thick ascending limb (TAL)** back into the cortex.
- In the cortex the **TAL** (also known as the **distal straight tubule**) contacts the arterioles at the vascular pole of its parent renal corpuscle and there thickens focally as the **macula densa**.
- Tall epithelial cells of the **macula densa** and specialized smooth muscle cells in the adjacent afferent arteriole called **juxtaglomerular cells**, which secrete **renin**, comprise a juxtaglomerular apparatus (JGA) that is an important regulator of blood pressure.
- Beyond the macula densa, the tubule continues as the **distal convoluted tubule (DCT)**, where electrolyte levels of the filtrate are adjusted further and which lead to short **connecting tubules**.
- **Connecting tubules** from several nephrons join to form the cortical **collecting ducts**, of simple cuboidal epithelium, which enter the medulla in parallel with the loops of Henle and vasa recta and become larger with more columnar cells.

Urinary Tract

- **Principal cells** of the **collecting ducts** are pale-staining, with relatively few mitochondria and distinct cell membranes that are rich in **aquaporins** (water channels) for passive water reabsorption.
- The largest collecting ducts deliver filtrate into the **minor calyces**, where it undergoes no further modification and is called **urine**.
- The calyces, renal pelvis, ureters, and urinary bladder are lined by **urothelium**, or **transitional epithelium**, which protects underlying cells from hypertonic or toxic effects of urine.
- Large, bulbous superficial cells of the urothelium, called **umbrella cells**, have apical membranes consisting of hinged regions with dense plaques of **uroplakin** proteins that protect the cytoplasm.
- As the **urinary bladder** fills its highly folded mucosa unfolds, the urothelium gets somewhat thinner by cell movements, and the hinged membrane plaques of umbrella cells partially unfold.
- The **urethra** drains the bladder and is lined by unusual **stratified columnar** and **pseudostratified columnar epithelium**.
- In males the urethra has three regions: the **prostatic urethra** in the prostate gland; the short **membranous urethra** passing through the urogenital diaphragm, and the long **penile urethra**.

20 Endocrine Glands

Secretory cells of endocrine glands release their products, signaling molecules called **hormones**, into the neighboring vascularized compartment for uptake by capillaries and distribution throughout the body. There is no secretory duct as in exocrine glands. Endocrine cells are typically epithelial, at least in origin, and aggregated as cords or clusters. Besides the specialized endocrine glands discussed in this chapter, many other organs specialized for other functions, such as the heart, thymus, gut, kidneys, testis, and ovaries, contain various endocrine cells (Figure 20–1).

Distribution by the circulation allows hormones to act on target cells with receptors for those hormones at a distance from the site of their secretion. As discussed briefly in Chapter 2, other endocrine cells produce hormones that act on target cells only a short distance away. This may involve **paracrine** secretion, with localized dispersal in interstitial fluid or through short loops of blood vessels, as when gastrin made by pyloric G cells reaches target cells in the fundic glands, or **juxtacrine** secretion, in which a signaling molecule remains on the secreting cell's surface or adjacent extracellular matrix and affects target cells when the cells make contact. Juxtacrine signaling is particularly important in embryonic and regenerative tissue interactions. In **autocrine** secretion, cells may produce molecules that act on themselves or on cells of the same type. For example, insulin-like growth factor (IGF) produced by several cell types may act on the same cells that produced it. Endocrine glands are often also target organs for other hormones that can establish a feedback mechanism to control hormone secretion and keep blood hormonal levels within strict limits.

Hormones, like neurotransmitters, are frequently hydrophilic molecules such as proteins, glycoproteins, peptides, or modified amino acids with receptors on the surface of target cells. Alternatively, hydrophobic steroid and thyroid hormones must circulate on transport proteins but can diffuse through the cell membranes and activate cytoplasmic receptors in target cells (see Chapter 2).

❯ PITUITARY GLAND (HYPOPHYSIS)

The **pituitary gland**, or **hypophysis** (Gr. *hypo*, under + *physis*, growth), weighs about 0.5 g in adults and has dimensions of about $10 \times 13 \times 6$ mm. It lies below the brain in a small cavity on the sphenoid bone, the sella turcica (Figure 20–2). The pituitary is formed in the embryo partly from the developing brain and partly from the developing oral cavity (Figure 20–3). The neural component is the neurohypophyseal bud growing down from the floor of the future diencephalon as a stalk (or infundibulum) that remains attached to the brain. The oral component arises as an outpocketing of ectoderm from the roof of the primitive mouth and grows cranially, forming a structure called the **hypophyseal** (**Rathke**) **pouch**. The base of this pouch eventually constricts and separates from the pharynx. Its anterior wall then thickens greatly, reducing the pouch's lumen to a small fissure (Figure 20–3).

Because of its dual origin, the pituitary actually consists of two glands—the posterior **neurohypophysis** and the anterior **adenohypophysis**—united anatomically but with different functions. The neurohypophysis retains many histologic features of brain tissue and consists of a large part, the **pars nervosa**, and the smaller **infundibulum** stalk attached to the hypothalamus at the median eminence (Figure 20–2 and 20–4). The **adenohypophysis**, derived from the oral

FIGURE **20–1** Locations of the major endocrine glands.

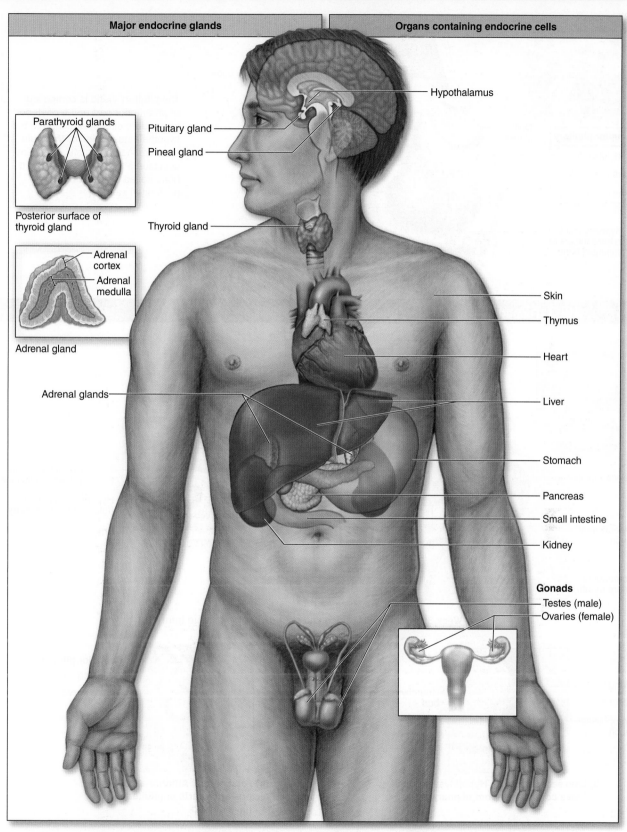

| Major endocrine glands | Organs containing endocrine cells |

Hypothalamus

Parathyroid glands

Pituitary gland

Pineal gland

Posterior surface of thyroid gland

Thyroid gland

Adrenal cortex

Adrenal medulla

Adrenal gland

Skin

Thymus

Heart

Adrenal glands

Liver

Stomach

Pancreas

Small intestine

Kidney

Gonads
Testes (male)
Ovaries (female)

In addition to the large endocrine glands shown at the left here, there are widely distributed endocrine cells as well as various other tissues in organs (right) throughout the body with endocrine functions. Not shown are adipocytes, which exert important endocrine functions, and the many tissues in which paracrine signalling is important.

FIGURE **20–2** Pituitary gland.

Hypothalamus

Mammillary body

Median eminence

Optic chiasm

Infundibulum

Anterior pituitary

Pars tuberalis

Pars intermedia

Pars distalis

Posterior pituitary

Infundibular stalk

Pars nervosa

Hypophyseal fossa in sella turcica of sphenoid bone

The pituitary gland is composed of an anterior part and a posterior part that is directly attached to the hypothalamus region of the brain by an infundibular stalk. The gland occupies a fossa of the sphenoid bone called the **sella turcica** (L. Turkish saddle).

FIGURE **20–3** Formation of the pituitary gland.

Diencephalon

Neuroectoderm

Neurohypophyseal bud

Oral ectoderm

Hypophyseal pouch

Stomodeum (future mouth)

Neurohypophyseal bud (future posterior pituitary)

Hypophyseal pouch (future anterior pituitary)

Pharynx

(a) Week 3: Hypophyseal pouch and neurohypophyseal bud form

Infundibulum

Neurohypophyseal bud

Hypophyseal pouch

(b) Late second month: Hypophyseal pouch loses contact with roof of pharynx

Anterior pituitary

Pars tuberalis

Pars intermedia

Pars distalis

Posterior pituitary

Median eminence

Pars nervosa

(c) Fetal period: Anterior and posterior parts of pituitary have formed

The pituitary gland forms from two separate embryonic structures. **(a)** During the third week of development, a hypophyseal pouch (or Rathke pouch, the future anterior pituitary) grows from the roof of the pharynx, while a neurohypophyseal bud (future posterior pituitary) forms from the diencephalon.

(b) By late in the second month, the hypophyseal pouch detaches from the roof of the pharynx and merges with the neurohypophyseal bud. **(c)** During the fetal period, the anterior and posterior parts of the pituitary complete development.

FIGURE **20–4** Pituitary gland.

Histologically the two parts of the pituitary gland reflect their origins, as seen in this low-magnification section of an entire gland. The infundibular stalk (**IS**) and pars nervosa (**PN**) of the neurohypophysis resemble CNS tissue, while the adenohypophysis' pars distalis (**PD**), pars intermediate (**PI**), and pars tuberalis (**PT**) are typically glandular in their level of staining. X30. H&E.

ectoderm, has three parts: a large **pars distalis** or **anterior lobe**; the **pars tuberalis**, which wraps around the infundibulum; and the thin **pars intermedia** adjacent to the posterior pars nervosa (Figures 20–2 and 20–4).

The Hypothalamic-Hypophyseal Tract & Blood Supply

The pituitary gland's neural connection to the brain and its blood supply are both of key importance for its function (Figures 20–4 and 20–5). Embryologically, anatomically, and functionally, the pituitary gland is connected to the hypothalamus at the base of the brain. In addition to the vascular portal system carrying small regulatory peptides from the hypothalamus to the adenohypophysis, a bundle of axons called the **hypothalamic-hypophyseal tract** courses into the neurohypophysis from two important hypothalamic nuclei. The peptide

hormones ADH (antidiuretic hormone) and oxytocin are synthesized by large neurons in the **supraoptic** and the **paraventricular nuclei**, respectively. Both hormones undergo axonal transport and accumulate temporarily in the axons of the hypothalamic-hypophyseal tract before their release and uptake by capillaries branching from the inferior arteries.

The blood supply derives from two groups of vessels coming off the internal carotid artery and drained by the hypophyseal vein. The **superior hypophyseal arteries** supply the median eminence and the infundibular stalk; the **inferior hypophyseal arteries** provide blood mainly for the neurohypophysis. The superior arteries divide into a **primary plexus** of fenestrated capillaries that irrigate the stalk and median eminence. These capillaries then rejoin to form venules that branch again as a larger secondary capillary plexus in the adenohypophysis (Figure 20–5). These vessels make up the **hypothalamic-hypophyseal portal system** that has great

FIGURE **20–5** The hypothalamic-hypophyseal tract and portal system.

Hypothalamus

Paraventricular nucleus
(produces oxytocin)

Supraoptic nucleus
(produces ADH)

Optic chiasm

Hypothalamic-hypophyseal
tract

Posterior pituitary
Infundibulum

Pars nervosa
(With axons storing
oxytocin and ADH)

(a)

Hypothalamus

Superior hypophyseal artery

Hypophyseal portal veins

Anterior pituitary

Hypophyseal vein

Secondary plexus of the
hypothalamic-hypophyseal
portal system

Hypophyseal vein

Infundibulum

Primary plexus of the
hypothalamic-hypophyseal
portal system

Hypophyseal veins

Posterior pituitary

Inferior hypophyseal
artery

(b)

(a) The **hypothalamic-hypophyseal tract** consists of axons extending from the hypothalamic supraoptic and paraventricular nuclei, through the infundibulum and into the pars nervosa of the posterior pituitary, where peptide hormones they carry are released for capillary uptake.

(b) The **hypothalamic-hypophyseal portal system**, with blood from the superior hypophyseal artery, consists of two capillary networks connected by the hypophyseal portal vein. The primary plexus surrounds the infundibulum and median eminence, and the second is throughout the pars distalis and drains into the hypophyseal veins.

importance because it carries neuropeptides from the median eminence the short distance to the adenohypophysis where they either stimulate or inhibit hormone release by the endocrine cells there.

Adenohypophysis (Anterior Pituitary)

The three parts of the adenohypophysis are derived embryonically from the hypophyseal pouch.

Pars Distalis

The **pars distalis** accounts for 75% of the adenohypophysis and has a thin fibrous capsule. The main components are cords of well-stained endocrine cells interspersed with fenestrated capillaries and supporting reticular connective tissue (Figures 20–4 and 20–6). Common stains suggest two broad groups of cells in the pars distalis with different staining affinities: **chromophils** and **chromophobes**. Chromophils are secretory cells in which hormone is stored

in cytoplasmic granules. They are also called **basophils** and **acidophils**, based on their affinities for basic and acidic dyes, respectively (Figure 20–6).

Subtypes of basophilic and acidophilic cells are identified by their granular morphology in the TEM or more easily by immunohistochemistry (Figure 20–7). Specific cells are usually named according to their hormone's target cells (Table 20–1). Acidophils secrete either growth hormone (somatotropin) or prolactin and are called **somatotrophs** and **lactotrophs** (or somatotropic cells and lactotropic cells), respectively. The basophilic cells are the **corticotrophs**, **gonadotrophs**, and **thyrotrophs**, with target cells in the adrenal cortex, gonads, and thyroid gland, respectively. Somatotrophs typically constitute about half the cells of the pars distalis in humans, with thyrotrophs the least abundant.

With two exceptions, each type of anterior pituitary cell makes one kind of hormone (see Table 20–1). Gonadotrophs secrete two different glycoproteins: **follicle-stimulating hormone (FSH)** and **luteinizing hormone (LH**; called interstitial

FIGURE **20–6** Pars distalis: Acidophils, basophils, and chromophobes.

(a, b) Most general staining methods simply allow the parenchymal cells of the pars distalis to be subdivided into acidophil cells (**A**), basophils (**B**), and chromophobes (**C**) in which the cytoplasm is poorly stained. Also shown are capillaries and sinusoids (**S**) in the second capillary plexus of the portal system. Cords of acidophils and basophils vary in distribution and number in different regions of the pars distalis, but they are always closely associated microvasculature that carries off secreted hormones into the general circulation. X400. H&E. **(c)** The same area is seen after staining with Gomori trichrome. X400.

cell-stimulating hormone [ICSH] in men). The main protein synthesized in corticotrophs is pro-opiomelanocortin (POMC), which is cleaved posttranslationally into the polypeptide hormones **adrenocortical trophic hormone (ACTH)** and β-**lipotropin** (β-**LPH**). Hormones produced by the pars distalis have widespread functional activities. They regulate almost all other endocrine glands, ovarian function and sperm production, milk production, and the metabolism of muscle, bone, and adipose tissue (see Table 20–1; Figure 20–8).

Chromophobes stain weakly, with few or no secretory granules, and also represent a heterogeneous group, including stem

and undifferentiated progenitor cells as well as any degranulated cells present.

Pars Tuberalis

The **pars tuberalis** is a smaller funnel-shaped region surrounding the infundibulum of the neurohypophysis (Figures 20–2 and 20–4). Most of the cells of the pars tuberalis are gonadotrophs.

Pars Intermedia

The **pars intermedia** is a thin zone of basophilic cells between the pars distalis and the pars nervosa of the neurohypophysis,

FIGURE **20–7** Ultrastructure and immunohistochemistry of somatotropic cells.

(a) Ultrastructurally, cytoplasm of all chromophil cells is shown to have well-developed Golgi complexes (**G**), euchromatic nuclei (**N**), and cytoplasm filled with secretory granules, as shown here for a somatotroph, the most common acidophil. The **arrow** indicates the cell membrane. Specific chromophils are more easily identified using immunohistochemistry and antibodies against the hormone products. X10,000. (b) The micrograph shows somatotrophs stained using an antibody against somatotropin. X400. Hematoxylin counterstain.

TABLE **20–1** | Major cell types of the anterior pituitary and their major functions.

Cell Type	% of Total Cells	Hormone Produced	Major Function
Somatotrophs	50	Somatotropin (growth hormone, GH), a 22-kDa protein	Stimulates growth in epiphyseal plates of long bones via insulin-like growth factors (IGFs) produced in liver
Lactotrophs (or mammotrophs)	15-20	Prolactin (PRL), a 22.5-kDa protein	Promotes milk secretion
Gonadotrophs	10	Follicle-stimulating hormone (FSH) and luteinizing hormone (LH; interstitial cell-stimulating hormone [ICSH] in men), both 28-kDa glycoprotein dimers, secreted from the same cell type	FSH promotes ovarian follicle development and estrogen secretion in women and spermatogenesis in men; LH promotes ovarian follicle maturation and progesterone secretion in women and interstitial cell androgen secretion in men
Thyrotrophs	5	Thyrotropin (TSH), a 28-kDa glycoprotein dimer	Stimulates thyroid hormone synthesis, storage, and liberation
Corticotrophs	15-20	Adrenal corticotropin (ACTH), a 4-kDa polypeptide	Stimulates secretion of adrenal cortex hormones
		Lipotropin (LPH)	Helps regulate lipid metabolism

FIGURE **20–8** Hormones of the pars distalis and their targets.

Regulatory hormones of hypothalamus
Tropic hormones of anterior pituitary

Hypothalamus

Releasing hormones: TRH, PRH, GnRH, CRH, GHRH
Inhibiting hormones: PIH, GIH

Infundibulum

Anterior pituitary — — Posterior pituitary

Thyroid-stimulating hormone (TSH) stimulates the thyroid gland to release thyroid hormone (TH).

TSH

Thyroid

Muscle

GH

Growth hormone (GH) acts on all body tissues, especially cartilage, bone, muscle, and adipose connective tissue to stimulate growth.

Bone   Adipose connective tissue

PRL

Mammary gland

Prolactin (PRL) acts on mammary glands to stimulate milk production.

ACTH

Adrenal cortex

Adrenocorticotropic hormone (ACTH) acts on the adrenal cortex to cause release of corticosteroids (eg, cortisol).

FSH and LH

Follicle-stimulating hormone (FSH) and **luteinizing hormone (LH)** act on gonads (testes and ovaries) to stimulate development of gametes (sperm and oocyte).

Testis   Ovary

Adrenal gland

The anterior pituitary secretes six major tropic hormones controlling the activities of their target organs. Release of these hormones is regulated primarily by hypothalamic factors carried by the hypothalamic-hypophyseal blood supply.

which is often invaded by basophils (Figure 20–9). The pars intermedia develops from the dorsal wall of the hypophyseal pouch and usually contains colloid-filled cysts of various sizes that represent remnants of that structure's lumen (Figure 20–9). During fetal life cells of this region, like corticotrophs of the pars distalis, express POMC. However, in these cells POMC is cleaved by different proteases to produce smaller peptide hormones, including two forms of melanocyte-stimulating hormone (MSH), γ-LPH, and β-endorphin. MSH increases melanocyte activity, but the overall functional significance of this region remains uncertain, especially in adults.

Control of Hormone Secretion in the Anterior Pituitary

The activities of the cells of the anterior pituitary are controlled primarily by peptide-related **hypothalamic hormones**

produced by small neurons near the third ventricle, discharged from axons in the median eminence, and transported by capillaries of the portal system throughout the anterior pituitary. As shown in Table 20–2, most of these hormones are **releasing hormones** that stimulate secretion by specific anterior pituitary cells. Two of the hypothalamic factors, however, are **inhibiting hormones** that block hormone secretion in specific cells of the adenohypophysis (Table 20–2). Because of the strategic position of the hypothalamic neurons and the control they exert on the hypophysis and therefore on many bodily functions, many sensory stimuli coming to the brain, as well as stimuli arising within the CNS, can affect the function of the pituitary gland and then quickly also affect the function of many other organs and tissues.

Another mechanism controlling activity of anterior pituitary cells is **negative feedback** by hormones from the target organs on secretion of the relevant hypothalamic

FIGURE **20–9** Pars intermedia.

The pars intermedia (**PI**) lies between the pars distalis (**PD**) and the pars nervosa (**PN**), with many of its basophilic cells (**B**) usually invading the latter. Remnants of the embryonic hypophyseal pouch's lumen are usually present in this region as colloid-filled cysts (**C**) of various sizes. Function of this region in humans is not clear. X56. H&E.

factors and on hormone secretion by the relevant pituitary cells. Figure 20–10 illustrates this mechanism, using the thyroid as an example, and shows the complex chain of events that begins with the action of neural stimuli in the hypothalamus and ends with the effects of hormones from the pituitary's target organs.

Finally, hormone secretion in the anterior pituitary is affected by other hormones from outside the feedback loop or even outside the major target tissues. Examples include the polypeptide ghrelin produced mainly in the stomach mucosa, which also acts as a releasing hormone for somatotropin secretion, and oxytocin, released in the posterior pituitary during breast-feeding, which increases secretion of prolactin.

All these mechanisms allow the fine tuning of hormone secretion by cells of the anterior pituitary.

>> **MEDICAL APPLICATION**

Benign **pituitary adenomas** often produce excessive numbers of functional acidophils or basophils. Adenomas involving somatotropic cells can cause **gigantism** if occurring in children before closure of the long bones' epiphyseal plates or **acromegaly** in adults, with musculoskeletal, neurologic, and other medical consequences.

Neurohypophysis (Posterior Pituitary)

The neurohypophysis consists of the pars nervosa and the infundibular stalk (Figures 20–2 and 20–4) and, unlike the adenohypophysis, does not contain the cells that synthesize its two hormones. It is composed of neural tissue, containing some 100,000 unmyelinated axons of large secretory neurons with cell bodies in the supraoptic and paraventricular nuclei of the hypothalamus (Figure 20–5). Also present are highly branched glial cells called **pituicytes** that resemble astrocytes and are the most abundant cell type in the posterior pituitary (Figure 20–11).

The secretory neurons have all the characteristics of typical neurons, including the ability to conduct an action potential, but have larger-diameter axons and well-developed synthetic components related to the production of the 9-amino acid peptide hormones **antidiuretic hormone** (**ADH**)—also called arginine vasopressin—and **oxytocin**. Transported axonally into the pars nervosa, these hormones accumulate in axonal dilations called **neurosecretory bodies** or **Herring bodies**, visible in the light microscope as faintly eosinophilic structures (Figure 20–11). The neurosecretory bodies contain membrane-enclosed granules with either oxytocin or ADH bound to 10-kDa carrier proteins called **neurophysin I** and **II**, respectively. The hormone-neurophysin complex is synthesized as a single protein and then cleaved to produce the peptide hormone and its binding protein. Nerve impulses along the axons trigger the release of the peptides from the neurosecretory bodies for uptake by the fenestrated capillaries of the pars nervosa, and the hormones are then distributed to the general circulation. Axons from the supraoptic and paraventricular nuclei mingle in the neurohypophysis but are mainly concerned with ADH and oxytocin secretion, respectively.

ADH is released in response to increased blood tonicity, sensed by osmoreceptor cells in the hypothalamus, which then stimulate ADH synthesis in supraoptic neurons. ADH increases the permeability of the renal collecting ducts to water (see Chapter 19) so that more water is reabsorbed from the filtrate in these tubules and osmotic balance of body fluids is restored (Table 20–3).

TABLE **20–2**	Hypothalamic hormones regulating cells of the anterior pituitary.	
Hormone	**Chemical Form**	**Functions**
Thyrotropin-releasing hormone (TRH)	3-amino acid peptide	Stimulates release of thyrotropin (TSH)
Gonadotropin-releasing hormone (GnRH)	10-amino acid peptide	Stimulates the release of both follicle-stimulating hormone (FSH) and luteinizing hormone (LH)
Somatostatin	14-amino acid peptide	Inhibits release of both somatotropin (GH) and TSH
Growth hormone–releasing hormone (GHRH)	40- or 44-amino acid polypeptides (2 forms)	Stimulates release of GH
Dopamine	Modified amino acid	Inhibits release of prolactin (PRL)
Corticotropin-releasing hormone (CRH)	41-amino acid polypeptide	Stimulates synthesis of pro-opiomelanocortin (POMC) and release of both β-lipotropin (β-LPH) and corticotropin (ACTH)

FIGURE **20–10** Negative feedback loops affecting anterior pituitary secretion.

① A stimulus (eg, low body temperature) causes the hypothalamus to secrete thyrotropin-releasing hormone (TRH), which acts on the anterior pituitary.

Hypothalamus

→ stimulatory
→ inhibitory

Negative feedback inhibition

⑤ Increased body temperature is detected by the hypothalamus, and secretion of TRH by the hypothalamus is inhibited. TH also blocks TRH receptors on the thyrotropic cells, inhibiting synthesis and release of TSH. Both effects indirectly dampen TH production in the thyroid.

② Thyrotropic cells in the anterior pituitary release thyroid-stimulating hormone (TSH).

Anterior pituitary

Target organs in body

④ TH stimulates target cells to increase metabolic activities, resulting in an increase in basal body temperature.

③ TSH stimulates follicular cells of the thyroid gland to release thyroid hormone (TH).

Relationship between the hypothalamus, the anterior pituitary, and its target organs is shown, using the thyroid as an example. Hypothalamic thyrotropin-releasing hormone (**TRH**) stimulates secretion of thyroid-stimulating hormone or thyrotropin (**TSH**), which stimulates synthesis and secretion of thyroid hormone (**TH**). In addition to their effects on target organs, TH inhibits TSH secretion from the pars distalis and TRH secretion from the hypothalamus by negative feedback.

›› MEDICAL APPLICATION

Posterior pituitary function can be adversely affected by heritable mutations in the gene for vasopressin (ADH)-neurophysin, by compression from a tumor in adjacent tissues, and by **head trauma**. By lowering levels of vasopressin, such conditions can produce **diabetes insipidus**, a disorder characterized by inability to concentrate urine, which leads to frequent urination (**polyuria**) and increased thirst (**polydipsia**).

FIGURE **20–11** Pars nervosa: neurosecretory bodies and pituicytes.

The pars nervosa of the posterior pituitary consists of modified neural tissues containing unmyelinated axons supported and ensheathed by glia cells called **pituicytes** (**P**), the most numerous cell present. The axons run from the supraoptic and paraventricular hypothalamic nuclei, and have swellings called **neurosecretory (Herring) bodies** (**NB**) from which either oxytocin or vasopressin is released upon neural stimulation. The released hormones are picked up by capillaries (**C**) for distribution. X400. H&E.

Oxytocin stimulates contraction of the myoepithelial cells of uterine smooth muscle during childbirth and of alveoli and ducts in the mammary glands (Table 20–3). A nursing infant induces oxytocin secretion by stimulating sensory tracts that act on the hypothalamus in a neurohormonal reflex producing rapid ejection of milk.

› ADRENAL GLANDS

The **adrenal** (or suprarenal) **glands** are paired organs lying near the superior poles of the kidneys, embedded in the perirenal adipose tissue (see Figure 20–1; Figure 20–12). They are flattened structures with a half-moon shape, about 4 to 6 cm long, 1 to 2 cm wide, and 4 to 6 mm thick in adults. Together, they weigh about 8 g, but their weight and size vary with the age and physiologic condition of the individual. Adrenal glands are each covered by a dense connective tissue capsule that sends thin trabeculae into the gland's parenchyma. The stroma consists mainly of reticular fibers supporting the

FIGURE **20–12** Location and blood supply of the adrenal glands.

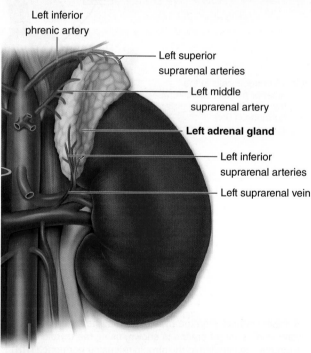

The paired adrenal glands are located at the superior pole of each kidney and each consists of an outer cortex that produces a variety of steroid hormones and an inner medulla that produces epinephrine and norepinephrine. This anterior view of the left adrenal gland and kidney shows the blood vessels supplying these glands.

TABLE **20–3**	Hormones of the posterior pituitary.
Hormone	**Function**
Vasopressin/antidiuretic hormone (ADH)	Increases water permeability of renal collecting ducts
Oxytocin	Stimulates contraction of mammary gland myoepithelial cells and uterine smooth muscle

secretory cells and microvasculature. Each gland has two concentric regions: a yellowish **adrenal cortex** and a reddish-brown central **adrenal medulla**.

The adrenal cortex and medulla can be considered two different organs with distinct embryonic origins, functions, and morphologic characteristics that become united during embryonic development. The cortex arises from mesoderm and the medulla from the neural crest. The general histologic appearance of the adrenal gland is typical of an endocrine gland in which cells of both cortex and medulla are grouped in cords along wide capillaries.

The adrenal glands are supplied by several arteries that enter at various points around their periphery (see Figure 20–12). The branches of these arteries form **cortical arterioles**, which branch as capillaries and sinusoids that irrigate the cortex and then join the medullary capillaries, and **medullary arterioles**, which penetrate directly to the medulla and form a network of fenestrated sinusoids there. The adrenal medulla thus has a dual blood supply with both arterial blood from the medullary arterioles and venous blood from capillaries of the cortex. The capillaries and sinusoids give rise to the central **medullary veins**, which join as the **suprarenal vein** leaving the gland (see Figure 20–12).

Adrenal Cortex

Cells of the adrenal cortex have characteristic features of steroid-secreting cells: acidophilic cytoplasm rich in lipid droplets, with central nuclei. Ultrastructurally their cytoplasm shows an exceptionally profuse smooth ER (SER) of interconnected tubules, which contain the enzymes for cholesterol synthesis and conversion of the steroid prohormone pregnenolone into specific active steroid hormones. The mitochondria are often spherical, with tubular rather than shelflike cristae (Figure 20–13). These mitochondria not only synthesize ATP but also contain the enzymes for converting cholesterol to pregnenolone and for some steps in steroid synthesis. The function of steroid-producing cells involves close collaboration between SER and mitochondria.

Steroid hormones are not stored in granules like proteins or undergo exocytosis. As small lipid-soluble molecules, steroids diffuse freely from cells through the plasma membrane.

The adrenal cortex has three concentric zones in which the cords of epithelial steroid-producing cells are arranged somewhat differently and which synthesize different classes of steroid hormones (Figure 20–14):

- The **zona glomerulosa**, immediately inside the capsule and comprising about 15% of the cortex, consists of closely packed, rounded or arched cords of columnar or pyramidal cells with many capillaries (Figure 20–15). The steroids made by these cells are called **mineralocorticoids** because they affect uptake of Na⁺, K⁺, and water by cells of renal tubules. The principal product is **aldosterone**, the major regulator of salt balance, which acts to stimulate Na⁺ reabsorption in the distal

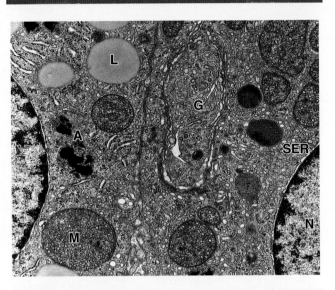

FIGURE **20–13** Ultrastructure of cortical adrenalocytes.

TEM of two adjacent steroid-secreting cells from the zona fasciculate shows features typical of steroid-producing cells: lipid droplets (**L**) containing cholesterol esters, mitochondria (**M**) with tubular and vesicular cristae, abundant **SER**, and autophagosomes (**A**), which remove mitochondria and SER between periods of active steroid synthesis. Also seen are the euchromatic nuclei (**N**), a Golgi apparatus (**G**), RER, and lysosomes. X25,700.

convoluted tubules (see Chapter 19). Aldosterone secretion is stimulated primarily by angiotensin II and also by an increase in plasma K⁺ concentration, but only weakly by ACTH.

- The middle **zona fasciculata**, occupies 65% to 80% of the cortex and consists of long cords of large polyhedral cells, one or two cells thick, separated by fenestrated sinusoidal capillaries (Figure 20–15). The cells are filled with lipid droplets and appear vacuolated in routine histologic preparations. These cells secrete **glucocorticoids**, especially **cortisol**, which affect carbohydrate metabolism by stimulating gluconeogenesis in many cells and glycogen synthesis in the liver. Cortisol also suppresses many immune functions and can induce fat mobilization and muscle proteolysis. Secretion is controlled by ACTH with negative feedback proportional to the concentration of circulating glucocorticoids (Figure 20–10). Small amounts of weak androgens are also produced here.

- The innermost **zona reticularis** comprises about 10% of the cortex and consists of smaller cells in a network of irregular cords interspersed with wide capillaries (Figure 20–15). The cells are usually more heavily stained than

FIGURE 20–14 Adrenal gland.

Inside the capsule of each adrenal gland is an adrenal cortex, formed from embryonic mesodermal cells, which completely surrounds an innermost adrenal medulla derived embryologically from neural crest cells. Both regions are very well vascularized with fenestrated sinusoidal capillaries. Cortical cells are arranged as three layers: the zona glomerulosa near the capsule, the zona fasciculata (the thickest layer), and the zona reticularis.

those of the other zones because they contain fewer lipid droplets and more lipofuscin pigment. Cells of the zona reticularis also produce cortisol but primarily secrete the **weak androgens**, including **dehydroepiandrosterone (DHEA)** that is converted to testosterone in both men and women. Secretion by these cells is also stimulated by ACTH with regulatory feedback.

> **›› MEDICAL APPLICATION**
>
> **Addison disease** or **adrenal cortical insufficiency** is a disorder, usually autoimmune in origin, which causes degeneration in any layer of adrenal cortex, with concomitant loss of glucocorticoids, mineralocorticoids, or androgen production.

Adrenal Medulla

The adrenal medulla is composed of large, pale-staining polyhedral cells arranged in cords or clumps and supported by a reticular fiber network (Figure 20–16). A profuse supply of sinusoidal capillaries intervenes between adjacent cords and a few parasympathetic ganglion cells are present. Medullary parenchymal cells, known as **chromaffin cells**, arise from neural crest cells, as do the postganglionic neurons of sympathetic and parasympathetic ganglia. Chromaffin cells can be considered modified sympathetic postganglionic neurons, lacking axons and dendrites and specialized as secretory cells.

> **›› MEDICAL APPLICATION**
>
> In the adrenal medulla, benign **pheochromocytomas** periodically secrete high levels of catecholamines that cause swings in blood pressure between hypertension and hypotension.

Unlike cells of the adrenal cortex, chromaffin cells contain many electron-dense granules, 150 to 350 nm in diameter, for storage and secretion of catecholamines, either **epinephrine** or **norepinephrine**. The granules of epinephrine-secreting cells are less electron-dense and generally smaller than those of norepinephrine-secreting cells (Figure 20–16). Both catecholamines, together with Ca^{2+} and ATP, are bound in granular storage complexes with 49-kDa proteins called **chromogranins**.

Norepinephrine-secreting cells are also found in paraganglia (collections of catecholamine-secreting cells adjacent to the autonomic ganglia) and in various viscera. The conversion of norepinephrine to epinephrine (adrenalin) occurs only in chromaffin cells of the adrenal medulla. About 80% of the catecholamine secreted from the adrenal is epinephrine.

Medullary chromaffin cells are innervated by cholinergic endings of preganglionic sympathetic neurons, which trigger hormone release. Epinephrine and norepinephrine are released to the blood in large quantities during intense emotional reactions, such as fright, and produce vasoconstriction, increased blood pressure, changes in heart rate, and elevated blood glucose levels. These effects facilitate various defensive

FIGURE **20–15** Adrenal cortex.

The steroid-secreting cells of the adrenal cortex are arranged differently to form three fairly distinct concentric layers, the zonae glomerulosa (**G**), fasciculata (**F**), and reticularis (**R**), surrounding the medulla (**M**). Shown here are sections from two adrenal glands, stained with H&E (left) and Mallory trichrome, in which the sparse collagen appears blue (right).

(a, b) Immediately beneath the capsule (**C**), the **zona glomerulosa** consists of rounded clusters of columnar cells principally secreting the mineral corticoid aldosterone.

(c, d) The thick middle layer, the **zona fasciculata**, consists of long cords of large, spongy-looking cells mainly secreting glucocorticoids such as cortisol.

(e, f) Cells of the innermost **zona reticularis**, next to the medulla (**M**), are small, better stained, arranged in a close network and secrete mainly sex steroids. Cells of all the layers are closely associated with sinusoidal capillaries.

Left: X20 H&E.; a, c, e: X200. H&E. b, d, f: X200. Mallory trichrome.

FIGURE **20–16** Adrenal medulla.

The hormone-secreting cells of the adrenal medulla are chromaffin cells, which resemble sympathetic neurons.
(a) The micrograph shows that they are large pale-staining cells, arranged in cords interspersed with wide capillaries. Faintly stained cytoplasmic granules can be seen in most chromaffin cells. X200. H&E.

(b) TEM reveals that the granules of norepinephrine-secreting cells (**NE**) are more electron-dense than those of cells secreting epinephrine (**E**), which is due to the chromogranins binding the catecholamines. Most of the hormone produced is epinephrine, which is only made in the adrenal medulla. X33,000.

reactions (the fight-or-flight response). During normal activity, the adrenal medulla continuously secretes small quantities of the hormones.

❯ PANCREATIC ISLETS

The **pancreatic islets** (islets of Langerhans) are compact spherical or ovoid masses of endocrine cells embedded within the acinar exocrine tissue of the pancreas (Figure 20–17). Most islets are 100 to 200 μm in diameter and contain several hundred cells, but some have only a few cells. The pancreas has more than 1 million islets, mostly in the gland's narrow tail region, but they only constitute 1% to 2% of the organ's total volume. A very thin reticular capsule surrounds each islet, separating it from the adjacent acinar tissue. Pancreatic islets have the same embryonic origin as the pancreatic acinar tissue: in epithelial outgrowths from endoderm of the developing gut.

The cells of islets are polygonal or rounded, smaller, and more lightly stained than the surrounding acinar cells, arranged in cords separated by fenestrated capillaries (Figure 20–17).

Routine stains or trichrome stains show that most islet cells are acidophilic or basophilic with fine cytoplasmic granules (Figure 20–17). Ultrastructural features are those of active polypeptide-secreting cells, with secretory granules that vary in size, morphology, and electron density from cell to cell.

The major islet cells are most easily identified and studied by immunohistochemistry:

- α or **A cells** secrete primarily **glucagon** and are usually located peripherally.
- β or **B cells** produce **insulin** (L. *insula*, island), are the most numerous, and are located centrally.
- δ or **D cells,** secreting **somatostatin**, are scattered and much less abundant.

❯❯ MEDICAL APPLICATION

Diabetes mellitus is characterized by loss of the insulin effect and a subsequent failure of cells to take up glucose, leading to elevated blood sugar or **hyperglycemia**. **Type 1 diabetes** or **insulin-dependent diabetes mellitus (IDDM)** is caused by loss of the β cells from autoimmune destruction and is treated by regular injections of insulin. In **type 2 diabetes** or **non–insulin-dependent diabetes mellitus (NIDDM)**, β cells are present but fail to produce adequate levels of insulin in response to hyperglycemia and the peripheral target cells "resist" or no longer respond to the hormone. Type 2 diabetes commonly occurs with obesity, and poorly understood, multifactorial genetic components are also important in this disease's onset.

FIGURE **20–17** Pancreatic islets.

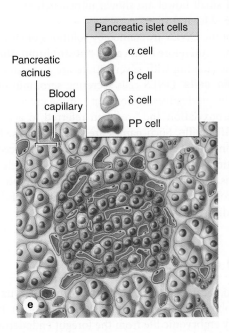

Pancreatic islets are clumped masses of pale-staining endocrine cells embedded in the exocrine acinar tissue of the pancreas. **(a)** The islets are clusters of cells smaller and lighter staining than cells of the surrounding tissue. X12.5. H&E.

(b) At higher magnification an islet's capillary system can be seen. Several arterioles enter each islet, branch into fenestrated capillaries (**C**) among the peripheral islet cells, then converge centrally before leaving the islet as efferent capillaries carrying blood to the acini surrounding the islet. This local vascular system allows specific islet hormones to help control secretion of other islet cells and the neighboring acini. X40. H&E.

(c) With H&E staining all cells of an islet appear similar, although slight differences in cell size and basophilia may be apparent. Capillaries (**C**) are also apparent. X55. H&E.

(d) An islet prepared with a modified aldehyde fuchsin stain shows that granules in the peripheral α cells are a deep brownish purple and the central β cells granules are brownish orange. Reticulin connective tissue of the islet capsule and along the capillaries stains green in this preparation. Immunohistochemistry with antibodies against the various islet polypeptide hormones allows definitive identification of each islet cell type. X300. Modified aldehyde fuchsin and light green.

(Figure 20-17d, with permission, from Dr Arthur A. Like, Department of Pathology, University of Massachusetts Medical School, Worcester.)

(e) The diagram shows the four major islet hormones and the cells secreting them: α cells making glucagon, β cells making insulin, δ cells making somatostatin, and PP cells making pancreatic polypeptide.

TABLE 20–4	Major cell types and hormones of pancreatic islets.			
Cell Type	Quantity (%)	Hormone Produced	Hormone Structure and Size	Hormone Function
α	~20	Glucagon	Polypeptide; 3500 Da	Acts on several tissues to make energy stored in glycogen and fat available through glycogenolysis and lipolysis; increases blood glucose content
β	~70	Insulin	Dimer of α and β chains with S-S bridges; 5700-6000 Da	Acts on several tissues to cause entry of glucose into cells and promotes decrease of blood glucose content
δ or D	5-10	Somatostatin	Polypeptide; 1650 Da	Inhibits release of other islet cell hormones through local paracrine action; inhibits release of GH and TSH in anterior pituitary and HCl secretion by gastric parietal cells
PP	Rare	Pancreatic polypeptide	Polypeptide; 4200 Da	Stimulates activity of gastric chief cells; inhibits bile secretion, pancreatic enzyme and bicarbonate secretion, and intestinal motility

A minor fourth cell type, more common in islets located within the head of the pancreas, are **PP cells**, which secrete **pancreatic polypeptide**. Table 20–4 summarizes the types, quantities, and main functions of the major pancreatic hormones. Pancreatic islets also normally contain a few enterochromaffin cells, like those of the digestive tract, which are also scattered in the pancreatic acini and ducts and which secrete other hormones affecting the digestive system.

Activity of α and β cells is regulated largely by blood glucose levels above or below the normal level of 70 mg/dL. Increased glucose levels stimulate β cells to release insulin and inhibit α cells from releasing glucagon; decreased glucose levels stimulate α cells to release glucagon. Opposing actions of these hormones help to precisely control blood glucose concentration, an important factor in homeostasis (see Table 20–4).

These hormones and somatostatin from the δ cells also act in a paracrine manner to affect hormone release within an islet as well as activity of the neighboring acinar cells. Sympathetic and parasympathetic nerve endings are closely associated with about 10% of α, β, and δ cells and can also function as part of the control system for insulin and glucagon secretion. Gap junctions transfer the autonomic neural stimulus to the other cells. Sympathetic fibers increase glucagon release and inhibit insulin release; parasympathetic fibers increase secretion of both glucagon and insulin.

> ## DIFFUSE NEUROENDOCRINE SYSTEM

The enterochromaffin cells scattered in both the islets and small ducts of the pancreas are similar to those of the digestive tract (see Chapter 15). Collectively these dispersed cells, as well as similar cells in the respiratory mucosa, make up the **diffuse neuroendocrine system** (**DNES**). Like the pancreatic islets, most of these cells are derived from endodermal cells of the embryonic gut or bronchial buds. These secretory cells are considered neuroendocrine because they produce many of the same polypeptides and neurotransmitter-like molecules, such as serotonin (5-hydroxytryptamine), also released by neurosecretory cells in the CNS. Several such cells, along with their hormones and major functions, are summarized in Table 15–1 with the digestive system. Most of these hormones are polypeptides and act in a paracrine manner, affecting primarily the activities of neighboring contractile cells and secretory cells (both exocrine and endocrine). Enteroendocrine cells of the stomach and small bowel are shown ultrastructurally in Figures 15–20, 15–24c, and 15–27.

Many cells of the DNES are stained by solutions of chromium salts and have therefore been called **enterochromaffin cells**, while those staining with silver nitrate are sometimes called **argentaffin cells**. DNES cells secreting serotonin or certain other amine derivatives demonstrate amine precursor uptake and decarboxylation and are often referred to acronymically as **APUD cells**. Such names are still widely used, but, as indicated in Table 15–1, they have been largely replaced by letter designations like those used for pancreatic islet cells. Whatever name is used, cells of the DNES are highly important due to their role in regulating motility and secretions of all types within the digestive system.

> ## THYROID GLAND

The thyroid gland, located anterior and inferior to the larynx, consists of two lobes united by an isthmus (Figure 20–18). It originates in early embryonic life from the foregut endoderm

FIGURE 20–18 Thyroid gland.

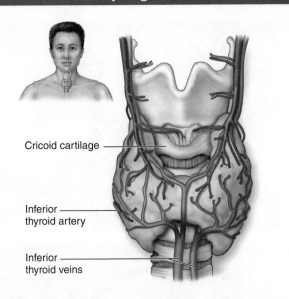

Cricoid cartilage

Inferior thyroid artery

Inferior thyroid veins

The thyroid is a highly vascular, butterfly-shaped gland surrounding the anterior surface of the trachea just below the larynx.

near the base of the developing tongue. It synthesizes the thyroid hormones **thyroxine** (tetra-iodothyronine or **T₄**) and **tri-iodothyronine** (**T₃**), which help control the basal metabolic rate in cells throughout the body, as well as the polypeptide hormone **calcitonin**.

The parenchyma of the thyroid is composed of millions of rounded epithelial **thyroid follicles** of variable diameter, each with simple epithelium and a central lumen densely filled with gelatinous acidophilic **colloid** (Figure 20–19). The thyroid is the only endocrine gland in which a large quantity of secretory product is stored. Moreover, storage is outside the cells, in the colloid of the follicle lumen, which is also unusual. There is sufficient hormone in follicles to supply the body for up to 3 months with no additional synthesis. Thyroid colloid contains the large glycoprotein **thyroglobulin** (660 kDa), the precursor for the active thyroid hormones.

The thyroid gland is covered by a fibrous capsule from which septa extend into the parenchyma, dividing it into lobules and carrying blood vessels, nerves, and lymphatics. Follicles are densely packed together, separated from one another only by sparse reticular connective tissue (Figure 20–19), although this stroma is very well vascularized with fenestrated capillaries for transfer of released hormone to the blood.

The follicular cells, or **thyrocytes**, range in shape from squamous to low columnar (Figure 20–19), their size and other features varying with their activity that is controlled by thyroid-stimulating hormone (TSH) from the anterior pituitary. Active glands have more follicles of low columnar epithelium; glands with mostly squamous follicular cells are hypoactive.

Thyrocytes have apical junctional complexes and rest on a basal lamina (Figure 20–20). The cells exhibit organelles indicating active protein synthesis and secretion, as well as phagocytosis and digestion. The nucleus is generally round and central. Basally the cells are rich in rough ER and apically, facing the follicular lumen, are Golgi complexes, secretory granules, numerous phagosomes and lysosomes, and microvilli.

Another endocrine cell type, the **parafollicular cell**, or **C cell**, is also found inside the basal lamina of the follicular epithelium or as isolated clusters between follicles (Figure 20–20). Derived from the neural crest, parafollicular cells are usually somewhat larger than follicular cells and stain less intensely. They have a smaller amount of rough ER, large Golgi complexes, and numerous small (100-180 nm in diameter) granules containing calcitonin (Figure 20–20). Secretion of calcitonin is triggered by elevated blood Ca²⁺ levels and it inhibits osteoclast activity, but this function in humans is less important than the roles of parathyroid hormone and vitamin D in the regulation of normal calcium homeostasis.

⟩⟩ MEDICAL APPLICATION

Chronic dietary iodine deficiencies inhibit thyroid hormone production, causing thyrotropic cells of the anterior pituitary gland to produce excess TSH. This leads to excessive growth of thyroid follicles and enlargement of the thyroid gland, a condition known as **goiter**.

Production of Thyroid Hormone & Its Control

Production, storage, and release of thyroid hormones involve an unusual, multistage process in the thyrocytes, with both an exocrine phase and an endocrine phase. Both phases are promoted by TSH and occur in the same cell, as summarized in Figure 20–21. The major activities of this process include the following:

1. The **production of thyroglobulin**, which is similar to that in other glycoprotein-exporting cells, with synthesis in the rough ER and glycosylation in the Golgi apparatus. Thyroglobulin has no hormonal activity itself but contains 140 tyrosyl residues critical for thyroid hormone synthesis. The glycoprotein is released as an exocrine product from apical vesicles of thyrocytes into the follicular lumen.

2. The **uptake of iodide** from blood by Na/I symporters (NIS) in the thyrocytes' basolateral cell membranes, which allows for 30-fold concentration of dietary iodide in thyroid tissue relative to plasma. Decreased levels of circulating iodide trigger synthesis of NIS, increasing iodide uptake and compensating for the lower plasma concentration. An apical iodide/chloride transporter (also called **pendrin**) pumps I⁻ from thyrocytes into the colloid.

FIGURE **20–19** Thyroid follicular cells and parafollicular cells.

(a) A low-power micrograph of thyroid gland shows the thin capsule (**C**), from which septa (**S**) with the larger blood vessels, lymphatics, and nerves enter the gland. The parenchyma of the organ is distinctive, consisting of colloid-filled epithelial follicles of many sizes. The lumen of each follicle is filled with a lightly staining colloid of a large gelatinous protein called **thyroglobulin**. X12. H&E.

(b) The lumen (**L**) of each follicle is surrounded by a simple epithelium of thyrocytes in which the cell height ranges from squamous to low columnar. Also present are large pale-staining parafollicular or C cells (**C**) that secrete calcitonin, a polypeptide involved with calcium metabolism. X200. H&E.

(c-e) C cells may be part of the follicular epithelium or present singly or in groups outside of follicles. Thyrocytes (**T**) can usually be distinguished from parafollicular C cells (**C**) by their smaller size and darker staining properties. Unlike thyrocytes, C cells seldom vary in their size or pale staining characteristics. C cells are somewhat easier to locate in or between small follicles. c and d: X400. H&E; e: X400. Mallory trichrome.

3. **Iodination of tyrosyl residues** in thyroglobulin with either one or two atoms occurs in the colloid after oxidation of iodide to iodine by membrane-bound thyroid peroxidase on the microvilli surfaces of thyrocytes.

4. **Formation of T_3 and T_4** (also called thyroxine) occurs as two iodinated tyrosines, still part of colloidal thyroglobulin, which are covalently conjugated in coupling reactions.

5. **Endocytosis of iodinated thyroglobulin** by the thyrocytes involves both fluid-phase pinocytosis and receptor-mediated endocytosis. The endocytic vesicles fuse with lysosomes, and the thyroglobulin is thoroughly degraded by lysosomal proteases, freeing active thyroid hormone as both T_3 and T_4.

6. **Secretion of T_4 and T_3** at the basolateral domains of thyrocytes occurs in an endocrine manner: both molecules are immediately taken up by capillaries.

Nearly all of both thyroid hormones are carried in blood tightly bound to thyroxine-binding globulin or albumen. T_4 is the more abundant compound, constituting 90% of the circulating thyroid hormone. Both molecules bind the same intracellular receptors of target cells, but T_3 is 2- to 10-fold more active than T_4. The half-life of T_3 is 1.5 days in comparison with a week for T_4. Both thyroid hormones increase the number and size of mitochondria and stimulate mitochondrial protein synthesis, helping to enhance metabolic activity.

(a) TEM of the follicular epithelium shows pseudopodia and microvilli extending from the follicular thyrocytes (**T**) into the colloid of the lumen (**L**). The cells have apical junctional complexes, much RER, well-developed Golgi complexes, and many lysosomes. Inside the basement membrane (**BM**) of the follicle, but often not contacting the colloid in the lumen, are occasional C cells (**C**). To the left and right of the two C cells

seen here are capillaries intimately associated with the follicular cells, but outside the basement membrane. X2000.

(b) A TEM of a C cell, with its large Golgi apparatus (**G**), extensive RER, and cytoplasm filled with small secretory granules containing calcitonin. X5000.

The major regulator of the anatomic and functional state of thyroid follicles is TSH (thyrotropin) from the anterior pituitary (see Figure 20–8). With TSH receptors abundant on the basal cell membrane of thyrocytes, this tropic hormone increases cell height in the follicular epithelium and stimulates all stages of thyroid hormone production and release. Thyroid hormones inhibit the release of TSH, maintaining levels of circulating T_4 and T_3 within the normal range (see Figure 20–10). Secretion of TSH in the pituitary is also increased by exposure to cold and decreased by heat and stressful stimuli.

>> **MEDICAL APPLICATION**

Graves disease is an autoimmune disorder in which antibodies produce chronic stimulation of the follicular cells and release of thyroid hormones (**hyperthyroidism**), which causes a hypermetabolic state marked by weight loss, nervousness, sweating, heat intolerance, and other features. **Hypothyroidism**, with reduced thyroid hormone levels, can be caused by local inflammation (**thyroiditis**) or inadequate secretion of TSH by the anterior pituitary gland

and is often manifested by tiredness, weight gain, intolerance of cold, and decreased ability to concentrate.

> **PARATHYROID GLANDS**

The **parathyroid glands** are four small ovoid masses—each 3 × 6 mm—with a total weight of about 0.4 g. They are located on the back of the thyroid gland, usually embedded in the larger gland's capsule (Figure 20–22). The microvasculature of each arises from the inferior thyroid arteries. Each parathyroid gland is contained within a thin capsule from which septa extend into the gland. A sparse reticular stroma supports dense elongated clusters of secretory cells.

The parathyroid glands are derived from the embryonic pharyngeal pouches—the superior glands from the fourth pouch and the inferior glands from the third pouch. Their migration to the developing thyroid gland is sometimes misdirected so that the number and locations of the glands are somewhat variable. Up to 10% of individuals may have parathyroid tissue attached to the thymus, which originates from the same pharyngeal pouches.

FIGURE **20–21** Thyrocyte activities in thyroid hormone synthesis.

The diagram shows the multistep process by which thyroid hormones are produced via the stored thyroglobulin intermediate. In an exocrine phase of the process, the glycoprotein **thyroglobulin** is made and secreted into the follicular lumen and iodide is pumped across the cells into the lumen. In the lumen **tyrosine residues** of thyroglobulin are iodinated, to form monoiodotyrosine (MIT) or diiodotyrosine (DIT), and then covalently coupled to form T_3 and T_4 still within the glycoprotein. The iodinated thyroglobulin is then endocytosed by thyrocytes and degraded by lysosomes, releasing **free active T_3 and T_4** to the adjacent capillaries in an endocrine manner. Detailed steps are given in the text. Both phases are promoted by TSH and may occur simultaneously in the same cell.

The endocrine cells of the parathyroid glands, called **principal (chief) cells**, are small polygonal cells with round nuclei and pale-staining, slightly acidophilic cytoplasm (Figure 20–23). Irregularly shaped cytoplasmic granules contain the polypeptide **parathyroid hormone (PTH)**, an important regulator of blood calcium levels. PTH has three major targets:

- Osteoblasts respond to PTH by producing an osteoclast-stimulating factor that increases the number and activity of osteoclasts. The resulting resorption of the calcified bone matrix and release of Ca^{2+} increase the concentration of circulating Ca^{2+}, which suppresses PTH production. The effect of PTH on blood levels of Ca^{2+} is thus opposite to that of calcitonin.

- In the distal convoluted tubules of the renal cortex, PTH stimulates Ca^{2+} reabsorption (and inhibits phosphate reabsorption in the proximal tubules).

- PTH also indirectly increases the Ca^{2+} absorption in the small intestine by stimulating vitamin D activation.

FIGURE 20–22 Parathyroid glands.

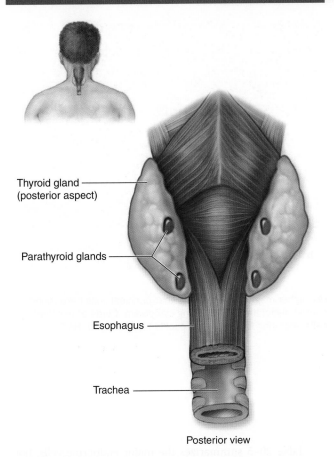

Thyroid gland
(posterior aspect)

Parathyroid glands

Esophagus

Trachea

Posterior view

The parathyroid glands are four small nodules normally embedded in the capsule on the posterior surface of the thyroid gland.

produced in **hyperparathyroidism** stimulates osteoclast number and activity, leading to increased levels of blood calcium that can be deposited pathologically in cartilage, arteries, or the kidneys.

› PINEAL GLAND

The **pineal gland**, also known as the **epiphysis cerebri**, regulates the daily rhythms of bodily activities. A small, pine cone-shaped organ, approximately 5-8 mm by 3-5 mm, the pineal gland develops from neuroectoderm in the posterior wall of the third ventricle and remains attached to the brain by a short stalk. The pineal gland is covered by connective tissue of the pia mater, from which septa containing small blood vessels emerge and subdivide variously sized lobules.

Prominent and abundant secretory cells called **pinealocytes** have slightly basophilic cytoplasm and irregular euchromatic nuclei (Figure 20–24). Ultrastructurally pinealocytes are seen to have secretory vesicles, many mitochondria, and long cytoplasmic processes extending to the vascularized septa, where they end in dilatations near capillaries, indicating an endocrine function. These cells produce **melatonin**, a low-molecular-weight tryptophan derivative. Unmyelinated sympathetic nerve fibers enter the pineal gland and end among pinealocytes, with some forming synapses.

Melatonin release from pinealocytes is promoted by darkness and inhibited by daylight. The resulting diurnal fluctuation in blood melatonin levels induces rhythmic changes in the activity of the hypothalamus, pituitary gland, and other endocrine tissues that characterize the circadian (24 hours, day/night) rhythm of physiological functions and behaviors. In humans and other mammals, the cycle of light and darkness is detected within the retinas and transmitted to the pineal via the retinohypothalamic tract, the suprachiasmatic nucleus, and the tracts of sympathetic fibers entering the pineal. The pineal gland acts, therefore, as a neuroendocrine transducer, converting sensory input regarding light and darkness into variations in many hormonal functions.

The pineal gland also has interstitial glial cells that are modified **astrocytes**, staining positively for glial fibrillary acidic protein, which represent about 5% of the cells. These have elongated nuclei more heavily stained than those of pinealocytes and are usually found in perivascular areas and between the groups of pinealocytes.

A characteristic feature of the pineal gland is the presence of variously sized concretions of calcium and magnesium salts called **corpora arenacea**, or brain sand, which form as extracellular protein deposits become mineralized. Such concretions appear during childhood and gradually increase in number and size with age, with no apparent effect on the gland's function.

With increasing age, many secretory cells are replaced with adipocytes, which may constitute more than 50% of the gland in older people.

Much smaller populations of **oxyphil cells**, often clustered, are sometimes also present in parathyroid glands, more commonly in older individuals. These are much larger than the principal cells and are characterized by very acidophilic cytoplasm filled with abnormally shaped mitochondria. Some oxyphil cells show low levels of PTH synthesis, suggesting that these cells are transitional derivatives of principal cells.

›› MEDICAL APPLICATION

In **hypoparathyroidism**, diminished secretion of PTH can cause bones to become more mineralized and denser and striated muscle to exhibit abnormal contractions due to inadequate calcium ion concentrations. Excessive PTH

FIGURE **20–23** Parathyroid principal cells.

(a) A small lobe of parathyroid gland, surrounded by connective tissue septa (**S**), shows mainly densely packed cords of small principal cells (**P**). Older parathyroid glands show increasing numbers of much larger and acidophilic nonfunctional oxyphil cells (**O**) that may occur singly or in clumps of varying sizes. X60. H&E.

(b) Higher magnification shows that principal cells have round central nuclei and pale-staining cytoplasm. Cords of principal cells secreting PTH surround capillaries (**C**). X200. H&E.

>> MEDICAL APPLICATION

Densely calcified corpora arenacea can be used as landmarks for the midline location of the pineal gland in a various **radiological examinations** of the brain. **Tumors** originating from pinealocytes are very rare, but they can be either benign or highly malignant.

Table 20–5 summarizes the major endocrine cells, hormones, and functions of the adrenal gland, pancreatic islets, thyroid, parathyroid, and pineal glands.

Endocrine Glands SUMMARY OF KEY POINTS

Pituitary Gland

- The **pituitary gland** has two major parts: the **posterior** part called the **pars nervosa** develops as a downgrowth of the developing brain and is attached in the **hypothalamus** by the **infundibulum**.
- The anterior pituitary includes the large **pars distalis**, the **pars tuberalis** that surrounds the infundibulum, and the thin **pars intermedia** adjacent to the pars nervosa.
- Blood vessels of the **hypothalamic hypophyseal portal system** are important in carrying peptide factors from hypothalamic neurons to cells of the anterior pituitary where they control cell secretion.
- This portal system includes a **primary capillary plexus** in the infundibulum and lower hypothalamus and a **secondary plexus** in the pars distalis, connected by **portal veins** and draining to the **hypophyseal vein.**

- Endocrine cells of the anterior pituitary can be called **acidophils, basophils,** or **chromophobes** based on their general staining properties; the latter lack secretory granules and stain poorly.
- Acidophils and basophils can be identified as to which pituitary hormone they produce using **immunohistochemistry** and antibodies against specific hormones.
  - Acidophils are primarily **somatotrophs** producing **somatotropin (growth hormone)**, or **lactotrophs** (or mammotrophs) producing **prolactin (PRL)**.
  - Basophils include **gonadotrophs** producing **follicle-stimulating hormone (FSH)** and **luteinizing hormone (LH)** and **thyrotrophs** making **thyroid-stimulating hormone (TSH)**.
  - A third type of basophil is the corticotroph, synthesizing **proopiomelanocortin (POMC)** that is cleaved by proteases to make

FIGURE **20–24** Pineal gland.

(a) The micrograph shows a group of pinealocytes surrounded by septa (**S**) containing venules (**V**) and capillaries (arrows). Also seen is an extracellular mineral deposit called a **corpus arenaceum** (**CA**) of unknown physiologic significance but an excellent marker for the pineal. X200. H&E.

(b) At higher magnification the numerous large pinealocytes (**P**) with euchromatic nuclei can be compared to much fewer astrocytes (**A**) that have darker, more elongated nuclei and are located mainly within septa and near small blood vessels (**V**). Capillaries (arrow) are not nearly as numerous as in other

endocrine glands. At the lower left is a port of a very large corpus arenaceum (**CA**), the calcified structures also known as **brain sand**. Along the septa run unmyelinated tracts of sympathetic fibers, associated indirectly with photoreceptive neurons in the retinas and running to the pinealocytes to stimulate melatonin release in periods of darkness. Levels of circulating melatonin are one factor determining the diurnal rhythms of hormone release and physiologic activities throughout the body. X400. H&E.

adrenocorticotropic hormone (**ACTH**) and **β-lipotropic hormone** (**LPH**).
- The **hypothalamic hypophyseal tract** includes bundles of nerve axons that run from **supraoptic nucleus** (**SON**) and **paraventricular nucleus** (**PVN**) in the hypothalamus to the posterior pituitary.
- Hypothalamic neurons in the SON synthesize **vasopressin/antidiuretic hormone** (**ADH**) and those of the PVN synthesize oxytocin, both of which are stored an axonal dilations called **Herring bodies** before release to capillaries in the posterior pituitary.

Adrenal Glands
- The **adrenal cortex** of each adrenal gland consists of three concentric zones, all histologically distinct but with cells producing steroid hormones and all drained by the same system of capillaries.
  - The most superficial **zona glomerulosa** has round clusters of cells producing **mineralocorticoids** such as **aldosterone** regulating electrolyte levels.

- The wider, middle **zona fasciculata** has elongated strands of cells producing **glucocorticoids** such as **cortisol**, which regulates several aspects of carbohydrate metabolism.
- The innermost zona reticularis has a network of cells making the **weak androgen dehydroepiandrosterone** (**DHEA**) that is converted to testosterone in men and women.
- The **adrenal medulla** contains neural crest-derived **chromaffin cells** synthesizing either **epinephrine** or **norepinephrine** that regulate the stress response.

Pancreatic Islets
- **Pancreatic islets of Langerhans** are small clusters of pale cells embedded within the exocrine tissue; they have primarily **β cells making insulin**, **α cell** (**glucagon**), and **δ cells** (**somatostatin**).

TABLE 20–5	Cells, important hormones, and functions of other major endocrine organs.		
Gland	**Endocrine Cells**	**Major Hormones**	**Major Functions**
Adrenal glands: Cortex	Cells of zona glomerulosa	Mineralocorticoids	Stimulate renal reabsorption of water and Na$^+$ and secretion of K$^+$ to maintain salt and water balance
	Cells of zona fasciculata	Glucocorticoids	Influence carbohydrate metabolism; suppress immune cell activities
	Cells of zona reticularis	Weak androgens	Precursors for testosterone or estrogen
Adrenal glands: Medulla	Chromaffin cells	Epinephrine	Increases heart rate and constricts vessels
		Norepinephrine	Dilates vessels and increases glucose release
Pancreatic islets	α Cells	Glucagon	Raises blood glucose levels
	β Cells	Insulin	Lowers blood glucose levels
	δ Cells	Somatostatin	Inhibits secretion of insulin, glucagon, and somatotropin
	PP cells	Pancreatic polypeptide	Inhibits secretion of pancreatic enzymes and HCO$_3^-$
Thyroid glands	Follicular cells	Thyroid hormones (T$_3$ and T$_4$)	Increase metabolic rate
	Parafollicular or C cells	Calcitonin	Lowers blood Ca^{2+} levels by inhibiting osteoclast activity
Parathyroid glands	Chief cells	Parathyroid hormone (PTH)	Raises blood Ca^{2+} levels by stimulating osteoclast activity
Pineal gland	Pinealocytes	Melatonin	Regulates circadian rhythms

Thyroid Gland

- The **thyroid gland** consists mainly of spherical **follicles** composed of simple epithelium of **thyrocytes** surrounding a lumen with **thyroglobulin**.
- **Thyroglobulin** is a large glycoprotein in which tyrosine residues are **iodinated** as precursors of the thyroid hormones **thyroxine** and **tri-iodothyronine**, which are released when the precursor is degraded.
- Thyroid follicles also contain a few smaller and paler cells called **parafollicular cells**, or **C cells**, which produce the polypeptide hormone **calcitonin**.

Parathyroid Glands

- On the posterior side of the thyroid glands are four small **parathyroid glands**, each consisting primarily of **principal cells** that secrete **parathyroid hormone** (**PTH**) that raises blood Ca^{2+} levels.

Pineal Gland

- The **pineal gland** develops from embryonic neuroectoderm, remains attached to the brain, and contains modified neurons called **pinealocytes** that secrete the amine **melatonin**.
- Pineal landmarks are the concretions called **corpora amylacea** (brain sand); neural connections from the retina to **pinealocytes** allow diurnal secretion of melatonin and rhythms in physiological activities.

21 The Male Reproductive System

The male reproductive system consists of the testes, genital ducts, accessory glands, and penis (Figure 21–1). Testes produce sperm but also contain endocrine cells secreting hormones such as testosterone, which drives male reproductive physiology. Testosterone is important for spermatogenesis, sexual differentiation during embryonic and fetal development, and control of gonadotropin secretion in the pituitary. A metabolite of testosterone, dihydrotestosterone, also begins to act on many tissues during puberty (eg, male accessory glands and hair follicles).

The genital ducts and accessory glands produce secretions required for sperm activity and contract to propel spermatozoa and the secretions from the penile urethra. These secretions provide nutrients for spermatozoa while they are confined to the male reproductive tract. Spermatozoa and the secretions of the accessory glands make up the **semen** (L, seed), which is introduced into the female reproductive tract by the penis.

› TESTES

Each **testis** (or testicle) is surrounded by a dense connective tissue capsule, the **tunica albuginea**, which thickens on the posterior side to form the **mediastinum testis**. From this fibrous region, septa penetrate the organ and divide it into about 250 pyramidal compartments or **testicular lobules** (Figures 21–2 and 21–3). Each lobule contains sparse connective tissue with endocrine **interstitial cells** (or **Leydig cells**) secreting testosterone, and one to four highly convoluted **seminiferous tubules** in which sperm production occurs.

The testes develop retroperitoneally in the dorsal wall of the embryonic abdominal cavity and are moved during fetal development to become suspended in the two halves of the scrotal sac, or scrotum, at the ends of the spermatic cords (Figure 21–2). During migration from the abdominal cavity, each testis carries with it a serous sac, the **tunica vaginalis**, derived from the peritoneum. This tunic consists of an outer parietal layer lining the scrotum and an inner visceral layer, covering the tunica albuginea on the anterior and lateral sides of the testis (Figure 21–2).

Having evolved in cold-blooded animals, certain molecular events in the process of sperm formation cannot occur at the core body temperature of 37°C. A permissive temperature of about 34°C is maintained in the scrotal sac by various mechanisms. Each testicular artery is surrounded by a rich **pampiniform venous plexus** containing cooler blood from the testis, which draws heat from the arterial blood by a countercurrent heat-exchange system. Evaporation of sweat from the scrotum also contributes to heat loss. Relaxation or contraction of the thin dartos muscle of the scrotum and the cremaster muscles of the spermatic cords move the testes away from or closer to the body, respectively, allowing further control on testicular temperature.

›› MEDICAL APPLICATION

An excessive accumulation of serous fluid in one or both sides of the scrotal sac, termed a **hydrocele**, is the most common cause of scrotal swelling and a condition easily corrected surgically.

Cryptorchidism (Gr. *kryptos*, hidden + *orchis*, testis), the failure of one or both testes to descend from the abdomen, occurs in about 4% of male neonates, but in most of these individuals the testes move to the scrotum during the first year. Bilateral cryptorchidism causes infertility if not surgically corrected by 2 to 3 years of age.

FIGURE **21–1** The male reproductive system.

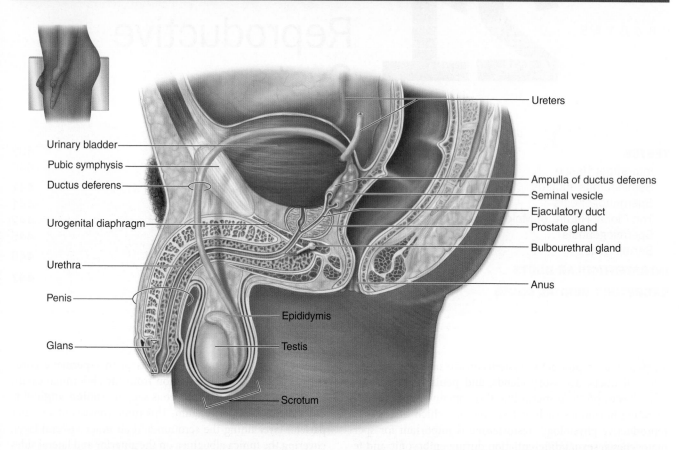

Ureters

Urinary bladder

Pubic symphysis

Ductus deferens

Urogenital diaphragm

Urethra

Penis

Glans

Epididymis

Testis

Scrotum

Ampulla of ductus deferens

Seminal vesicle

Ejaculatory duct

Prostate gland

Bulbourethral gland

Anus

The diagram shows the locations and relationships of the testes, epididymis, glands, and the ductus deferens running from the scrotum to the urethra. The ductus deferens is located along the anterior and superior sides of the bladder as a result of the testes descending into the scrotum from the abdominal cavity during fetal development.

Interstitial Tissue

The interstitial tissue of the testis between the seminiferous tubules consists of sparse connective tissue containing fibroblasts, lymphatics, and blood vessels including fenestrated capillaries. During puberty **interstitial cells**, or **Leydig cells**, develop as large round or polygonal cells with central nuclei and eosinophilic cytoplasm rich in small lipid droplets (Figures 21–2b and 21–4). These cells produce the steroid hormone **testosterone**, which promotes development of the secondary male sex characteristics. Testosterone is synthesized by enzymes present in the smooth ER and mitochondria similar to the system in adrenal cortical cells.

Testosterone secretion by interstitial cells is triggered by the pituitary gonadotropin, **luteinizing hormone** (**LH**), which is also called **interstitial cell stimulating hormone** (**ICSH**). Testosterone synthesis thus begins at puberty, when the hypothalamus begins producing gonadotropin-releasing hormone. In the late embryonic testes gonadotropin from the placenta stimulates interstitial cells to synthesize the testosterone needed for development of the ducts and glands of the male reproductive system. These fetal interstitial cells are very active during the third and fourth months of pregnancy, then regress and become quiescent cells resembling fibroblasts until puberty when they resume testosterone synthesis in response to the pituitary gonadotropin.

>> **MEDICAL APPLICATION**

Both **interstitial cell tumors** and **Sertoli cell tumors** are rare. Most (95%) **testicular cancer** involves **germ cell tumors**, which only appear after puberty and are much more likely to develop in men with untreated cryptorchidism.

Seminiferous Tubules

Sperm are produced in the seminiferous tubules at a rate of about 2×10^8 per day in the young adult. Each testis has from 250 to 1000 such tubules in its lobules, and each tubule measures 150 to 250 μm in diameter and 30 to 70 cm in length.

FIGURE **21–2** Testes and seminiferous tubules.

The anatomy of a testis is shown. **(a)** The diagram shows a partially cutaway sagittal section of the testis. **(b)** A seminiferous tubule cross section shows spermatogonia (**SG**) near the periphery, near nuclei of Sertoli cells (**SC**), primary spermatocytes (**PS**), and late spermatids (**LS**) near the lumen, with interstitial cells (**IC**) in the surrounding connective tissue. X400. H&E.

The combined length of the tubules of one testis totals about 250 m. Each tubule is actually a loop linked by a very short, narrower segment, the **straight tubule**, to the **rete testis**, a labyrinth of epithelium-lined channels embedded in the mediastinum testis (see Figures 21–2a and 21–3). About 10-20 **efferent ductules** connect the rete testis to the head of the epididymis (Figure 21–2a).

Each seminiferous tubule is lined with a complex, specialized stratified epithelium called **germinal** or **spermatogenic epithelium** (Figure 21–2b). The basement membrane of this epithelium is covered by fibrous connective tissue, with an innermost layer containing flattened, smooth muscle-like **myoid cells** (Figure 21–2b), which allow weak contractions of the tubule. The germinal epithelium consists of two types of cells:

- Large nondividing **Sertoli cells** (Figure 21–4c,d), which physically and metabolically support developing sperm cell precursors.
- Dividing cells of the **spermatogenic lineage** (Figure 21–5a).

The cells of the spermatogenic lineage comprise four to eight concentric cell layers and produce the cells that become sperm. As shown in Figure 21–5, **spermatogenesis** is the first part of sperm production, including stem cell mitosis and meiosis, and **spermiogenesis** is the final differentiation process occurring in the haploid male germ cells.

Spermatogenesis

Spermatogenesis begins at puberty with proliferation of stem and progenitor cells called **spermatogonia** (Gr. *sperma* + *gone*, generation), small round cells about 12 μm in diameter. These cells occupy a basal niche in the epithelial wall of the tubules, next to the basement membrane and closely associated with Sertoli cell surfaces (Figures 21–5, 21–6 and 21–7).

Different stages of spermatogonia development can be recognized by subtle changes in shape and staining properties of their nuclei. Spermatogonia with dark, ovoid nuclei act as stem cells, dividing infrequently and giving rise both to new stem cells and to cells with more pale-staining, ovoid nuclei that divide more rapidly as transit amplifying (progenitor) cells (Figure 21–7).

FIGURE **21–3** Lobules converging at rete testis.

The dense capsule of the testis, the tunica albuginea, thickens on the posterior side as the mediastinum (**M**) testis, from which many thin septa (**S**) subdivide the organ into about 250 lobules. Each lobule contains one to four convoluted seminiferous tubules (**ST**) in a sparse connective tissue interstitium.

Each tubule is a loop attached by means of a short straight tubule to the rete testis (**RT**), a maze of channels embedded in the mediastinum testis. From the rete testis the sperm move into the epididymis. X60. H&E.

These **type A spermatogonia** each undergo several unique clonal divisions that leave most of the cells interconnected as a syncytium. These become **type B spermatogonia**, which have more spherical and pale nuclei.

Each type B spermatogonium then undergoes a final mitotic division to produce two cells that grow in size and become **primary spermatocytes**, which are spherical cells with euchromatic nuclei (Figures 21–6 and 21–7). Primary spermatocytes replicate their DNA, so each chromosome consists of duplicate chromatids, and enter meiosis, during which homologous chromosomes come together in synapsis, DNA recombination occurs, and two rapid cell divisions produce haploid cells (see Chapter 3).

The primary spermatocyte has 46 (44 + XY) chromosomes, the diploid number, and a DNA content of 4N. (The letter *N* denotes either the haploid number of chromosomes, 23 in humans, or the amount of DNA in this set.) Soon after their formation, these cells enter the first meiotic prophase that lasts about 3 weeks. Most spermatocytes seen in sections of testis are in this phase of meiosis. The primary spermatocytes are the largest cells of the spermatogenic lineage and are characterized by the presence of partially condensed chromosomes in various stages of synapsis and recombination (Figure 21–6).

Homologous chromosomes separate in the first meiotic division, which produces smaller cells called **secondary spermatocytes** (Figures 21–5a and 21–7) with only 23 chromosomes (22 + X or 22 + Y), but each still consists of two chromatids so the amount of DNA is 2N (see Chapter 3). Secondary spermatocytes are rare in testis sections because they are very short-lived cells that remain in interphase only briefly and quickly undergo the second meiotic division.

Division of each secondary spermatocyte separates the chromatids of each chromosome and produces two haploid cells called **spermatids** each of which contains 23 chromosomes (Figures 21–5a, 21–6, and 21–7). Because no S phase (DNA replication) occurs between the first and second meiotic divisions, the amount of DNA per cell is reduced by half when the chromatids separate and the cells formed are haploid

FIGURE **21–4** Seminiferous tubule and interstitial cells.

(a) Seminiferous tubules are surrounded by connective tissue containing many large interstitial cells (**IC**) that secrete androgens. The tubule wall is a unique epithelium composed of columnar Sertoli cells (**SC**), with oval or pyramidal nuclei and distinct nucleoli, and dividing spermatogenic stem cells with round nuclei (**arrow**). Also numerous are flattened peritubular myoid cells (**M**) whose contractions help move fluid in the tubules. X400. H&E.

(b) A plastic section shows lipid droplets filling the cytoplasm of the clumped interstitial cells (**IC**), or Leydig cells, in the connective tissue (**CT**) between tubules. Such cytoplasm is typical of steroid-secreting endocrine cells. The epithelium of a nearby seminiferous tubule is immediately surrounded by myoid cells (**M**). X400. PT.

(c) Immunohistochemistry of seminiferous tubule wall shows the full height of Sertoli cells (**S**) and the dendritic nature of their cytoplasm. Spermatogenic cells are intimately associated with Sertoli cell surfaces. 400X.

(d) Lower magnification of the same preparation shows the distribution and density of Sertoli cells (**S**) in the seminiferous tubules. 100X. Both with fluorescent antibody against sulfated glycoprotein-1 (prosaposin).

(*Figure 21–4c, d used, with permission, of Dr Richard Sharpe, Medical Research Council/University of Edinburgh Centre for Reproductive Health, UK.*)

FIGURE **21–5** Spermatogenesis and spermiogenesis.

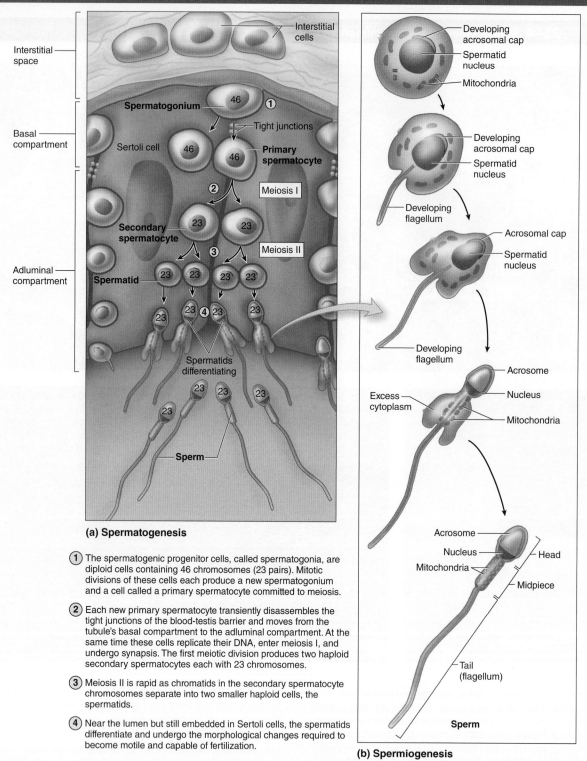

(a) Spermatogenesis

① The spermatogenic progenitor cells, called spermatogonia, are diploid cells containing 46 chromosomes (23 pairs). Mitotic divisions of these cells each produce a new spermatogonium and a cell called a primary spermatocyte committed to meiosis.

② Each new primary spermatocyte transiently disassembles the tight junctions of the blood-testis barrier and moves from the tubule's basal compartment to the adluminal compartment. At the same time these cells replicate their DNA, enter meiosis I, and undergo synapsis. The first meiotic division produces two haploid secondary spermatocytes each with 23 chromosomes.

③ Meiosis II is rapid as chromatids in the secondary spermatocyte chromosomes separate into two smaller haploid cells, the spermatids.

④ Near the lumen but still embedded in Sertoli cells, the spermatids differentiate and undergo the morphological changes required to become motile and capable of fertilization.

(b) Spermiogenesis

(a) The diagram shows two large, columnar Sertoli cells with their surfaces binding many germ cells in various stages of spermatogenesis. Near the basement membrane are **spermatogonia,** which divide by mitosis to produce both more spermatogonia and also **primary spermatocytes** that undergo meiosis to produce haploid spermatids that differentiate as sperm. Newly formed spermatocytes temporarily disassemble the tight junctions between Sertoli cells that act as the "blood-testis barrier" in order to move from the **basal compartment** to the **adluminal compartment** of the tubule.

(b) Spermiogenesis is the process of cell differentiation by which spermatids become sperm. The major changes that occur during spermiogenesis are shown here. These involve flattening of the nucleus, formation of an **acrosome** that resembles a large lysosome, growth of a **flagellum** (tail) from the basal body, reorganization of the mitochondria in the **midpiece** region, and shedding of unneeded cytoplasm.

FIGURE **21–6** Seminiferous tubules: Sertoli cells and spermatogenesis.

(**a, b**) In these cross sections of seminiferous tubules, most of their cell types can be seen. Outside the tubules are myoid cells (**M**) and fibroblasts (**F**). Inside near the basement membrane are many prominent spermatogonia (**SG**), small cells that divide mitotically but give rise to a population that enters meiosis. The primary spermatocytes (**PS**) remain for 3 weeks in prophase of the first meiotic division during which recombination occurs. Primary spermatocytes are the largest spermatogenic cells and are usually abundant at all levels between the basement membrane and the lumen. Each divides to form

two secondary spermatocytes, which are rarely seen because they undergo the second meiotic division almost immediately to form two haploid spermatids. Newly formed round, early spermatids (**ES**) differentiate and lose volume in becoming late spermatids (**LS**) and finally highly specialized sperm cells. All stages of spermatogenesis and spermiogenesis occur with the cells intimately associated with the surfaces of adjacent Sertoli cells (**SC**) that perform several supportive functions. Both X750. H&E.

(1N). With fertilization, a haploid ovum and sperm produced by meiosis unite and the normal diploid chromosome number is restored.

The Clonal Nature of Male Germ Cells

The stem cells produced by mitotic divisions of spermatogonia remain as separate cells. However, all subsequent divisions of the daughter cells that become transit amplifying progenitor cells have incomplete cytokinesis after telophase and the cells

remain attached to one another by **intercellular bridges** of cytoplasm (Figure 21–7). These allow free cytoplasmic communication among the cells during their remaining mitotic and meiotic divisions. Although some cells degenerate without completing spermatogenesis and some cells may separate, clones of approximately a hundred cells may remain linked through meiosis. The complete significance of this **spermatogenic syncytium** is not clear, but the cytoplasmic bridges allow the haploid cells to be supplied with products of the complete diploid genome, including proteins and RNA encoded by genes

> # FIGURE **21–7** Clonal nature of spermatogenesis.

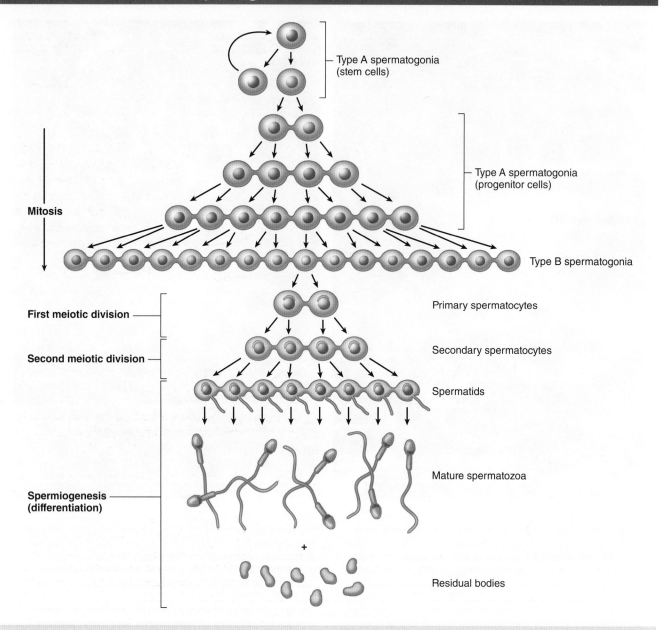

A subpopulation called **type A spermatogonia** act as stem cells, dividing to produce new stem cells and other type A spermatogonia that undergo transit amplification as progenitor cells. Mitosis in these cells occurs with incomplete cytokinesis, leaving the cytoplasm of most or all of these cells connected by cytoplasmic bridges. Type A spermatogonia divide mitotically two or three more times, then differentiate as **type B spermatogonia** that undergo a final round of mitosis to form the cells that then enter meiosis and become **primary**

spermatocytes (only two are shown), still interconnected. The intercellular bridges persist during the **first and second meiotic divisions**, but they are lost as the haploid **spermatids** differentiate into **sperm** (spermiogenesis) and shed excess cytoplasm as **residual bodies**. The interconnections of the cells allow free cytoplasmic communication among the cells and help coordinate their progress through meiosis and spermiogenesis.

on the X or Y chromosome missing in their haploid nuclei. The germ cells finally become separated from one another during differentiation (Figure 21–7).

The cellular events and changes between the final mitoses of spermatogonia and the formation of spermatids take

about 2 months. The spermatogenic cells are not randomly distributed in the spermatogenic epithelium. Cells at different stages of development are typically grouped together along the tubule, with the intercellular bridges helping to coordinate their divisions and differentiation.

Spermiogenesis

Spermiogenesis, the final phase of sperm production, is the temperature-sensitive process by which spermatids differentiate into spermatozoa, which are highly specialized to deliver male DNA to the ovum. No cell division occurs during this process, and as with spermatogenesis the cells involved remain associated with Sertoli cells.

The haploid spermatids are small (7-8 μm in diameter) cells near the lumen of the seminiferous tubules (Figures 21–5a and 21–6b). Spermiogenesis includes formation of the **acrosome** (Gr. *akron*, extremity + *soma*, body), condensation and elongation of the nucleus, development of the **flagellum** (L, whip), and the loss of much of the cytoplasm. The end result is the mature spermatozoon, which is released from the Sertoli cell surface into the tubule's lumen. Spermiogenesis is commonly divided into four phases:

- In the **Golgi phase** the cytoplasm contains a prominent Golgi apparatus near the nucleus, mitochondria, paired centrioles, and free ribosomes. Small **proacrosomal**

vesicles from the Golgi apparatus coalesce as a single membrane-limited **acrosomal cap** close to one end of the nucleus (Figures 21–5b and 21–8). The centrioles migrate to a position farthest from the acrosomal cap and one acts as a basal body, organizing the axoneme of the flagellum which is structurally and functionally similar to that of a cilium (see Chapter 2).

- In the **cap phase** the acrosomal cap spreads over about half of the condensing nucleus (Figures 21–5b and 21–8). The acrosome is a specialized type of lysosome containing hydrolytic enzymes, mainly hyaluronidase and a trypsin-like protease called **acrosin**. These enzymes are released when a spermatozoon encounters an oocyte and the acrosomal membrane fuses with the sperm's plasma membrane. They dissociate cells of the corona radiata and digest the zona pellucida, both structures that surround the egg (see Chapter 22). This process, the **acrosomal reaction**, is one of the first steps in fertilization.
- In the **acrosome phase** the **head** of the developing sperm, containing the acrosome and the condensing

FIGURE **21–8** Differentiating spermatid.

The head of a late spermatid during spermiogenesis is completely enclosed by Sertoli cell cytoplasm. As shown by TEM, the sperm nucleus (**N**) is half covered by the thin Golgi-derived acrosomal cap (**A**). The flagellum (**F**) can be seen emerging from a basal body near the nucleus on the side opposite the acrosome. A perinuclear bundle of microtubules and actin filaments called the **manchette** (**M**) transports vesicles, mitochondria, and keratins into position as the spermatid elongates. X7500.

nucleus, remains embedded in the Sertoli cell while the growing axoneme extends into the lumen of the tubule (Figure 21–6b). Nuclei become more elongated and very highly condensed, with the histones of nucleosomes replaced by small basic peptides called **protamines**. Flagellum growth continues as the tail and mitochondria aggregate around its proximal region to form a thickened **middle piece** where the ATP for flagellar movements is generated (Figure 21–5).

▪ In the **maturation phase** of spermiogenesis, unneeded cytoplasm is shed as a **residual body** from each spermatozoon and remaining intercellular bridges are lost. Mature but not yet functional sperm (Figure 21–5) are released into the lumen of the tubule.

> ## >> MEDICAL APPLICATION

Decreased semen quality, which is frequently idiopathic (arising from unknown causes), is a major cause of **male infertility**. Common features of poor semen quality include **oligospermia** (ejaculate volume >2 mL), sperm cell density less than 10-20 million/mL, abnormal sperm morphology, and flagellar defects that impair sperm motility.

Sertoli Cells

The **Sertoli cells**, named after Enrico Sertoli (1842-1910) who first demonstrated their physiologic significance, are tall columnar or pyramidal epithelial cells that form the basal lamina of the seminiferous tubules (Figure 21–4c). All cells of the spermatogenic lineage are closely associated with the extended surfaces of Sertoli cells and depend on them for metabolic and physical support.

Sertoli cells adhere to the basal lamina and their apical ends extend to the lumen, as shown immunohistochemically in Figure 21–4c,d. In routine preparations the outlines of Sertoli cells surrounding the spermatogenic cells are very poorly defined (Figures 21–6 and 21–8). Each Sertoli cell supports 30 to 50 developing germ cells. Ultrastructurally Sertoli cells are seen to contain abundant SER, some rough ER, well-developed Golgi complexes, numerous mitochondria, and lysosomes (Figure 21–8). Their nuclei are typically ovoid or triangular, euchromatic, and have a prominent nucleolus, features that allow Sertoli cells to be distinguished from the neighboring germ cells (Figure 21–6).

Important in Sertoli cell function are elaborate tight occluding junctions between their basolateral membranes that form a **blood-testis barrier** within the seminiferous epithelium (Figure 21–5a). The tightest blood-tissue barrier in mammals, this physical barrier is one part of a system that prevents autoimmune attacks against the unique spermatogenic cells, which first appear after the immune system is mature and central self-tolerance is well established.

Spermatogonia lie in a **basal compartment** of the tubule, below the tight junctions and not sealed off from the vascularized interstitial tissue containing lymphocytes and other immune cells. Newly formed primary spermatocytes temporarily disassemble the adhesion molecules of the local occluding junctions and move into the tubule's **adluminal compartment** while still adhering to Sertoli cells (Figure 21–5a). Like the spermatogonia, all spermatocytes and spermatids lie within invaginations of the Sertoli cells surfaces. Adluminal migration occurs without compromising the blood-testis barrier, which is all the more impressive when one remembers that the germ cells remain linked by intercellular bridges. Sertoli cells are also connected and coupled ionically by gap junctions, which may help regulate the transient changes in the occluding junctions and synchronize activities in the spermatogenic cells. As the flagellar tails of the spermatids develop, they appear as tufts extending from the apical ends of the Sertoli cells.

Related to their role in establishing the blood-testis barrier, Sertoli cells have three general functions:

▪ **Support, protection, and nutrition of the developing spermatogenic cells:** Because spermatocytes, spermatids, and developing sperm are isolated from plasma proteins and nutrients by the blood-testis barrier, they depend on Sertoli cells for production or transport into the lumen of metabolites and nutritive factors such as the iron-transport protein transferrin. Thus, while protecting spermatogenic cells from circulating immune components, Sertoli cells supply many plasma factors needed for cell growth and differentiation.

▪ **Exocrine and endocrine secretion:** Sertoli cells continuously release into the seminiferous tubules water that carries new sperm out of the testis. Production of nutrients and **androgen-binding protein** (**ABP**), which concentrates testosterone to a level required for spermiogenesis, is promoted by follicle-stimulating hormone (FSH). As endocrine cells, they secrete the 39-kDa glycoprotein **inhibin**, which feeds back on the anterior pituitary gland to suppress FSH synthesis and release. In the fetus Sertoli cells also secrete a 140-kDa glycoprotein called **müllerian-inhibiting substance** (**MIS**) that causes regression of the embryonic müllerian (paramesonephric) ducts; in the absence of MIS these ducts persist and become parts of the female reproductive tract.

▪ **Phagocytosis:** During spermiogenesis, excess cytoplasm shed as residual bodies is phagocytosed and digested by Sertoli cell lysosomes. No proteins from sperm normally pass back across the blood-testis barrier.

> ## >> MEDICAL APPLICATION

Acute or chronic inflammation of the testis, **orchitis**, frequently involves the ducts connecting this organ to the epididymis. Common forms of orchitis are produced by infective agents and occur secondarily to a **urinary tract infection** or a **sexually transmitted pathogen** such as *Chlamydia* or *Neisseria gonorrhoeae* entering the testis from the epididymis or via the lymphatics.

Acute **epididymitis** is a result of **sexually transmitted infections** such as gonorrhea or *Chlamydia* infection and causes intrascrotal pain and tenderness. Persistent inflammation of the epididymis, such as that associated with **gonorrhea** infections, includes massive invasion by leukocytes into the infected duct, stimulating fibrosis that obstructs the epididymis and is a common cause of **male infertility.**

› INTRATESTICULAR DUCTS

The intratesticular ducts are the **straight tubules** (or tubuli recti), the **rete testis**, and the **efferent ductules** (Figure 21–2), all of which carry spermatozoa and liquid from the seminiferous tubules to the duct of the epididymis (Table 21–1).

The loops of seminiferous tubules join the rete testis by the short straight tubules, which are lined initially only by Sertoli cells (Figure 21–9). These empty into the rete testis, an interconnected network of channels lined with cuboidal epithelium and supported by connective tissue of the mediastinum (Figure 21–9).

The rete testis drains into about 20 efferent ductules lined by an unusual epithelium in which groups of nonciliated cuboidal cells alternate with groups of taller ciliated cells and give the tissue a characteristic scalloped appearance (Figure 21–10). The nonciliated cells absorb most of the fluid secreted by the Sertoli cells of seminiferous tubules. This absorption and the ciliary activity create a fluid flow that carries sperm out of the testis toward the epididymis. A thin layer of circularly oriented smooth muscle cells in the walls of efferent ductules aids sperm movement into the duct of the epididymis.

› EXCRETORY GENITAL DUCTS

The excretory genital ducts are those of the **epididymis**, the **ductus** (or **vas**) **deferens**, and the **urethra**. They transport sperm from the scrotum to the penis during ejaculation.

Epididymis

The long, coiled duct of the epididymis, surrounded by connective tissue, lies in the scrotum along the superior and posterior sides of each testis (see Figure 21–2). About 4 to 5 m in length, it includes a **head** region where the efferent ductules enter, a **body**, and a **tail** opening into the ductus deferens.

TABLE **21–1**	Summary of histology and functions of male genital ducts.			
Duct	Location	Epithelium	Support Tissues	Function(s)
Seminiferous tubules	Testicular lobules	Spermatogenic, with Sertoli cells and germ cells	Myoid cells and loose connective tissue	Produce sperm
Straight tubules (tubuli recti)	Periphery of the mediastinum testis	Sertoli cells in proximal portions, simple cuboidal in distal portions	Connective tissue	Convey sperm into the rete testis
Rete testis	In mediastinum testis	Simple cuboidal	Dense irregular connective tissue	Channels with sperm from all seminiferous tubules
Efferent ductules	From rete testis to head of epididymis	Alternating patches of simple cuboidal nonciliated and simple columnar ciliated	Thin circular layer of smooth muscle and vascular loose connective tissue	Absorb most fluid from seminiferous tubules; convey sperm into the epididymis
Epididymal duct	Head, body, and tail of the epididymis	Pseudostratified columnar, with small basal cells and tall principal cells bearing long stereocilia	Circular smooth muscle initially, with inner and outer longitudinal layers in the tail	Site for sperm maturation and short-term storage; expels sperm at ejaculation
Ductus (vas) deferens	Extends from epididymis to ejaculatory ducts in prostate gland	Pseudostratified columnar, with fewer stereocilia	Fibroelastic lamina propria and three very thick layers of smooth muscle	Carries sperm by rapid peristalsis from the epididymis to the ejaculatory ducts
Ejaculatory ducts	In prostate, formed by union of ductus deferens and ducts of the seminal vesicles	Pseudostratified and simple columnar	Fibroelastic tissue and smooth muscle of the prostate stroma	Mix sperm and seminal fluid; deliver semen to urethra, where prostatic secretion is added

FIGURE **21–9** Seminiferous tubules, straight tubules and rete testis.

(a) The seminiferous tubules (**S**) drain into short, much narrower straight tubules (**T**), which connect to the rete testis (**R**), a network of channels embedded along with blood vessels (**V**) in the connective tissue (**CT**) of the mediastinum testis. X120. H&E.

(b) At higher magnification the enclosed portion of part **a** shows the transition from wide seminiferous tubule (**S**) to the straight tubule (**T**). Initially the straight tubule wall has only tall Sertoli cells devoid of germ cells. The wall becomes a simple cuboidal epithelium near its connection to the rete testis (**R**), which is also lined with simple cuboidal epithelium. X300. H&E.

While passing through this duct, sperm become motile and their surfaces and acrosomes undergo final maturation steps. Fluid within the epididymis contains glycolipid **decapacitation factors** that bind sperm cell membranes and block acrosomal reactions and fertilizing ability until the factors are removed as part of the capacitation process in the female reproductive tract.

The epididymal duct is lined with pseudostratified columnar epithelium consisting of columnar **principal cells**, with characteristic long **stereocilia**, and small round stem cells (Figure 21–11). The principal cells secrete glycolipids and glycoproteins, but also absorb water and remove residual bodies or other debris not removed earlier by Sertoli cells. The duct

epithelium is surrounded by a few layers of smooth muscle cells, arranged as inner and outer longitudinal layers as well as a circular in the tail of the epididymis. Peristaltic contractions move the sperm along the duct and empty the body and tail regions at ejaculation.

Ductus or Vas Deferens

From the epididymis the **ductus** (or **vas**) **deferens**, a long straight tube with a thick, muscular wall and a relatively small lumen, continues toward the prostatic urethra where it empties (see Figure 21–1). As shown in Figure 21–12, its mucosa is slightly folded longitudinally, the lamina propria contains

FIGURE 21–10 Rete testis and efferent ductules.

(a) Rete testis (**R**) channels have simple cuboidal epithelium and are usually embedded in dense connective tissue. X350. Mallory trichrome.

(b) The efferent ductules (**E**) that drain the rete testis have a lining with a characteristic scalloped appearance in section, consisting of patches of simple cuboidal cells with water-absorbing microvilli alternating with patches of taller cells with cilia (**arrows**). X350. H&E.

many elastic fibers, and the epithelial lining is pseudostratified with some cells having sparse stereocilia. The very thick muscularis consists of longitudinal inner and outer layers and a middle circular layer. The muscles produce strong peristaltic contractions during ejaculation, which rapidly move sperm along this duct from the epididymis.

The ductus (vas) deferens forms part of the spermatic cord, which also includes the testicular artery, the pampiniform plexus, and nerves (see Figure 21–2). Following the general path along which the embryonic testes descend, each ductus passes over the urinary bladder where it enlarges as an **ampulla** (L. a small bottle) where the epithelium is thicker and more extensively folded (Figure 21–13). Within the prostate gland, the ends of the two ampullae merge with the ducts of the two seminal vesicles, joining these ducts to form the **ejaculatory ducts** which open into the **prostatic urethra**.

The histology of the intratesticular and excretory ducts is summarized in Table 21–1.

> ACCESSORY GLANDS

The accessory glands of the male reproductive tract produce secretions that are mixed with sperm during ejaculation to produce semen and that are essential for reproduction. The accessory genital glands are the **seminal vesicles** (or glands), the **prostate gland**, and the **bulbourethral glands** (Figure 21–13).

Seminal Vesicles

The two **seminal vesicles** consist of highly tortuous tubes, each about 15 cm long, enclosed by a connective tissue capsule. The unusual mucosa of the tube displays a great number of thin, complex folds that fill much of the lumen (Figure 21–14). The folds are lined with simple or pseudostratified columnar epithelial cells rich in secretory granules. The lamina propria contains elastic fibers and is surrounded by smooth muscle with inner circular and outer longitudinal layers that empty the gland during ejaculation. The seminal vesicles are exocrine glands in which production of their viscid, yellowish secretion depends on testosterone. Fluid from seminal vesicles typically makes up about 70% of the ejaculate and its components include the following:

- **Fructose,** a major energy source for sperm, as well as inositol, citrate, and other metabolites;

FIGURE **21-11** Epididymis.

(a) The long, coiled duct of the epididymis (**DE**), where sperm undergo maturation and short-term storage, is enclosed by connective tissue with many blood vessels (**V**) and covered by a capsule and the tunica vaginalis (**TV**). The duct is lined by a pseudostratified columnar epithelium with long stereocilia (**arrows**). X140. H&E.

(b) The columnar epithelium of the epididymal duct is surrounded by a thin circular layer of smooth muscle (**SM**)

cells and its lumen contains sperm (**S**). The smooth muscle becomes thicker and a longitudinal layer develops in the body and tail of the epididymis. X400. H&E.

(c) The inset photo shows the epithelium with tall principal cells (**P**) with stereocilia and fewer small basal stem cells (**B**). Intraepithelial lymphocytes are also commonly seen in the epididymal duct. X500. H&E.

- **Prostaglandins,** which stimulate activity in the female reproductive tract; and
- **Fibrinogen,** which allows semen to coagulate after ejaculation.

Prostate Gland

The **prostate gland** is a dense organ that surrounds the urethra below the bladder. It is approximately 2 cm × 3 cm × 4 cm in size and weighs about 20 g. The prostate is a collection of 30 to 50 tubuloacinar glands embedded in a dense fibromuscular stroma in which smooth muscle contracts at

ejaculation (Figure 21–13b). Ducts from individual glands may converge but all empty directly into the prostatic urethra, which runs through the center of the prostate. As shown in Figure 21–15, the glands are arranged in three major zones around the urethra:

- The **transition zone** occupies only about 5% of the prostate volume, surrounds the superior portion of the urethra, and contains the periurethral **mucosal gland**s.
- The **central zone** comprises 25% of the gland's tissue and contains the periurethral **submucosal glands** with longer ducts.

FIGURE **21–12** Ductus deferens.

(a) A cross section of the vas deferens shows the mucosa (**M**), a thick muscularis with inner and outer layers of longitudinal smooth muscle (**L-SM**) and an intervening layer of circular smooth muscle (**C-SM**), and an external adventitia (**A**). The muscularis is specialized for powerful peristaltic movement of sperm at ejaculation. X60. H&E.

(b) The lamina propria (**LP**) is rich in elastic fibers and the thick epithelial lining (**E**) shows longitudinal folds. X150. Mallory trichrome.

(c) Higher magnification of the mucosa shows that the epithelium is pseudostratified with basal cells and many columnar cells, some with stereocilia. X400. H&E.

- The **peripheral zone**, with about 70% of the organ's tissue, contains the prostate's **main glands** with still longer ducts (Figure 21–16).

The tubuloacinar glands of the prostate are all lined by a simple or pseudostratified columnar epithelium and produce fluid that contains various glycoproteins, enzymes, and small molecules such as prostaglandins and is stored until ejaculation. A clinically important product of the prostate is prostate-specific antigen (PSA), a 34-kDa serine protease that helps liquefy coagulated semen for the slow release of sperm after ejaculation. Small amounts of PSA also leak normally into the prostatic vasculature; elevated levels of circulating PSA indicate abnormal glandular mucosa typically due to prostatic carcinoma or inflammation.

Small spherical concretions, 0.2 to 2 mm in diameter and often partially calcified, are normally present in the lumens of many prostatic tubuloacinar glands (Figure 21–16). These concretions, called **corpora amylacea**, containing primarily deposited glycoproteins and keratan sulfate, may become more numerous with age but seem to have no physiologic or clinical significance. The prostate is surrounded by a fibroelastic capsule, from which septa extend and divide the gland into indistinct lobes. Like the seminal vesicles, the prostate's structure and function depend on the level of testosterone.

FIGURE 21–13 Accessory glands of the male reproductive tract.

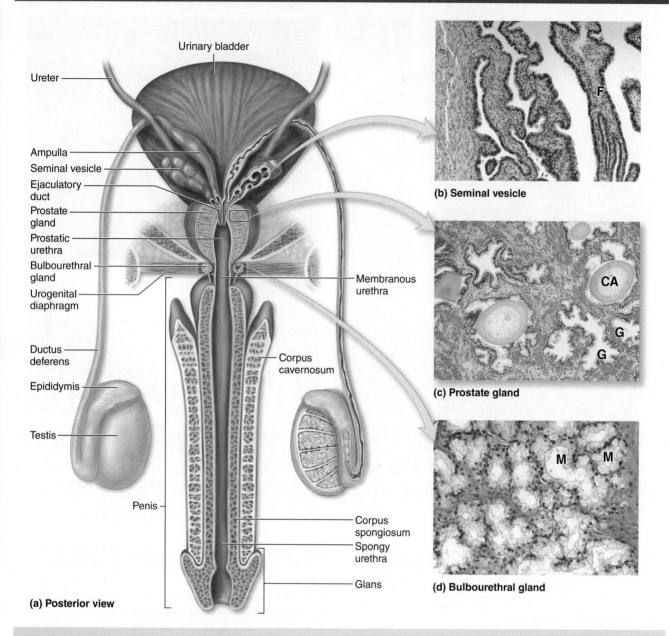

(a) Posterior view

(b) Seminal vesicle

(c) Prostate gland

(d) Bulbourethral gland

Labels on diagram (a): Urinary bladder, Ureter, Ampulla, Seminal vesicle, Ejaculatory duct, Prostate gland, Prostatic urethra, Bulbourethral gland, Urogenital diaphragm, Ductus deferens, Epididymis, Testis, Penis, Membranous urethra, Corpus cavernosum, Corpus spongiosum, Spongy urethra, Glans

(a) Three sets of glands connect to the ductus deferens or urethra: the paired **seminal vesicles**, the **prostate**, and the paired **bulbourethral glands**. The first two types of glands contribute the major volume to semen and the latter produces a secretion that lubricates the urethra before ejaculation.

(b) Seminal vesicles have a characteristic thin mucosal folds (**F**) with a large surface area.

(c) The prostate gland has many individual tubuloacinar glands (**G**), some containing concretions called corpora amylacea (**CA**).

(d) The small, paired bulbourethral glands consist mainly of mucous acini (**M**). a,b,c all X80. H&E.

>> **MEDICAL APPLICATION**

The prostate gland is prone to three common problems: (1) **chronic prostatitis**, usually involving bacteria or other infectious agents; (2) **nodular hyperplasia** or **benign prostatic hypertrophy**, occurring mainly in the periurethral mucosal glands where it often leads to compression of the urethra and problems with urination; and (3) **prostate cancer** (adenocarcinoma), the most common cancer in nonsmoking men, occurring mainly in glands of the peripheral zone.

FIGURE **21–14** Seminal vesicles.

The seminal vesicles are paired exocrine glands that secrete most seminal fluid, including sperm nutrients. **(a)** A low-power micrograph shows that each consists of a coiled duct with a mucosa organized with many thin folds (**arrows**) in the lumen (**L**) and surrounded by two layers of smooth muscle (**SM**). X20. H&E.

(b, c) The mucosal folds include smooth muscle (**SM**), a thin lamina propria (**LP**), and a simple columnar epithelium of principal secretory cells. Both: X300. b: H&E; c: PSH.

FIGURE **21–15** Organization of the prostate gland.

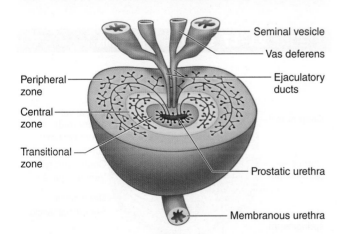

Seminal vesicle

Vas deferens

Ejaculatory ducts

Peripheral zone

Central zone

Transitional zone

Prostatic urethra

Membranous urethra

The prostate consists of 30-50 branched tubuloacinar glands organized into three layers, shown here schematically. Around the prostatic urethra is the **transition zone** containing mucosal glands. Surrounding most of that zone is the intermediate **central zone**, which contains the submucosal glands. The outermost and largest layer is the **peripheral zone**, which contains the most numerous main glands.

Bulbourethral Glands

The paired round **bulbourethral glands** (or Cowper glands), 3-5 mm in diameter, are located in the urogenital diaphragm (Figure 21–13) and empty into the proximal part of the penile urethra. Each gland has several lobules with tubuloacinar secretory units surrounded by smooth muscle cells and lined by a mucus-secreting simple columnar epithelium that is also testosterone-dependent (Figure 21–13d). During erection the bulbourethral glands, as well as numerous, very small, and histologically similar urethral glands along the penile urethra, release a clear mucus-like secretion that coats and lubricates the urethra in preparation for the imminent passage of sperm.

❭ PENIS

The penis consists of three cylindrical masses of erectile tissue, plus the penile urethra, surrounded by skin (see Figure 21–1). Two of the erectile masses—the **corpora cavernosa**—are dorsal; the ventral **corpus spongiosum** surrounds the urethra (Figure 21–17). At its end the corpus spongiosum expands, forming the **glans** (Figure 21–13a). Most of the penile urethra is lined with pseudostratified columnar epithelium. In the glans, it becomes stratified squamous epithelium

FIGURE **21–16** Prostate gland.

(a) The prostate has a dense fibromuscular stroma (**S**) in which are embedded a large number of small tubuloalveolar glands (**G**). X20. H&E.

(b) A micrograph of one prostatic gland, showing a corpus amylaceum (**CA**) concretion and the secretory epithelium (**E**)

surrounded by a thin lamina propria (**LP**) and thick smooth muscle (**M**). X122. H&E.

(c) Higher magnification shows the lamellar nature of a corpus amylaceum (**CA**) and the pseudostratified columnar epithelium underlain by lamina propria (**LP**). X300. Mallory trichrome.

continuous with that of the thin epidermis covering the glans surface. Small mucus-secreting **urethral glands** are found along the length of the penile urethra. In uncircumcised men the glans is covered by the **prepuce** or foreskin, a retractable fold of thin skin with sebaceous glands on the internal surface.

The corpora cavernosa are each surrounded by a dense fibroelastic layer, the **tunica albuginea** (Figures 21–17 and 21–18). All three erectile tissues consist of many venous **cavernous spaces** lined with endothelium and separated by trabeculae with smooth muscle and connective tissue continuous with the surrounding tunic (Figure 21–19).

Central arteries in the corpora cavernosa branch to form nutritive arterioles and small coiling **helicine arteries**, which lead to the cavernous vascular spaces of erectile tissue. Arteriovenous shunts are present between the central arteries and the dorsal veins.

Penile **erection** involves blood filling the cavernous spaces in the three masses of erectile tissue. Triggered by external stimuli to the CNS, erection is controlled by autonomic nerves in these vascular walls. Parasympathetic stimulation relaxes the trabecular smooth muscle and dilates the

FIGURE **21–17** Structure of the penis.

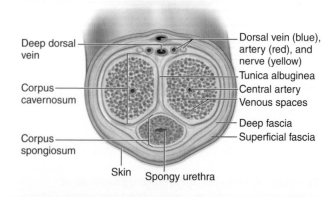

A diagram of the penis in transverse section shows the relationships of the three **erectile bodies,** the **tunica albuginea,** and **major blood vessels**. Compare this section to the longitudinal diagram in Figure 21–13.

FIGURE **21–18** Penis.

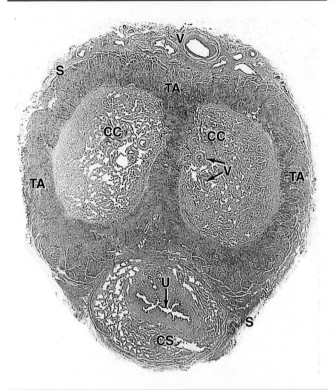

The corpus spongiosum (**CS**) is on the ventral side of the penis and surrounds the urethra (**U**). Two corpora cavernosa (**CC**) occupy most of the dorsal side and are surrounded by dense, fibrous tunica albuginea (**TA**). Along the dorsal side run the major blood vessels (**V**) and deep in each corporal mass of erectile tissue are smaller blood vessels (**V**), including the central arteries. The penis is covered loosely by skin (**S**), which distally forms the large foreskin fold and becomes thin over the glans. X15. H&E.

helicine arteries, allowing increased blood flow and filling the cavernous spaces. This enlarges the corpora cavernosa and causes them to compress the dorsal veins against the dense tunica albuginea, which blocks the venous outflow and produces tumescence and rigidity in the erectile tissue. Beginning at ejaculation, sympathetic stimulation constricts the helicine arteries and trabecular muscle, decreasing blood flow into the spaces, lowering the pressure there, and allowing the veins to drain most blood from the erectile tissue.

≫ MEDICAL APPLICATION

At the beginning of an erection acetylcholine from parasympathetic nerves causes the vascular endothelial cells of the helicine arteries and cavernous tissue to release nitric oxide (NO). NO diffuses into the surrounding smooth muscle cells and activates guanylate cyclase to produce cyclic GMP, which causes these cells to relax and promotes blood flow for the erection.

Erectile dysfunction, or **impotence**, can result from diabetes, anxiety, vascular disease, or nerve damage during prostatectomy. The drug **sildenafil** may alleviate the problem by inhibiting the phosphodiesterase that degrades cyclic GMP in the smooth muscle cells of helicine arteries and erectile tissue. The subsequent higher level of cGMP promotes relaxation of these cells and enhances the neural effect to produce or maintain an erection.

The Male Reproductive System SUMMARY OF KEY POINTS

Testes

- In each **testis** approximately each of 250 **lobules** contains one or more very long, convoluted **seminiferous tubules** in a sparse, vascular stroma containing testosterone-producing **interstitial cells (of Leydig)**.
- **Seminiferous tubules** consist of spermatogenic epithelium containing columnar **Sertoli cells**, each of which supports and nourishes many germ cells embedded at its surface.
- **Tight junctions** between Sertoli cells establish two compartments within seminiferous tubules: a **basal compartment** with spermatogonia and an **adluminal compartment** with spermatocytes and spermatids.
- **Sertoli cells** also produce **androgen-binding protein**, which concentrates testosterone, **phagocytose** shed debris from differentiating spermatids, and **secrete fluid** that carries sperm along the tubules.

- Stem cells called **spermatogonia** undergo mitosis and give rise to **primary spermatocytes**, which undergo a first meiotic division to form haploid **secondary spermatocytes**.
- After a very short interval, **secondary spermatocytes** undergo the second meiotic division to produce small, round **spermatids**, which differentiate while still associated with Sertoli cells.
- A spermatid undergoes **spermiogenesis** by greatly condensing its **nucleus**, forming a long **flagellum** with a surrounding mitochondrial **middle piece**, and forming a perinuclear **acrosomal cap**.
- From the seminiferous tubules, sperm enter the short **straight tubules** that lead to channels of the **rete testis** in the mediastinum testis, then move via 15 or 20 **efferent ductules** where fluid is absorbed.

Excretory Genital Ducts

- From efferent ductules sperm move into and through **epididymal ducts** in the head, body, and tail of **epididymis**, also located in the scrotum, for their final maturation and short storage prior to ejaculation.

FIGURE **21–19** Penile urethra and erectile tissue.

(a) The corpus spongiosum (**CS**) surrounds the longitudinally folded wall of the penile urethra (**PU**). Small urethral glands (**UG**) with short ducts to the urethra release mucus during erection, supplementing the similar secretion from the bulbourethral glands. The two dorsal corpora cavernosa (**CC**) are ensheathed by dense, fibrous tunica albuginea (**TA**) and in one here a small helicine artery (**HA**) is shown. X100. H&E.

(b) A higher magnification of erectile tissue is shown with a small portion of tunica albuginea (**TA**) and fibrous, elastic connective tissue containing smooth muscle (**SM**) and many small, cavernous spaces (**CS**) lined by vascular endothelium. Very little blood normally passes through this vasculature due to constriction of the helicine arteries (**HA**) serving them. During erection the vascular smooth muscle relaxes, allowing rapid blood flow into the cavernous spaces, filling them and causing compression of their venous drainage, which makes the masses of erectile tissue much larger and turgid. X200. H&E.

▪ The **epididymis** is lined by **pseudostratified columnar epithelium** containing **principal cells** that have long **stereocilia**; along its length the number of surrounding **smooth muscle** layers increases.

▪ At ejaculation the body and tail of the **epididymis** are emptied into the **ductus (vas) deferens**, also lined by **pseudostratified columnar epithelium** with three thick layers of **smooth muscle** for peristalsis.

Accessory Glands

▪ Most semen is produced by the paired **seminal vesicles** (glands), characterized by numerous thin folds of secretory mucosa; a duct from each seminal vesicle joins a ductus deferens as an **ejaculatory duct**.

▪ Inside the medial **prostate gland** the two **ejaculatory ducts** and dozens of ducts from **tubuloacinar prostatic glands** merge with the **urethra** that transports semen through the penis.

▪ **Semen** components from the seminal vesicles nourish sperm (eg, **fructose**), activate ciliary and muscle activity in the female reproductive tract (**prostaglandins**), and control the product's viscosity for sperm release.

Penis

▪ The **penis** contains two dorsal **corpora cavernosa** and a periurethral **corpus spongiosum**, all composed of vascular **cavernous tissue** and small amounts of surrounding **smooth muscle** and **helicine arteries**.

▪ For erection **parasympathetic** stimulation relaxes muscle of the small **helicine arteries** and adjacent tissues, allowing vessels of the **cavernous tissue** to fill with blood; the enlarging corpora compress the venous drainage, producing further enlargement and turgidity in the three corpora masses.

▪ The **sympathetic** stimulation at ejaculation constricts blood flow through the **helicine** arteries, allowing blood to empty from the cavernous tissues.

22 The Female Reproductive System

The female reproductive system consists of the paired ovaries and oviducts (or uterine tubes), the uterus, the vagina, and the external genitalia (Figure 22–1). This system produces the female gametes (**oocytes**), provides the environment for fertilization, and holds the embryo during its complete development through the fetal stage until birth. As with male gonads, the ovaries produce steroidal sex hormones that control organs of the reproductive system and influence other organs. Beginning at **menarche**, when the first menses occurs, the reproductive system undergoes monthly changes in structure and function that are controlled by neurohormonal mechanisms. **Menopause** is a variably timed period during which the cyclic changes become irregular and eventually disappear. In the postmenopausal period the reproductive organs slowly involute. Although the mammary glands do not belong to the genital system, they are included here because they undergo changes directly connected to the functional state of the reproductive organs.

> OVARIES

Ovaries are almond-shaped bodies approximately 3 cm long, 1.5 cm wide, and 1 cm thick. Each ovary is covered by a simple cuboidal epithelium, the **surface** (or germinal) **epithelium**, continuous with the mesothelium and overlying a layer of dense connective tissue capsule, the **tunica albuginea**, like that of the testis. Most of the ovary consists of the **cortex**,

a region with a stroma of highly cellular connective tissue and many **ovarian follicles** varying greatly in size after menarche (Figure 22–1). The most internal part of the ovary, the **medulla**, contains loose connective tissue and blood vessels entering the organ through the hilum from mesenteries suspending the ovary (Figures 22–1 and 22–2). There is no distinct border between the ovarian cortex and medulla.

Early Development of the Ovary

In the first month of embryonic life, a small population of **primordial germ cells** migrates from the yolk sac to the gonadal primordia. There the cells divide and differentiate as **oogonia**. In developing ovaries of a 2-month embryo, there are about 600,000 oogonia that produce more than 7 million by the fifth month. Beginning in the third month, oogonia begin to enter the prophase of the first meiotic division but arrest after completing synapsis and recombination, without progressing to later stages of meiosis (see Chapter 3). These cells arrested in meiosis are called **primary oocytes** (Gr. *oon*, egg + *kytos*, cell). Each primary oocyte becomes surrounded by flattened support cells called **follicular cells** to form an ovarian follicle. By the seventh month of development, most oogonia have transformed into primary oocytes within follicles. Many primary oocytes, however, are lost through a slow, continuous degenerative process called **atresia**, which continues through a woman's reproductive life. At puberty the ovaries contain about 300,000 oocytes. Because generally only one

FIGURE **22–1** **The female reproductive system and overview of ovary.**

(a) Posterior view

(b) Lateral sectional view

(c)

(a) The diagram shows the internal organs of the female reproductive system, which includes as the principal organs the **ovaries**, **uterine tubes**, **uterus**, and **vagina**. **(b)** A lateral sectional view of an ovary shows the ovary and the relationship of its main supporting mesenteries, the mesovarium and the mesosalpinx of the broad ligament. **(c)** A sectioned ovary, indicating the medulla and cortex, with follicles of several different sizes in the cortex. X15. H&E.

oocyte resumes meiosis with ovulation during each menstrual cycle (average duration, 28 days) and the reproductive life of a woman lasts about 30 to 40 years, only about 450 oocytes are liberated from ovaries by ovulation. All others degenerate through atresia.

Ovarian Follicles

An ovarian follicle consists of an oocyte surrounded by one or more layers of epithelial cells within a basal lamina. The follicles that are formed during fetal life—**primordial follicles**—consist of a primary oocyte enveloped by a single layer of the flattened follicular cells (Figure 22–2b; Figures 22–3 and 22–4). These follicles occur in the superficial ovarian cortex. The oocyte in the primordial follicle is spherical and about 25 μm in diameter, with a large nucleus containing chromosomes in the first meiotic prophase. The organelles tend to be concentrated near the nucleus and include numerous mitochondria, several Golgi complexes, and extensive RER. The basal lamina surrounds the follicular cells, marking a clear boundary between the follicle and the vascularized stroma.

FIGURE **22–2** Follicle development and changes within the ovary.

(b) Primordial follicles

Primordial follicles | Primary oocyte | Follicle cells

500x

(c) Primary follicle

Primary oocyte | Follicle cells

Primary follicle

500x

(d) Secondary or antral follicle

Zona pellucida

Primary oocyte | Corona radiata | Antrum | Follicle cells

Secondary follicle

50x

(a) Cross section of ovary

Primordial follicles | Primary oocyte | Granulosa cells | Secondary follicle | Zona pellucida | Antrum | Suspensory ligament of ovary

Primary follicles

Medulla

Primordial follicles

Tunica albuginea

Surface epithelium

Ovarian ligament

Corpus albicans | **Corpus luteum** | Developing corpus luteum | Cortex

Vesicular follicle
Antrum
Secondary oocyte
Zona pellucida

Corona radiata
Zona pellucida
Ovulated secondary oocyte

(g) Corpus albicans

Corpus albicans

80x

(f) Corpus luteum

Corpus luteum

25x

(e) Mature, preovulatory, or graafian follicle

Antrum | Corona radiata | Zona pellucida | Secondary oocyte

100x

The ovary produces both oocytes and sex hormones. A diagram of a sectioned ovary **(a)** shows the **different stages of follicle maturation**, **ovulation**, and **corpus luteum formation and degeneration**. All of the stages and structures shown in this diagram actually would appear at different times during the ovarian cycle and do not occur simultaneously. Follicles are arranged here for easy comparisons. The **primordial follicles** shown are greatly enlarged. The histologic sections identify primordial follicles **(b)**, a primary follicle **(c)**, a secondary follicle **(d)**, and a large vesicular follicle **(e)**. After ovulation, the portion of the follicle left behind forms the corpus luteum **(f)**, which then degenerates into the corpus albicans **(g)**. All H&E.

FIGURE **22–3** Stages of ovarian follicles, from primordial to mature.

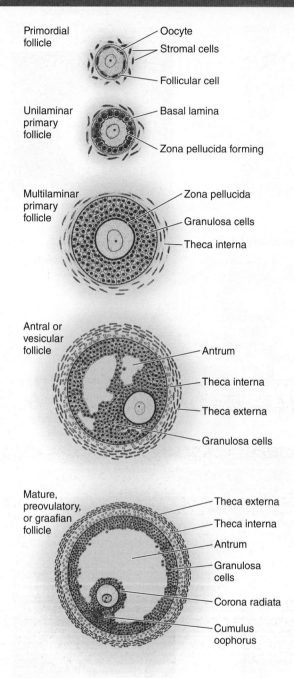

Diagrams of sectioned ovarian follicles show the changing size and morphology of follicular/granulosa cells at each stage and the disposition of the surrounding thecal cells. However, the relative proportions of the follicles are not maintained in the series of drawings: mature follicles are much larger relative to the early follicles. Deep within each follicle is a single large, growing oocyte with a large nucleus and prominent nucleolus. Follicular or granulosa cells around the oocyte support that cell's rapid growth.

FIGURE **22–4** Primordial follicles.

The cortical region of an ovary is surrounded by the surface epithelium (**SE**), a mesothelium with usually cuboidal cells. This layer is sometimes called the germinal epithelium because of an early erroneous view that it was the source of oogonia precursor cells. Underlying the epithelium is a connective tissue layer, the tunica albuginea (**TA**). Groups of primordial follicles, each formed by an oocyte (**O**) surrounded by a layer of flat epithelial follicular cells (**arrows**), are present in the ovarian connective tissue (stroma). X200. H&E.

Follicular Growth & Development

Beginning in puberty with the release of follicle-stimulating hormone (FSH) from the pituitary, a small group of primordial follicles each month begins a process of follicular growth. This involves growth of the oocyte, proliferation and changes in the follicular cells, as well as proliferation and differentiation of the stromal fibroblasts around each follicle. Selection of the primordial follicles that undergo growth and recruitment early in each cycle and of the dominant follicle destined to ovulate that month both involve complex hormonal balances and subtle differences among follicles in FSH receptor numbers, aromatase activity, estrogen synthesis, and other variables.

Prompted by FSH, an oocyte grows most rapidly during the first part of follicular development, reaching a diameter of about 120 μm. Oocyte differentiation includes the following:

- Growth of the cell and nuclear enlargement;
- Mitochondria becoming more numerous and uniformly distributed;
- RER becoming much more extensive and Golgi complexes enlarging and moving peripherally; and
- Formation of specialized secretory granules called **cortical granules** containing various proteases. These lie just inside the oocyte's plasma membrane and undergo exocytosis early in fertilization.

Follicular cells undergo mitosis and form a simple cuboidal epithelium around the growing oocyte. The follicle

FIGURE **22–5** Primary follicles.

(a) A micrograph of ovarian cortex shows several primordial follicles (**PF**) and their flattened follicle cells (**arrows**), and two unilaminar primary follicles (**UF**) in which the follicle cells or granulosa cells (**G**) form a single cuboidal layer around the large primary oocyte (**O**). X200. PT.

(b) This micrograph taken at the same magnification shows a larger multilayered primary follicle. Granulosa cells (**G**) have now proliferated to form several layers. Between them and the oocyte (**O**) is the 5- to 10-μm-thick zona pellucida (**ZP**), a glycoprotein layer produced by the oocyte that is required for sperm binding and fertilization. The primary oocyte is now a very large cell. With this stain, the basement membrane (**BM**) that separates the follicle from the surrounding stroma can also be seen. X200. PSH.

is now called a **unilaminar primary follicle** (Figures 22–3 and 22–5a). The follicular cells continue to proliferate, forming a stratified follicular epithelium, the **granulosa**, in which the cells communicate through gap junctions. Follicular cells are now termed **granulosa cells** and the follicle is a **multilaminar primary follicle** (Figures 22–3 and 22–5b) still surrounded by a basement membrane.

Between the oocyte and the first layer of granulosa cells of the growing primary follicle, extracellular material accumulates as the **zona pellucida**, 5 to 10 μm thick and containing four glycoproteins secreted by the oocyte (Figures 22–5b and 22–6). The zona pellucida components ZP3 and ZP4 are important sperm receptors, binding specific proteins on the sperm surface and inducing acrosomal

activation. Filopodia of granulosa cells and microvilli of the oocyte penetrate the zona pellucida, allowing communication between these cells via gap junctions.

›› MEDICAL APPLICATION

Growing primary follicles can become involved in **polycystic ovary syndrome** (**PCOS**) that is characterized by enlarged ovaries with numerous cysts and an anovulatory state (with no follicles completing maturation successfully.) The clinical presentation of this disorder is variable and the etiology is unclear, although increased androgen production by the ovaries or adrenals is likely involved. PCOS is a common cause of **infertility** in women.

FIGURE 22–6 Ultrastructure of primary follicle and zona pellucida.

An SEM of a fractured primary follicle shows the oocyte surrounded by granulosa cells (**GC**). Between the very large oocyte surface and the granulosa cells is a layer of extracellular material, the zona pellucida (**ZP**), which contains four related glycoproteins that bind sperm and form an irregular meshwork. X3000.

Stromal cells immediately outside each growing primary follicle differentiate to form the **follicular theca** (Gr. *theca*, outer covering). This subsequently differentiates further as two distinct tissues around the follicle (see Figure 22–3; Figures 22–7 and 22–8):

- A well-vascularized endocrine tissue, the **theca interna**, with typical steroid-producing cells secreting androstenedione. This precursor molecule diffuses into the follicle through the basement membrane, and in the granulosa cells the enzyme aromatase converts it to estradiol, an FSH-dependent function. This estrogen returns to the thecae and stroma around the follicle, enters capillaries, and is distributed throughout the body.
- A more fibrous **theca externa** with fibroblasts and smooth muscle merges gradually with the surrounding stroma.

As the primary follicles grow, they move deeper in the ovarian cortex. Within such follicles small spaces appear between the granulosa layers as the cells secrete **follicular fluid** (or **liquor folliculi**). This fluid accumulates, the spaces enlarge and gradually coalesce, and the granulosa cells reorganize themselves around a larger cavity called the **antrum** (Figures 22–3 and 22–7a), producing follicles now called **vesicular** or **antral follicles**. Follicular fluid contains the large GAG hyaluronic acid, growth factors, plasminogen,

fibrinogen, the anticoagulant heparan sulfate proteoglycan, and high concentrations of steroids (progesterone, androstenedione, and estrogens) with binding proteins.

As the antrum develops, the granulosa cells around the oocyte form a small hillock, the **cumulus oophorus**, which protrudes into the antrum (Figures 22–3 and 22–7b). Those granulosa cells that immediately surround the zona pellucida make up the **corona radiata** and accompany the oocyte when it leaves the ovary at ovulation.

The single large antrum of a **mature** or **preovulatory follicle** (or **graafian follicle** named after the 17th-century reproductive biologist Regnier De Graaf) accumulates follicular fluid rapidly and expands to a diameter of 2 cm or more. A preovulatory follicle forms a bulge at the ovary surface visible with ultrasound imaging. The granulosa layer becomes thinner at this stage because its cells do not multiply in proportion to the growth of the antrum. A mature follicle has thick thecal layers and normally develops from a primordial follicle over a period of about 90 days.

Follicular Atresia

Most ovarian follicles undergo the degenerative process called **atresia**, in which follicular cells and oocytes die and are disposed of by phagocytic cells. Follicles at any stage of development, including nearly mature follicles, may become atretic (Figure 22–9). Atresia involves apoptosis and detachment of the granulosa cells, autolysis of the oocyte, and collapse of the zona pellucida. Early in this process, macrophages invade the degenerating follicle and phagocytose the debris, followed later by fibroblasts. Although follicular atresia takes place from before birth until a few years after menopause, it is most prominent just after birth, when levels of maternal hormones decline rapidly, and during both puberty and pregnancy, when qualitative and quantitative hormonal changes occur again.

During a typical menstrual cycle, one follicle becomes dominant and develops farther than the others. The **dominant follicle** usually reaches the most developed stage of follicular growth and undergoes ovulation, while the other primary and antral follicles undergo atresia. Although their oocytes are never directly used, the large growing follicles produce much estrogen before becoming **atretic follicles** each month. As described later, this estrogen stimulates preparation of the reproductive tract to transport and sustain the embryo if the oocyte from the dominant follicle is fertilized.

>> **MEDICAL APPLICATION**

Late primary or antral follicles can produce **follicular cysts**, which are thin-walled, fluid-filled structures with both granulosa and thecal endocrine cells. Follicular cysts are common and usually benign, but can produce high estrogen levels and lead to menstrual irregularities. If cyst formation disrupts blood vessels blood enters the fluid, often rapidly, and produces a **hemorrhagic cyst**.

FIGURE **22–7** Antral follicle and preovulatory follicle.

(a) An antral follicle shows the large, fluid-filled antral cavities or vesicles (**A**) that form within the granulosa layer as the cells produce follicular fluid. The oocyte (**O**) is surrounded by the zona pellucida (**ZP**) and granulosa cells (**G**), which also line the wall of the follicle. Fibroblastic cells immediately outside the growing follicles have developed as a steroid-secreting theca interna (**TI**) and a covering theca externa (**TE**). X100. H&E.

(b) A slightly more developed preovulatory follicle shows a very large single antrum (**A**) filled with follicular fluid in which the

proteins formed a thin film during fixation. The oocyte (**O**) now projects into this fluid-filled cavity, still surrounded by granulosa cells that now make up the corona radiata (**CR**). The corona radiata and oocyte are attached to the side of the follicle within a larger mass of granulosa cells called the **cumulus oophorus** (**CO**) which is continuous with the cells of the granulosa layer (**G**). Thecae interna (**TI**) and externa (**TE**) surround the whole follicle. X100. PT.

Ovulation & Its Hormonal Regulation

Ovulation is the hormone-stimulated process by which the oocyte is released from the ovary. Ovulation normally occurs midway through the menstrual cycle, that is, around the 14th day of a typical 28-day cycle. In the hours before ovulation, the mature dominant follicle bulging against the tunica albuginea develops a whitish or translucent ischemic area, the **stigma**, in which tissue compaction has blocked blood flow. In humans usually only one oocyte is liberated during each cycle, but sometimes either no oocyte or two or more simultaneous oocytes may be expelled.

Just before ovulation the oocyte completes the first meiotic division, which it began and arrested in prophase during fetal life (Figure 22–10). The chromosomes are equally divided between the two daughter cells, but one of these retains almost all of the cytoplasm. That cell is now the **secondary oocyte** and the other becomes the **first polar body**, a very small nonviable cell containing a nucleus and a minimal amount of cytoplasm. Immediately after expulsion of the first polar body, the nucleus of the oocyte begins the second meiotic division but arrests at metaphase and never completes meiosis unless fertilization occurs (Figure 22–10).

FIGURE **22–8** Wall of antral follicle.

At higher magnification, a small part of the wall of an antral follicle shows the cell layers of the granulosa (**G**) next to the antrum (**A**), in which proteins have aggregated on cells in contact with the follicular fluid. The theca interna (**TI**) surrounds the follicle, its cells appearing vacuolated and lightly stained because of their cytoplasmic lipid droplets, a characteristic of steroid-producing cells. The overlying theca externa (**TE**) contains fibroblasts and smooth muscle cells and merges with the stroma (**S**). A basement membrane (**BM**) separates the theca interna from the granulosa, blocking vascularization of the latter. X400. PT.

FIGURE **22–9** Atresia.

Atresia or degeneration of a follicle can occur at any stage of its development and is shown here in a follicle that had developed a large antrum. Atresia is characterized by apoptosis of granulosa cells (**G**) and autolysis of the oocyte, with macrophages entering the degenerating structure to clean up debris. Many apoptotic cells are seen loose in the antrum (**A**) here and the cells of the corona radiata have already disappeared, leaving the degenerative oocyte (**O**) free within the antrum. X200. PT.

As mentioned before, follicular development depends on FSH from pituitary gonadotrophs, whose secretion is stimulated by gonadotropin-releasing hormone (GnRH) from the hypothalamus. Figure 22–11 summarizes the main hormonal interactions that regulate follicular growth as well as the ovulation and formation of the corpus luteum. Note that negative feedback of estrogen and progesterone on the hypothalamus and anterior pituitary is reinforced by a polypeptide hormone, **inhibin**, also produced by granulosa and luteal cells. In the days preceding ovulation, the dominant vesicular follicle secretes higher levels of estrogen which stimulate more rapid pulsatile release of GnRH from the hypothalamus.

The increased level of GnRH causes a surge of LH release from the pituitary gland that rapidly triggers a sequence of major events in and around the dominant follicle:

- **Meiosis I is completed** by the primary oocyte, yielding a secondary oocyte and the first polar body which degenerates (Figure 22–10).
- Granulosa cells are stimulated to produce much greater amounts of both **prostaglandin** and extracellular **hyaluronan**. This hydrophilic GAG loosens these cells and rapidly increases the volume, pressure, and viscosity of the follicular fluid.
- Ballooning at the stigma, the **ovarian wall weakens** as activated plasminogen (plasmin) from broken capillaries degrades collagen in the tunica albuginea and surface epithelium.
- **Smooth muscle contractions** begin in the theca externa, triggered by prostaglandins diffusing from follicular fluid.

The increasing pressure with the follicle and weakening of the wall lead to rupture of the ovarian surface at the stigma. The oocyte and corona radiata, along with follicular fluid, are expelled by the local smooth muscle contractions. The ovulated secondary oocyte adheres loosely to the ovary surface in the viscous follicular fluid and, as described later, is drawn into the opening of the uterine tube where fertilization may occur. If not fertilized within about 24 hours, the secondary oocyte begins to degenerate. Cells of the ovulated follicle that remain in the ovary redifferentiate under the influence of LH and give rise to the corpus luteum (Figure 22–11).

Corpus Luteum

After ovulation, the granulosa cells and theca interna of the ovulated follicle reorganize to form a larger temporary endocrine gland, the **corpus luteum** (L., yellowish body), in the ovarian cortex. Ovulation is followed immediately by the collapse and folding of the granulosa and thecal layers of the follicle's wall, and blood from disrupted capillaries typically accumulates as a clot in the former antrum (Figure 22–12). The granulosa is now invaded by capillaries. Cells of both the granulosa and theca interna change histologically and functionally under the influence of LH, becoming specialized for

FIGURE **22–10** Oogenesis.

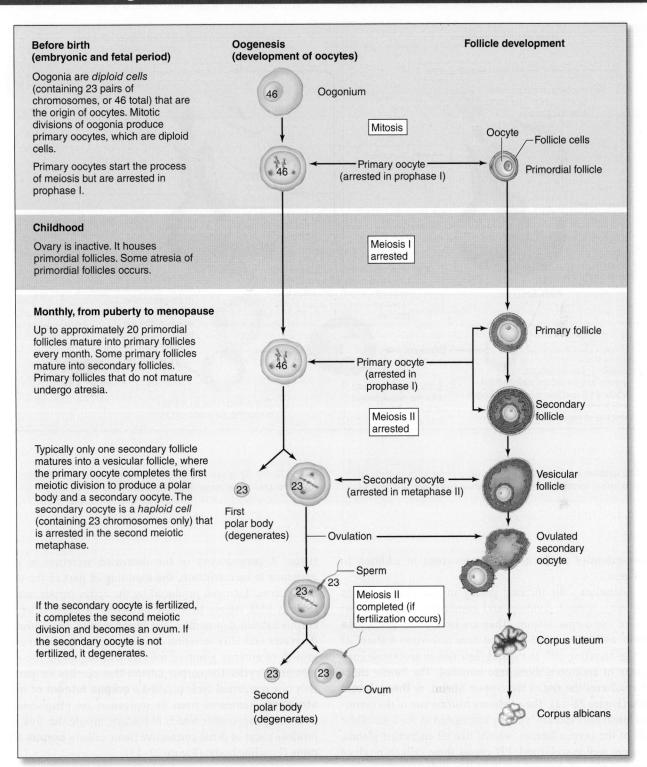

Before birth (embryonic and fetal period)

Oogonia are *diploid cells* (containing 23 pairs of chromosomes, or 46 total) that are the origin of oocytes. Mitotic divisions of oogonia produce primary oocytes, which are diploid cells.

Primary oocytes start the process of meiosis but are arrested in prophase I.

Childhood

Ovary is inactive. It houses primordial follicles. Some atresia of primordial follicles occurs.

Monthly, from puberty to menopause

Up to approximately 20 primordial follicles mature into primary follicles every month. Some primary follicles mature into secondary follicles. Primary follicles that do not mature undergo atresia.

Typically only one secondary follicle matures into a vesicular follicle, where the primary oocyte completes the first meiotic division to produce a polar body and a secondary oocyte. The secondary oocyte is a *haploid cell* (containing 23 chromosomes only) that is arrested in the second meiotic metaphase.

If the secondary oocyte is fertilized, it completes the second meiotic division and becomes an ovum. If the secondary oocyte is not fertilized, it degenerates.

Oogenesis (development of oocytes)

Oogonium — 46
Mitosis
Primary oocyte (arrested in prophase I) — 46
Meiosis I arrested
Primary oocyte (arrested in prophase I) — 46
Meiosis II arrested
First polar body (degenerates) — 23 / 23 — Secondary oocyte (arrested in metaphase II)
Sperm — 23 / 23
Meiosis II completed (if fertilization occurs)
Second polar body (degenerates) — 23 / 23 — Ovum

Follicle development

Oocyte — Follicle cells
Primordial follicle
Primary follicle
Secondary follicle
Vesicular follicle
Ovulation — Ovulated secondary oocyte
Corpus luteum
Corpus albicans

Oogenesis begins in the female fetus, with primary oocytes arresting at prophase I in primordial follicles, which remain inactive during childhood. At puberty, a population of primordial follicles begins to develop each month. Typically one per month produces a female gamete (a secondary oocyte).

FIGURE 22–11 Hormonal regulation of ovarian function.

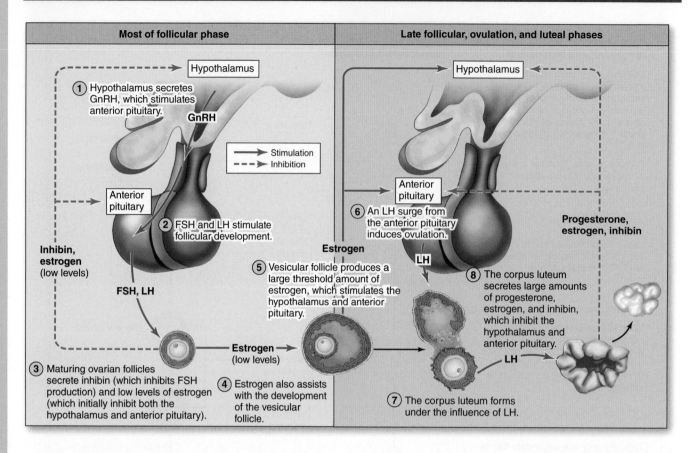

| Most of follicular phase | Late follicular, ovulation, and luteal phases |

(1) Hypothalamus secretes GnRH, which stimulates anterior pituitary.

→ Stimulation
- - - → Inhibition

(2) FSH and LH stimulate follicular development.

Inhibin, estrogen (low levels)

(5) Vesicular follicle produces a large threshold amount of estrogen, which stimulates the hypothalamus and anterior pituitary.

Estrogen (low levels)

(3) Maturing ovarian follicles secrete inhibin (which inhibits FSH production) and low levels of estrogen (which initially inhibit both the hypothalamus and anterior pituitary).

(4) Estrogen also assists with the development of the vesicular follicle.

(6) An LH surge from the anterior pituitary induces ovulation.

Progesterone, estrogen, inhibin

(8) The corpus luteum secretes large amounts of progesterone, estrogen, and inhibin, which inhibit the hypothalamus and anterior pituitary.

(7) The corpus luteum forms under the influence of LH.

The **ovarian cycle** of follicular growth, followed by ovulation and luteal formation, is initiated when the hypothalamus se-cretes GnRH. This stimulates the anterior pituitary to secrete FSH and LH, in the cycle depicted here.

---

more extensive production of progesterone in addition to estrogens.

Granulosa cells increase greatly in size (20-35 μm in diameter), without dividing, and eventually comprise about 80% of the corpus luteum. They are now called **granulosa lutein cells** (Figure 22–12) and have lost many features of protein-secreting cells to expand their role in aromatase conversion of androstenedione into estradiol. The former theca interna forms the rest of the corpus luteum, as **theca lutein cells** (Figure 22–12). These cells are half the size of the granulosa lutein cells and are typically aggregated in the folds of the wall of the corpus luteum, which, like all endocrine glands, becomes well vascularized. LH causes these cells to produce large amounts of progesterone as well as androstenedione.

The short-term fate of the corpus luteum depends on whether a pregnancy occurs. The ovulatory LH surge causes the corpus luteum to secrete progesterone for 10 to 12 days. Without further LH stimulation and in the absence of pregnancy, both major cell types of the corpus luteum cease steroid production and undergo apoptosis, with regression of the

tissue. A consequence of the decreased secretion of progesterone is menstruation, the shedding of part of the uterine mucosa. Estrogen produced by the active corpus luteum inhibits FSH release from the pituitary. However, after the corpus luteum degenerates, the blood steroid concentration decreases and FSH secretion increases again, stimulating the growth of another group of follicles and beginning the next menstrual cycle. The corpus luteum that persists for part of only one menstrual cycle is called a **corpus luteum of menstruation**. Remnants from its regression are phagocytosed by macrophages, after which fibroblasts invade the area and produce a scar of dense connective tissue called a **corpus albicans** (L., white body) (Figure 22–13).

If pregnancy occurs, the uterine mucosa must not be allowed to undergo menstruation because the embryo would be lost. To prevent the drop in circulating progesterone, trophoblast cells of the implanted embryo produce a glycoprotein hormone called **human chorionic gonadotropin (HCG)** with targets and activity similar to that of LH. HCG maintains and promotes further growth of the corpus luteum, stimulating

FIGURE **22–12** Corpus luteum.

The corpus luteum is a large endocrine structure formed from the remains of the large dominant follicle after it undergoes ovulation. **(a)** A low-power micrograph shows the corpus luteum (**CL**), characterized by folds of the former granulosa that collapses as the theca externa contracts at ovulation. The former antrum often contains a blood clot (**BC**) from vessels in the thecal layers disrupted during ovulation. Cells of the granulosa and theca interna become reorganized under the influence of pituitary LH and their names are changed. X15. H&E.

(b) Granulosa lutein cells (**GL**), seen at higher magnification here, undergo significant hypertrophy, producing most of the corpus luteum's increased size, and begin producing progesterone. The theca lutein cells (**TL**) increase only slightly in size, are somewhat darker-staining than the granulosa lutein cells, and continue to produce estrogens. Theca lutein cells, derived from the theca interna, are typically located within the folds that comprise the bulk of this tissue. X100. H&E.

secretion of progesterone to maintain the uterine mucosa. This **corpus luteum of pregnancy** becomes very large and is maintained by HCG for 4 to 5 months, by which time the placenta itself produces progesterone (and estrogens) at levels adequate to maintain the uterine mucosa. It then degenerates and is replaced by a large corpus albicans.

› UTERINE TUBES

The paired **uterine tubes**, or **oviducts**, supported by ligaments and mesenteries that allow considerable mobility, each measure about 10 to 12 cm in length (Figure 22–14). Each opens into the peritoneal cavity near the ovary, with regions in the following sequence:

- The **infundibulum**, a funnel-shaped opening fringed with fingerlike extensions called **fimbriae** (L., fringes) next to the ovary;
- The **ampulla**, the longest and expanded region where fertilization normally occurs;
- The **isthmus**, a more narrow portion nearer the uterus;
- The **uterine** or **intramural part**, which passes through the wall of the uterus and opens into the interior of this organ.

The wall of the oviduct consists of a folded mucosa, a thick, well-defined muscularis with interwoven circular (or spiral) and longitudinal layers of smooth muscle (Figure 22–15a), and a thin serosa covered by visceral peritoneum with mesothelium.

FIGURE **22–13** Corpus albicans.

A corpus albicans (**CA**) is the scar of connective tissue that forms at the site of a corpus luteum after its involution. It contains mostly collagen, with few fibroblasts or other cells, and gradually becomes very small and lost in the ovarian stroma. Involution of the corpus luteum does not involve atresia. X60. H&E.

The numerous branching, longitudinal folds of the mucosa are most prominent in the ampulla, which in cross section resembles a labyrinth (Figure 22–14b). These mucosal folds become smaller in the regions closer to the uterus and are absent in the intramural portion of the tube.

Along its entire length, the mucosa is lined by simple columnar epithelium on a lamina propria of loose connective tissue (Figure 22–15b). The epithelium contains two interspersed, functionally important cell types:

- **Ciliated cells** in which ciliary movements sweep fluid toward the uterus,
- **Secretory peg cells**, nonciliated and often darker staining, often with an apical bulge into the lumen, which secrete glycoproteins of a nutritive mucus film that covers the epithelium.

Triggered primarily by estrogens, the cilia elongate and both cell types undergo hypertrophy during the follicular growth phase of the ovarian cycle and undergo atrophy with loss of cilia during the late luteal phase.

At the time of ovulation, mucosal hypertrophy and increased local blood flow have enlarged and moved the uterine tubes. The fringed infundibulum lies very close to the ovary and the fimbriae partially surround that organ. This favors the transport of the ovulated secondary oocyte into the tube. Promoted by sweeping muscular contractions of the fimbriae and ciliary activity, the oocyte enters the infundibulum and moves to the ampulla. The secretion covering the mucosa has nutritive and protective functions for both the oocyte and the sperm, including **capacitation factors** that activate sperm and make those cells able to fertilize an oocyte.

› MAJOR EVENTS OF FERTILIZATION

Fertilization, the union of the female and male gametes, normally occurs in the ampulla of a uterine tube, a site usually reached by only a few hundred of the millions of ejaculated sperm. Only sperm that have undergone capacitation in the female reproductive tract are capable of fertilization, a process with the following major steps:

- Upon contact with cells of the corona radiata, sperm undergo the **acrosomal reaction** in which **hyaluronidase** is released by exocytosis at multiple locations around the sperm head. This allows sperm to move more easily to the zona pellucida.
- Specific proteins on the sperm surface bind the receptors ZP3 and ZP4, activating the protease **acrosin** on the acrosomal membrane to degrade the zona pellucida locally.
- The first sperm penetrating the zona pellucida fuses with the oocyte plasmalemma and triggers Ca^{2+} release from vesicles, which induces exocytosis of proteases from the cortical granules. This **cortical reaction** quickly spreads like a wave across the entire surface of the oocyte, with the proteases converting the zona pellucida to the impenetrable **perivitelline barrier** that constitutes a permanent block to polyspermy.
- The nucleus of the secondary oocyte immediately completes meiosis II, producing a second polar body and the **female pronucleus** of the haploid **ovum**. The haploid nucleus of the single penetrating sperm head undergoes decondensation, becoming the **male pronucleus**. Fusion of the two pronuclei yields the new diploid cell, the **zygote** (Gr. *zygotos*, yoked together).

Cell division occurs while the embryo is transported by contractions of the oviduct muscularis and ciliary movements to the uterus, which takes about 5 days. This transport occurs normally in women with immotile ciliary syndrome, indicating a more important role for muscle contractions in moving the embryo.

›› MEDICAL APPLICATION

Tubal ligation is a common surgical type of contraception. The uterine tube mucosa can become inflamed if infectious agents ascend from the lower genital tract, producing a condition named **salpingitis** after another name for these tubes, the **salpinges**. Mucosal damage or adhesions caused by chronic salpingitis can lead to **infertility** or an **ectopic (tubal) pregnancy** if there is blockage of oocyte or embryo transport to the uterus.

In tubal pregnancies, the lamina propria may react like the uterine endometrium and form decidual cells. But because of its small diameter and inability to expand, the tube cannot contain the growing embryo and will rupture, causing potentially fatal hemorrhage.

FIGURE **22–14** Uterine tubes and uterus.

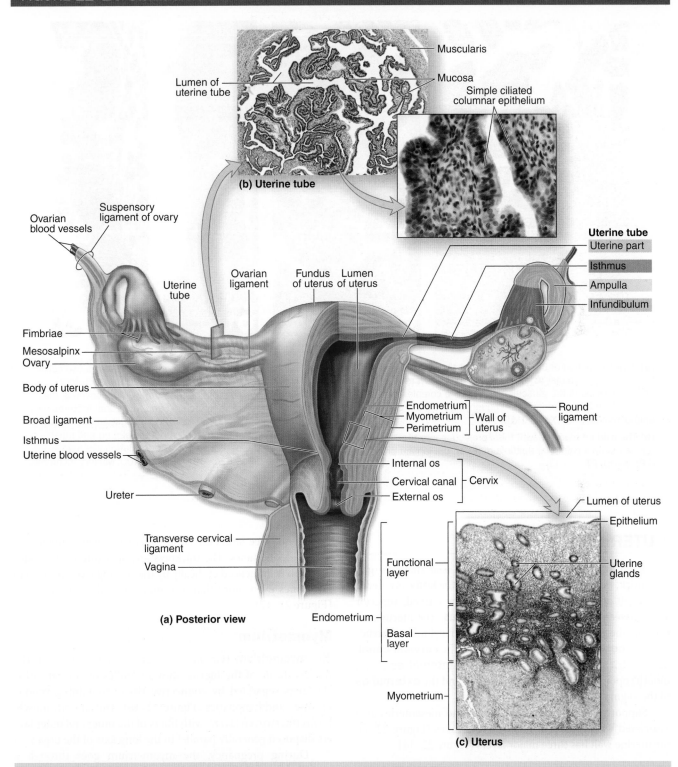

(b) Uterine tube

(a) Posterior view

(c) Uterus

The uterine tubes or oviducts are paired ducts that catch the ovulated secondary oocyte, nourish both the oocyte and sperm, provide the microenvironment for fertilization, and transport the embryo undergoing cleavage to the uterus.
(a) The diagram shows the relationship between the uterine tubes and the uterus in an intact posterior view (left) and in a cutaway view (right).

(b) Shown here is a cross section of uterine tube with a high magnification of the mucosa. X35 and 400. H&E.

(c) Shown here is the uterine wall with the myometrium and the two layers of the endometrium. X45. H&E.

FIGURE **22–15** Mucosa of the uterine tube wall.

(a) A cross section of the uterine tube at the ampulla shows the interwoven circular (**C**) and longitudinal (**L**) layers of smooth muscle in the muscularis and in the complex of folded mucosa, the lamina propria (**LP**) underlying a simple columnar epithelium (arrows). X140. H&E.

(b) The oviduct mucosa, with folds projecting into the lumen (**L**), has simple columnar epithelium (**E**) on the lamina propria (**LP**). X200. PT.

(c, d) Higher magnification of the epithelium shows two cell types: ciliated cells (**CC**) interspersed with the secretory peg cells (**PC**), which produce the nutritive fluid covering the epithelium. These cells' histologic and functional features vary during the ovarian cycle due to hormonal fluctuations. In **(d)** the peg cells shown are at their most developed and most active state in the period shortly after ovulation when an embryo might be present. c: X400, PT; d: X400, Mallory trichrome.

❯ UTERUS

As shown in Figure 22–14, the uterus is a pear-shaped organ with thick, muscular walls. Its largest part, the **body**, is entered by the left and right uterine tubes and the curved, superior area between the tubes is called the **fundus**. The uterus narrows in the **isthmus** and ends in a lower cylindrical structure, the **cervix**. The lumen of the cervix, the **cervical canal**, has constricted openings at each end: the **internal os** (L. *os*, mouth) opens to the main uterine lumen and the **external os** to the vagina (Figure 22–14).

Supported by the set of ligaments and mesenteries also associated with the ovaries and uterine tubes (Figure 22–1), the uterine wall has three major layers (Figure 22–14):

- An outer connective tissue layer, the **perimetrium**, continuous with the ligaments, which is adventitial in some areas, but largely a serosa covered by mesothelium;
- A thick tunic of highly vascularized smooth muscle, the **myometrium** (Figure 22–16); and
- A mucosa, the **endometrium**, lined by simple columnar epithelium.

These three layers are continuous with their counterparts in the uterine tubes. The thickness and structure of the endometrium is influenced cyclically by the shifting levels of ovarian hormones even more than the mucosa of the uterine tubes (Figure 22–17).

Myometrium

The **myometrium** (Gr. *myo*, muscle + *metra*, uterus), the thickest tunic of the uterus, shows bundles of smooth muscle fibers separated by connective tissue containing venous plexuses and lymphatics (Figure 22–16). The smooth muscle forms interwoven layers, with fibers of the inner and outer layers disposed generally parallel to the long axis of the organ.

During pregnancy, the myometrium goes through a period of extensive growth involving both **hyperplasia** (increasing the number of smooth muscle cells), cell hypertrophy, and increased collagen production by the muscle cells, which strengthens the uterine wall. This well-developed uterine myometrium contracts very forcefully during **parturition** to expel the infant from the uterus. After pregnancy, uterine smooth muscle cells shrink and many undergo apoptosis, with

FIGURE **22–16** Uterus.

(a) The basal layer (**B**) of the endometrium, bordering the myometrium (**M**), contains the basal ends of the uterine glands (**G**) and many small arteries (**A**) embedded in a distinctive connective tissue stroma with many fibroblasts, ground substance and primarily fine type III collagen, but no adipocytes. X100. Mallory trichrome.

(b) Superficial to the basal layer of the endometrium is its functional layer, the part that changes histologically and functionally depending on estrogen levels. This micrograph shows

only the functional layer and includes parts of the long uterine glands (**G**) as well as one spiral artery (**A**). X100. Mallory trichrome.

(c) The surface epithelium (**SE**) lining the endometrium is simple columnar, with many cells having cilia. The underlying stroma (**S**) has an extensive microvasculature, much ground substance, and fibroblastic cells with large, active nuclei. X400. Mallory trichrome.

removal of unneeded collagen, and the uterus returns almost to its prepregnancy size.

Endometrium

The lamina propria or stroma of the **endometrium** contains primarily nonbundled type III collagen fibers with abundant fibroblasts and ground substance. Its simple columnar epithelial lining has both ciliated and secretory cells, and the latter line the numerous tubular **uterine glands** that penetrate the full thickness of the endometrium (Figures 22–16 and 22–18).

The endometrium has two concentric zones:

- The **basal layer** adjacent to the myometrium has a more highly cellular lamina propria and contains the deep basal ends of the uterine glands (Figure 22–16a).
- The superficial **functional layer** has a spongier lamina propria, richer in ground substance, and includes most of the length of the glands, as well as the surface epithelium (Figure 22–16b,c).

The functional layer undergoes profound changes during the menstrual cycles, but the basal layer remains relatively unchanged (Figure 22–17).

The blood vessels supplying the endometrium have special significance in the periodic sloughing of the functional layer during menses. Arcuate arteries in the middle layers of the myometrium send two sets of smaller arteries into the endometrium (Figure 22–18): **straight arteries**, which supply only the basal layer, and long, progesterone-sensitive **spiral arteries**, which extend farther and bring blood throughout the functional layer. Spiral arteries branch with numerous arterioles supplying a rich, superficial capillary bed that includes many dilated, thin-walled **vascular lacunae** drained by venules.

Menstrual Cycle

Throughout the female reproductive system, estrogens and progesterone control growth and differentiation of epithelial cells and associated connective tissue. Even before birth, these cells are influenced by circulating maternal estrogen and progesterone that reach the fetus through the placenta. After menopause, diminished synthesis of these hormones results in a general involution of tissues in the reproductive tract.

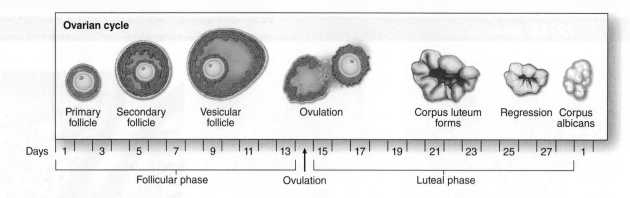

Ovarian cycle

Primary follicle · Secondary follicle · Vesicular follicle · Ovulation · Corpus luteum forms · Regression · Corpus albicans

Days: 1 · 3 · 5 · 7 · 9 · 11 · 13 · 15 · 17 · 19 · 21 · 23 · 25 · 27 · 1

Follicular phase — Ovulation — Luteal phase

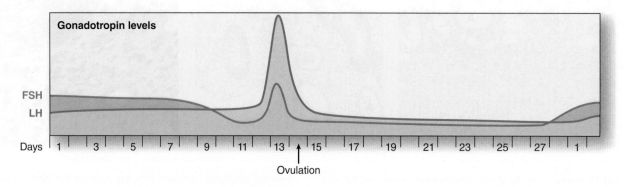

Gonadotropin levels

FSH
LH

Days: 1 · 3 · 5 · 7 · 9 · 11 · 13 · 15 · 17 · 19 · 21 · 23 · 25 · 27 · 1

Ovulation

Ovarian hormone levels

Estrogen
Progesterone

Days: 1 · 3 · 5 · 7 · 9 · 11 · 13 · 15 · 17 · 19 · 21 · 23 · 25 · 27 · 1

Uterine cycle

Menstrual flow

Functional layer
Basal layer

Days: 1 · 3 · 5 · 7 · 9 · 11 · 13 · 15 · 17 · 19 · 21 · 23 · 25 · 27 · 1

Menstrual phase — Proliferative phase — Secretory phase

The cyclic development of **ovarian follicles** and the **corpus luteum**, controlled by the pituitary **gonadotropins** FSH and LH, lead to cyclic shifts in the levels of the major ovarian hormones: steroidal **estrogens and progesterone**. Estrogen stimulates the proliferative phase of the uterine cycle and its level peaks near the day of ovulation, which marks the midpoint of the ovarian cycle. After ovulation the corpus luteum forms and produces both progesterone and estrogens, which together promote growth and development of the endometrial **functional layer.** Unless fertilization and implantation of an embryo occur, regression of the corpus luteum leads to declining levels of the steroid hormones and failure of the new endometrial tissue to be maintained. This tissue sloughs off as the menstrual flow, the first day of which is taken to mark day 1 of both the ovarian cycle and the uterine cycle. The basal layer of endometrium is not sensitive to the loss of progesterone and is retained during menstruation, serving to regenerate the functional layer during the ensuing proliferative phase.

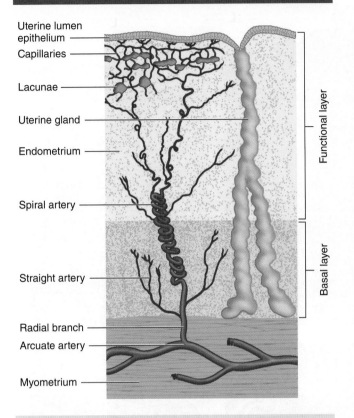

FIGURE 22–18 Arterial supply to the endometrium.

Uterine lumen epithelium
Capillaries
Lacunae
Uterine gland
Endometrium
Spiral artery
Straight artery
Radial branch
Arcuate artery
Myometrium

Functional layer
Basal layer

The **basal and functional layers** of the endometrium are supplied by different sets of small arteries emerging from the uterine arcuate arteries in the myometrium: the **straight arteries** and **spiral arteries**, respectively. The spiral arteries are uniquely sensitive to progesterone, growing rapidly in a spiral fashion as the functional layer thickens under the influence of that luteal steroid and providing blood to a microvasculature that includes many lacunae lined by thin endothelium. This blood supply brings oxygen and nutrients to cells of the functionalis and to an embryo implanting itself into that tissue. If no embryo is present to produce the gonadotropin replacing LH, the corpus luteum undergoes regression 8-10 days after ovulation. The rapid decline in the level of progesterone causes constriction of the spiral arteries and other changes that quickly lead to local ischemia in the functional layer and its separation from the basal layer during menstruation.

›› MEDICAL APPLICATION

Viable endometrial cells frequently undergo menstrual reflux into or through the uterine tubes. In some women this can lead to **endometriosis**, a disorder with pelvic pain due to endometrial tissue growing on the ovaries, oviducts, or elsewhere. Under the influence of estrogen and progesterone, the ectopic tissue grows and degenerates monthly but cannot be removed effectively from the body. In addition to pain endometriosis can produce inflammation, ovarian cysts, adhesions, and scar tissue that can cause infertility.

From puberty until menopause at about age 45 to 50, pituitary gonadotropins produce cyclic changes in ovarian hormone levels, which cause the endometrium to undergo cyclic modifications during the menstrual cycle (Figures 22–17 and 22–19). The duration of the menstrual cycle may be variable but averages 28 days. Because menstrual cycles are a consequence of ovarian follicle changes related to oocyte production, a woman is fertile only during the years when she is having menstrual cycles.

Day 1 of the menstrual cycle is usually taken as the day when menstrual bleeding appears. The menstrual discharge consists of degenerating endometrium mixed with blood from its ruptured microvasculature. The **menstrual period** lasts 3 to 4 days on average. The next phase of the cycle, the **proliferative phase**, is of variable length, 8 to 10 days on average, and the **secretory phase** begins at ovulation and lasts about 14 days (Figure 22–17). The cyclic structural changes occur gradually and the activities characterizing these phases overlap to some extent.

Proliferative Phase

After the menstrual phase, the uterine mucosa is relatively thin (~0.5 mm). The beginning of the **proliferative phase**, also called the **follicular** or **estrogenic phase**, coincides with the rapid growth of a small group of ovarian follicles growing as vesicular follicles. With development of their thecae interna, these follicles actively secrete estrogen and increase its plasma concentrations (Figure 22–17).

Estrogens act on the endometrium, inducing regeneration of the functional layer lost during menstruation. Cells in the basal ends of glands proliferate, migrate, and form the new epithelial covering over the surface exposed during menstruation. During the proliferative phase, the endometrial lining is a simple columnar surface epithelium and the uterine glands are relatively straight tubules with narrow, nearly empty lumens (Figure 22–19a,d). Mitotic figures can be found among both the epithelial cells and fibroblasts. Spiral arteries lengthen as the functional layer is reestablished and grows (Figure 22–16) and extensive microvasculature forms near the surface of the functional layer. At the end of the proliferative phase, the endometrium is 2 to 3 mm thick.

Secretory Phase

After ovulation, the **secretory** or **luteal phase** starts as a result of the progesterone secreted by the corpus luteum. Progesterone stimulates epithelial cells of the uterine glands that formed during the proliferative phase and these cells begin to secrete and accumulate glycogen, dilating the glandular lumens and causing the glands to become coiled (Figure 22–19b,e). The superficial microvasculature now includes thin-walled, blood-filled lacunae (Figures 22–18 and 22–19e). The endometrium reaches its maximum thickness (5 mm) during the secretory phase as a result of the accumulation of secretions and edema in the stroma.

If fertilization occurred during the day after ovulation, the embryo has been transported to the uterus by about

FIGURE **22–19** Proliferative, secretory, and premenstrual phases in the uterus.

The major phases of the uterine cycle overlap but produce distinctly different and characteristic changes in the functional layer (**F**) closest to the lumen (**L**) with little effect on the basal layer (**B**) and myometrium (**M**). Characteristic features of each phase include the following. During most of the proliferative phase (**a, d**), the functional layer is still relatively thin, the stroma is more cellular, and the glands (**G**) are relatively straight, narrow, and empty.

In the secretory phase (**b, e**) the functional layer is less heavily cellular and perhaps four times thicker than the basal layer. The tubular glands have wider lumens containing

secretory product and coil tightly up through the stroma, giving a zigzag or folded appearance histologically. Superficially in the functional layer, lacunae (**La**) are widespread and filled with blood.

The short premenstrual phase (**c, f**) begins with constriction of the spiral arteries, which produces hypoxia that causes swelling and dissolution of the glands (**G**). The stroma of the peripheral functionalis is more compact and that near the basal layer typically appears more sponge-like during this time of blood stasis, apoptosis, and breakdown of the stromal matrix. a: X20; b and c: X12; d, e, and f: X50. All H&E.

TABLE 22–1	Summary of events of the menstrual cycle.			
	Stage of Cycle			
	Proliferative	**Secretory or Luteal**		**Menstrual**
Main actions of pituitary hormones	Follicle-stimulating hormone stimulates rapid growth of ovarian follicles	Peak of luteinizing hormone at the beginning of secretory stage, secreted after estrogen stimulation, induces ovulation and development of the corpus luteum		
Main events in the ovary	Growth of ovarian follicles; dominant follicle reaches preovulatory stage	Ovulation	Development of the corpus luteum	Degeneration of the corpus luteum
Dominant ovarian hormone	Estrogens, produced by the growing follicles, act on vagina, tubes, and uterus	Progesterone, produced by the corpus luteum, acts mainly on the uterus	Progesterone production ceases	
Main events in the endometrium	Growth of the mucosa after menstruation	Further growth of the mucosa, coiling of glands, secretion		Shedding of part of the mucosa about 14 days after ovulation

5 days later and now attaches to the uterine epithelium when the endometrial thickness and secretory activity are optimal for embryonic implantation and nutrition. The major nutrient source for the embryo before and during implantation is the uterine secretion. In addition to promoting this secretion, progesterone inhibits strong contractions of the myometrium that might interfere with embryo implantation.

Menstrual Phase

When fertilization of the oocyte and embryonic implantation do not occur, the corpus luteum regresses and circulating levels of progesterone and estrogens begin to decrease 8 to 10 days after ovulation, causing the onset of menstruation (Figure 22–17). The drop-off in progesterone produces (1) spasms of muscle contraction in the small spiral arteries of the functional layer, interrupting normal blood flow, and (2) increased synthesis by arterial cells of prostaglandins, which produce strong vasoconstriction and local hypoxia. Cells undergoing hypoxic injury release cytokines that increase vascular permeability and immigration of leukocytes. The leukocytes release collagenase and several other matrix metalloproteinases (MMPs) that degrade basement membranes and other ECM components (Figure 22–19c,f).

The basal layer of the endometrium, not dependent on the progesterone-sensitive spiral arteries, is relatively unaffected by these activities. However, major portions of the functional layer, including the surface epithelium, most of each gland, the stroma and blood-filled lacunae, detach from the endometrium and slough away as the menstrual flow or **menses**. Arterial constriction normally limits blood loss during menstruation, but some blood does emerge from the open ends of venules. The amount of endometrium and blood lost in menstruation varies among women and in the same woman at different times.

At the end of the menstrual phase, the endometrium is usually reduced to a thin layer and is ready to begin a new cycle as its cells begin dividing to reconstitute the mucosa. Table 22–1 summarizes the main events of the menstrual cycle.

› EMBRYONIC IMPLANTATION, DECIDUA, & THE PLACENTA

The zygote produced by fertilization undergoes mitotic cleavages as it is moved toward the uterus, with its cells called **blastomeres** (Gr. *blastos*, germ + *meros*, part) in a compact aggregate called the **morula** (L. *morum*, mulberry). No growth occurs during the period of cell cleavage, with blastomeres becoming smaller at each division, and the morula is about the same size as the oocyte at fertilization.

About 5 days after fertilization the embryo reaches the uterine cavity, by which time blastomeres have moved to form a central cavity in the morula and the embryo enters the **blastocyst** stage of development. The blastomeres then arrange themselves as a peripheral layer called the **trophoblast** around the cavity, while a few cells just inside this layer make up the **embryoblast** or **inner cell mass** (Figure 22–20). The blastocyst remains in the lumen of the uterus for about 2 days, immersed in the endometrial glands' secretion on the mucosa.

Implantation, or nidation, involves attachment of the blastocyst to the surface epithelial cells of the endometrium and its proteolytic penetration through this epithelium into the underlying stroma (Figure 22–20), a process that lasts about 3 days. Cells of the trophoblast drive the events of implantation, during which time cells of the embryoblast rearrange around

FIGURE **22–20** Embryo implantation.

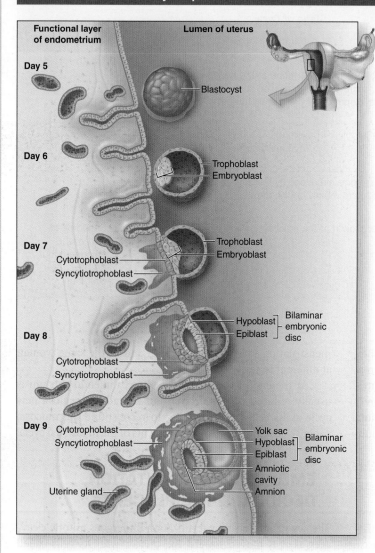

Functional layer of endometrium

Lumen of uterus

Day 5 — Blastocyst

Day 6 — Trophoblast / Embryoblast

Day 7 — Trophoblast / Embryoblast; Cytotrophoblast / Syncytiotrophoblast

Day 8 — Hypoblast / Epiblast — Bilaminar embryonic disc; Cytotrophoblast / Syncytiotrophoblast

Day 9 — Cytotrophoblast / Syncytiotrophoblast; Yolk sac / Hypoblast / Epiblast — Bilaminar embryonic disc; Amniotic cavity / Amnion; Uterine gland

The embryo enters the uterus as a blastocyst about 5 days after ovulation or fertilization, when the uterus is in the secretory phase and best prepared for implantation. To begin implantation, receptors on cells of the outer embryonic trophoblast bind glycoprotein ligands on the endometrial epithelium. The trophoblast forms an invasive, outer syncytial layer called the **syncytiotrophoblast**. Proteases are activated and/or released locally to digest stroma components, which allows the developing embryo to embed itself within the stroma. The newly implanted embryo absorbs nutrients and oxygen from the endometrial tissue and blood in the lacunae.

two new cavities, the **amnion** and the **yolk sac**. Where the cells lining these cavities make contact, the **bilaminar embryonic disc** develops with its **epiblast** layer continuous with the amnion and its **hypoblast** layer continuous with the yolk sac (Figure 22–20).

All parts of the embryo develop from this early embryonic disc. The yolk sac and amnion form extraembryonic structures, but only the latter persists throughout pregnancy. As shown in Figure 22–20, the trophoblast differentiates during implantation into the following:

- The **cytotrophoblast**, a layer of mitotically active cells immediately around the amnion and yolk sac; and
- The **syncytiotrophoblast**, a more superficial, nonmitotic mass of multinucleated cytoplasm which invades the surrounding stroma.

By about the ninth day after ovulation, the embryo is totally implanted in the endometrium and derives nutrients

primarily from blood there. Cytotrophoblast cells synthesize anti-inflammatory cytokines to prevent an adverse uterine reaction to the implanted embryo and these are supplemented later by various embryonic factors that produce local immune tolerance for the embryo throughout the pregnancy.

The endometrial stroma undergoes histologic changes in the period following implantation. Fibroblasts become enlarged, polygonal, more active in protein synthesis, and are now called **decidual cells**. The whole endometrium is now called the **decidua** (L. *deciduus*, falling off, shedding) and includes three areas (Figure 22–21):

- The **decidua basalis** between the implanted embryo and the myometrium;
- The **decidua capsularis**, the region between the embryo and the uterine lumen which thins as the embryo gets larger; and
- The **decidua parietalis**, on the side of the uterus away from the embryo.

FIGURE **22–21** Extraembryonic membranes, decidua and placenta.

(a)

(b)

Chorion
Amnion

Placenta
Myometrium
Decidua basalis
Chorionic villi
Yolk sac
Decidua capsularis
Decidua parietalis
Chorionic cavity
(extraembryonic celom)
Uterine cavity

Cervical mucous plug

Umbilical cord

Maternal artery
Maternal vein

Maternal blood

Umbilical vein
Umbilical arteries

Umbilical vein
(carries oxygenated
blood to embryo)

Umbilical artery
(carries deoxygenated
blood to placenta)

(c)

(a) The membranous extraembryonic **amnion, chorion**, and **yolk sac** appear during the second week of development, with the embryonic disc between the amnion and yolk sac.

(b) After implantation the endometrium changes histologically and is called the **decidua**. It develops three different regions: **decidua basalis, capsularis**, and **parietalis**. **Chorionic villi** develop most profusely in the decidua basalis, which becomes the major portion of the **placenta**.

(c) Each of the many **chorionic stem villi** in the placenta contains a branch of the umbilical artery and vein, which form loops of microvasculature into smaller villus branches. The entire stem villus is bathed in maternal blood circulated by endometrial arteries and veins.

›› MEDICAL APPLICATION

The initial attachment of the embryo usually occurs on the ventral or dorsal walls of the body of the uterus. Sometimes the embryo attaches close to the internal os. In this case the placenta will be interposed between the fetus and the vagina, obstructing the passage of the fetus at parturition. This situation, called **placenta previa**, must be recognized by the physician, and the fetus must be delivered by cesarean section. Otherwise, obstructed parturition can lead to death of the fetus.

The **placenta** is the site of exchange for nutrients, wastes, O_2, and CO_2 between the mother and the fetus and contains tissues from both individuals. The embryonic part is the **chorion**, derived from the trophoblast and the maternal part is from the decidua basalis. Exchange occurs between embryonic blood in chorionic villi outside the embryo and maternal blood in lacunae of the decidua basalis. Chorionic villi of the developing placenta go through three stages:

- **Primary villi** appear 2 days after implantation as simple cords of proliferating cytotrophoblast cells covered by syncytiotrophoblast extend into lacunae containing maternal blood.
- **Secondary villi** begin to form on about the 15th day of embryonic development as the primary villi are invaded by extraembryonic mesenchyme.
- **Tertiary villi** develop within a few more days as mesenchyme in the secondary villi differentiates to form capillary loops continuous with the embryonic circulatory system.

By the end of the first month of the pregnancy, the placenta contains thousands of tertiary chorionic villi, each branching many times and each branch having one or more capillary loops (Figure 22–21c). Suspended in pools of maternal blood in the decidua, the chorionic villi provide an enormous surface area for metabolite exchange (Figure 22–22). Exchange of gases, nutrients, and wastes occurs between fetal blood in the capillaries and maternal blood bathing the villi, with diffusion occurring across the trophoblast layer and the capillary endothelium.

The placenta is also an endocrine organ, producing HCG, a lactogen, relaxin, and various growth factors, in addition to estrogen and progesterone. More detailed information on the developing embryo and placenta should be sought in embryology textbooks.

› CERVIX

As noted earlier the **cervix** is the lower, cylindrical part of the uterus (see Figure 22–1). The cervix differs histologically from the rest of the uterus. The **endocervical mucosa** is a simple columnar epithelium on a thick lamina propria, with many large, branched, mucus-secreting **cervical glands**. It lacks

---

FIGURE 22–22 Term placenta.

The placenta contains chorionic villi of the fetus and maternal blood pooled in the decidua. **(a)** A full-term placenta has many villus stems, containing arteries (**A**) and (**V**) of the extraembryonic vasculature, and hundreds of smaller villus branches (**arrows**) that contain connective tissue and microvasculature. Maternal blood (**MB**) fills the space around the villi. X50. H&E.

(b) Higher magnification of villus branches surrounded by maternal blood (**MB**) each containing capillaries (**C**) or sinusoids (**S**) with fetal blood. By the end of pregnancy cytotrophoblast cells have greatly decreased in number in many areas, leaving only a thin syncytiotrophoblast and basement membrane covering the villus in these regions (**arrows**). The extraembryonic blood vessels become closely associated with these areas of thin trophoblast for maximal diffusion of material between the two pools of blood. X400. H&E.

spiral arteries, does not change its 2-3 mm thickness during the ovarian cycle, and is not shed during menstruation.

The cervical region around the external os projects slightly into the upper vagina and is covered by the **exocervical mucosa** with nonkeratinized stratified squamous epithelium continuous with that of the vagina. The junction between this squamous epithelium and the mucus-secreting columnar epithelium of the endocervix occurs in the **transformation zone**, an area just outside the external os that shifts slightly with the cyclical changes in uterine size (Figure 22–23). Periodic exposure of the squamous-columnar junction to the vaginal environment can stimulate reprogramming of epithelial stem cells, which occasionally leads to intraepithelial neoplasia at that site.

Under the influence of progesterone, the consistency of **cervical mucus** changes cyclically and plays a significant role in fertilization and early pregnancy. At ovulation, mucous secretion is abundant and watery, facilitating sperm movements into the uterus. In the luteal phase mucus is more viscous and hinders the passage of sperm. During pregnancy, the cervical glands proliferate and secrete highly viscous mucus that forms a plug in the cervical canal (Figure 22–21b).

The deeper wall of the cervix consists mainly of dense connective tissue, with much less smooth muscle than the rest of the uterus (Figure 22–23). The cervix becomes relatively rigid during pregnancy and helps retain the fetus in the uterus. Before parturition a process of **cervical effacement** occurs in which its connective tissue undergoes extensive remodeling and significant collagen removal, mediated in part by macrophages. As a result the cervix softens, the cervical canal dilates, and birth occurs more easily.

>> **MEDICAL APPLICATION**

The incidence of **cervical cancer** worldwide has been greatly reduced by widespread, routine screening by **exfoliative cytology** to examine for dysplasia of the cervical epithelium (Figure 22-23c). The test called the **Pap smear** after its developer George Papanicolaou, who introduced this diagnostic technique in the 1920s, uses cells that have been lightly scraped from cervix. Abnormal cells suggestive of precancerous changes in the epithelium are then detected microscopically. The epithelial dysplasia that precedes **squamous cell neoplasia**, the most common type of cervical cancer, occurs in metaplastic cells of the transformation zone at a mean age of 54 years. The **human papillomas virus** (HPV) is strongly implicated in the pathogenesis of this cancer.

❯ VAGINA

The wall of the **vagina** (L., *vagina*, sheath, scabbard) lacks glands and consists of a **mucosa**, a **muscular layer**, and an **adventitia**.

The epithelium of the vaginal mucosa is stratified squamous, with a thickness of 150-200 μm in adults (Figure 22–24). Stimulated by estrogens, the epithelial cells synthesize and accumulate glycogen. When the cells desquamate, bacteria metabolize glycogen to lactic acid, causing a relatively low pH within the vagina, which helps provide protection against pathogenic microorganisms. The lamina propria of the mucosa is rich in elastic fibers, with numerous narrow papillae projecting into the overlying epithelium (Figure 22–24). The mucosa normally contains lymphocytes and neutrophils in relatively large quantities.

Mucus in the vagina is produced by the cervical glands. During sexual arousal lubricating mucus is also provided by glands at the vaginal vestibule, including the paired **greater vestibular glands** (of Bartholin), which are homologous to the male bulbourethral glands.

The muscular layer of the vagina is composed mainly of two indistinct layers of smooth muscle, disposed as circular bundles next to the mucosa and as thicker longitudinal bundles near the adventitial layer (Figure 22–24). The dense connective tissue of the adventitia is rich in elastic fibers, making the vaginal wall strong and elastic while binding it the surrounding tissues. This outer layer also contains an extensive venous plexus, lymphatics, and nerves.

>> **MEDICAL APPLICATION**

Atrophic vaginitis involves thinning or atrophy of the vaginal epithelium caused by diminished estrogen levels and occurs most often in postmenopausal woman. This change allows the more frequent inflammation and infections characteristic of this condition. Primary **squamous cell carcinoma** of the vagina occurs rarely, with most vaginal malignancies having spread secondarily from the cervix or vulva.

❯ EXTERNAL GENITALIA

The female **external genitalia**, or **vulva**, include several structures, all covered by stratified squamous epithelium:

- The **vestibule**, a space whose wall includes the tubulo-acinar vestibular glands;
- The paired **labia minora**, folds of skin lacking hair follicles but with numerous sebaceous glands;
- The paired **labia majora**, homologous and histologically similar to the skin of the scrotum; and
- The **clitoris**, an erectile structure homologous to the penis with paired corpora cavernosa.

The mucosa of these structures, abundantly supplied with sensory nerves and tactile receptors also found in skin (see Chapter 18), is important in the physiology of sexual arousal.

FIGURE **22–23** Cervix.

(a) The mucosa of the cervical canal (**CC**) is continuous with the endometrium and like that tissue is lined by simple columnar epithelium (**SC**). This endocervical mucosa includes many large branched cervical mucous glands (**arrows**). At the external os, the point at which the cervical canal opens into the vagina (**V**), there is an abrupt junction (**J**) between the columnar epithelium and the stratified squamous epithelium (**SS**) covering the exocervix and vagina. Deeper, the cervical wall is primarily fibromuscular tissue (**F**). X15. H&E.

(b) The epithelial junction (**arrow**) is seen more clearly. X50. H&E.

(c) Exfoliative cytology of epithelial cells from the exocervical mucosa in a routine cervical smear. The squamous cells,

stained on a slide by the Papanicolaou procedure using hematoxylin, orange G, and eosin, stain differently according to their content of keratins. Cells with atypical nuclei or other abnormalities can be detected by this method that is used routinely to check for cervical carcinoma. X200. Papanicolaou stain.

(d) The endocervical mucosa is exposed to a relatively high population of microorganisms and normally has a large number of neutrophils and other leukocytes. Such cells occur in the lamina propria and epithelium (**arrows**), but they are also numerous and readily apparent in the layer of mucus (**M**) that was fixed in place here. X400. H&E.

❯ MAMMARY GLANDS

The **mammary glands** of the breasts develop embryologically as invaginations of surface ectoderm along two ventral lines, the milk lines, from the axillae to the groin. In humans one set of glands resembling highly modified apocrine sweat

glands persists on each side of the chest. Each mammary gland consists of 15-25 **lobes** of the compound tubuloalveolar type whose function is to secrete nutritive milk for newborns. Each lobe, separated from the others by dense connective tissue with much adipose tissue, is a separate gland with its own excretory **lactiferous duct** (Figure 22–25). These ducts, each 2-4.5 cm

FIGURE 22–24 Vagina.

The vagina has mucosal, muscular, and adventitial layers. **(a)** The lamina propria (**L**) is highly cellular and extends narrow papillae into the thick, nonkeratinized stratified squamous epithelium (**E**). The muscular layer (**M**) has bundles of smooth muscle arranged in a circular manner near the mucosa and longitudinally near the adventitia. X60. H&E.

(b) Higher magnification of the epithelium and lamina propria (**LP**) shows invasion of leukocytes (**arrows**) between epithelial cells from the connective tissue. X200. PSH.

long, emerge independently in the **nipple**, which has 15 to 25 pore-like openings, each about 0.5 mm in diameter. The histologic structure of the mammary glands varies according to sex, age, and physiologic status.

Breast Development During Puberty

Before puberty, the mammary glands in both sexes are composed only of **lactiferous sinuses** near the nipple, with very small, branching ducts emerging from these sinuses. In girls undergoing puberty, higher levels of circulating estrogens cause the breasts to grow as a result of adipocyte accumulation and elongation of the duct system.

In nonpregnant adult women each mammary gland lobe consists of many **lobules**, sometimes called **terminal duct lobular units** (**TDLU**). Each lobule has several small, branching ducts, but the attached secretory units are small and rudimentary (Figure 22–25). Lactiferous sinuses are lined with stratified cuboidal epithelium, and the lining of the lactiferous ducts and terminal ducts is simple cuboidal epithelium covered by closely packed myoepithelial cells. Sparse fibers of smooth muscle also encircle the larger ducts. The duct system is embedded in loose, vascular connective tissue, and a denser, less cellular connective tissue separates the lobes. In the premenstrual phase of the reproductive cycle connective tissue of

the breast becomes somewhat edematous, making the breasts slightly larger.

The **areola**, or skin covering the nipple, is thin skin with sebaceous glands and abundant sensory nerves, continuous with the mucosa of the lactiferous sinuses. The areola contains more melanin than skin elsewhere on the breast and darkens further during pregnancy. Connective tissue of the nipple is rich in smooth muscle fibers that run parallel to the lactiferous sinuses and produce nipple erection when they contract.

Breasts During Pregnancy & Lactation

The mammary glands undergo growth during pregnancy as a result of the synergistic action of several hormones, mainly estrogen, progesterone, prolactin, and the placental lactogen. These cause cell proliferation in secretory **alveoli** at the ends of the intralobular ducts (Figures 22–25 and 22–26). The spherical alveoli are composed of cuboidal epithelium, with stellate myoepithelial cells between the secretory cells and the basal lamina. The degree of glandular development varies among lobules and even within a single lobule.

While the alveoli and duct system grow and develop during pregnancy in preparation for lactation, the stroma becomes less prominent (Figures 22–26 and 22–27). The loose connective tissue within lobules is infiltrated by lymphocytes and plasma cells, the latter becoming more numerous late in pregnancy.

FIGURE **22–25** Mammary gland.

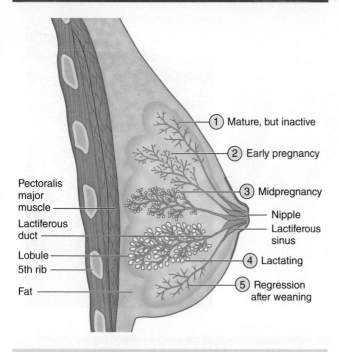

1 Mature, but inactive
2 Early pregnancy
3 Midpregnancy
Nipple
Lactiferous sinus
4 Lactating
5 Regression after weaning

Pectoralis major muscle
Lactiferous duct
Lobule
5th rib
Fat

Shown here is the sequence of changes that occur in the alveolar secretory units and duct system of mammary glands before, during, and after pregnancy and lactation. (**1**) Before pregnancy, the gland is inactive, with small ducts and only a few small secretory alveoli. (**2**) Alveoli develop and begin to grow early in a pregnancy. (**3**) By midpregnancy, the alveoli and ducts have become large and have dilated lumens. (**4**) At parturition and during the time of lactation, the alveoli are greatly dilated and maximally active in production of milk components. (**5**) After weaning, the alveoli and ducts regress with apoptotic cell death.

Late in pregnancy the glandular alveoli and ducts are dilated by an accumulation of **colostrum**, a fluid rich in proteins and containing leukocytes, that is produced under the influence of prolactin. Immunoglobulin A (IgA) antibodies are synthesized abundantly by plasma cells and transferred into colostrum, from which passive acquired immunity is conferred on the breast-fed newborn.

Following parturition, the alveoli of mammary glands start active milk production, or **lactation**, stimulated primarily by prolactin from the anterior pituitary (see Chapter 20). Epithelial cells of the alveoli enlarge and activate various processes involved in lactation:

- Large amounts of **protein** are synthesized, packaged into secretory vesicles, and undergo **merocrine secretion** into the lumen (Figure 22–28). Human milk contains about 1 g of protein per deciliter, including aggregated caseins (44% of the total protein), as well as soluble

β-lactoglobulin and α-lactalbumin, all of which are a source of amino acids by the infant. Less abundant proteins in milk include many factors that assist digestion, several such as lactoferrin with antimicrobial activity, and various mitogenic growth factors important for gut development in the newborn.

- **Lipid droplets** form initially from short-chain fatty acids synthesized in the epithelial cells and grow by accretion of longer fatty acids and cholesterol originating from the diet or fat stores. They eventually undergo **apocrine secretion**, during which the droplets become enveloped with a portion of the apical cell membrane (see Figure 22–28). Milk contains 4 or 5 g of total fat per deciliter.

- **Lactose**, the major carbohydrate and energy source in milk, is synthesized in the Golgi apparatus and secreted with lactalbumin. Human milk contains over 7 g of lactose per deciliter, more than the combined total of proteins and lipids. Lactose is also responsible for generating the osmotic gradient that draws water and Ca^{2+} into the alveolar lumen.

Throughout lactation, secretion of proteins, membrane-bound lipid droplets, lactose, iron, and calcium is ongoing, with the products accumulating as milk in the lumens of the duct system (Figure 22–27).

Postlactational Regression in the Mammary Glands

When breast-feeding is stopped (weaning), most alveoli that developed during pregnancy and lactation degenerate. Epithelial cells undergo apoptosis, autophagy, or sloughing (Figure 22–29), with dead cells and debris removed by macrophages. The duct system of the gland returns to its general appearance in the inactive state (Figure 22–25). After menopause, alveoli and ducts of the mammary glands are reduced further in size and there is loss of fibroblasts, collagen, and elastic fibers in the stroma.

FIGURE **22–26** Alveolar development in the breast during pregnancy.

(a) The mammary glands of adult, nonpregnant women are inactive, with small ducts and few lobules (**L**) having secretory alveoli which are not well-developed. The structure with the large lumen in each lobule is part of the duct; the smaller structures are the small, undeveloped alveoli. The breasts are composed largely of connective tissue (**CT**), having considerable fat.

(b) The glands become active during pregnancy, with the duct system growing rapidly and the secretory units of each lobule

becoming much larger and more extensively branched. In this micrograph adipocytes (**A**) are included, but these are only a small fraction of those present.

(c) During lactation, the lobules are greatly enlarged and the lumens of both the numerous glandular alveoli (**A**) and the excretory ducts (**D**) are filled with milk. The intralobular connective tissue is more sparse and difficult to see, except for small septa (arrows). All X60, H&E.

›› MEDICAL APPLICATION

Breast cancer is almost always derived from epithelial cells in the terminal lobules of the glands. The most common form is invasive **ductal carcinoma** in which neoplastic cells of intralobular ducts or small branches of lactiferous ducts invade the surrounding stroma, forming a fixed, palpable mass. Cell spreading (or metastasizing) from the carcinoma via the circulatory or lymphatic vessels to critical organs such as the lungs or brain is responsible for the mortality associated with breast cancer. If the treatment is **mastectomy**, axillary lymph nodes are usually

also removed surgically and examined histologically for the presence of metastatic mammary carcinoma cells. Early detection (eg, through self-examination, mammography, ultrasound, and other techniques) and consequent early treatment have significantly reduced the mortality rate.

Bacterial infection of a mammary gland, or acute mastitis, may occur in the lactating or involuting breast, usually after obstruction by milk left within small components of the duct system.

FIGURE **22–27** Actively developing and lactating alveoli.

Glandular alveoli develop completely only during pregnancy and begin milk production near the end of pregnancy. **(a)** Alveoli (**A**) develop as spherical structures composed of cuboidal epithelial cells surrounded by the contractile processes of myoepithelial cells (**M**). Development occurs at different rates throughout the breast. Late in pregnancy lymphocytes (**L**) leave venules (**V**), accumulate in the intralobular connective tissue, and differentiate as plasma cells (**P**) secreting IgA. Intralobular ducts (**D**) are lined by epithelium containing secretory cells,

nonsecretory cells, and plasma cells; larger lumens may show milk (**arrow**). X400. H&E.

(b) Secretory cells of the lactating gland are more columnar and contain variously sized lipid droplets, which are also visible in the milk (**LD**). Connective tissue (**CT**) contains small blood vessels (**V**). Secretory cells in the enclosed area are shown diagrammatically in Figure 22–28. X400. PT.

FIGURE **22–28** Secretion in the mammary gland.

Alveolar cells of the lactating mammary gland are highly active in protein synthesis and lipid synthesis. Most proteins are packaged into secretory vesicles in the Golgi apparatus and secreted at the apical end of the cells by typical exocytosis or merocrine secretion. Lipids coalesce as free cytoplasmic droplets and eventually undergo apocrine secretion, in which they are extruded from the cell along with a portion of the apical cell membrane (and often a small amount of attached cytoplasm.) Both types of secretion are shown here in a sequence moving from left to right.

FIGURE 22–29 Apoptosis during postlactational mammary gland regression.

After weaning, all glandular alveoli of the breast regress, as shown in this plastic section of a single alveolus. The secretory cells have undergone autophagy and are now squamous. Many apoptotic cells have sloughed into the lumen. Milk with lipid droplets is also still present there. The dead cells and other tissue debris are removed by invading macrophages. X400. PT.

The Female Reproductive System SUMMARY OF KEY POINTS

Ovaries, Follicles and Oocytes

- The female gonads, the paired **ovaries**, each have an outer **cortex** containing many hundreds of **ovarian follicles** and an inner **medulla** of dense connective tissue and large blood vessels.
- The ovary's cortex is covered by a cuboidal mesothelium, the **surface epithelium** (or germinal epithelium) that overlies a layer of connective tissue, the **tunica albuginea**.
- Before puberty all follicles are **primordial follicles**, formed in the developing fetal gonad, with each having one **primary oocyte** arrested in **meiotic prophase I** and a surrounding layer of squamous **follicular epithelial cells**.
- After puberty some primordial follicles develop each month as growing **primary follicles**, with an enlarging primary oocyte surrounded by larger epithelial cells now called **granulosa cells**.
- During follicular growth the **granulosa cells**, surrounded by a basement membrane, become stratified and actively engage in fluid secretion and steroid hormone metabolism.
- Between the oocyte and the granulosa cells a thin layer forms called the **zona pellucida**, which contains glycoproteins (**ZO proteins**) to which the sperm surface must bind to reach the oocyte at fertilization.
- **Antral** or **vesicular follicles** are larger and have developed fluid-filled spaces among their granulosa cells, but the growing oocyte is still in prophase I.
- While the primary follicle grows, mesenchymal cells immediately around it form the highly vascular layer, the **theca interna**, and a more fibrous **theca externa**, with smooth muscle cells.
- Endocrine cells of the **theca interna** secrete both **progesterone** and estrogen precursors, which are converted by **granulosa cells** into **estrogen**.
- Antral follicles continue developing as **mature, graafian follicles**, which have a large antrum filled with fluid, with the large primary oocyte enclosed by granulosa cells of the **cumulus oophorus**.

- Each month only one graafian follicle becomes a **dominant follicle** and undergoes **ovulation**; most other developing follicles arrest and degenerate with apoptosis in a process called **atresia**.

Ovulation and the Corpus Luteum

- **Ovulation** involves movement of a very large, dominant graafian follicle to the ovary surface to form a bulge, completion of meiosis I, and release of a **polar body** from the oocyte.
- Rupture of the follicle and ovarian coverings releases the **secondary oocyte**, arrested now in **metaphase II**, and a layer of attached granulosa cells that make up the **corona radiata**.
- Cells of the granulosa and thecal layers left in the ovary after ovulation are reorganized under the influence of **luteinizing hormone** (**LH**) to form the endocrine gland called the **corpus luteum**.
- The cells of the **corpus luteum** are **granulosa lutein cells**, producing estrogen and comprising 80% of the gland, and **theca lutein cells** producing progesterone.
- LH levels drop about 2 weeks after ovulation, causing the **corpus luteum** to lose activity, degenerate, and be removed by macrophages, leaving a temporary collagen-filled region called a **corpus albicans**.

Uterine Tubes or Oviducts

- The **ovulated secondary oocyte** is swept into the large open **infundibulum** of the **uterine tube**, or **oviduct**, and enters that organ's **ampulla** region where it degenerates if it is not fertilized.
- **Fertilization** involves **sperm capacitation** in the oviduct, **acrosomal activation** and sperm penetration of the corona radiata, and the following events at the oocyte surface:
  - Surface ligands on one sperm first attach to ZO proteins around the oocyte, allowing penetration.
  - **Cortical granules** of the oocyte undergo exocytosis, releasing proteases that convert the zona pellucida to the **vitelline barrier** which prevents **polyspermic fertilization**.
  - The oocyte completes meiosis II, producing the second **polar body** and the female pronucleus of the haploid **ovum**.

- The **female pronucleus** and the **male pronucleus** from the sperm fuse, yielding a diploid cell, the **zygote**.
- The **oviduct mucosa** is **highly folded** in the ampulla region and lined by a **simple columnar epithelium** of **ciliated cells** and **secretory cells** producing nutritive mucus that bathes the sperm (and zygote).
- The thick oviduct **muscularis**, organized for peristaltic contractions of the tube, is mainly responsible for moving the developing embryo to the **uterus**.

Uterus

- The **uterine mucosa** or **endometrium** is lined by **simple columnar epithelium**, from which numerous large **uterine glands** extend into underlying connective tissue.
- This connective tissue is vascular, lacks fat, and consists of a highly cellular **basal layer** next to the uterine muscularis or **myometrium**, and a more superficial **functional layer**.
- Changing levels of estrogen and progesterone from the **ovarian follicles** and **corpus luteum** produce cyclic changes in the thickness, glandular activity, and vascular status of the endometrial **functional layer**.
- A **blastocyst** stage embryo arriving in the uterus attaches to the endometrial surface and implants itself into the **functional layer** when that layer's secretory activity and vascular supply are maximal.
- If no embryo implants, degeneration of the **corpus luteum** causes collapse of the progesterone-dependent **spiral arteries** that bring blood to the **functional layer**.

- Spiral artery degeneration produces ischemia in the **functional layer**, causing this layer to be sloughed off during **menses**, after which it regenerates from the **basal layer** under the influence of estrogen.
- The **placenta** consists mainly of **chorionic villi**, which form as highly vascularized projections of the extraembryonic **trophoblast** into the **vascular lacunae** of the endometrium.
- **Placental exchange** of nutrients, wastes, O_2, and CO_2 occurs between **fetal blood** in the **chorionic villi** and **maternal blood** bathing the villi in the **lacunae**.

Cervix, Vagina, and Mammary Glands

- The mucosa of the narrow, inferior end of the uterus, the **cervix**, does not change cyclically under hormone influence; at its **external os** columnar epithelium changes abruptly to stratified squamous.
- The mucosa of the **vagina** is lined by **stratified squamous epithelium**, surrounded by a muscularis.
- In the **mammary glands**, **alveolar secretory units** develop after puberty on a branching duct system with **lactiferous sinuses** converging at the **nipple**.
- **Milk secretion** (lactation), which begins in late pregnancy and continues until weaning, involves both protein exocytosis and apocrine secretion of lipid droplets.

Information about the external world is conveyed to the central nervous system (CNS) from **sensory receptors**. Chemoreceptive cells for the senses of taste and smell were discussed with the digestive and respiratory system (see Chapters 15 and 17, respectively) and the various mechanoreceptors that mediate the sense of touch were presented with the skin (see Chapter 18). This chapter describes the eye, both its photoreceptors and auxiliary structures, and the ear which mediates the senses of equilibrium and hearing via mechanoreceptors in the vestibulocochlear apparatus.

› EYES: THE PHOTORECEPTOR SYSTEM

Eyes (Figure 23–1) are highly developed photosensitive organs for analyzing the form, intensity, and color of light reflected from objects and providing the sense of sight. Protected within the orbits of the skull which also contain adipose cushions, each eyeball consists externally of a tough, fibrous globe that maintains its overall shape. Internally the eye contains transparent tissues that refract light to focus the image, a layer of photosensitive cells, and a system of neurons that collect, process, and transmit visual information to the brain.

Each eye is composed of three concentric tunics or layers (Table 23–1):

- A tough external **fibrous layer** consisting of the **sclera** and the transparent **cornea**;
- A middle **vascular layer** that includes the **choroid, ciliary body**, and **iris**; and
- An inner sensory layer, the **retina**, which communicates with the cerebrum through the posterior **optic nerve** (Figure 23–1).

Not part of these layers, the **lens** is a perfectly transparent biconvex structure held in place by a circular system of **zonular fibers** that attach it to the **ciliary body** and by close apposition to the posterior vitreous body (Figure 23–1). Partly covering the anterior surface of the lens is an opaque pigmented extension of the middle layer called the **iris**, which surrounds a central opening, the **pupil** (Figure 23–1).

Located in the anterior portion of the eye, the iris and lens are bathed in clear **aqueous humor** that fills both the **anterior chamber** between the cornea and iris and the **posterior chamber** between the iris and lens (Figure 23–1). Aqueous humor flows through the pupil that connects these two chambers.

The posterior **vitreous chamber**, surrounded by the retina, lies behind the lens and its zonular fibers and contains a large gelatinous mass of transparent connective tissue called the **vitreous body**.

Important aspects of embryonic eye formation are shown in Figure 23–2 and include the following:

- In the 4-week embryo epithelial **optic vesicles** bulge bilaterally from the forebrain, then elongate as the optic stalks bearing **optic cups** (Figure 23–2a).
- Inductive interactions between the optic cups and the overlying surface ectoderm cause the latter to invaginate and eventually detach as the initially hollow **lens vesicles** (Figure 23–2b).
- The optic stalk develops as the **optic nerve** and in an inferior groove called the **choroid fissure** encloses the **hyaloid vessels** that supply blood for the developing lens and optic cup (Figure 23–2c).
- In the ensuing weeks, head mesenchyme differentiates to form most of the tissue in the eye's two outer layers and the vitreous. Ectoderm of the optic cup differentiates as the retina and surface ectoderm forms the corneal epithelium

FIGURE **23–1** Internal anatomy of the eye.

The sagittal section of an eye shows the interrelationships among the major ocular structures, the three major layers or tunics of the wall, important regions within those layers, and the refractive elements (cornea, lens, and vitreous).

(Figure 23–2d). When the lens is fully formed, the distal hyaloid artery and vein disappear, leaving only the blood supply to the retina.

Fibrous Layer

This layer includes two major regions, the posterior sclera and anterior cornea, joined at the limbus.

Sclera

The fibrous, external layer of the eyeball protects the more delicate internal structures and provides sites for muscle insertion (Table 23–1). The white posterior five-sixths of this layer is the **sclera** (Figure 23–1), which encloses a portion of the eyeball about 22 mm in diameter in adults. The sclera averages 0.5 mm in thickness and consists mainly of dense connective tissue, with flat bundles of type I collagen parallel to the organ surface but intersecting in various directions; microvasculature is present near the outer surface.

Tendons of the **extraocular muscles** which move the eyes insert into the anterior region of the sclera. Posteriorly the sclera thickens to approximately 1 mm and joins with the epineurium covering the optic nerve. Where it surrounds the choroid, the sclera includes an inner **suprachoroid lamina**, with less collagen, more fibroblasts, elastic fibers, and melanocytes.

Cornea

In contrast to the sclera, the anterior one-sixth of the eye—the **cornea**—is transparent and completely avascular (Figure 23–1). A section of the cornea shows five distinct layers:

- An external **stratified squamous epithelium**;
- An **anterior limiting membrane (Bowman's membrane)**, which is the basement membrane of the external stratified epithelium;
- The thick **stroma**;
- A **posterior limiting membrane (Descemet's membrane)**, which is the basement membrane of the endothelium; and
- An inner simple squamous **endothelium**.

TABLE **23-1**	Tunics of the eye.

Structures	Components	Function
Fibrous Tunic (External Layer)		
Sclera	Dense irregular connective tissue	Supports eye shape
		Protects delicate internal structures
		Extrinsic eye muscle attachment site
Cornea	Two layers of epithelium with organized connective tissue in between	Protects anterior surface of the eye
		Refracts (bends) incoming light
Vascular Tunic (Middle Layer)		
Choroid	Areolar connective tissue; highly vascularized	Supplies nourishment to retina
		Pigment absorbs extraneous light
Ciliary body	Ciliary smooth muscle and ciliary processes; covered with a secretory epithelium	Holds suspensory ligaments that attach to the lens and change lens shape for far and near vision
		Epithelium secretes aqueous humor
Iris	Two layers of smooth muscle (sphincter pupillae and dilator pupillae) and connective tissue, with a central pupil	Controls pupil diameter and thus the amount of light entering the eye
Retina (Internal Layer)		
Pigmented layer	Pigmented epithelial cells	Absorbs extraneous light
		Provides vitamin A for photoreceptor cells
Neural layer	Photoreceptors, bipolar neurons, ganglion cells, and supporting Müller cells	Detects incoming light rays; light rays are converted to nerve signals and transmitted to the brain

Diagram labels:
Fibrous tunic — Sclera, Cornea
Vascular tunic — Iris, Ciliary body, Choroid
Retina — Pigmented layer, Neural layer

The stratified surface epithelium is nonkeratinized, five or six cell layers thick, and comprises about 10% of the corneal thickness (Figure 23–3). The basal cells have a high proliferative capacity important for renewal and repair of the corneal surface and emerge from stem cells in the **corneoscleral limbus** that encircles the cornea. The flattened surface cells have microvilli protruding into a protective tear film of lipid, glycoprotein, and water. As another protective adaptation, the corneal epithelium also has one of the richest sensory nerve supplies of any tissue.

The basement membrane of this epithelium, often called **Bowman's membrane**, is very thick (8-10 μm) and contributes to the stability and strength of the cornea, helping to protect against infection of the underlying stroma.

The **stroma**, or substantia propria, makes up 90% of the cornea's thickness and consists of approximately 60 layers of parallel collagen bundles aligned at approximately right angles to each other and extending almost the full diameter of the cornea. The uniform orthogonal array of collagen fibrils contributes to the transparency of this avascular tissue. Between the collagen lamellae are cytoplasmic extensions of flattened fibroblast-like cells called **keratocytes** (Figure 23–3). The ground substance around these cells contains proteoglycans such as lumican, with keratan sulfate and chondroitin sulfate, which help maintain the precise organization and spacing of the collagen fibrils.

›› MEDICAL APPLICATION

The shape or curvature of the cornea can be changed surgically to improve certain visual abnormalities involving the ability to focus. In the common ophthalmologic procedure, laser-assisted in situ keratomileusis (LASIK) surgery, the corneal epithelium is displaced as a flap and the stroma reshaped by an excimer laser which vaporizes collagen and keratocytes in a highly controlled manner with no damage to adjacent cells or ECM. After reshaping the stroma, the epithelial flap is repositioned and a relatively rapid regenerative response reestablishes normal corneal physiology. LASIK surgery is used to correct myopia

FIGURE **23–2** Development of eye.

(a) Early week 4: Optic vesicle forms a two-layered optic cup; overlying ectoderm forms a lens pit.

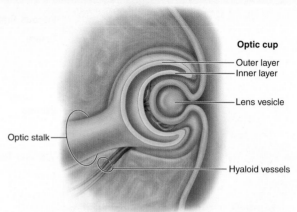

(b) Late week 4: Optic cup deepens and forms inner and outer layers; lens pit forms lens vesicle.

(c) Week 6: Lens becomes an internal structure; corneas, sclera, and choroid start to form.

(d) Week 20: Three tunics of the eye have formed.

Eyes begin to form early in development as the two **optic vesicles** bulge bilaterally from the forebrain (prosencephalon). These grow, remaining connected to the developing brain by the **optic stalks**, and approach the surface ectoderm. At this point each vesicle folds in on itself to form the inner and outer layers of the **optic cup** and inducing surface ectoderm to invaginate into the cup as the **lens vesicle**, which soon detaches from the surface and lies in the opening of the optic cup.

Blood vessels, called the **hyaloid vessels**, grow along the optic stalk, enter the optic cup, and grow toward the developing lens. Head mesenchyme associates with the developing optic cup as it forms the two major layers of the retina. The mesenchymal cells differentiate around the pigmented layer of the developing retina as the iris, ciliary body and choroid of the vascular layer, and as the more external fibrous layer. The hyaloid vessels regress, leaving a space called the **hyaloid canal**, in the vitreous body. Folds of skin develop features of the eyelids and conjunctiva, the latter developing in continuity with the surface epithelium of the cornea and sclera.

(near-sightedness), hyperopia (far-sightedness), or astigmatism (irregular curvature of the cornea).

Corneal grafts (transplants) between unrelated individuals can usually be accomplished successfully without immune rejection due in part to this tissue's lack of both a vascular supply and lymphatic drainage and to local immune tolerance produced by ocular antigen-presenting cells and immunomodulatory factors in aqueous humor.

FIGURE **23–3** Cornea.

The anterior structure of the eye, the cornea has five layers. **(a)** The external stratified squamous epithelium (**E**) is nonkeratinized, five or six cells thick, and densely supplied with sensory-free nerve endings that trigger the blinking reflex. The stroma (**S**) comprises approximately 90% of the cornea's thickness, consisting of some 60 layers of long type I collagen fibers arranged in a precise orthogonal array and alternating with flattened cells called **keratocytes**. The stroma is lined internally by endothelium (**EN**). X100. H&E.

(b) The corneal epithelium (**E**) rests firmly on the thick homogeneous Bowman's membrane (**B**). The stroma (**S**) is completely avascular, and nutrients reach the keratocytes and epithelial cells by diffusion from the surrounding limbus and aqueous humor behind the cornea. X400. H&E. **(c)** The posterior surface of the cornea is covered by simple squamous epithelium (**EN**) that rests on another thick, strong layer called Descemet's membrane (**D**) adjacent to the stroma (**S**). X400. H&E.

The posterior surface of the stroma is bounded by another thick basement membrane, called **Descemet's membrane**, which supports the internal simple squamous corneal endothelium (Figure 23–3).

This endothelium maintains Descemet's membrane and includes the most metabolically active cells of the cornea. Na⁺/K⁺ ATPase pumps in the basolateral membranes of these cells are largely responsible for regulating the proper hydration state of the corneal stroma to provide maximal transparency and optimal light refraction.

Limbus

Encircling the cornea is the **limbus**, a transitional area where the transparent cornea merges with the opaque sclera (Figures 23–1 and 23–4). Here Bowman's membrane ends and the surface epithelium becomes more stratified as the **conjunctiva** that covers the anterior part of the sclera (and lines the eyelids). As mentioned previously, epithelial stem cells located at the limbus surface give rise to rapidly dividing progenitor cells that move centripetally into the corneal epithelium. The stroma becomes vascular and less well-organized at the limbus, as the collagen bundles merge with those of the sclera.

Also at the limbus Descemet's membrane and its simple endothelium are replaced with a system of irregular endothelium-lined channels called the **trabecular meshwork** (Figure 23–5). These penetrate the stroma at the corneoscleral junction and allow slow, continuous drainage of aqueous humor from the anterior chamber. This fluid moves from these channels into the adjacent larger space of the **scleral venous sinus**, or **canal of Schlemm** (Figures 23–1, 23–4, and 23–5), which encircles the eye. From this sinus aqueous humor drains into small blood vessels (veins) of the sclera.

FIGURE **23–4** Corneoscleral junction (limbus) and ciliary body.

FIGURE 23–4 Corneoscleral junction (limbus) and ciliary body.

At the circumference of the cornea is the limbus or corneoscleral junction (**CSJ**), where the transparent corneal stroma merges with the opaque, vascular sclera (**S**). The epithelium of the limbus is slightly thicker than the corneal epithelium, containing stem cells for the latter, and is continuous with the conjunctive (**C**) covering the anterior sclera and lining the eyelids. The stroma of the limbus contains the scleral venous sinus (**SVS**), or canal of Schlemm, which receives aqueous humor from an adjacent trabecular meshwork at the surface of the anterior chamber (**AC**).

Internal to the limbus, the middle layer of the eye consists of the ciliary body and its anterior extension, the iris (**I**). The thick ring of the ciliary body includes loose connective tissue containing melanocytes, smooth ciliary muscle (**CM**), numerous extensions covered by epithelium called the ciliary processes (**CP**), and the ciliary zonule (**CZ**), a system of fibrillin-rich fibers that attach to the capsule of the lens (**L**) in the center of the ciliary body. Pieces of one zonular fiber can be seen (**arrow**). Projecting into the posterior chamber (**PC**), the ciliary processes produce aqueous humor that then flows into the anterior chamber through the pupil. Behind the ciliary zonule and lens, a thin, transparent membrane (not shown) surrounds the vitreous body and separates the posterior chamber from the vitreous chamber (**VC**). X12.5. H&E.

Vascular Layer

The eye's more vascular middle layer, known as the **uvea**, consists of three parts, from posterior to anterior: the **choroid**, the **ciliary body**, and the **iris** (Table 23–1).

Choroid

Located in the posterior two-thirds of the eye, the **choroid** consists of loose, well-vascularized connective tissue and contains numerous melanocytes (Figure 23–6). These form a characteristic black layer in the choroid and prevent light from entering the eye except through the pupil. Two layers make up the choroid (Figure 23–6):

- The inner **choroido-capillary lamina** has a rich microvasculature important for nutrition of the outer retinal layers.
- **Bruch's membrane**, a thin extracellular sheet, is composed of collagen and elastic fibers surrounding the adjacent microvasculature and basal lamina of the retina's pigmented layer.

Ciliary Body

The **ciliary body**, the anterior expansion of the uvea that encircles the lens, lies posterior to the limbus (Figures 23–1 and 23–4). Like the choroid, most of the ciliary body rests on the sclera. Important structures associated with the ciliary body include the following:

- **Ciliary muscle** makes up most of the ciliary body's stroma and consists of three groups of smooth muscle fibers. Contraction of these muscles affects the shape of the lens and is important in visual accommodation (see Lens).
- **Ciliary processes** are a radially arranged series of about 75 ridges extending from the inner highly vascular region of the ciliary body. These provide a large surface area covered by a double layer of low columnar epithelial cells, the ciliary epithelium (Figure 23–7). The epithelial cells directly covering the stroma contain much melanin and correspond to the anterior projection of the pigmented retina epithelium. The surface layer of cells lacks melanin and is contiguous with the sensory layer of the retina.

  Cells of this dual epithelium have extensive basolateral folds with Na⁺/K⁺-ATPase activity and are specialized for secretion of **aqueous humor**. Fluid from the stromal microvasculature moves across this epithelium as aqueous humor, with an inorganic ion composition similar to that of plasma but almost no protein. As shown in Figure 23–8, aqueous humor is secreted by ciliary processes into the posterior chamber, flows through the pupil into the anterior chamber, and drains at the angle formed by the cornea and the iris into the channels of the trabecular meshwork and the scleral venous sinus, from which it enters venules of the sclera.

- The **ciliary zonule** is a system of many radially oriented fibers composed largely of fibrillin-1 and 2 produced by the nonpigmented epithelial cells on the ciliary processes. The fibers extend from grooves between the ciliary processes and attach to the surface of the lens (Figure 23–9), holding that structure in place.

FIGURE **23–5** Trabecular meshwork and scleral venous sinus.

(a) At the corneoscleral junction (**CSJ**), or limbus, encircling the cornea, the posterior endothelium and its underlying Descemet's membrane are replaced by a meshwork of irregular channels lined by endothelium and supported by trabeculae of connective tissue. At the iridocorneal angle between limbus and iris (**I**), aqueous humor moves from the anterior chamber (**AC**) into

channels of this trabecular meshwork (**TM**) and is pumped by endothelial cells into the adjacent scleral venous sinus (**SVS**). X50. H&E.

(b) Scanning electron microscopy (SEM) shows the transition from corneal endothelium (**CE**) surface to the channels of the trabecular meshwork (**TM**). X300.

›› MEDICAL APPLICATION

Aqueous humor is produced continuously. If its drainage from the anterior chamber is impeded, typically by obstruction of the trabecular meshwork or scleral venous sinus, intraocular pressure can increase, causing the condition called **glaucoma**. Untreated glaucoma can cause pressing of the vitreous body against the retina, affecting visual function and possibly leading to neuropathy in that tissue.

When the iridocorneal angle is more narrow than usual, the thickening of the peripheral iris that occurs with dilation of the pupil can occlude the angle and obstruct drainage of aqueous humor at the trabecular meshwork. This can result in the rapid development of intraocular hypertension known as **angle closure glaucoma**, **acute glaucoma**, or **closed (narrow) angle glaucoma**. This condition usually affects both eyes and causes blurred vision, eye pain, and headache. Treatment of this type of glaucoma usually includes some form of surgical intervention.

Iris

The **iris** is the most anterior extension of the middle uveal layer which covers part of the lens, leaving a round central **pupil** (Figure 23–1). The anterior surface of the iris, exposed to aqueous humor in the anterior chamber, consists of a dense layer of fibroblasts and melanocytes with interdigitating processes and is unusual for its lack of an epithelial covering (Figure 23–10a,b). Deeper in the iris, the stroma consists of loose connective tissue with melanocytes and sparse microvasculature.

The posterior surface of the iris has a two-layered epithelium continuous with that covering the ciliary processes, but very heavily filled with melanin. The highly pigmented posterior epithelium of the iris blocks all light from entering the eye except that passing through the pupil. **Myoepithelial cells** form a partially pigmented epithelial layer and extend contractile processes radially as the very thin **dilator pupillae muscle** (Figure 23–10). Smooth muscle fibers form a circular bundle near the pupil as the **sphincter pupillae muscle**. The dilator and sphincter muscles of the iris have sympathetic and parasympathetic innervation, respectively, for enlarging and constricting the pupil.

FIGURE **23–6** Sclera, choroid, and retina.

The lateral wall of an eye includes dense connective tissue of the sclera (**S**) and the loose, vascular connective tissue of the choroid (**C**). Melanocytes are prominent in the choroid, especially in its outer region, the suprachoroidal lamina (**SCL**). The choroid's inner region, the choroidocapillary lamina (**CCL**), has a rich microvasculature that helps provide O$_2$ and nutrients to the adjacent retina. Between the choroid and the retina is a thin layer of extracellular material known as **Bruch's layer** (**B**).

The outer layer of the retina is the pigmented layer (**P**) of cuboidal epithelium containing melanin. Adjacent to this are the packed photoreceptor components of the rods and cones (**R&C**), whose cell bodies make up the outer nuclear layer (**ONL**). Junctional complexes between these cells and glia are aligned and can be seen as a thin line called the **outer limiting layer** (**OLL**). Axons of the rods and cones extend into the outer plexiform layer (**OPL**) forming synapses there with dendrites of the neurons in the inner nuclear layer (**INL**). These neurons send axons into the inner plexiform layer (**IPL**), where they synapse with dendrites of cells in the ganglionic layer (**GL**). Axons from these cells fill most of the nerve fiber layer (**NFL**) which is separated by the inner limiting layer (**ILL**) from the gelatin-like connective tissue of the vitreous body (**VB**). X200. H&E.

Melanocytes of the iris stroma provide the color of one's eyes. In individuals with very few lightly pigmented cells in the stroma, light with a blue color is reflected back from the black pigmented epithelium on the posterior iris surface. As the number of melanocytes and density of melanin increase in the stroma, the iris color changes through various shades of green, gray, and brown. Individuals with albinism have almost no pigment and the pink color of their irises is due to the reflection of incident light from the blood vessels of the stroma.

FIGURE **23–7** Epithelium of ciliary processes.

The surface epithelium of ciliary processes is a double layer of pigmented (**PE**) and nonpigmented epithelial (**NE**) low columnar or cuboidal cells. The two layers are derived developmentally from the folded rim of the embryonic optic cup, so that the exposed surface of the nonpigmented layer is actually the basal surface of the cells. No true basal lamina is present, but instead these cells produce the components that give rise to the fibers of the ciliary zonule in the embryo. Beneath the double epithelium is a core of connective tissue with many small blood vessels (**V**). Fluid from these vessels is pumped by the epithelial cells out of the ciliary processes as aqueous humor. X200. PT.

Lens

The **lens** is a transparent biconvex structure suspended immediately behind the iris, which focuses light on the retina (see Figure 23–1). Derived from an invagination of the embryonic surface ectoderm (see Figure 23–2), the lens is a unique avascular tissue and is highly elastic, a property that normally decreases with age. The lens has three principal components:

■ A thick (10-20 μm), homogeneous **lens capsule** composed of proteoglycans and type IV collagen surrounds the lens (Figure 23–11) and provides the place of attachment for the fibers of the ciliary zonule (Figure 23–10). This layer originates as the basement membrane of the embryonic lens vesicle.

■ A subcapsular **lens epithelium** consists of a single layer of cuboidal cells present only on the anterior surface of the lens (Figure 23–11). The epithelial cells attach basally to the surrounding lens capsule and their apical surfaces bind to the internal lens fibers. At the posterior

FIGURE **23–8** Production and removal of aqueous humor.

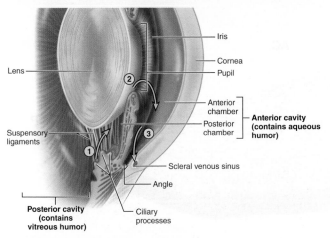

(1) Aqueous humor is secreted by the ciliary processes into the posterior chamber.

(2) Aqueous humor moves from the posterior chamber, through the pupil, to the anterior chamber.

(3) Excess aqueous humor is resorbed via the scleral venous sinus.

Aqueous humor is a continuously flowing liquid that carries metabolites to and from cells and helps maintain an optimal microenvironment within the **anterior cavity** of the eye. As shown here, it is secreted from **ciliary processes** into the posterior chamber of the anterior cavity, flows into the anterior chamber through the **pupil**, and drains into the **scleral venous sinus (canal of Schlemm)**.

FIGURE **23–9** Ciliary zonule fibers.

The structure of the ciliary zonule is best studied by SEM. **(a)** The surface of the ciliary body (**CB**) has projecting ciliary processes, between which emerge delicate zonular fibers (**ZF**). An array of these fibers constitutes the zonule that anchors the lens in the center of the ciliary body. X400.

(b) Zonular fibers (**ZF**) attach tangentially to the fibrous ECM of the lens capsule (**LC**). X500.

edge of this epithelium, near the equator of the lens, the epithelial cells divide to provide new cells that differentiate as lens fibers. This process allows for growth of the lens and continues at a slow, decreasing rate near the equator of the lens throughout adult life.

▪ **Lens fibers** are highly elongated, terminally differentiated cells that appear as thin, flattened structures (Figure 23–11). Developing from cells in the lens epithelium, lens fibers typically become 7 to 10 mm long, with cross-section dimensions of only 2 by 8 μm. The cytoplasm becomes filled with a group of proteins called **crystallins**, and the organelles and nuclei undergo autophagy. Lens fibers are packed tightly together and form a perfectly transparent tissue highly specialized for light refraction.

The lens is held in place by fibers of the **ciliary zonule**, which extend from the lens capsule to the ciliary body (Figures 23–1 and 23–9). Together with the ciliary muscles, this structure allows the process of visual **accommodation**, which permits focusing on near and far objects by changing the curvature of the lens (Figure 23–12). When the eye is at rest or gazing at distant objects, ciliary muscles relax and the resulting shape of

the ciliary body puts tension on the zonule fibers, which pulls the lens into a flatter shape. To focus on a close object the ciliary muscles contract, causing forward displacement of the ciliary body, which relieves some of the tension on the zonule and allows the lens to return to a more rounded shape and keep the object in focus. In the fourth decade of life **presbyopia** (Gr. *presbyter*, elder + L. *opticus*, relating to eyes) normally causes the lenses to lose elasticity and their ability to undergo accommodation.

▶▶ MEDICAL APPLICATION

Presbyopia is corrected by wearing glasses with convex lenses (reading glasses). In older individuals, denaturation of crystallins commonly begins to occur in lens fibers, making them less transparent. When areas of the lens become opaque or cloudy and vision is impaired, the condition is termed a **cataract**. Causes of cataract include excessive exposure to ultraviolet light or other radiation, trauma, and as secondary effects in diseases such as diabetes mellitus and hypertension.

FIGURE 23–10 Iris.

The iris regulates the amount of light to which the retina is exposed. **(a)** The low-power micrograph shows a section of the central iris, near the pupil (**P**). The anterior surface, exposed to aqueous humor in the anterior chamber (**AC**), has no epithelium and consists only of a matted layer of interdigitating fibroblasts and melanocytes. Cells of the external pigmented epithelium (**PE**) are very rich in melanin granules to protect the eye's interior from an excess of light. Cells of the other layer are myoepithelial, less heavily pigmented, and comprise the dilator pupillae muscle (**DPM**) that extends along most of the iris. Near the pupil, fascicles of smooth muscle make up the sphincter pupillae muscle (**SPM**). X140. H&E. The underlying stroma (**S**) contains many melanocytes with varying amounts of melanin.

(b) SEM reveals the nonepithelial anterior surface of the iris. X900. **(c)** The deep stroma also is richly vascularized (**arrows**). The myoepithelial dilator pupillae muscle (**DPM**) is more easily seen here, in relation to the sphincter pupillae muscle (**SPM**) and posterior pigmented epithelium (**PE**). X100. PT.

In modern cataract surgery the lens is removed by aspiration of the lens substance while it is emulsified by a vibrating probe. The posterior side of the lens capsule and its inserted zonular fibers are left in place at the posterior chamber. The concave posterior capsule, or capsular bag, is then used as the site for implantation of an acrylic **intraocular lens** (**IOL**) prosthesis. Research is under way to develop IOLs capable of natural accommodation.

FIGURE **23–11** Lens.

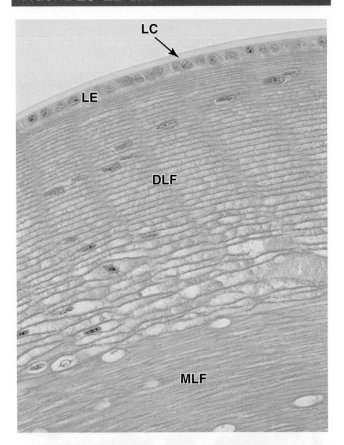

The lens is a transparent, elastic tissue that focuses light on the retina. Surrounding the entire lens is a thick, homogenous external lamina called the **lens capsule** (**LC**). The anterior surface of the lens, beneath the capsule, is covered by a simple columnar lens epithelium (**LE**). Because of its origin as an embryonic vesicle pinching off of surface ectoderm, the basal ends of the lens epithelial cells rest on the capsule and the apical regions are directed into the lens interior.

At the equator of the lens, near the ciliary zonule, the epithelial cells proliferate and give rise to cells that align parallel to the epithelium and become the lens fibers. Differentiating lens fibers (**DLF**) still have their nuclei but are greatly elongating and filling their cytoplasm with proteins called **crystallins**. The mature lens fibers (**MLF**) have lost their nuclei and become densely packed to produce a unique transparent structure. The lens is difficult to process histologically and sections usually have cracks or blebs among the lens fibers. X200. H&E.

Vitreous Body

The **vitreous body** occupies the large vitreous chamber behind the lens (see Figure 23–1). It consists of transparent, gel-like connective tissue that is 99% water (vitreous humor), with collagen fibrils and hyaluronate, contained within an external lamina called the vitreous membrane. The only cells in the vitreous body are a small mesenchymal population near the membrane called **hyalocytes**, which synthesize the hyaluronate and collagen, and a few macrophages.

FIGURE **23–12** Accommodation of the lens.

Continuous changes in the shape of the lens keep images focused on the retina. **(a)** The lens flattens for distant vision when the ciliary muscles are relaxed and the shape of the ciliary body holds the ciliary zonule taut. **(b)** To see closer objects, the ciliary muscle fibers contract, changing the shape of the ciliary body, relaxing tension on the ciliary zonule, and allowing the lens to assume the more rounded shape.

Retina

The **retina**, the innermost tunic of the eye, develops with two fundamental sublayers from the inner and outer layers of embryonic optic cup (see Figure 23–2 and Table 23–1):

- The outer **pigmented layer** is a simple cuboidal epithelium attached to Bruch's membrane and the choroidocapillary lamina of the choroid (see Figure 23–6). This heavily pigmented layer forms the other part of the dual epithelium covering the ciliary body and posterior iris.
- The inner retinal region, the **neural layer**, is thick and stratified with various neurons and photoreceptors. Although its neural structure and visual function extend anterior only as far as the **ora serrata** (see Figure 23–1), this layer continues as part of the dual cuboidal epithelium that covers the surface of the ciliary body and posterior iris.

The pigmented epithelium and the photoreceptor layer of the retina, derived from the two layers of the optic cup, are not firmly joined to each other. Head trauma or other conditions can cause the two layers to separate with an intervening space. In such regions of **detached retina**, the photoreceptor cells no longer have access to metabolic support from the pigmented layer and choroid and will eventually die. Prompt repositioning of the retina and reattaching it with laser surgery is an effective treatment.

Retina Pigmented Epithelium

The pigmented epithelial layer consists of cuboidal or low columnar cells with basal nuclei and surrounds the neural layer of the retina. The cells have well-developed junctional complexes, gap junctions, and numerous invaginations of the basal membranes associated with mitochondria. The apical ends of the cells extend processes and sheath-like projections that surround the tips of the photoreceptors. Melanin granules are numerous in these extensions and in the apical cytoplasm (Figure 23–13). This cellular region also contains numerous phagocytic vacuoles and secondary lysosomes, peroxisomes, and abundant smooth ER (SER) specialized for **retinal** (vitamin A) isomerization. The diverse functions of the retinal pigmented epithelium include the following:

- The pigmented layer **absorbs scattered light** that passes through the neural layer, supplementing the choroid in this regard.
- With many tight junctions, cells of the pigmented epithelium form an important part of the protective **blood-retina barrier** isolating retina photoreceptors from the highly vascular choroid and regulating **ion transport** between these compartments.
- The cells play key roles in the visual cycle of **retinal regeneration**, having enzyme systems that isomerize all-*trans*-retinal released from photoreceptors and produce 11-*cis*-retinal that is then transferred back to the photoreceptors.
- **Phagocytosis** of shed components from the adjacent photoreceptors and degradation of this material occurs in these epithelial cells.
- Cells of pigmented epithelium **remove free radicals** by various protective antioxidant activities and **support the neural retina** by secretion of ATP, various polypeptide growth factors, and immunomodulatory factors.

Neural Retina

True to its embryonic origin, the neural retina functions as an outpost of the CNS with glia and several interconnected neuronal subtypes in well-organized strata. Nine distinct layers

FIGURE 23–13 Pigmented epithelium of retina.

The two distinct layers of the retina are the pigmented epithelium and the photosensitive neural layer, which are derived from the outer and inner layers of the optic cup, respectively. Shown here is the interface between the two layers. The pigmented epithelium (**PE**) is of simple cuboidal cells resting on Bruch's membrane inside the choroid (**C**). Rod cells and cone cells are neurons with their nuclei collected in the outer nuclear layer (**ONL**) and with axons of one end forming synapses in an area called the outer plexiform layer (**OPL**) and modified dendrites at the other end serving as photosensitive structures. These structures have mitochondria-rich inner segments (**IS**) and photosensitive outer segments (**OS**) with stacks of folded membranes where the visual pigments are located.

The inner segments of the rod and cone cells are attached to elongated glial cells called **Müller cells**, which are modified astrocytes of the retina. The junctional complexes of these attachments can be seen in light micrographs as the outer limiting layer (**OLL**). X500. H&E.

comprise the neural retina, described here with their functional significance.

Three major layers contain the nuclei of the interconnected neurons (see Figure 23–6; Figures 23–14 and 23–15):

- Near the pigmented epithelium, the **outer nuclear layer** (**ONL**) contains cell bodies of photoreceptors (the rod and cone cells).
- The **inner nuclear layer** (**INL**) contains the nuclei of various neurons, notably the bipolar cells, amacrine cells, and horizontal cells, all of which make specific connections with other neurons and integrate signals from rods and cones over a wide area of the retina.
- Near the vitreous, the **ganglionic layer** (**GL**) has neurons (ganglion cells) with much longer axons. These axons make up the **nerve fiber layer** (**NFL**) and converge to form the **optic nerve** which leaves the eye and passes to the brain. The GL is thickest near the central, macular region of the retina (Figure 23–15), but it thins peripherally to only one layer of cells (see Figure 23–6).

Between the three layers with cell nuclei are two fibrous or "plexiform" regions containing only axons and dendrites connected by synapses (Figures 23–14 and 23–15):

- The **outer plexiform layer** (**OPL**) includes axons of the photoreceptors and dendrites of association neurons in the INL.
- The **inner plexiform layer** (**IPL**) consists of axons and dendrites connecting neurons of the INL with the ganglion cells

The rod and cone cells, named for the shape of their outer segments, are polarized neurons with their photosensitive portions aligned in the retina's **rod and cone layer** (**RCL**) and their axons in the IPL (Figure 23–15). As shown schematically in Figure 23–16, both rod and cone cells have highly specialized outer and inner segments.

All neurons of the retina are supported physically by glial cells called **Müller cells**. With their nuclei in the INL, Müller cells extend fine processes and branching lamellae that serve as a scaffold for the neurons and their fibers. Müller cells also organize two boundaries that appear as very thin layers within the retina:

FIGURE 23–14 General structure and organization of the retina.

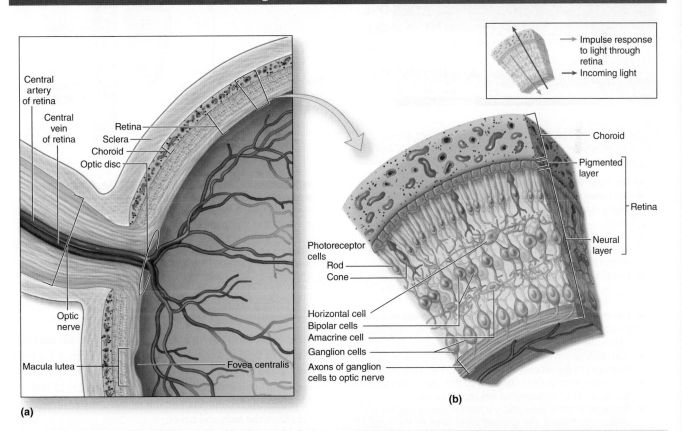

(a)

(b)

The retina is the thick layer of the eye inside the choroid. **(a)** The central retinal artery and vein pass through the optic nerve and enter the eye at the optic disc. These vessels initially lie between the vitreous body and the ILL of the retina, but their smaller lateral branches penetrate this layer and enter the retina, forming capillaries that extend as far as the INL. Nutrients and O_2 for the outer retinal layers diffuse from capillaries in the choroid. **(b)** The layers and major neurons of the retina and their general organization are shown schematically here and the Müller support cells are omitted.

FIGURE 23–15 Layers of the retina.

Between the vitreous body (**VB**) and the choroid (**C**), the retina can usually be seen to consist of nine neural layers and a pigmented layer. Following the path of the light, these are:

- The inner limiting layer (**ILL**)
- The nerve fiber layer (**NFL**), containing the ganglionic cell axons that converge at the optic disc and form the optic nerve
- The ganglionic layer (**GL**), containing cell bodies of the ganglion cells and thicker near the retina's center than its periphery
- The inner plexiform layer (**IPL**), containing fibers and synapses of the ganglion cells and the bipolar neurons of the next layer
- The inner nuclear layer (**INL**), with the cell bodies of several types of bipolar neurons which begin to integrate signals from the rod and cone cells
- The outer plexiform layer (**OPL**), containing fibers and synapses of the bipolar neurons and rod and cone cells
- The outer nuclear layer (**ONL**), with the cell bodies and nuclei of the photosensitive rod and cone cells
- The outer limiting layer (**OLL**), a line formed by junctional complexes holding the rod and cone cells to the intervening Müller cells
- The rod and cone layer (**RCL**), which contains the outer segments of these cells where the photoreceptors are located
- The non-neural pigmented layer (**PL**), which has several supportive functions important for the function and maintenance of the neural retina. X150. H&E

FIGURE 23–16 Rod and cone cells.

Rod cells (right) and cone cells (left) all have the general shapes and important cytoplasmic features shown diagrammatically here. The outer limiting layer is the line of adherent junctions that attach the rod and cone inner segments to the distal ends of the Müller glial cells (not shown). The membranous discs of the cone outer segments are continuous with the cell membrane; those of the rods are not.

- The **outer limiting layer** (**OLL**) is a faint but well-defined series of tight and adherent junctions that form at the level of the rod and cone inner segments between the photoreceptors and Müller cell processes (Figures 23–15 and 23–16). The OLL forms one side of the compartment that encloses the rods and cones.
- The **inner limiting layer** (**ILL**) consists of terminal expansions of other Müller cell processes that cover the collagenous membrane of the vitreous body.

All these layers of the retina can be seen by routine light microscopy, as shown in Figures 23–6 and 23–15. It is important to note that light must pass through all the layers of the neural retina before reaching the layer of rods and cones. Branches of the central retinal artery and vein (see Figure 23–1) run mainly within the nerve fiber and GLs, surrounded by perivascular feet of astrocytes located there. In some retina regions capillaries extend as deeply as the INL. A few scattered microglial cells occur throughout the neural retina.

Rod Cells

The human retina has on average 92 million **rod cells**. They are extremely sensitive to light, responding to a single photon, and allow some vision even with light low levels, such as at dusk or nighttime. Rod cells are thin, elongated cells (50 μm × 3 μm), composed of two functionally distinct segments (Figure 23–16). The **outer segment** is a modified primary cilium, photosensitive and shaped like a short rod; the inner segment contains glycogen, mitochondria, and polyribosomes for the cell's biosynthetic activity.

The rod-shaped segment consists mainly of 600 to 1000 flattened **membranous discs** stacked like coins and surrounded by the plasma membrane (Figure 23–16). Proteins on the cytoplasmic surface of each disc include abundant **rhodopsin** (or **visual purple**) which is bleached by light and initiates the visual stimulus. Between this outer segment and the cell's inner segment is a constriction, the **connecting stalk**, which is part of the modified primary cilium arising from a basal body (Figure 23–17).

The membranous discs form by repetitive in-folding of the plasma membrane near the connecting stalk and insertion of rhodopsin and other proteins transported there from the inner segment. In rod cells the newly assembled discs detach from the plasma membrane and are displaced distally as new discs form. Eventually the discs arrive at the end of the rod, where they are shed, phagocytosed, and digested by the cells of the pigmented epithelium (Figure 23–13). Each day approximately 90 membranous discs are lost and replaced in each rod, with the process of assembly, distal movement, and apical shedding taking about 10 days.

Cone Cells

Less numerous and less light-sensitive than rods, the average 4.6 million **cone cells** in the human retina produce color vision in adequately bright light. There are three morphologically similar classes of cones, each containing one type of the visual pigment **iodopsin** (or photopsins). Each of the three iodopsins has maximal sensitivity to light of a different wavelength, in the red, blue, or green regions of the visible spectrum, respectively. By mixing neural input produced by these visual pigments, cones produce a color image.

Like rods cone cells (Figure 23–16) are elongated, with outer and inner segments, a modified cilium connecting stalk, and an accumulation of mitochondria and polyribosomes. The outer segments of cones differ from those of rods in their shorter,

FIGURE 23–17 Connection between inner and outer segments.

TEM of a sectioned retina shows the inner segments (**IS**) with mitochondria in the upper part of the figure and the outer photosensitive segment (**OS**) consisting of flat, parallel membranous discs. The cell in the middle of the figure shows a basal body giving rise to a primary cilium that forms the connecting stalk (**CS**) and is further modified distally as the outer segment. The stacked membranes of the discs are very distinct and electron-dense due to the high density of proteins they contain. X24,000.

more conical form and in the structure of their stacked membranous discs, which in cones remain as continuous invaginations of the plasma membrane along one side (Figure 23–16). Also, newly synthesized iodopsins and other membrane proteins are distributed uniformly throughout the cone outer segment and, although iodopsin turns over, discs in cones are shed much less frequently than in rods.

Phototransduction

The stacked membranous discs of rod and cone outer segments are parallel with the retinal surface, which maximizes their exposure to light. The membranes are very densely packed with rhodopsin or one of the iodopsin proteins; one rod contains about a billion rhodopsin molecules. Each of these visual pigments contains a transmembrane protein, the **opsin**, with a small, light-sensitive **chromophore** molecule bound to it. The vitamin A derivative called **retinal** acts as the chromophore of rhodopsin in rods.

Phototransduction involves a cascade of changes in the cells triggered when light hits and activates the chromophore, a basically similar process in both rods and cones. As diagrammed for a rod in Figure 23–18, in darkness rhodopsin is not active and cation channels in the cell membrane are open. The cell is depolarized and continuously releases neurotransmitter at the synapse with the bipolar neurons. When retinal on rhodopsin absorbs a photon of light, it isomerizes within one picosecond from 11-*cis*-retinal to all-*trans*-retinal. This causes a configuration change in the opsin, which in turn activates the adjacent membrane-associated protein **transducin**, a heterotrimeric G protein to which opsin is coupled. Transducin activity then indirectly closes cGMP-gated Na$^+$ channels, causing hyperpolarization which reduces the synaptic release of neurotransmitter. This change in turn depolarizes sets of bipolar neurons, which send action potentials to the ganglion cells of the optic nerve.

The conformation change induced by light in retinal which initiates this cascade of events also causes the chromophore to dissociate from the opsin, a process called **bleaching** (Figure 23–18). The free all-*trans*-retinal is transported from the rod into the adjacent pigmented epithelial cell where it is converted back to 11-*cis*-retinal, then transported back into a photoreceptor for reuse. This cycle of retinal regeneration and rhodopsin recovery from bleaching may take a minute or more and is part of the slow adaptation of the eyes that occurs when moving from bright to dim light.

Specialized Areas of the Retina

The blind spot of the retina, or **optic disc**, lacks photoreceptors and all conducting neurons. It occurs in the posterior area of the retina where axons in the NFL converge to produce the optic nerve which leaves the retina. The central artery and vein of the retina enter at the optic disc (Figure 23–14).

Near the optic disc, within the portion of retina directly opposite the pupil, lies a specialized area about 1.5 mm in diameter called the **fovea centralis** (see Figure 23–1), where visual acuity or sharpness is maximal. The fovea (L. *fovea*, a small pit) is a shallow depression with only cone cells at its center; ganglion cells and other conducting neurons are located only at its periphery. Cone cells in the fovea are long, narrow, and closely packed. Blood vessels do not cross the fovea and light falls directly on its cones. The locations and structural adaptations of the fovea together account for the extremely precise visual acuity of this region.

Surrounding the fovea centralis is the **macula lutea** (L. *macula*, spot; *lutea*, yellow), or simply macula, 5 mm in diameter (Figure 23–14). Here all layers of the retina are present and the two plexiform layers are rich in various carotenoids, which give this area its yellowish color. The carotenoids have antioxidant properties and filter potentially damaging short-wavelength light, thus helping to protect the cone cells of the fovea.

Within the GL of the entire retina a subset of ganglion cells serve as **nonvisual photoreceptors**. These neurons contain 11-*cis*-retinal bound to the protein **melanopsin** and serve to detect changes in light quantity and quality during each 24-hour dawn/dusk cycle. Signals from these cells pass via axons of the retinohypothalamic tract to the suprachiasmatic nuclei and the pineal gland, where they help establish the body's physiologic circadian rhythms (see Chapter 20).

Accessory Structures of the Eye

Conjunctiva

The **conjunctiva** is a thin, transparent mucosa that covers the exposed, anterior portion of the sclera and continues as the lining on the inner surface of the eyelids. It consists of a stratified columnar epithelium, with numerous small goblet cells, supported by a thin lamina propria of loose vascular connective tissue (Figure 23–19). Mucous secretions from conjunctiva cells are added to the tear film that coats this epithelium and the cornea.

FIGURE 23–18 Rod cell phototransduction.

In the dark:

Pigmented epithelium cell

Disc

Inactive rhodopsin (opsin and retinal)

Transducin

Phosphodiesterase

High cGMP levels

Na⁺

K⁺

Cell depolarized

Rod

Continuous (tonic) release of neurotransmitter to bipolar neurons

When light enters:

Activated retinal

Opsin (bleached)

Decreased cGMP

Closed

K⁺

Na⁺

Cell hyperpolarized

Light

Reduced release of neurotransmitter to bipolar neurons

Phototransduction involves a series of changes in **rod and cone cells** that begins when light hits the stacked **membranous discs**. The main parts of the process are similar in both rods and cones but have been better studied in the more abundant rod cells, as shown here. Membranes of the discs are densely packed with proteins, although only one of each major type is shown here. In the dark, **rhodopsin** and its **11-*cis*-retinal** are inactive and the intracellular concentration of the second messenger cyclic GMP (**cGMP**) is high. One effect of cGMP is to keep open the abundant cGMP-gated sodium channels in the cell membrane and therefore the cell is depolarized, continuously releasing its **neurotransmitter** (glutamate) at the synapse with the bipolar neurons.

When photons of light are absorbed by the retinal of rhodopsin, the molecule isomerizes from 11-*cis*-retinal to **all-*trans*-retinal** and this change activates the opsin. This in turn activates the adjacent peripheral membrane protein **transducin**, a heterotrimeric **G protein**, allowing it to release its α subunit, which moves laterally and stimulates another membrane protein, **phosphodiesterase**, to hydrolyze cGMP. With less cGMP, many of the sodium channels now close, producing hyperpolarization of the cell which decreases the release of neurotransmitter at the synapses. This change at the synapse depolarizes sets of bipolar neurons, which then send action potentials to the various ganglion cells of the optic nerve that will allow the brain to produce an image. When retinal is activated by light, it also dissociates from rhodopsin, leaving a more pale-colored (bleached) opsin. The free retinal moves into the surrounding **pigmented epithelial cells**, where the all-*trans*-isomer is regenerated. It is then transported back into a rod or cone cell to again bind opsin and be used in another round of phototransduction.

›› MEDICAL APPLICATION

Conjunctivitis, or **pink eye**, is a condition in which the conjunctiva is inflamed usually due to bacterial or viral infection or to allergies. The inflammation increases the discharge of mucus and enlarges the microvasculature of the sclera, causing the white sclera to have a reddish appearance. Bacterial and viral conjunctivitis are contagious but have little effect on vision.

Eyelids

Eyelids (Figure 23–19) are pliable structures containing skin, muscle, and conjunctiva that protect the eyes. The skin is loose and elastic, lacks fat, and has only very small hair follicles and fine hair, except at the distal edge, where large follicles with eyelashes are present. Associated with the follicles of eyelashes are sebaceous glands and modified apocrine sweat glands.

Beneath the skin are striated fascicles of the orbicularis oculi and levator palpebrae muscles that fold the eyelids. Adja-

FIGURE **23–19** Eyelid.

a

b

(a) The eyelid is a pliable tissue with skin (**S**) covering its external surface and smooth conjunctiva (**C**) lining its inner surface. At the outer rim of the eyelid are a series of large hair follicles (**F**) for the eyelashes. Associated with these hair follicles are small sebaceous glands and modified apocrine sweat glands. Internally eyelids contain fascicles of striated muscle (**M**) comprising the orbicularis oculi muscle and closer to the conjunctiva a thick plate of fibroelastic connective tissue called the tarsus (**T**). This tarsal plate provides structural support for the eyelid and surrounds a series of large sebaceous glands, the tarsal glands (**TG**) (aka Meibomian glands),

with acini secreting into long central ducts (**D**) that empty at the free edge of the eyelids. X12.5. H&E.

(b) At higher magnification, only the inner aspect of the eyelid is seen, and it shows that the conjunctiva (**C**) is a mucous membrane consisting of a stratified columnar epithelium with small cells resembling goblet cells and resting on a thin lamina propria (**LP**). Large cells undergoing typical holocrine secretion are shown in the tarsal gland acini (**TG**), and the fibrous connective tissue in the tarsus (**T**) surrounding the acini. Sebum from these glands is added to the tear film and helps lubricate the ocular surface. X200. H&E.

cent to the conjunctiva is a dense fibroelastic plate called the **tarsus** that supports the other tissues. The tarsus surrounds a series of 20 to 25 large sebaceous glands, each with many acini secreting into a long central duct that opens among the eyelashes

(Figure 23–19). Oils in the sebum produced by these **tarsal glands**, also called **Meibomian glands**, form a surface layer on the tear film, reducing its rate of evaporation, and help lubricate the ocular surface.

>> **MEDICAL APPLICATION**

Infections near an opening of the tarsal gland ducts, generally caused by *Staphylococcus aureus*, are called **styes**. They are most common in infants but can occur at any age and can be quite painful. Like certain other infections, styes can occur in periods of immunosuppression caused by poor nutrition or stress.

Lacrimal Glands

The **lacrimal glands** produce fluid continuously for the tear film that moistens and lubricates the cornea and conjunctiva and supplies O_2 to the corneal epithelial cells. Tear fluid also contains various metabolites, electrolytes, and proteins of innate immunity such as lysozyme. The main lacrimal glands are located in the upper temporal portion of the orbit and have several lobes that drain through individual excretory ducts into the superior fornix, the conjunctiva-lined recess between the eyelids and the eye.

The lacrimal glands have acini composed of large serous cells filled with lightly stained secretory granules and surrounded by well-developed myoepithelial cells and a sparse, vascular stroma (Figure 23–20).

Tear film moves across the ocular surface and collects in other parts of the bilateral **lacrimal apparatus**: flowing through two small round openings (0.5 mm in diameter) to canaliculi at the medial margins of the upper and lower eyelids, then passing into the lacrimal sac, and finally draining into the nasal cavity via the nasolacrimal duct. The canaliculi are lined by stratified squamous epithelium, but the more distal sac and duct are lined by pseudostratified ciliated epithelium like that of the nasal cavity.

› EARS: THE VESTIBULOAUDITORY SYSTEM

Tissues of the ear mediate the senses of equilibrium and hearing. Each ear consists of three major parts (Figure 23–21):

- The **external ear**, which receives sound waves;
- The **middle ear**, in which sound waves are transmitted from air to fluids of the internal ear via a set of small bones;
- The **internal ear**, in which these fluid movements are transduced to nerve impulses that pass via the acoustic nerve to the CNS. In addition to the auditory organ, or cochlea, the internal ear also contains the vestibular organ that allows the body to maintain equilibrium.

Most structures of the middle and internal ear develop in the embryo and are enclosed within the temporal bone as it forms from head mesenchyme.

External Ear

The **auricle**, or **pinna** (L. *pinna*, wing) is an irregular, funnel-shaped plate of elastic cartilage, covered by tightly adherent skin, which directs sound waves into the ear.

FIGURE 23–20 Lacrimal gland.

Lacrimal glands secrete most components of the tear film that moisturizes, lubricates, and helps protect the eyes. The glands have acini (**A**) composed of secretory cells filled with small, light-staining granules and myoepithelial cells (**M**). Connective tissue surrounding the acini contains blood vessels (**V**) of the microvasculature and intra- and interlobular ducts (**D**) converging as excretory ducts that empty into the superior conjunctival fornix between the upper eyelid and the eye. X400. H&E.

Sound waves enter the **external acoustic meatus** (L. passage), a canal lined with stratified squamous epithelium that extends from the auricle to the middle ear. Near its opening hair follicles, sebaceous glands, and modified apocrine sweat glands called **ceruminous glands** are found in the submucosa (Figure 23–22). **Cerumen**, the waxy material formed from secretions of the sebaceous and ceruminous glands, contains various proteins, saturated fatty acids, and sloughed keratinocytes and has protective, antimicrobial properties. The wall of the external auditory meatus is supported by elastic cartilage in its outer third, while the temporal bone encloses the inner part (Figure 23–21).

Across the deep end of the external acoustic meatus lies a thin, somewhat transparent sheet called the **tympanic membrane** or **eardrum**. This membrane consists of fibroelastic

FIGURE 23–21 Major divisions of the ear.

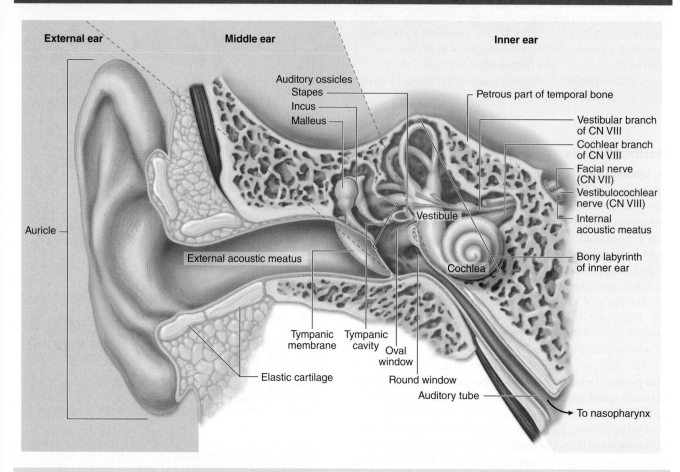

The external, middle, and internal regions of the right ear are shown here, with the major structures of each region.

connective tissue covered externally with epidermis and internally by the simple cuboidal epithelium of the mucosa that lines the middle ear cavity. Sound waves cause vibrations of the tympanic membrane, which transmit energy to the middle ear (Figure 23–21).

Middle Ear

The **middle ear** contains the air-filled **tympanic cavity**, an irregular space that lies within the temporal bone between the tympanic membrane and the bony surface of the internal ear (Figure 23–21). Anteriorly, this cavity communicates with the pharynx via the **auditory tube** (also called the **eustachian** or **pharyngotympanic tube**) and posteriorly with the smaller, air-filled mastoid cavities of the temporal bone. The simple cuboidal epithelium lining the cavity rests on a thin lamina propria continuous with periosteum. Entering the auditory tube, this simple epithelium is gradually replaced by the ciliated pseudostratified columnar epithelium that lines the tube. Below the

temporal bone this tube is usually collapsed; swallowing opens it briefly, which serves to balance the air pressure in the middle ear with atmospheric pressure. In the medial bony wall of the middle ear are two small, membrane-covered regions devoid of bone: the **oval** and **round windows** with the internal ear behind them (Figure 23–21).

The tympanic membrane is connected to the oval window by a series of three small bones, the **auditory ossicles**, which transmit the mechanical vibrations of the tympanic membrane to the internal ear (Figure 23–23). The three ossicles are named for their shapes the **malleus**, **incus**, and **stapes**, the Latin words for "hammer," "anvil," and "stirrup," respectively. The malleus is attached to the tympanic membrane and the stapes to the membrane across the oval window. The ossicles articulate at synovial joints, which along with periosteum are completely covered with simple squamous epithelium. Two small skeletal muscles, the tensor tympani and stapedius, insert into the malleus and stapes, respectively, restricting ossicle movements and

FIGURE 23–22 External acoustic meatus.

The external acoustic meatus leads from the opening in the auricle to the tympanic membrane (or eardrum). This section of the wall in the outer third of the acoustic meatus shows the lining of skin containing small hair follicles (**F**), sebaceous glands (**SG**), and modified apocrine sweat glands called **ceruminous glands** (**CG**). Secretions from these two glands form a yellowish, waxy product called **cerumen** (**C**). X50. H&E.

protecting the oval window and inner ear from potential damage caused by extremely loud sound.

›› MEDICAL APPLICATION

The middle ear tympanic cavity may show inflammation (**otitis media**) when viral or bacterial infections extend there from the upper respiratory tract via the auditory tubes. Otitis media is most common in young children, where the short auditory tubes facilitate infection of the tympanic cavity.

Internal Ear

The **internal ear** is located completely within the temporal bone, where an intricate set of interconnected spaces, the **bony**

FIGURE 23–23 Middle ear.

Three **auditory ossicles**, with joints and striated muscles, span the tympanic cavity of the middle ear, which is enclosed by the **temporal bone** and the **tympanic membrane**.

labyrinth, houses the smaller **membranous labyrinth**, a set of continuous fluid-filled, epithelium-lined tubes and chambers (Figure 23–21). The membranous labyrinth is derived from an ectodermal vesicle, the otic vesicle, which invaginates into subjacent mesenchyme during the fourth week of embryonic development, loses contact with the surface ectoderm, and becomes embedded in rudiments of the developing temporal bone. Components of the bony and membranous labyrinths and their functions are summarized in Table 23–2.

The embryonic otic vesicle, or otocyst, forms the membranous labyrinth with its major divisions:

- Two connected sacs called the **utricle** and the **saccule,**
- Three **semicircular ducts** continuous with the utricle,
- The **cochlear duct**, which provides for hearing and is continuous with the saccule.

Mediating the functions of the inner ear, each of these structures contains in its epithelial lining large areas with columnar mechanoreceptor cells, called **hair cells**, in specialized sensory regions:

- Two **maculae** of the utricle and saccule,
- Three **cristae ampullares** in the enlarged ampullary regions of each semicircular duct,
- The long **spiral organ of Corti** in the cochlear duct.

The entire membranous labyrinth is within the bony labyrinth, which includes the following regions (Figure 23–24):

TABLE 23–2	Structure and function of internal ear components.		
Bony Labyrinth Component (Containing Perilymph and the Membranous Labyrinth)	**Membranous Labyrinth Component (Within Bony Labyrinth and Containing Endolymph)**	**Structures with Sensory Receptors**	**Major Function**
Vestibule	Utricle, saccule	Maculae	Detect linear movements and static position of the head
Semicircular canals	Semicircular ducts	Cristae ampullares	Detect rotational movements of the head
Cochlea	Cochlear duct	Spiral organ	Detect sounds

- An irregular central cavity, the **vestibule** (L. *vestibulum*, area for entering) houses the saccule and the utricle.
- Behind this, three osseous **semicircular canals** enclose the semicircular ducts.

- On the other side of the vestibule, the **cochlea** (L. snail, screw) contains the cochlear duct (Figure 23–24). The cochlea is about 35 mm long and makes 2¾ turns around a bony core called the **modiolus** (L. hub of wheel). The

FIGURE 23–24 Internal ear.

The internal ear consists of a cavity in the temporal bone, the **bony labyrinth**, which houses a fluid-filled **membranous labyrinth**. The membranous labyrinth includes the vestibular organs for the sense of equilibrium and balance (the **saccule, utricle,** and **semicircular ducts**) and the **cochlea** for the sense of hearing.

modiolus contains blood vessels and surrounds the cell bodies and processes of the acoustic branch of the eighth cranial nerve in the large **spiral** or **cochlear ganglion**.

The bony and membranous labyrinths contain two different fluids (Figure 23–24). The separation and ionic differences between these fluids are important for inner ear function.

- **Perilymph** fills all regions of the bony labyrinth and has an ionic composition similar to that of cerebrospinal fluid and the extracellular fluid of other tissues, but it contains little protein. Perilymph emerges from the microvasculature of the periosteum and drains via a perilymphatic duct into the adjoining subarachnoid space. Perilymph suspends and supports the closed membranous labyrinth, protecting it from the hard wall of the bony labyrinth.
- **Endolymph** fills the membranous labyrinth and is characterized by a high-K^+ (150 mM) and low-Na^+ (16 mM) content, similar to that of intracellular fluid. Endolymph is produced in a specialized area in the wall of the cochlear duct (described below) and drains via a small endolymphatic duct into venous sinuses of the dura mater.

Utricle and Saccule

The interconnected, membranous **utricle** and the **saccule** are composed of a very thin connective tissue sheath lined with simple squamous epithelium and are bound to the periosteum of the bony labyrinth by strands of connective tissue containing microvasculature. The maculae in the walls of the utricle and saccule are small areas of columnar neuroepithelial cells innervated by branches of the vestibular nerve (Figure 23–25). The macula of the saccule lies in a plane perpendicular to that of the utricle, but both are similar histologically. Each consists of a thickening of the wall containing several thousand columnar hair cells, each with surrounding supporting cells and synaptic connections to nerve endings.

Hair cells act as mechanoelectrical transducers, converting mechanical energy into the electrical energy of nerve action potentials. Each has an apical hair bundle consisting of one rigid cilium, the **kinocilium**, up to 40 μm long, and a bundle of 30-50 rigid, unbranched **stereocilia**. The base of each stereocilium is tapered and connected to an actin-rich region of apical cytoplasm, the cuticular plate, which returns these rigid projecting structures to a normal upright position after bending. They are arranged in rows of decreasing length, with the longest adjacent to the kinocilium (Figure 23–25). The tips of the stereocilia and kinocilium are embedded in a thick, gelatinous layer of proteoglycans called the **otolithic membrane**. The outer region of this layer contains barrel-shaped crystals of $CaCO_3$ and protein called **otoliths** (or otoconia) typically 5-10 μm in diameter (Figure 23–25b).

All hair cells have basal synapses with afferent (to the brain) nerve endings but are of two types (Figure 23–26a):

- Type I hair cells have rounded basal ends completely surrounded by an afferent terminal calyx (L, cup).

- The more numerous type II hair cells are cylindrical, with bouton endings from afferent nerves.

Synaptic connections with *efferent* (from the brain) fibers are also present on hair cells of both types, or on their afferents, to modulate the sensitivity of these mechanoreceptors (Figure 23–26a). The supporting cells provide metabolic and physical support for the mechanoreceptors.

Sensory information from the utricle and saccule allows the brain to monitor the **static position** and **linear acceleration** of the head. This information, along with that provided visually and by musculoskeletal proprioceptors, is important for maintaining equilibrium and allowing the eyes to remain fixed on the same point while moving the head. The head's position determines the position of the otolithic membrane in contact with hair cells of the two maculae. Because the otoliths are heavier than endolymph, the hair bundles are deflected by gravity when the head is not moving, when the head is tilted, and when the individual is moving in a straight line and inertia causes drag on the otolithic membrane.

Deflection or bending of the stereocilia changes the hair cells' resting potential and their rate of neurotransmitter release to the afferent nerves, which is the basis for mechanoelectrical transduction (Figure 23–26b). When the hair bundle is deflected *toward* the kinocilium, protein fibrils called **tip links** connecting the stereocilia are pulled and mechanically gated channels open to allow an influx of K^+ ions (the major cation in endolymph). The resulting depolarization of the hair cell opens voltage-gated Ca^{2+} channels in the basolateral membrane, and Ca^{2+} entry stimulates release of neurotransmitter and generates an impulse in the afferent nerve (Figure 23–27a).

When the head stops moving, the stereocilia straighten and hair cells quickly repolarize and reestablish the resting potential. Head movements that bend the stereocilia *away from* the kinocilium cause the tip links to be slack, allowing closure of the apical cation channels and hyperpolarization of the cell. This in turn closes Ca^{2+} channels and reduces neurotransmitter release (Figure 23–27b).

> **>> MEDICAL APPLICATION**
>
> Problems of the vestibular system can result in **vertigo**, or dizziness, a sense of bodily rotation and lack of equilibrium. Spinning the body produces vertigo due to overstimulation of the cristae ampullares of the semicircular ducts. Overstimulation of the maculae of the utricle caused by repetitive changes in linear acceleration and directional changes can normally lead to **motion sickness** (seasickness).

Sensory impulses from the maculae of the vestibular complex move toward the CNS via branches of the eighth cranial nerve and are interpreted along with input from the semicircular ducts and other sources to help maintain equilibrium.

FIGURE 23–25 Vestibular maculae.

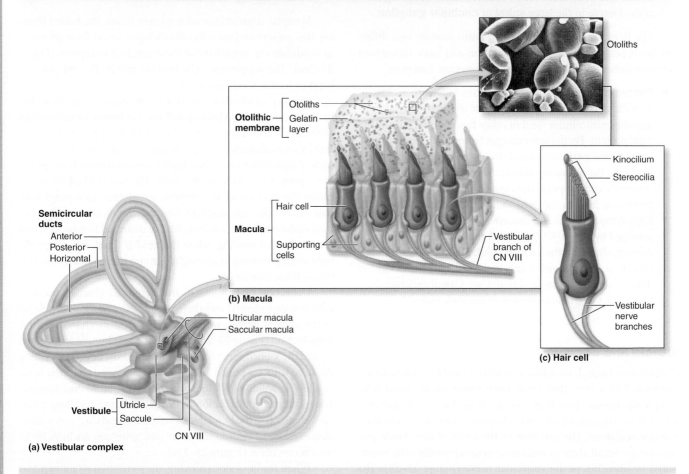

(a) Vestibular complex

(b) Macula

(c) Hair cell

(a) Two sensory areas called **maculae** occur in the **membranous labyrinth** of the vestibular **utricle** and **saccule**, both specialized for detecting gravity and endolymph movements.

(b) A more detailed diagram of a macular wall shows that it is composed of **hair cells**, **supporting cells**, and endings of the **vestibular branch** of the eighth cranial nerve. The apical surface of the hair cells is covered by a gelatinous otolithic layer or membrane and the basal ends of the cells have synaptic connections with the nerve fibers. The SEM shows **otoliths** embedded in this membrane. These mineralized structures make the otolithic membrane heavier than endolymph alone, which facilitates bending of the kinocilia and stereocilia by gravity or movement of the head.

   (SEM, with permission, from David J. Lim, House Ear Institute and Department of Cell & Neurobiology, University of Southern California, Los Angeles, CA.)

(c) A diagram of a single generalized hair cell shows the numerous straight **stereocilia**, which contain bundled actin, and a longer single **kinocilium**, a modified cilium whose tip may be slightly enlarged.

❯❯ MEDICAL APPLICATION

The sensation of **vertigo** associated with rapid head movements can also be produced by internal ear inflammation (**vestibular neuritis**) or neurologic conditions that cause dysfunctional activity of the vestibular system. **Ménière disease** involves episodes of vertigo accompanied by hearing loss and ringing in the ears (**tinnitus**) and is caused when increased pressure within the membranous labyrinth (**endolymphatic hydrops**) leads to rupture and leakage of endolymph into the perilymph.

Semicircular Ducts

The three **semicircular ducts** extend from and return to the wall of the utricle. They lie in three different spatial planes, at approximately right angles to one another (Figure 23–24).

Each semicircular duct has one enlarged ampulla end containing hair cells and supporting cells on a crest of the wall called the **crista ampullaris** (Figure 23–28). Each crista ampullaris is perpendicular to the long axis of the duct. Cristae are histologically similar to maculae, but the proteoglycan layer called the **cupola** attached to the hair cells apically lacks otoliths and is thicker. The cupola extends completely across the ampulla, contacting the opposite nonsensory wall (Figure 23–28).

FIGURE 23–26 Hair cells and hair bundles.

(a)

(b)

(a) This diagram shows the two types of hair cells in the maculae and cristae ampullares. Basal ends of **type I hair** cells are rounded and enclosed within a nerve calyx on the afferent fiber. **Type II hair cells** are columnar and associated with typical bouton synaptic connections to their afferents. Both types are also associated with efferent fibers.

(b) A more detailed diagram shows that **stereocilia** occur in rows of increasing height, with the tallest next to the single **kinocilium** on one side of the cell. By TEM the end of each stereocilium shows an electron-dense region containing cation channels and proteins involved in **mechanoelectrical transduction** (MET) that converts mechanical activity of the stereocilia to electrical activity. Neighboring stereocilia are connected by proteins of various side links; the best understood of these are the **tip links** that connect the tips of stereocilia and contain very long cadherin proteins. Changes in the tension of the tip links caused by bending of the hair bundle open or close the adjacent mechanically gated K^+ channels and change the afferent synaptic activity of the hair cells.

The hair cells of the cristae ampullares act as mechanoelectrical transducers like those of the maculae in the utricle and saccule, signaling afferent axons by pulsed transmitter release determined by depolarization and hyperpolarization states (Figure 23–27). Here the mechanoreceptors detect **rotational movements** of the head as they are deflected by endolymph movement in the semicircular ducts. The cells are oriented with opposite polarity on each side of the side, so that turning the head causes hair cell depolarization on one side and hyperpolarization on the other. Neurons of the **vestibular nuclei** in the CNS receive input from the sets of semicircular ducts on each side simultaneously and interpret head rotation on the basis of the relative transmitter discharge rates of the two sides.

Inputs from the semicircular ducts travel together with those from the utricle and saccule along the eighth cranial nerve to vestibular nuclei in the CNS. There they are interpreted together with inputs from mechanoreceptors of the musculoskeletal system to provide the basis for perceiving movement and orientation in space and for maintaining equilibrium or balance.

>> MEDICAL APPLICATION

Brief periods of vertigo produced by sudden changes in position of head, such as standing up quickly or sitting up after lying in bed, may be examples of **benign paroxysmal positional vertigo** (**BPPV**). BPPV also results when one or more of the dense otoliths (or otoconia) detach from the otolithic membrane and move into an ampulla of the posterior semicircular duct as **canaliths** that may also

FIGURE **23–27** Mechanotransduction in hair cells.

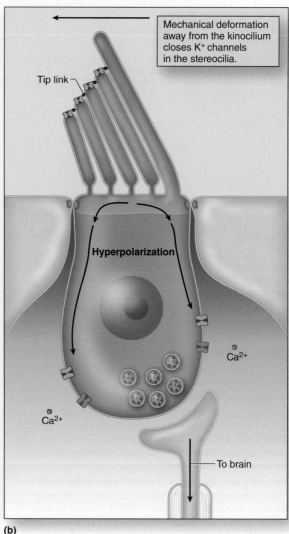

Hair cells and **supporting cells** are part of an epithelium with tight junctions. The *apical* ends of the cells are exposed to endolymph with a high concentration of K^+, and perilymph with a much lower K^+ concentration bathes their *basolateral* surface. At rest, hair cells are polarized with a small amount of K^+ entry and a low level of neurotransmitter release to afferent nerve fibers at the basal ends of the cells.

(a) As shown here, head movements that cause the stereocilia bundle to be deflected *toward* the kinocilium produce tension in the tip links, which is transduced to electrical activity by opening of adjacent cation channels. Entry of K^+ *depolarizes* the cell, opening voltage-gated basolateral Ca^{2+} channels,

which stimulates release of neurotransmitter. When this movement stops, the cells quickly repolarize.

(b) Movements in the opposite direction, *away from* the kinocilium, produce slackness on the tip links, allowing the mechanically gated apical K^+ channels to close completely, producing *hyperpolarization*, and inhibiting transmitter release. With different numbers of afferent and efferent fibers on the hair cells and with various hair cells responding differently to endolymph movements due to their positions within the maculae and cristae ampullares, the sensory information produced collectively by these cells can be processed by the vestibular regions of the brain and used to help maintain equilibrium.

adhere to the cupula. Being heavy, canaliths make that crista ampullaris gravity-sensitive. When that semicircular canal is aligned with gravity during head movements, sensory impulses are produced which the brain interprets incorrectly as continuous head rotations. A specific series

of slow head movements that make up the **canalith repositioning procedure**, or **Epley maneuver**, can be used to return the otoliths to the utricle and relieve the sensation of dizziness and unsteadiness.

FIGURE 23–28 Ampullae and cristae of the semicircular ducts.

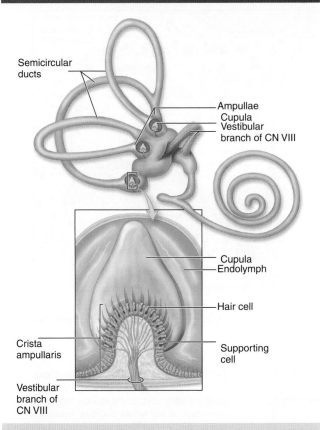

Semicircular ducts

Ampullae
Cupula
Vestibular branch of CN VIII

Cupula
Endolymph

Hair cell

Crista ampullaris

Supporting cell

Vestibular branch of CN VIII

Each of the semicircular ducts has an expanded end called the **ampulla**. The wall of each ampulla is raised as a ridge called the **crista ampullaris**, a section of which is shown here diagrammatically. Hair cells of the crista epithelium resemble the two types found in the maculae, with hair bundles projecting into a dome-shape overlying layer of proteoglycan called the **cupula**. The cupula is attached to the wall opposite the crista and is moved by endolymph movement within the semicircular duct.

Cochlear Duct

The **cochlear duct**, a part of the membranous labyrinth shaped as a spiral tube, contains the hair cells and other structures that allow auditory function. Held in place within the bony cochlea, this duct is one of three parallel compartments, or scalae (L., ramps or ladders) which coil 2¾ turns within the cochlea (Figure 23–29):

- The cochlear duct itself forms the middle compartment, or **scala media**, filled with endolymph. It is continuous with the saccule and ends at the apex of the cochlea.
- The larger **scala vestibuli** contains perilymph and is separated from the scala media by the very thin **vestibular membrane (Reissner's membrane)** lined on each side by simple squamous epithelium (Figure 23–30). Extensive tight junctions between cells of this membrane block ion diffusion between perilymph and endolymph.

- The scala tympani also contains perilymph and is separated from the scala media by the fibroelastic **basilar membrane** (Figure 23–29b).

The scalae tympani and vestibuli communicate with each other at the apex of the cochlea via a small opening called the **helicotrema**. Thus these two spaces with perilymph are actually one long tube; the scala vestibuli begins near the vestibular oval window and the scala tympani ends at the round window (Figure 23–24).

The **stria vascularis**, located in the lateral wall of the cochlear duct (scala media) (Figures 23–29b and 23–30), produces the endolymph with high levels of K^+ that fills the entire membranous labyrinth. Stratified epithelial cells of the stria vascularis extend cytoplasmic processes and folds around the capillaries of an unusual intraepithelial plexus. K^+ released from the capillaries is transported across tightly joined cells at the strial surface into the endolymph, which bathes the stereocilia of hair cells and produces conditions optimal for these cells' depolarization.

The **organ of Corti**, or **spiral organ**, where sound vibrations of different frequencies are detected, consists of hair cells and other epithelial structures supported by the basilar membrane (Figure 23–29). Here the sensory hair cells have precisely arranged V-shaped bundles of rigid stereocilia (Figure 23–31); each loses its single larger kinocilium during development. Two major types of hair cells are present (Figure 23–29c, d):

- **Outer hair cells**, about 12,000 in total, occur in three rows near the saccule, increasing to five rows near the apex of the cochlea. Each columnar outer hair cell bears a V-shaped bundle of stereocilia (Figure 23–31).
- **Inner hair cells** are shorter and form a single row of about 3500 cells, each with a single more linear array of shorter stereocilia (Figure 23–31).

≫ MEDICAL APPLICATION

Deafness can result from many factors, which usually fall into two categories: (1) **Conductive hearing loss** involves various problems in the middle ear which can reduce conduction of vibrations by the chain of ossicles from the tympanic membrane to the oval window. A common example is otosclerosis, in which scar-like lesions develop on the bony labyrinth near the stapes which inhibit its movement of the oval window. Infection of the middle ear (otitis media) is common in young children and can reduce sound conduction due to fluid accumulation in that cavity. (2) **Sensorineural deafness** can be congenital or acquired and due to defects in any structure or cell from the cochlea to the auditory centers of the brain, but it commonly involves loss of hair cells or nerve degeneration.

Both outer and inner hair cells have synaptic connections with afferent and efferent nerve endings, with the inner row of cells more heavily innervated. The cell bodies of the

FIGURE **23–29** Cochlea and spiral organ (of Corti).

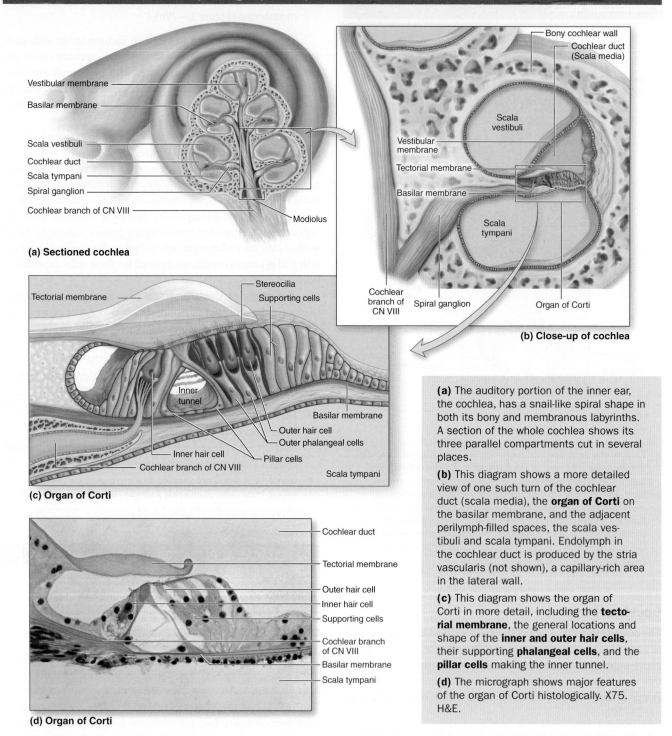

(a) Sectioned cochlea

(b) Close-up of cochlea

(c) Organ of Corti

(d) Organ of Corti

(a) The auditory portion of the inner ear, the cochlea, has a snail-like spiral shape in both its bony and membranous labyrinths. A section of the whole cochlea shows its three parallel compartments cut in several places.

(b) This diagram shows a more detailed view of one such turn of the cochlear duct (scala media), the **organ of Corti** on the basilar membrane, and the adjacent perilymph-filled spaces, the scala vestibuli and scala tympani. Endolymph in the cochlear duct is produced by the stria vascularis (not shown), a capillary-rich area in the lateral wall.

(c) This diagram shows the organ of Corti in more detail, including the **tectorial membrane**, the general locations and shape of the **inner and outer hair cells**, their supporting **phalangeal cells**, and the **pillar cells** making the inner tunnel.

(d) The micrograph shows major features of the organ of Corti histologically. X75. H&E.

afferent bipolar neurons constitute the **spiral ganglion** located in the bony core of the modiolus and (Figures 23–29 and 23–30).

Two major types of columnar supporting cells are attached to the basilar membrane in the organ of Corti (Figure 23–29c):

■ Inner and outer **phalangeal cells** extend apical processes that intimately surround and support the basolateral parts of both inner and outer hair cells and the synaptic nerve endings. The apical ends of phalangeal cells are joined to those of the hair cells by tight zonulae occludens, forming an apical plate across the spiral organ through which

FIGURE **23–30** Cochlear duct and spiral ganglion.

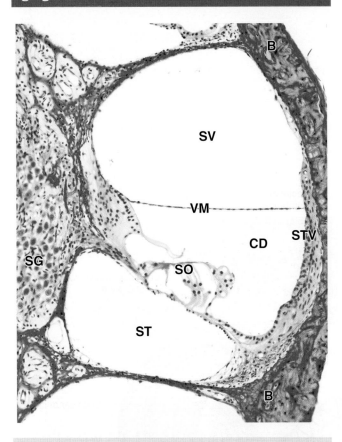

The spiral organ (**SO**) or organ of Corti lies within the cochlear duct (**CD**), or scala media. This duct is filled with endolymph produced in the stria vascularis (**STV**), an unusual association of epithelial cells and the capillaries in the periosteum of the bone (**B**). On either side of the cochlear duct are the scala vestibuli (**SV**) and scala tympani (**ST**), which are filled with perilymph and are continuous at the apex of the cochlea. The vestibular membrane (**VM**) separates perilymph in the scala vestibuli from endolymph in the cochlear duct. Cell bodies of bipolar neurons in the spiral ganglion (**SG**) send dendrites to the hair cells of the spiral organ and axons to the cochlear nuclei of the brain. X25. H&E.

FIGURE **23–31** Stereocilia hair bundles of cochlear hair cells.

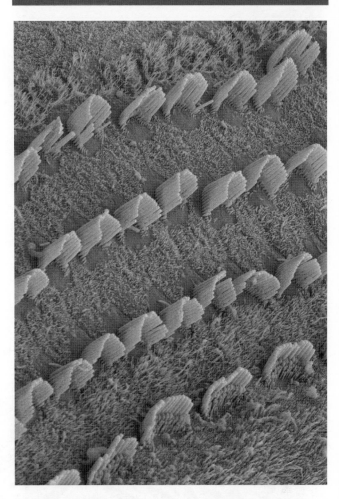

With the tectorial membrane removed, SEM shows the **apical plate** of the rat spiral organ through which rigid **stereocilia bundles** project into endolymph. Shown are hair bundles from three rows of **outer hair cells** and the single row of **inner hair cells** (bottom) in the middle turn of the cochlea. X3000.

(*With permission, from Dr Bechara Kachar and Dr Leonardo Andrade, Laboratory of Cell Structure and Dynamics, National Institutes of Health, Bethesda, MD.*)

the stereocilia bundles project into endolymph (Figure 23–31).

▪ **Pillar cells** are stiffened by heavy bundles of keratin and outline a triangular space, the inner tunnel, between the outer and inner complexes of hair cells and phalangeal cells. The stiff inner tunnel also plays a role in sound transmission.

On the outer hair cells the tips of the tallest stereocilia are embedded in the gel-like **tectorial membrane**, an acellular layer that extends over the organ of Corti from the connective tissue around the modiolus (Figure 23–29). The tectorial

membrane consists of fine bundles of collagen (types II, V, IX, and XI) associated with proteoglycans and forms during the embryonic period from secretions of cells lining this region.

By detecting minute movements of the stereocilia, hair cells in the spiral organ of Corti act as mechanoelectrical transducers very much like those of the vestibular maculae described previously and mediate the sense of hearing. As shown in Figure 23–32, sound waves collected by the external ear cause the tympanic membrane to vibrate, which moves the chain of middle ear ossicles and the oval window. The large size of the tympanic membrane compared to the oval window and the mechanical

FIGURE **23–32** Path of sound waves through the ear.

① Sound waves enter ear and cause the tympanic membrane to vibrate.

② Tympanic membrane vibration moves auditory ossicles; sound waves are amplified.

③ The stapes at the oval window generates pressure waves in the perilymph within the scala vestibuli.

④ Pressure waves cause the vestibular membrane to move, resulting in pressure wave formation in the endolymph within the cochlear duct and displacement of a specific region of the basilar membrane. Hair cells in the organ of Corti are distorted, initiating a nerve signal in the cochlear branch of CN VIII.

⑤ Remaining pressure waves are transferred to the scala tympani and exit the inner ear via the round window.

properties of the ossicle chain amplify the movements and allow optimal transfer of energy between air and perilymph, from sound waves to vibrations of the tissues and fluid-filled chambers.

Pressure waves within the perilymph begin at the oval window and move along the scala vestibuli. Each pressure wave causes momentary displacement of the vestibular and/or basilar membranes and the endolymph surrounding the organ of Corti (Figure 23–32).

The width, rigidity, thickness, and other physical properties of the basilar membrane and its organ of Corti all vary in precise gradients along its length. This allows the region of maximal displacement to vary with the sound waves' frequency, that is, the number of waves moving past a point per unit of time (measured in *hertz*). High-frequency sounds displace the basilar membrane maximally near the oval window. Sounds of progressively lower frequency produce pressure waves that move farther along the scala vestibuli and displace the spiral organ at points farther from the oval window (Figure 23–33). The sounds of the lowest

frequency that can be detected produce movement of the basilar membrane at the apex or helicotrema of the cochlea. After crossing the cochlear duct (scala media) and organ of Corti, pressure waves are transferred to the scala tympani and exit the inner ear at the round window (Figure 23–32).

FIGURE **23–33** Interpretation of sound waves in the cochlea.

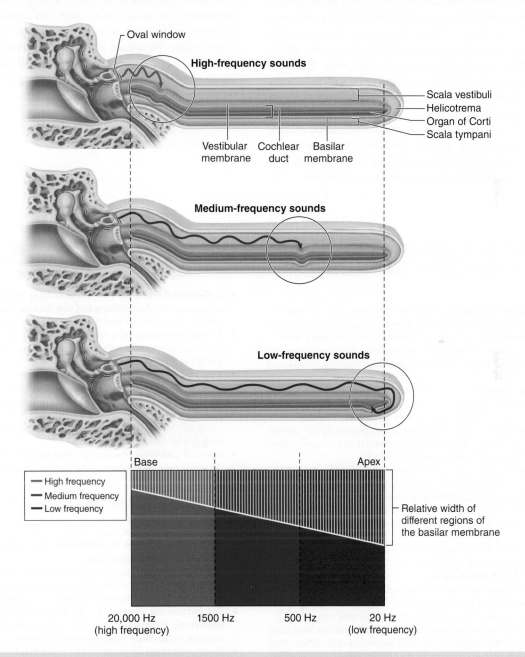

The cochlea is completely straightened in this diagram to more easily show how sound waves are interpreted according to their frequency at specific sites along the organ of Corti. High-frequency sound waves (red arrow) generate pressure waves that displace the basilar membrane near the base of the cochlea, close to the oval window. Medium-frequency sound

waves (green arrow) generate pressure waves that displace the membrane at different points along the central region of the cochlea. Low-frequency sound waves (blue arrow) generate waves that displace the membrane near the helicotrema, at the apical end of the cochlea.

The main mechanoreceptors for the sense of hearing are the more heavily innervated inner hair cells in the organ of Corti. The outer hair cells, with their stereocilia tips embedded in the tectorial membrane, are depolarized when stereocilia are deformed, as described previously, for vestibular hair cells (Figure 23–27). In the organ of Corti, however, hair cell activities are more complex, allowing greater control on sensory reception.

Depolarization of the outer hair cells causes these columnar cells to shorten very rapidly, an effect mediated by an unusual 80-kD transmembrane protein called **prestin** (It. *presto*, very fast) abundant in the lateral cell membranes. Prestin undergoes a voltage-dependent conformational change that affects the cytoskeleton, rapidly shortening the cells when the membrane is depolarized and elongating them again with membrane hyperpolarization. Piston-like movements of the outer hair cells pull down the tectorial membrane against the stereocilia of the inner hair cells (Figure 23–29c), causing depolarization of these cells which then send the signals to the brain for processing as sounds. This sequential role for outer and inner hair cells produces further cochlear amplification of the sound waves.

>> **MEDICAL APPLICATION**

Some types of **sensorineural deafness** can be treated by a **cochlear implant**. A small cable with a series of electrodes is threaded into the scala tympani, with the electrodes along the wall containing branches of the cochlear nerve. A device containing a microphone, a speech processor to filter extraneous sounds, and a transmitter is worn behind the external ear. Sounds of various frequencies transmit signals to a receiver implanted in a bone of the skull and attached to the array of electrodes that stimulate nerve branches appropriate for those frequencies. The neural impulses are interpreted in the brain as sounds. Cochlear implants do not restore normal hearing but can provide a range of sounds that allows understanding of speech.

The Eye & Ear: Special Sense Organs SUMMARY OF KEY POINTS

Eye

- The eye has **three tunics**: the **sclera** and **cornea** form the outer fibrous tunic; the middle **vascular layer** (or uvea) consists of the **choroid**, **ciliary body**, and **iris**; and the **retina** forms the **inner tunic**.
- The transparent **cornea** consists of an anterior **stratified squamous epithelium** on **Bowman's membrane**, a thick avascular **stroma**, and an inner **endothelium** on **Descemet's membrane**.
- **Aqueous humor** is secreted by **ciliary processes** into the **posterior chamber**, flows through the **pupil** into the **anterior chamber**, and is drained by the **scleral venous sinus** in the **limbus**.
- The **iris** stroma contains **melanocytes** and posteriorly has smooth muscle fibers of the **sphincter pupillae muscle** and the **myoepithelial cells** forming the **dilator pupillae muscle**.
- The **lens** is a unique avascular tissue composed of long **lens fibers**, covered on its anterior side by cuboidal **lens epithelium**, and surrounded by a thick acellular layer called the **lens capsule**.
- The **lens** is suspended behind the **iris** and its central **pupil** by the **ciliary zonule** of fibrillin fibers produced by epithelial cells covering the encircling **ciliary body**.
- The **retina** has the two major parts derived from the embryonic optic cup: the **pigmented epithelium** next to the vascular **choroid** layer and the thicker **neural retina**.
- Cells of the **pigmented epithelium** absorb **scattered light**, form part of a **blood-retina barrier**, regenerate **11-*cis*-retinal**, **phagocytose** shed discs from rods, and support the rod and cone cells.
- **Rod cells** are **photoreceptors** detecting **light intensity** with short rod-shaped outer segments; less numerous **cone cells**, with conical outer segments, are receptors for the primary **colors** (light of different wavelengths).
- **Rods** have stacked **membrane discs** in which the membranes are densely packed with the protein **rhodopsin** with bound **retinal**.
- Photons of light convert 11-*cis*-retinal to all-*trans*-retinal, causing rhodopsin to release the retinal (**bleaching**), and activate the adjacent G protein **transducin**, which causes a nerve impulse.

- In the **neural retina** the **rod and cone layer** (**RCL**) is nearest to the **retina pigmented epithelium** and near the **inner nuclear layer** (**INL**) which contains the cell bodies of these photoreceptors.
- An **outer plexiform layer** (**OPL**) contains the photoreceptor's axons connected in synapses with dendrites of various integrating neurons whose cell bodies form the **INL**.
- Axons from cells in the INL form synapses in the **inner plexiform layer** (**IPL**) with neurons of **ganglionic layer** (**GL**), which send axons through the **nerve fiber layer** (**NFL**) to the **optic nerve**.
- Eyelids are lined by **conjunctiva**, a stratified columnar epithelium with goblet cells, which also covers the anterior part of the sclera and is continuous with the corneal epithelium.
- **Lacrimal glands** continuously produce the tear film that drains into the nasal cavity via the ducts of the **lacrimal apparatus**.

Ear

- The **acoustic meatus** of the **external ear** ends at the **tympanic membrane** and its mucosa contains sebaceous and **ceruminous glands** that produce an antimicrobial substance, cerumen.
- The **tympanic cavity** of the **middle ear** opens to the nasopharynx via the **auditory (eustachian) tube**.
- Within the **tympanic cavity**, an articulated series of three small bony **ossicles** (malleus, incus, and stapes) connects the **tympanic membrane** with the **oval window** in the wall of the **internal ear**.
- The **internal ear** consists of a **membranous labyrinth** containing **endolymph**; the membranous labyrinth is enclosed by the temporal bone's **bony labyrinth** which contains perilymph.
- The **membranous labyrinth** has a central **vestibule** with two subdivisions: the **utricle** connects to the three **semicircular ducts** and the **saccule** connects to the **cochlear duct**.
- The walls of the **utricle** and **saccule** each have a thickened area, the **macula**, which contains both sensory **hair cells** with synaptic connections to sensory nerves and **supporting cells**.

- A bundle of rigid **stereocilia** and one rigid **kinocilium** project apically from each **hair cell** and are surrounded by endolymph containing a gel-like matrix with mineralized crystals called **otoliths**.
- Head movements cause **endolymph** and the **otolithic membrane** to move, deforming the rigid apical structures of the **hair cells**, depolarizing them and producing nerve impulses.
- Each of the **semicircular ducts**, oriented 90 degrees from one another, has a terminal **ampulla** region with a thickened **crista ampullaris** containing **hair cells** that contact a gel-like **cupola**.
- **Head movements** displace endolymph and stereocilia of hair cells in the **utricle, saccule,** and **semicircular ducts** which together produce signals that contribute to the sense of equilibrium.

- The **cochlear duct** is the middle compartment (**scala media**) of the **cochlea** and runs between two other long compartments that contain perilymph: the **scala vestibuli** and the **scala tympani**.
- Along the base of the cochlear duct, the **basilar membrane** supports the **spiral organ of Corti**, which consists largely of **hair cells** connected to sensory fibers of cranial nerve VIII.
- The cochlear hair cells include three to five rows of **outer hair cells** with stereocilia embedded in a gel-like **tectorial membrane** and one row of more heavily innervated **inner hair cells**.
- Sound waves transmitted by the **ossicles** move the oval window and produce pressure waves in the cochlear **perilymph** which deflect the **basilar membrane** and **organ of Corti**, causing nerve impulses which the brain interprets as sounds.

Appendix | *Light Microscopy Stains*

Hematoxylin and Eosin (H&E)

Hematoxylin stains cellular regions rich in basophilic macromolecules (DNA or RNA) a purplish blue color. It is the most common stain for demonstrating cell nuclei and cytoplasm rich in rough ER. Usually used as the contrasting "counterstain" with hematoxylin, **eosin** is an acidic stain that binds to basic macromolecules such as collagen and most cytoplasmic proteins, especially those of mitochondria. Eosin stains regions rich in such structures a pinkish red color. Tissue sections showing only structures with shades of purple and pink are most likely stained with H&E.

Pararosaniline-Toluidine Blue (PT)

This dye combination stains chromatin shades of purple and cytoplasm and collagen a lighter violet. These stains penetrate plastic sections more readily than H&E and are used in this atlas primarily with acrylic resin-embedded sections to provide better detail of cell and tissue structures. Toluidine blue is also commonly used for differential staining of cellular components, particularly cytoplasmic granules.

Mallory Trichrome

This procedure employs a combination of stains applied in series which results in nuclei staining purple; cytoplasm, keratin, and erythrocytes staining bright red or orange; and collagen bright or light blue. **Mallory trichrome** is particularly useful in demonstrating cells and small blood vessels of connective tissue. Similar stains, such as **Masson trichrome** and Gomori trichrome, yield comparable results except that collagen stains blue-green or green.

Picro-Sirius-Hematoxylin (PSH)

The dye Sirius red in a solution of picric acid stains collagen red and cytoplasm a lighter violet or pink, with nuclei purple if first stained with hematoxylin. Under the polarizing microscope, collagen stained with **picro-sirius red** is birefringent and can be detected specifically.

Periodic Acid–Schiff Reaction (PAS)

This histochemical procedure stains complex carbohydrate-containing cell components, which become magenta (shades of purplish pink). **PAS** is used most commonly to demonstrate cells filled with mucin granules, glycogen deposits, or the glycocalyx.

Wright-Giemsa Stain

These are two similar combinations of stains that are widely used on fixed cells of blood or bone marrow smears to demonstrate types of blood cells. Granules in leukocytes are seen to have differential affinity for the stain components. Nuclei stain purple and erythrocytes stain uniformly pink or pinkish orange.

Silver or Gold Stains

Various procedures employing solutions of **silver or gold salts** have been developed to demonstrate filamentous structures in neurons and fibers of reticulin (type III collagen). By these "metal impregnation" techniques these filaments stain dark brown or black. Such stains have been largely replaced now by immunohistochemical procedures.

Stains for Elastin

Several staining methods have been developed to distinguish elastic structures from collagen, most of which stain the elastin-rich structures brown or shades of purple. Examples of such stains are Weigert's **resorcin fuchsin**, **aldehyde fuchsin**, and **orcein**.

Stains for Lipid

When special preparation techniques are used to retain lipids of cells, such as in frozen sections, lipophilic dyes are used to demonstrate lipid droplets and myelin. **Oil red O** and **Sudan black** stains lipid-rich structures as their names suggest. **Osmium tetroxide** (osmic acid), which is used as a fixative for TEM, is reduced to a black substance by unsaturated fatty acids and is also used to demonstrate lipids, including those of myelin and cell membranes.

Other Common Stains

Many basic aniline dyes, including azures, cresyl violet, brilliant cresyl blue, luxol fast blue, and light green, are used because of the permanence and brightness of the colors they impart to cellular and extracellular structures in paraffin sections. Many such stains were initially developed for use in the textile industry.

Figure Credits

Figure numbers in boldface indicate those appearing for the first time in this text; figure numbers in lightface indicate those taken from other sources.

Berman I. *Color Atlas of Basic Histology*. 3rd ed. New York, NY: McGraw-Hill; 2003.

Eckel CM. *Human Anatomy Lab Manual*. New York, NY: McGraw-Hill; 2008.

Fitzpatrick TB, et al. *Dermatology in General Medicine*. New York, NY: McGraw-Hill; 1971.

Hartwell L, Hood L, Goldberg M., et al. *Genetics: From Genes to Genomes*. 4th ed. New York, NY: McGraw-Hill; 2010.

Kaushansky K, Lichtman M, Beutler E, et al. *Williams Hematology*. 8th ed. New York, NY: McGraw-Hill; 2010.

Lewis R, Gaffin D, Hoefnagels M, et al. *Life*. 5th ed. New York, NY: McGraw-Hill; 2004.

Lichtman MA, Shafer MS, Felgar RE, Wang N: *Lichtman's Atlas of Hematology*. New York, NY: 2007. http://www.accessmedicine.com.

McKinley M, O'Loughlin VD. *Human Anatomy*. 2nd ed. New York, NY: McGraw-Hill; 2008.

McKinley M, O'Loughlin VD. *Human Anatomy*. 3rd ed. New York, NY: McGraw-Hill; 2012.

McKinley MP, O'Loughlin VD, Bidle TS. *Anatomy & Physiology: An Integrative Approach*. New York, NY: McGraw-Hill; 2013.

Murray RK, Bender DA, Botham KM, et al. *Harper's Illustrated Biochemistry*. 28th ed. New York, NY: McGraw-Hill; 2009.

Raven P, Johnson GB, Losos JB, et al. *Biology*. 7th ed. New York, NY: McGraw-Hill; 2005.

Weiss L, Greep RO. *Histology*. 4th ed. New York, NY: McGraw-Hill; 1977.

Widmaier EP, Raff H, Strang KT. *Vander's Human Physiology*. 11th ed. New York, NY: McGraw-Hill; 2008.

Chapter 1
1-14: McKinley et al 1-5.

Chapter 2
2-3: McKinley et al 4-5a; **2-6:** McKinley, O'Loughlin (2nd ed) 2-7; **2-8:** McKinley et al 4-19; **2-10a:** McKinley, O'Loughlin 2-8; **2-10b:** McKinley, O'Loughlin 2-8; **2-13a (left side):** McKinley, O'Loughlin 2-9; **2-16b:** McKinley, O'Loughlin 2-10; **2-16c:** McKinley, O'Loughlin 2-10; **2-20 (top part):** McKinley, O'Loughlin (2nd ed) 2-12; **2-21b:** McKinley, O'Loughlin 2-11; **2-24:** McKinley, O'Loughlin (2nd ed) 2-35.

Chapter 3
3-2: McKinley, O'Loughlin 2-17; **3-10:** Hartwell et al 17-22b; **3-12 (right):** McKinley, O'Loughlin 2-19; **3-18:** Lewis et al 9-10.

Chapter 4
4-4: Raven 7-13; **4-5:** Weiss 3-12; **4-20:** McKinley, O'Loughlin (2nd ed) 4-4; **4-15d:** Berman 1-16; **4-21a:** McKinley, O'Loughlin 4-6; **4-21b:** McKinley, O'Loughlin 4-6; **4-21c:** McKinley, O'Loughlin 4-6c; **4-27:** McKinley et al 4-14.

Chapter 5
5-2: McKinley et al 16-3; **5-3a:** Berman 2-6; **5-8a:** Berman 2-7; **5-12b:** Berman 2-24; **5-17b:** Murray et al 48-6.

Chapter 6
6-1c: Berman 2-20; **6-1d:** Berman 2-19.

Chapter 7
7-1: McKinley, O'Loughlin (2nd ed) 6-1; **7-5a:** Berman 3-4.

Chapter 8
8-1: McKinley et al 7-7; **8-9:** Berman 4-4; **8-13a:** Berman 5-7; **8-14:** McKinley, O'Loughlin (2nd ed) 6-11; **8-16:** McKinley, O'Loughlin (2nd ed) 6-12a,b; **8-17a:** Berman 5-3; **8-17b:** Berman 5-4; **8-18:** McKinley, O'Loughlin (2nd ed) 6-16; **8-19a:** McKinley, O'Loughlin (2nd ed) 9-4.

Chapter 9
9-1: McKinley, O'Loughlin (2nd ed) 14-1; **9-2:** McKinley, O'Loughlin (2nd ed) 14-16; **9-3:** McKinley et al 12-2; **9-4:** McKinley et al 12-1 (table); **9-5:** Berman 6-8; **9-6a:** McKinley, O'Loughlin (2nd ed) 14-14b; **9-7:** McKinley, O'Loughlin (2nd ed) 14-13c; **9-8b:** Eckel 4-28b; **9-9:** McKinley, O'Loughlin (2nd ed) 14-7; **9-10a:** Berman 9-11a; **9-17:** Eckel 16-1c; **9-18a:** McKinley, O'Loughlin (2nd ed) 16-2b; **9-19:** McKinley, O'Loughlin 15-4; **9-20c:** McKinley, O'Loughlin (2nd ed) 15-7a; **9-21a:** McKinley, O'Loughlin (2nd ed) 14-8(1); **9-21b:** McKinley, O'Loughlin (2nd ed) 14-8(2); **9-21c:** McKinley, O'Loughlin (2nd ed) 14-8(3); **9-21d:** McKinley, O'Loughlin (2nd ed) 14-8(4); **9-22:** Berman 6-21; **9-25:** McKinley, O'Loughlin (2nd ed) 14-10a; **9-26a:** McKinley, O'Loughlin (2nd ed) 14-12a; **9-26b:** Berman 6-15; **9-26d:** McKinley, O'Loughlin (2nd ed) 14-12b; **9-28b:** Berman 6-19; **9-28d:** Berman 6-18; **9-29a:** Berman 6-10; **9-29c:** Berman 6-12.

Chapter 10
10-1: Widmaier 9-1; **10-2:** McKinley, O'Loughlin (2nd ed) 10-4; **10-3:** McKinley et al 10-1; **10-7a:** Berman 7-2; **10-7c:** Berman 7-4; **10-8:** McKinley, O'Loughlin (2nd ed) 10-6; **10-9:** McKinley et al 10-4; McKinley, O'Loughlin 10-9; **10-12:** McKinley et al 10-12; **10-13:** Widmaier 9-14; **10-14a:** Widmaier 10-4; Berman 7-6; **10-14b:** Berman 7-7; **10-15:** McKinley, O'Loughlin (2nd ed) 10-12; **10-16:** McKinley, O'Loughlin (2nd ed) 22-10a; **10-17a:** Berman 7-10; **10-17b:** Berman 7-11; **10-19a:** Berman 7-12; **10-21a:** McKinley, O'Loughlin (2nd ed) 10-16.

Chapter 11
11-1: McKinley, O'Loughlin 22-1; **11-2:** McKinley, O'Loughlin (2nd ed) 22-11; **11-5:** Berman 11-2; **11-6:** McKinley, O'Loughlin (2nd ed) 23-1; **11-8a:** Berman 11-11; **11-8b:** Berman 11-12; **11-13:** McKinley et al 20-5; **11-14a:** Berman 11-20; **11-14b:** Berman 11-22; **11-15:** McKinley et al 20-8; **11-16:** Berman 11-25; **11-21b:** Berman 11-21; **11-22b:** Berman 11-18; **11-22c:** Berman 11-13; **11-22d:** Berman 11-19; **11-24b:** McKinley, O'Loughlin (2nd ed) 24-2b.

Chapter 12
12-1: McKinley, O'Loughlin (2nd ed) 21-2; **12-3:** McKinley et al 18-2; **12-4a:** Widmaier 12-67; **12-4b,c:** McKinley, O'Loughlin (2nd ed) 21-4; **12-8:** Lichtman II.A.4; **12-10d:** Lichtman II.E.7; **12-11b:** Berman 8-5; **12-12c:** Berman 8-6; **12-12d:** Berman 8-1; **12-13a:** Berman 8-9; **12-14:** McKinley, O'Loughlin (2nd ed) 21-10.

Chapter 13
13-1: Kaushansky et al 4-1; **13-5:** McKinley et al 18-4b; **13-7a:** Berman 9-6 through 9-9; **13-7b:** Berman 8-8; **13-10 top, bottom, insets:** Berman 9-2, 9-1; 9-4, 9-5; **13-13a:** Berman 9-11; **13-13b:** Berman 9-13; **13-14:** Berman 9-14.

Chapter 14

14-1: McKinley et al 21-1; **14-2:** McKinley et al 22-17; **14-3:** McKinley et al 22-18a; **14-5:** McKinley et al 22-9; **14-6:** McKinley et al 22-18; **14-8a:** McKinley et al 21-5; **14-8c:** McKinley et al 21-5; **14-11:** McKinley et al 22-14; **14-13a:** Berman 10-5; **14-16:** McKinley et al 21-6.

Chapter 15

15-1: McKinley, O'Loughlin (2nd ed) 26-1; **15-2:** McKinley, O'Loughlin (2nd ed) 26-9; **15-4:** McKinley et al 16-7; **15-5a:** Berman 12-10; **15-5b:** Berman 12-12; **15-6a:** McKinley, O'Loughlin 26-6c; **15-6b:** McKinley/O'Loughlin (2nd ed) 26-5; **15-10a:** Berman 12-1; **15-10b:** Berman 12-4; **15-12:** McKinley, O'Loughlin 26-10; **15-13a:** Berman 12-16; **15-14a:** McKinley et al 26-9a; **15-14b:** McKinley et al 26-10; **15-15:** Berman 12-22; **15-17d:** McKinley et al 26-10c; **15-22:** McKinley, O'Loughlin (2nd ed) 26-15; **15-31:** McKinley, O'Loughlin (2nd ed) 26-26; **15-32a:** McKinley et al 26-23a; **15-32b:** McKinley et al 26-23b; **15-33a:** Berman 12-41; **15-33b:** Berman 12-43.

Chapter 16

16-1: McKinley, O'Loughlin (2nd ed) 26-4a; **16-3b:** Berman 13-26; **16-5a:** Berman 13-29; **16-5b:** Berman 13-32; **16-7:** McKinley, O'Loughlin 26-20; **16-8:** Berman 13-17; **16-9a:** Berman 13-21; **16-11a,b:** McKinley, O'Loughlin 26-19; **16-12a:** Berman 13-3; **16-12b:** Berman 13-4; **16-13b:** Berman 13-7; **16-19:** McKinley et al 26-17; **16-20a:** Berman 13-15.

Chapter 17

17-1: McKinley, O'Loughlin (2nd ed) 25-1; **17-3:** McKinley et al 16-6; **17-4:** Berman 14-1; **17-6:** McKinley, O'Loughlin (2nd ed) 25-8; **17-7:** Berman 14-10; **17-8a:** Berman 14-11; **17-8b:** Berman 14-12; **17-9a:** Berman 14-13; **17-9c:** Berman 14-14; **17-11a:** McKinley et al 26-11; **17-11b,c:** McKinley, O'Loughlin (2nd ed) 25-9; **17-12:** Berman 14-18; **17-13a:** McKinley et al 23-12; **17-13b:** McKinley,

O'Loughlin (2nd ed) 25-10; **17-14:** Berman 14-20; **17-18a:** McKinley, O'Loughlin (2nd ed) 25-11.

Chapter 18

18-1: McKinley et al 6-6; **18-2:** McKinley, O'Loughlin (2nd ed) 5-2; **18-3:** Berman 15-4; **18-5:** Berman 15-3; **18-6a:** Berman 15-2; **18-6b:** McKinley, O'Loughlin (2nd ed) 5-4a; **18-7b:** Fitzpatrick 70-9; **18-9:** Fitzpatrick 7-6; **18-10:** McKinley, O'Loughlin (2nd ed) 19-5; **18-11:** McKinley et al 16-3; **18-12:** Eckel 17-2; **18-13a:** McKinley et al 6-9; **18-13c:** McKinley, O'Loughlin (2nd ed) 5-9; **18-14a:** Berman 15-15; **18-14b:** Berman 15-14; **18-14c:** Berman 15-13; **18-15a,b:** McKinley, O'Loughlin (2nd ed) 5-8; **18-16:** McKinley et al 6-10a; **18-17a:** Berman 15-10; **18-19:** Fitzpatrick 81-2; **18-20:** McKinley et al 6-12.

Chapter 19

19-1: McKinley et al 24-3 (right side); **19-2:** McKinley et al 24-4; **19-3:** McKinley et al 24-8; **19-4:** Berman 16-4; **19-5a:** McKinley, O'Loughlin (2nd ed) 27-6; **19-5c:** McKinley et al 24-11a; **19-5d:** McKinley, O'Loughlin (2nd ed) 27-6; **19-6b:** Berman 16-11; **19-6c:** McKinley et al 24-11b; **19-8a:** Berman 16-8; **19-9a,b,c:** McKinley, O'Loughlin (2nd ed) 27-7; **19-13:** McKinley et al 24-9; **19-16:** McKinley, O'Loughlin (2nd ed) 27-8; **19-17a:** Berman 16-18.

Chapter 20

20-1: McKinley et al 17-3; **20-2:** McKinley, O'Loughlin (2nd ed) 20-4; **20-3:** McKinley, O'Loughlin (2nd ed) 20-15; **20-4:** Berman 17-1; **20-5a:** McKinley, O'Loughlin 20-8; **20-5b:** McKinley, O'Loughlin 20-6; **20-6:** Berman 17-3; **20-8:** McKinley et al 17-4; **20-9:** Berman 17-4, McKinley, O'Loughlin (2nd ed) 20-10; **20-12:** McKinley, O'Loughlin (2nd ed) 20-13a; **20-14:** McKinley, O'Loughlin (2nd ed) 20-13c,d; **20-17c:** Berman 17-13; **20-17e:** McKinley, O'Loughlin (2nd ed) rt qt; **20-18:** McKinley, O'Loughlin (2nd ed) 20-9; **20-19:** Berman 17-15; **20-21 (upper**

right): McKinley et al 17-18; **20-22:** McKinley, O'Loughlin (2nd ed) 20-11a; **20-23:** Berman 17-17.

Chapter 21

21-1: McKinley, O'Loughlin (2nd ed) 28-11; **21-2:** McKinley, O'Loughlin (2nd ed) 28-13; **21-3:** Berman 18-2; **21-4a:** Berman 18-5; **21-5:** McKinley et al 28-18; **21-6a:** Berman 18-7; **21-6b:** Berman 18-8; **21-9a:** Berman 18-10; **21-9b:** Berman 18-11; **21-10b:** Berman 18-13; **21-11a:** Berman 18-14; **21-12a:** Berman 18-16; **21-13a:** McKinley et al 28-19; **21-14a:** Berman 18-18; **21-16a:** Berman 18-20; **21-16b:** Berman 18-21; **21-17:** McKinley, O'Loughlin (2nd ed) 18-17b; **21-18:** Berman 18-23.

Chapter 22

22-1a,b: McKinley, O'Loughlin (2nd ed) 28-11; **22-2:** McKinley, O'Loughlin (2nd ed) 28-4; **22-9:** McKinley, O'Loughlin (2nd ed) 3-7; **22-10:** McKinley et al 28-6; **22-11:** McKinley et al 28-8; **22-13:** Berman 19-8; **22-14:** McKinley, O'Loughlin (2nd ed) 28-7; **22-15a:** Berman 19-16; **22-17:** McKinley, O'Loughlin (2nd ed) 28-6; **22-19a:** Berman 19-19; **22-19b:** Berman 19-20; **22-19c:** Berman 19-21; **22-20:** McKinley, O'Loughlin (2nd ed) 2-6; **22-21c:** McKinley et al 29-7 **22-23a:** Berman 19-22; **22-24a:** Berman 19-23; **22-26a:** Berman 19-24; **22-26b:** Berman 19-25; **22-26c:** Berman 19-26; **22-27a:** Berman 19-27.

Chapter 23

23-1: McKinley 19-12b; **23-2:** McKinley, O'Loughlin (2nd ed) 19-19; **23-8:** McKinley et al 16-16; **23-10a:** Berman 20-4; **23-14:** McKinley, O'Loughlin (2nd ed) 19-14a,b; **23-15:** Berman 20-9; **23-21:** McKinley, O'Loughlin (2nd ed) 19-20; **23-23:** McKinley et al 16-25; **23-24:** McKinley et al 26-26; **23-25:** McKinley et al 16-32; **23-28:** McKinley, O'Loughlin (2nd ed) 19-25; **23-29a,b:** McKinley et al 16-27a,b; **23-29c:** McKinley 19-27; **23-29d:** McKinley et al 16-27d; **23-32:** McKinley et al 16-28; **23-33:** McKinley et al 16-29.

Index

Note: Page numbers followed by *f* indicate figures; and page numbers followed by *t* indicate tables